NURSE'S 5-MINUTE CLINICAL CONSULT

Procedures

 Wolters Kluwer | Lippincott Williams & Wilkins
Health

Philadelphia · Baltimore · New York · London
Buenos Aires · Hong Kong · Sydney · Tokyo

STAFF

Executive Publisher
Judith A. Schilling McCann, RN, MSN

Editorial Director
H. Nancy Holmes

Clinical Director
Joan M. Robinson, RN, MSN

Art Director
Elaine Kasmer

Editorial Project Manager
Jennifer Kowalak

Clinical Project Manager
Beverly Ann Tscheschlog, RN, BS

Editors
Naina D. Chohan, Julie Munden

Clinical Editor
Kathryn Henry, RN, MSN

Copy Editors
Kimberly Bilotta (supervisor), Jane Bradford,
Amy Furman, Elizabeth Mooney,
Dona Perkins, Dorothy P. Terry,
Pamela Wingrod

Designer
Matie Anne Patterson

Digital Composition Services
Diane Paluba (manager), Joyce Rossi Biletz

Manufacturing
Beth J. Welsh

Editorial Assistants
Megan L. Aldinger, Karen J. Kirk,
Linda K. Ruhf

Design Assistant
Georg W. Purvis IV

Indexer
Barbara Hodgson

Library of Congress
Cataloging-in-Publication Data

Nurse's 5-minute clinical consult. Procedures.
    p. ; cm.
  Includes bibliographical references and index.
  1. Nurse practitioners—Handbooks, manuals, etc.
2. Nursing —Handbooks, manuals, etc. I.
Lippincott Williams & Wilkins. II. Title: Nurse's five-minute clinical consult. Procedures. III. Title:
Procedures.
  [DNLM: 1. Nursing Care—methods—Handbooks.
2. Clinical Medicine—Handbooks. WY 49 N97428
2007]
RT82.8.N874 2007
610.7306'92—dc22
ISBN13: 978-1-58255-513-3
ISBN10: 1-58255-513-3 (alk. paper)   2006032412

Contents

Contributors and consultants

Marsha Conroy, RN, MSN, APN
Nurse Educator
Cuyahoga Community College
Cleveland

Kim Cooper, RN, MSN
Nursing Department Program Chair
Ivy Tech Community College
Terre Haute, Ind.

Arlene M. Coughlin, RN, MSN
Nursing Faculty
Holy Name Hospital School of Nursing
Teaneck, N.J.

Donna Headrick, RN, MSN, FNP
Professor
Bakersfield (Calif.) Community College

Christine Kennedy, RN, MSN
Nursing Instructor
Eli Whitney Technical School
Hamden, Conn.

Theresa M. Leonard, RN, BSN, CCRN
Unit Educator
Stony Brook (N.Y.) University Hospital

Grace G. Lewis, RN, MS, BC
Assistant Professor of Nursing
Georgia Baptist College of Nursing of
Mercer University
Atlanta

Sherry Rogman, RN
Registered Nurse
BryanLGH Memorial Hospital
Lincoln, Neb.

Kelley Straub, RN, BSN, CCRN, RCIS
Interventional Radiology Nurse Manager
Mercy Suburban Hospital
Norristown, Pa.

Kimberly Such-Smith, RN, BSN, LNC
Legal Nurse Consultant/Healthcare
Advocate/Nurse Case Manager
Nursing Analysis and Review, LLC
Byron, Minn.

Colleen R. Walsh, RN, MSN, ACNP-BC, CS, ONC
Faculty, Graduate Nursing
University of Southern Indiana
Evansville

Procedures

Admixture of drugs in a syringe

DESCRIPTION

- Combining two drugs in one syringe alleviates the discomfort of two injections.
- Drugs usually can be mixed in a syringe:
- from two multidose vials (for example, regular and long-acting insulin)
- from one multidose vial and one ampule
- from two ampules
- from a cartridge-injection system combined with either a multidose vial or ampule.

CONTRAINDICATIONS

- Combining drugs if their compatibility isn't known
- Combining more than two compatible drugs in the same injection system

---

EQUIPMENT

Prescribed drugs ◆ patient's drug record and chart ◆ alcohol pads ◆ syringe and needle ◆ safety needle (optional) ◆ cartridge-injection system ◆ filter needle ◆ gauze pad

PREPARATION

- The type and size of syringe and needle depend on:
- drugs prescribed
- patient's build
- route and site of administration.

KEY STEPS

⚡ **WARNING** *Drugs that come in prefilled cartridges require a cartridge-injection system. (See* Cartridge-injection system.)

- Verify that the drugs match the patient's drug record and the prescriber's orders.
- Calculate the dose.
- Wash your hands.

MIXING DRUGS FROM TWO MULTIDOSE VIALS

- Before you insert the first needle, wipe the vial's rubber stopper with an alcohol pad.
- Pull back the syringe plunger until the volume of air drawn into the syringe equals the volume to be withdrawn from the drug vial.
- Without inverting the vial, insert the needle into the top of the vial, making sure that the needle's bevel tip doesn't touch the solution.
- Inject the air into the vial and then withdraw the needle. The air replaces the liquid in the vial and prevents the creation of a partial vacuum when the drug is withdrawn.
- Repeat the above steps for the second vial.
- After injecting air into the second vial, invert the vial, withdraw the prescribed dose, and withdraw the needle.
- Wipe the rubber stopper of the first vial again and insert the needle, taking care not to depress the plunger.
- Invert the vial, withdraw the prescribed dose, and withdraw the needle.

MIXING DRUGS FROM A MULTIDOSE VIAL AND AN AMPULE

- Clean the vial's rubber stopper with an alcohol pad.
- Pull back on the syringe plunger until the volume of air drawn into the syringe equals the volume to be withdrawn from the drug vial.
- Insert the needle into the top of the vial and inject the air.

- Invert the vial and keep the needle's bevel tip below the level of the solution as you withdraw the prescribed dose.
- Put the sterile needle cover over the needle.
- Wrap a sterile gauze pad or alcohol pad around the ampule's neck to protect you from injury (in case the glass splinters).
- Break open the ampule, directing the force away from you.
- If desired, switch to the filter needle to filter glass splinters.
- Insert the needle into the ampule.

⚡ **WARNING** *Be careful not to touch the outside of the ampule with the needle.*

- Draw the correct dose into the syringe.
- If you switched to a filter needle, change back to a safety needle to give the injection.

MIXING DRUGS FROM TWO AMPULES IN A SYRINGE

- Know that an opened ampule doesn't contain a vacuum.
- Calculate the prescribed doses.
- Open both ampules using aseptic technique.
- If desired, use a filter needle to draw up drugs.
- If a filter needle is used, change to a safety needle to give the injection.

Cartridge-injection system

A cartridge-injection system, such as Tubex or Carpuject, is a convenient, easy-to-use injection method that facilitates accuracy and sterility. The device consists of a plastic cartridge-holder syringe and a prefilled drug cartridge with needle attached. The drug in the cartridge is premixed and premeasured, which saves time and helps ensure an exact dose. The drug remains sealed in the cartridge and sterile until the injection is given to the patient.

The disadvantage of this system is that not all drugs are available in cartridge form. However, compatible drugs can be added to partially filled cartridges.

SPECIAL CONSIDERATIONS

◆ Insert the needle through the vial's rubber stopper at a slight angle, bevel up, and exert slight lateral pressure to avoid cutting a piece of rubber out of the stopper, which could be pushed into the vial.
◆ Be careful not to contaminate one drug with the other when mixing drugs from multidose vials.
◆ The needle should be changed after drawing the first drug into the syringe. This isn't always possible because many disposable syringes don't have removable needles.
◆ Some drugs are compatible only briefly after combining and should be given within 10 minutes after mixing.
◆ After 10 minutes, temperature and exposure to light and humidity may alter compatibility.
◆ Parenteral drugs are usually dispensed in single-dose vials to avoid contamination.
◆ When combining a cartridge-injection system and multidose vial, use a separate needle and syringe to inject air into the multidose vial to prevent contamination by the cartridge-injection system.

MIXING INSULINS

◆ Insulin is one of few drugs still packaged in multidose vials.
◆ Check facility policy before mixing insulins.
◆ Be careful when mixing regular and long-acting insulins.
◆ Draw up regular insulin first to avoid contamination by long-acting suspension.
◆ Know that if a small amount of regular insulin is accidentally mixed with long-acting insulin, it won't change the effect of the long-acting insulin.

COMPLICATIONS

None known

PATIENT TEACHING

◆ Tell the patient what drugs are in the injection system.
◆ Explain the drugs' purpose.
◆ Describe the expected outcomes.
◆ Instruct the patient to inform you of adverse reactions.

DOCUMENTATION

◆ Record the drugs given.
◆ Note the injection site.
◆ Document the time of administration.
◆ Record adverse drug effects.
◆ Note how the patient tolerated the injection.

SELECTED REFERENCES

Paparella, S. "Death by Syringe," *Journal of Emergency Nursing* 30(6):552-55, December 2004.

Preston, S.T., and Hegadoren, K. "Glass Contamination in Parenterally Administered Medication," *Journal of Advanced Nursing* 48(3):266-70, November 2004.

Prot, S., et al. "Drug Administration Errors and Their Determinants in Pediatric In-patients," *International Journal for Quality in Health Care* 17(5):381-89, October 2005.

Thomas, M., et al. "I.V. Admixture Contamination Rates: Traditional Practice Site Versus a Class 1000 Cleanroom," *American Journal of Health-System Pharmacy* 62(22):2386-392, November 2005.

Airborne precautions

DESCRIPTION

◆ Used with standard precautions, airborne precautions prevent the spread of infectious diseases transmitted by airborne pathogens that are breathed, sneezed, or coughed. (See *Diseases requiring airborne precautions.*)

◆ Airborne precautions include the former categories of acid-fast bacillus isolation and respiratory isolation.

◆ They require a negative-pressure room with the door closed to maintain air pressure balance between the isolation room and adjoining anteroom, hallway, or corridor.

◆ Everyone entering the room must wear respiratory protection.

◆ Negative air pressure must be monitored, and air must be either vented to the outside of the building or filtered through a high-efficiency particulate air (HEPA) filtration system before recirculation.

◆ Protection is provided by using a disposable or reusable respirator.

⚡ **WARNING** *The respirator must be fit to the face properly each time it's worn, regardless of what type is used.*

◆ The patient needs to wear a surgical mask over his nose and mouth when leaving the room.

CONTRAINDICATIONS

None known

Respirators (either disposable N95 or HEPA respirators, or reusable HEPA respirators or powered air purifying respirators ◆ surgical masks ◆ isolation door card ◆ thermometer ◆ stethoscope ◆ blood pressure cuff ◆ personal protective equipment as needed

PREPARATION

◆ Keep airborne precaution supplies on the cart outside of the isolation room.

◆ Situate the patient in the negative-pressure room with the door closed (there should be an anteroom if possible).

◆ Put an airborne precautions sign on the door to notify anyone entering the room.

◆ Keep the patient's door (and anteroom door) closed to maintain negative pressure and contain airborne pathogens.

◆ Monitor negative pressure.

◆ Put on the respirator according to the manufacturer's directions.

◆ Adjust the straps for a firm, comfortable fit.

◆ Check the fit and respiratory seal. (See *Respirator seal check.*)

◆ Tape an impervious bag to the patient's bedside for disposal of facial tissues.

◆ Make sure that visitors wear respiratory protection while in the room.

◆ Limit the patient's movement from his room.

◆ Make sure that the patient wears the surgical mask over his nose and mouth when leaving the room.

◆ Notify the receiving department of isolation precautions so they can be maintained and the patient can be returned to his room promptly.

Diseases requiring airborne precautions

DISEASE	PRECAUTIONARY PERIOD
Chickenpox (varicella)	Until lesions are crusted and no new lesions appear
Herpes zoster (disseminated)	Duration of illness
Herpes zoster (localized in an immunocompromised patient)	Duration of illness
Measles (rubeola)	Duration of illness
Smallpox	Duration of illness
Tuberculosis (TB) (pulmonary or laryngeal, confirmed or suspected)	Depends on clinical response; patient must be on effective therapy, be improving clinically (decreased cough and fever and improved findings on chest X-ray), and have three consecutive negative sputum smears collected on different days, or TB must be ruled out.

◆ Before leaving the room, remove your gloves (if worn) and wash your hands.

WARNING *Strict hand washing is required after contact with the patient or items contaminated with respiratory secretions.*

◆ Remove the respirator outside of the room after closing the door.

◆ Discard the respirator or clean and store it until next use; follow facility policy and the manufacturer's recommendations.

◆ To prevent microbial growth, store nondisposable respirators in a dry, well-ventilated place (not a plastic bag).

◆ Two patients with the same infection may share a room if necessary.

COMPLICATIONS

None known

◆ Explain isolation precautions to the patient and his family.

◆ Instruct the patient to cover his nose and mouth with a tissue when coughing or sneezing, to properly dispose of soiled tissues, and to wash his hands frequently.

◆ Record the need for precautions on the care plan, as indicated by your facility.

◆ Document the precaution period.

◆ Describe the patient's tolerance of the procedure.

◆ Document patient or family teaching.

◆ Record the date precautions were discontinued.

◆ Document microbiology and virology specimens obtained and the results of laboratory tests if available.

SELECTED REFERENCES

Coffey, C.C., et al. "Errors Associated with Three Methods of Assessing Respirator Fit," *Journal of Occupational and Environmental Hygiene* 3(1):44-52, January 2006.

Gamage, B., et al. "Protecting Health Care Workers from SARS and Other Respiratory Pathogens: A Review of the Infection Control Literature," *American Journal of Infection Control* 33(2):114-21, March 2005.

Leonard, M.K., et al. "Increased Efficiency in Evaluating Patients with Suspected Tuberculosis by Use of a Dedicated Airborne Infection Isolation Unit," *American Journal of Infection Control* 34(2):69-72, March 2006.

Muller, M.P., and McGeer, A. "Febrile Respiratory Illness in the Intensive Care Unit Setting: An Infection Control Perspective," *Current Opinion in Critical Care* 12(1):37-42, February 2006.

Stirling, B., et al. "Nurses and the Control of Infectious Disease. Understanding Epidemiology and Disease Transmission Is Vital to Nursing Care," *The Canadian Nurse* 100(9):16-29, November 2004.

Thrupp, L. "Tuberculosis Prevention and Control in Long–Term-Care Facilities for Older Adults," *Infection Control and Hospital Epidemiology* 25(12):1097-108, December 2004.

Respirator seal check

Before using a respirator, always check the respirator seal. To do this, place your hands over the respirator and exhale. If air leaks around your nose, adjust the nosepiece. If air leaks at the respirator's edges, adjust the straps along the side of your head. Recheck the respirator's fit after this adjustment.

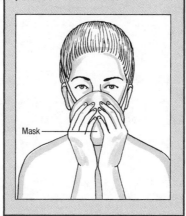

Mask

Alignment and pressure-reducing devices

DESCRIPTION

- These devices are used to maintain correct body positioning and prevent complications that result from prolonged bed rest.
- Equipment includes alignment and pressure-reducing devices, such as:
  - boots that help protect heels and help prevent skin breakdown and footdrop
  - abduction pillows that help prevent internal hip rotation after femoral fracture, hip fracture, or surgery
  - trochanter rolls that help prevent external hip rotation
  - hand rolls that help prevent hand contractures.
- Protective boots, trochanter rolls, and hand rolls are useful when caring for patients who have a loss of sensation, mobility, or consciousness.

CONTRAINDICATIONS
None known

EQUIPMENT

Protective boots ◆ abduction pillow ◆ trochanter rolls ◆ hand rolls (see *Common preventive devices*)

KEY STEPS

- Confirm the patient's identity using two patient identifiers according to facility policy.
- Explain the purpose and steps of the procedure to the patient.

APPLYING A PROTECTIVE BOOT
- Open the slit on the superior surface of the boot.
- Place the patient's foot in the boot and fasten the ankle and foot straps.
- If he's positioned laterally, apply the boot only to the bottom foot and support the flexed top foot with a pillow.
- Insert the other foot in the second boot, if needed.

Common preventive devices

Equipment is available to reduce pressure or help maintain positioning, depending on the patient's needs.

Boot — Prevents footdrop and skin breakdown

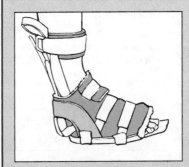

Abduction pillow — Prevents internal hip rotation

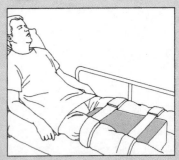

Trochanter roll — Prevents external hip rotation

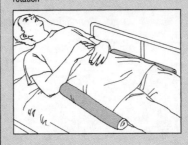

Hand roll — Prevents hand contractures

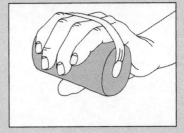

◆ Position his legs in proper alignment to prevent strain on hip ligaments and pressure on bony prominences.

APPLYING AN ABDUCTION PILLOW
◆ Put the patient in the supine position and place a pillow between his legs.
◆ Slide the pillow toward his groin so it touches the legs along their entire length.
◆ Place the upper part of both legs in the pillow's lateral indentations.
◆ Secure the straps to prevent the pillow from slipping.

APPLYING TROCHANTER ROLLS
◆ Position one roll along the outside of the thigh, from the iliac crest to mid-thigh.
◆ Place another roll along the other thigh in the same manner.

WARNING *To avoid peroneal nerve compression and palsy, which can lead to footdrop, make sure that neither roll extends as far as the knee.*

◆ If you've made trochanter rolls from a towel or rolled-up sheet, leave several inches unrolled and tuck this under the patient's thigh to hold the device in place and maintain the patient's position.

APPLYING HAND ROLLS
◆ Place one roll in each of the patient's hands to maintain a neutral position.
◆ Secure the straps, if present, or apply roller gauze and secure it with nonallergenic adhesive tape.

SPECIAL CONSIDERATIONS

◆ If using a device that's available in different sizes, select the appropriate size for the patient.
◆ Use of assistive devices doesn't preclude regularly scheduled patient positioning, range-of-motion exercises, and skin care.
◆ Some protective boots are made of soft material that cradles the heel and prevents pressure.
◆ Other boots have aluminum frames with a fleece lining and a toe extension that protects toes and prevents hip adduction.
◆ High-top sneakers may be used to help prevent footdrop, but they don't prevent external hip rotation or heel pressure.
◆ An abduction pillow is a wedge-shaped piece of sponge rubber with lateral indentations for the patient's thighs. The straps wrap around the thighs to maintain correct positioning.
◆ A properly shaped bed pillow may be temporarily substituted for a commercial abduction pillow, but it's difficult to apply and doesn't maintain correct lateral alignment.
◆ Trochanter rolls are made of sponge rubber, but can be improvised with a rolled blanket or towel.
◆ Hand rolls, available in hard and soft materials, are held in place by fixed or adjustable straps.
◆ Hand rolls can be improvised with a rolled washcloth secured with roller gauze and adhesive tape.

COMPLICATIONS
◆ Hand rolls and other assistive devices causing contractures and pressure ulcers (To avoid problems, remove a soft hand roll every 4 hours or every 2 hours if the patient has hand spasticity; remove a hard hand roll every 2 hours.)

PATIENT TEACHING

◆ Explain the use of appropriate devices to the patient and his caregiver.
◆ Demonstrate how to use the devices; emphasize proper alignment of the extremities.
◆ Have the patient or his caregiver demonstrate the technique to verify proper use.
◆ Emphasize how to prevent pressure ulcers.

DOCUMENTATION

◆ Record use of the devices in the patient's chart and care plan.
◆ Indicate assessment for complications.
◆ Reevaluate patient care goals as needed.
◆ Record patient and caregiver teaching and their understanding of the teaching in the patient's chart.

SELECTED REFERENCES
Defloor, T., et al. "The Effect of Various Combinations of Turning and Pressure Reducing Devices on the Incidence of Pressure Ulcers," *International Journal of Nursing Studies* 42(1):37-46, January 2005.

Feuchtinger, J., et al. "A 4-cm Thermoactive Viscoelastic Foam Pad on the Operating Room Table to Prevent Pressure Ulcer during Cardiac Surgery," *Journal of Clinical Nursing* 15(2):162-67, February 2006.

Marklew, A. "Body Positioning and Its Effect on Oxygenation — A Literature Review," *Nursing in Critical Care* 11(1):16-22, January-February 2006.

Moody, P., et al. "The Effect of Body Position and Mattress Type on Interface Pressure in Quadriplegic Adults: A Pilot Study," *Dermatology Nursing* 16(6):507-12, December 2004.

Schaum, K.D. "Pressure-Reducing Support Surfaces," *Ostomy/Wound Management* 51(2):36, 96, February 2005.

Ambulation, progressive

DESCRIPTION

◆ After surgery or period of bed rest, the patient must begin gradual return to full ambulation.

◆ If begun promptly, progressive ambulation prevents many complications of prolonged inactivity.

◆ Complications that can be prevented include respiratory stasis and hypostatic pneumonia; circulatory stasis, thrombophlebitis, and emboli; urine retention, urinary tract infection, urinary stasis, and calculus formation; abdominal distention, constipation, and decreased appetite; and sensory deprivation.

◆ Progressive ambulation helps restore the patient's equilibrium and enhances confidence and self-image.

◆ Progressive ambulation begins with dangling the patient's feet over the edge of the bed and progresses to seating him in an armchair or wheelchair, walking around the room, then assisted walking until he can walk by himself.

◆ Progress depends on his physical condition and tolerance.

◆ Procedures require correct body mechanics, careful patient observation, and open communication among the patient, physician, and nurse.

CONTRAINDICATIONS
None known

EQUIPMENT

Robe ◆ chair or wheelchair ◆ slippers (for sitting) ◆ hard-soled shoes (for walking) ◆ assistive device (cane, crutches, walker) if necessary

⚠ **WARNING** *Patients with orthostatic hypotension may have special requirements, such as elastic stockings, to maintain adequate circulation and prevent fainting.*

KEY STEPS

◆ Confirm the patient's identity using two patient identifiers according to facility policy.

◆ If the patient requires an assistive device, the physical therapist usually selects it and provides instruction.

◆ Check the patient's history, diagnosis, and therapeutic regimen.

◆ Ask him whether he's in pain or feels weak; if necessary, give an analgesic and wait 30 to 60 minutes before trying ambulation.

◆ A medicated patient may develop hypotension, dizziness, or drowsiness.

◆ Explain the goal of ambulation. (See *Helping the patient regain mobility*.)

◆ Provide encouragement if he's hesitant or fearful.

◆ Reassure him that he shouldn't do more than he can reasonably do.

◆ If he has pain in an incision, show him how to splint the incision, or splint the incision for him.

◆ Provide a clear path to enable safe movement and prevent falls.

◆ Lock the wheels on the bed or chair, if appropriate.

DANGLING THE PATIENT'S LEGS

◆ Position the bed horizontally and the patient laterally, facing you.

◆ You can raise the head of the bed to a 45-degree angle to allow easier elevation of the patient. Don't use this method if the patient has trouble balancing while sitting.

◆ Move the patient's legs over the side of bed and grasp his shoulders, standing with your feet apart to provide a wide base of support.

◆ Ask him to help by pushing up from the bed with his arms.

◆ Shift your weight from the foot closest to his head to your other foot as you raise him to a sitting position.

◆ Pull with your whole body, not just your arms, to avoid straining your back and jostling the patient.

◆ Ask a coworker for assistance when needed.

◆ While the patient adjusts to an upright position, continue to stand facing him to keep him from falling.

Helping the patient regain mobility

DANGLING LEGS
To help the patient support himself while dangling his legs, move an overbed table in front of him and place a pillow on it. Remain next to the patient in case he becomes dizzy.

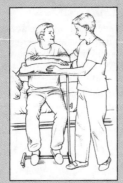

SITTING
Seat the patient in a chair with armrests and a straight back with his lower back against the rear of the chair, his feet flat on the floor, his hips and knees at right angles, and his upper body straight. Have him rest his forearms on the armrests.

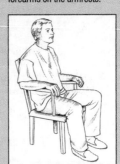

WALKING
Provide a path clear of equipment and other objects, and avoid overexertion. If necessary, hold the patient so you can control his upper and lower body and any lateral movements.

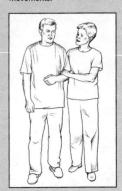

● **WARNING** *Be alert for signs and symptoms of orthostatic hypotension, such as fainting, dizziness, and complaints of blurred vision.*
◆ Check the patient's pulse rate and blood pressure.
◆ If his pulse rate increases more than 20 beats/minute, allow him to rest before progressing slowly.

● **WARNING** *If the patient's balance is impaired, he may need support while sitting for leg dangling to avoid injury.*

HELPING THE PATIENT STAND

◆ After the patient can dangle his legs, have him attempt to stand.
◆ Help him put on a robe and nonskid slippers.
◆ Don't allow the robe, drainage tube, or anything else to dangle around his feet.
◆ If he's alert and fairly strong, have him place his feet flat on the floor and stand by himself.
◆ As he stands, place one hand under his axilla and your other hand around his waist to prevent falls.
◆ Help him stand fully erect.
◆ Encourage him to look forward and not at floor to help him maintain his balance.
◆ If he needs help standing, face him and position your knees at either side of his.
◆ Bend your knees, put your arms around his waist, and tell him to push up from the bed with his arms.
◆ Straighten your knees and pull him with you while rising to an erect position.

HELPING THE PATIENT SIT OR WALK

◆ After the patient stands, you can pivot and lower him into a chair or wheelchair, or begin to walk with him.
◆ If you've decided to seat him, make sure that the chair is secure and won't slip as you lower him into it.
◆ Place his lower back against the rear of the chair and his feet flat on floor.
◆ Position his hips and knees at right angles; keep his upper body straight.

◆ Flex his elbows and place his forearms on the chair's arms.
◆ If he can only walk safely with assistance, stand to the side and slightly behind him, placing one hand under his axilla and the other around his waist.
◆ If he has weakness or paralysis on one side, stand on the affected side and stabilize him by putting one arm around his waist.
◆ If necessary, ask a coworker to help. Stand on opposite sides of the patient and place one hand under his arms or on his elbows.
◆ Give him spoken and tactile cues to encourage him.
◆ Stay close to a railed wall or other supportive structure and, if necessary, allow him to rest in a chair before attempting to walk back to his room.
◆ If he can't walk back, tell him to remain seated while you summon help or get a wheelchair.

● **WARNING** *Never leave the patient unattended if you have reason to think he may fall.*
◆ If you can't find a chair, have him lean against the wall and call for help as you support him.
◆ If necessary, steady him as he slides down the wall to sit on the floor.

SPECIAL CONSIDERATIONS

● **WARNING** *The patient taking a drug, such as a beta-adrenergic blocker or a vasodilator, may be subject to episodes of bradycardia and hypotension.*
◆ If early ambulation is impossible, encourage bed exercises.
◆ Don't let the use of catheters and infusion bottles prevent ambulation. Secure devices so they're portable.
◆ Measure the patient's pulse, respiratory rate, and blood pressure, as appropriate.
◆ Make certain he has a call button or signal device when leaving him sitting up in a chair.
◆ If he's confused, consider using safety devices, according to facility policy.

◆ After ambulation, check dressings and tubes for proper position and changes in drainage.

COMPLICATIONS
◆ Dyspnea
◆ Diaphoresis
◆ Orthostatic hypotension

PATIENT TEACHING

◆ Instruct the patient to use as much muscle power as possible to increase strength.
◆ Teach the patient to roll on one side and use his arm strength to change from a lying position to sitting.

DOCUMENTATION

◆ Record the type of transfer and assistance needed.
◆ Report the patient's duration of sitting, standing, or walking.
◆ Note the distance walked, if appropriate.
◆ Describe the patient's response to ambulation.
◆ Note significant changes in blood pressure, pulse, and respiration.
◆ Document measures taken to correct changes in blood pressure, pulse, and respiration.

SELECTED REFERENCES

Dobkin, B., et al. "Weight-Supported Treadmill vs. Over-ground Training for Walking after Acute Incomplete SCI," *Neurology* 66(4):484-93, February 2006.

Iwanczyk, L., et al. "Orthostatic Hypotension in the Nursing Home Setting," *Journal of the American Medical Directors Association* 7(3):163-67, May-June 2006.

Komara, F.A. "The Slippery Slope: Reducing Fall Risk in Older Adults," *Primary Care* 32(3):683-97, September 2005.

Wilson, D.J., et al. "Ambulation Training With and Without Partial Weight-bearing after Traumatic Brain Injury: Results of a Randomized, Controlled Trial," *American Journal of Physical Medicine & Rehabilitation* 85(1):68-74, January 2006.

Antiembolism stockings

DESCRIPTION

- Antiembolism stockings help prevent deep vein thrombosis (DVT) and pulmonary embolism by compressing superficial leg veins.
- They increase venous return by forcing blood into the deep venous system rather than allowing it to pool in the legs and form clots.
- Antiembolism stockings can provide equal pressure over the entire leg or graded pressure that's greatest at the ankle and decreases over the length of the leg.
- They're usually indicated for postoperative, bedridden, or elderly patients, patients at risk for DVT, and patients with chronic venous problems.
- Intermittent pneumatic compression stockings may be used during surgery and postoperatively.

CONTRAINDICATIONS

- Dermatoses or open skin lesions
- Gangrene
- Severe arteriosclerosis or other ischemic vascular diseases
- Pulmonary or massive edema
- Recent vein ligation
- Vascular or skin grafts

EQUIPMENT

Tape measure ◆ talcum powder ◆ antiembolism stockings of correct size and length

PREPARATION

Before applying a knee-length stocking

- Confirm the patient's identity using two patient identifiers according to facility policy.
- Measure the circumference of the patient's calf at its widest point and the leg length from the bottom of the heel to the back of the knee. (See *Measuring for antiembolism stockings*.)

Before applying a thigh-length stocking

- Measure the circumference of the calf and thigh at the widest points and leg length from the bottom of the heel to the gluteal fold.

Before applying a waist-length stocking

- Measure the circumference of the calf and thigh at the widest points and leg length from the bottom of the heel to the waist.
- Obtain the correct size stocking according to the manufacturer's specifications.
- If the patient's measurements are outside the range indicated by the manufacturer or if his legs are deformed or edematous, ask the practitioner if he wants to order custom-made stockings.

KEY STEPS

- Check the practitioner's orders and assess the patient's condition.

  WARNING *If the patient's legs are cold or cyanotic, notify the practitioner before proceeding.*

- Explain the procedure to patient, provide privacy, and wash your hands before beginning the procedure.
- Have the patient lie down.
- Dust his ankles with talcum powder to ease application.

APPLYING A KNEE-LENGTH STOCKING

- Insert your hand into the stocking from the top and grasp the heel pocket from inside.
- Holding the heel, turn the stocking inside out so the foot is inside the stocking leg. This is easier than gathering the entire stocking and working it up over the foot and ankle.
- With the heel pocket down, hook two fingers of both your hands into the foot section.
- Facing the patient, ease the stocking over his toes, stretching it sideways as you move it up the foot.
- Support his ankle with one hand and use the other to pull the heel pocket under the heel.

Measuring for antiembolism stockings

Measure the patient carefully to make sure that his antiembolism stockings provide enough compression for adequate venous return.

To choose the correct *knee-length* stocking, measure the circumference of the calf at its widest point (top left) and leg length from the bottom of the heel to the back of the knee (bottom left).

To choose a *thigh-length* stocking, measure the calf, as before, and thigh at its widest point (top right). Then measure leg length from the bottom of the heel to the gluteal fold (bottom right).

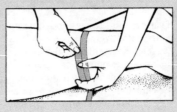
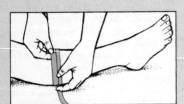
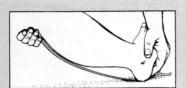
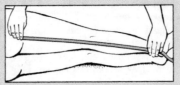

- Center the heel in pocket.
- Supporting his ankle with one hand, use the other to stretch the stocking toward the knee, front, and back to distribute the material evenly.
- The stocking top should be 1″ to 2″ (2.5 to 5 cm) below the bottom of the patella.
- Gently snap the fabric around the ankle to ensure a tight fit and eliminate gaps that could reduce pressure.
- Adjust the foot section for fabric smoothness and toe comfort by tugging on the toe section. Properly position the toe window, if one is there.
- Repeat the procedure for the second stocking, if ordered.

APPLYING A THIGH-LENGTH STOCKING
- Follow the procedure for applying a knee-length stocking.
- Take care to distribute the fabric evenly below the knee before continuing the procedure.
- With the patient's leg extended, stretch the rest of the stocking over the knee.
- Flex the patient's knee and pull the stocking over the thigh until the top is 1″ to 3″ (2.5 to 7.5 cm) below the gluteal fold.
- Stretch the stocking from the top, front, and back to distribute the fabric evenly over the thigh.
- Gently snap the fabric behind the knee to eliminate gaps that could reduce pressure.

APPLYING A WAIST-LENGTH STOCKING
- Follow the same procedure and extend the stocking top to the gluteal fold.
- Fit the patient with the belt that accompanies the stockings.
- ⚡ **WARNING** *Make sure that the waistband and fabric don't interfere with an incision, drainage tube, catheter, or other device.*

SPECIAL CONSIDERATIONS
- To minimize the risk of edema, apply stockings in the morning, if possible.
- If the patient has been ambulating, ask him to lie down and elevate his legs for 15 to 30 minutes before applying the stockings to facilitate venous return.
- Don't allow the stockings to roll or turn down at the top or toe because excess pressure could cause venous strangulation.
- Have him wear the stockings while in bed and during ambulation to provide continuous protection against thrombosis.
- Check his toes at least once every 4 hours — more often if he has a faint pulse or edema.
- Note the skin color and temperature, sensation, swelling, and ability to move his toes.
- Watch for allergic reactions because some patients can't tolerate the sizing of new stockings.
- Reduce the risk of an allergic reaction to sizing by laundering stockings before applying.
- Remove the stockings at least once daily to bathe skin and check for irritation and breakdown.
- Wash the stockings when soiled using warm water and mild soap.
- Keep a second pair of stockings for the patient to wear while the other pair is laundered.

COMPLICATIONS
- May cause obstruction of arterial blood (Obstruction is characterized by cold and bluish toes, dusky toenail beds, decreased or absent pedal pulses, and leg pain or cramps.)
- Allergic reaction
- Skin irritation
- ⚡ **WARNING** *If complications occur, remove the stockings and notify the practitioner immediately.*

PATIENT TEACHING
- If the patient requires antiembolism stockings after discharge, explain why it's important that he wear them.
- Teach the patient or a family member how to apply them correctly.
- Instruct the patient or a family member to care for the stockings properly and replace them if elasticity is lost.

DOCUMENTATION
- Record the date and time of the stocking application and removal.
- Document stocking length and size.
- Document the condition of the leg before and after treatment.
- Note the condition of the toes during treatment.
- Report complications and the patient's tolerance.
- Document patient teaching and the patient's understanding of what was taught.

SELECTED REFERENCES
"Applying Antiembolism Stockings Isn't Just Pulling on Socks," *Nursing* 34(8): 48-49, August 2004.

Howard, A., et al. "Randomized Clinical Trial of Low Molecular Weight Heparin with Thigh-length or Knee-length Antiembolism Stockings for Patients Undergoing Surgery," *British Journal of Surgery* 91(7):842-47, July 2004.

Ingram, J.E. "A Review of Thigh-length vs. Knee-length Antiembolism Stockings," *British Journal of Nursing* 12(14):845-51, July-August 2003.

Iwama, H., et al. "Changes in Femoral Vein Blood Flow Velocity by Intermittent Pneumatic Compression: Calf Compression Device Versus Plantar-calf Sequential Compression Device," *Journal of Anesthesia* 18(3):232-33, August 2004.

Morris, R.J., and Woodcock, J.P. "Evidence-Based Compression: Prevention of Stasis and Deep Vein Thrombosis," *Annals of Surgery* 239(2):162-71, February 2004.

Parnaby, C. "A New Anti-embolism Stocking. Use of Below-knee Products and Compliance," *British Journal of Perioperative Nursing* 14(7):302-304, 306-307, July 2004.

Arterial pressure monitoring, invasive

OVERVIEW

DESCRIPTION
- Monitoring permits direct continuous measurement of systolic, diastolic, and mean pressures and allows arterial blood sampling.
- Known also as *intra-arterial pressure monitoring*, the procedure is generally more accurate than indirect methods based on blood flow alone (such as palpation and auscultation of blood pressure). Accuracy is increased because systemic vascular resistance is also reflected.
- Monitoring is indicated when highly accurate or frequent blood pressure measurements are required in patients with low cardiac output and high systemic vascular resistance or when an intra-aortic balloon pump is used.
- Procedure is used when frequent blood sampling is required or when patients receive titrated doses of vasoactive drugs.

CONTRAINDICATIONS
- Severe injury to the extremity
- Positive Allen's test
- Injury proximal to vessel
- Local skin compromise

EQUIPMENT

CATHETER INSERTION
Preassembled preparation kit (if available) ◆ sterile gloves ◆ sterile gown ◆ mask ◆ protective eyewear ◆ 16G to 20G catheter (type and length depend on insertion site, patient's size, and other anticipated uses of line) ◆ sterile drapes ◆ sheet protector ◆ prepared pressure transducer system ◆ ordered local anesthetic ◆ sterile marker ◆ sterile labels ◆ sutures ◆ syringe and needle (21G to 25G, 1″) ◆ I.V. pole ◆ tubing and drug labels ◆ site care kit ◆ arm board and soft wrist restraint (for femoral site, ankle restraint) ◆ scissors (to clip, rather than shave hair, if needed), optional (for femoral artery insertion)

BLOOD SAMPLE COLLECTION: OPEN SYSTEM
Gloves ◆ gown ◆ mask ◆ protective eyewear ◆ sterile 4″×4″ gauze pads ◆ sheet protector ◆ 500-ml I.V. bag ◆ 5- to 10-ml syringe for discard sample ◆ syringes of appropriate size and number for ordered laboratory tests ◆ laboratory request forms and labels ◆ needleless device (depending on facility policy) ◆ specimen tubes

BLOOD SAMPLE COLLECTION: CLOSED SYSTEM
Gloves ◆ gown ◆ mask ◆ protective eyewear ◆ syringes of appropriate size and number for ordered laboratory tests ◆ laboratory request forms and labels ◆ alcohol pads ◆ blood transfer unit ◆ specimen tubes

ARTERIAL LINE TUBING CHANGES
Gloves ◆ gown ◆ mask ◆ protective eyewear ◆ sheet protector ◆ preassembled arterial pressure tubing with flush device and disposable pressure transducer ◆ sterile gloves ◆ 500-ml bag of I.V. flush solution (such as dextrose 5% in water or normal saline solution) ◆ 500 or 1,000 units of heparin ◆ syringe and needle (21G to 25G, 1″) ◆ sterile label ◆ pressure bag ◆ site care kit ◆ sterile marker

ARTERIAL CATHETER REMOVAL
Gloves ◆ mask ◆ gown ◆ protective eyewear ◆ 2 sterile 4″×4″ gauze pads ◆ sheet protector ◆ sterile suture removal set ◆ dressing ◆ hypoallergenic tape

FEMORAL LINE REMOVAL
Sterile 4″×4″ gauze pads ◆ small sandbag ◆ adhesive bandage ◆ gloves

CATHETER-TIP CULTURE
Sterile scissors ◆ sterile container ◆ sterile gloves

PREPARATION
- Wash your hands.
- Maintain asepsis throughout procedures.
- Set up and prime the monitoring system.
- Assemble equipment, maintaining sterile technique.
- Set alarms on the bedside monitor according to facility policy.

KEY STEPS
- Confirm the patient's identity using two patient identifiers according to facility policy.
- Explain the procedure to the patient and his family.
- Make sure that a consent form was signed.
- Wear personal protective equipment throughout the procedures.
- Check the patient's history for allergy or hypersensitivity to iodine or the ordered local anesthetic.
- Position him for easy access to the catheter insertion site.
- Place a sheet protector under the site.
- If the catheter will be inserted into the radial artery, perform Allen's test to assess the collateral circulation in the hand and document the results.
- Label all medication syringes, medication containers, and solution containers on and off the sterile field.

WARNING *Ischemic injury of the hand is rare if there's adequate ulnar collateral flow, even though thrombosis of the radial artery at the catheter site is common.*

INSERTING AN ARTERIAL CATHETER

◆ The physician prepares and anesthetizes the insertion site and covers the surrounding area with sterile drapes.

⚡ **WARNING** *Cannulation of the brachial artery isn't recommended because of the potential for thrombosis and ischemia of the lower arm and hand.*

◆ The physician inserts the catheter into the artery and attaches it to the fluid-filled pressure tubing.
◆ While the physician holds the catheter in place, activate the fast-flush release (flushing 1 to 3 seconds) to flush blood from the catheter.
◆ After each fast flush, observe the drip chamber to verify a correct continuous flush rate.
◆ Observe the bedside monitor for a waveform.
◆ The physician may suture the catheter in place or secure it with hypoallergenic tape.
◆ Cover the insertion site with a sterile dressing.
◆ With a radial or brachial site, immobilize the insertion site according to facility policy.
◆ With a femoral site, assess the need for immobilization of the lower extremity and maintain the patient on bed rest, with the head of the bed raised no more than 30 degrees, to prevent the catheter from kinking.
◆ Level the zeroing stopcock of the transducer with the phlebostatic axis, and then zero the transducer system to atmospheric pressure.
◆ Activate monitor alarms, as appropriate.

OBTAINING A BLOOD SAMPLE FROM AN OPEN SYSTEM

◆ Turn off or temporarily silence the monitor alarms, according to facility policy.
◆ Open a sterile 4″ × 4″ gauze pad.
◆ Remove the dead-end cap from the stopcock nearest the patient and place it on the gauze pad.
◆ Connect the syringe for the discard sample to the stopcock, turn off the stopcock to the flush solution, and

withdraw 5 to 10 ml, according to facility policy.

⚡ **WARNING** *Don't use the discarded sample for laboratory tests because it's diluted with flushing solution.*

◆ If you feel resistance upon withdrawal or if you don't get a blood return, reposition the affected extremity, check the insertion site for obvious problems, and resume blood withdrawal.
◆ Turn the stopcock halfway back to the open position to close the system in all directions.
◆ Remove the discard sample syringe and dispose of the blood, observing universal precautions.
◆ Place the laboratory sample syringe in the stopcock, turn off the stopcock to the flush solution, and slowly withdraw the required amount of blood.
◆ Repeat the procedure for each sample required.

⚡ **WARNING** *Obtain blood for coagulation tests from the final syringe to prevent dilution from the flush device.*

◆ After you've obtained the blood samples, turn off the stopcock to the syringe and remove it.
◆ Activate the fast-flush release to clear the tubing, turn off the stopcock to the patient, and repeat the fast flush to clear the stopcock port.
◆ Turn off the stopcock to the stopcock port and replace the dead-end cap.
◆ Reactivate the monitor alarms.
◆ Attach the needleless device to the filled syringes and transfer the blood samples to the appropriate specimen tubes.
◆ Label the tubes and send them to the laboratory.
◆ Check the monitor for return of the arterial waveform and pressure reading.

OBTAINING A BLOOD SAMPLE FROM A CLOSED SYSTEM

◆ Locate the closed-system reservoir and blood-sampling site.
◆ Deactivate or temporarily silence the monitor alarms, according to facility policy.

◆ Clean the sampling site with an alcohol pad.
◆ Holding the reservoir upright, grasp the flexures and slowly fill the reservoir with blood to be discarded over 3 to 5 seconds.
◆ If you feel resistance, reposition the affected extremity, check the catheter site for obvious problems, and resume blood withdrawal.
◆ Turn off the one-way valve to the reservoir by turning the handle perpendicular to the tubing.
◆ Insert the cannula into the sampling site, using a syringe with the attached cannula, making sure that the plunger is depressed to the bottom of the syringe barrel.
◆ Slowly fill the syringe, grasp the cannula near the sampling site, and remove the syringe and cannula as one unit.
◆ Repeat the procedure, as needed.
◆ After filling the syringes, turn the one-way valve parallel to the tubing.
◆ Smoothly push down on the plunger until the flexures lock in place in the fully closed position and all fluid has been reinfused over a 3- to 5-second period.
◆ Activate the fast-flush release to clear blood from the tubing and reservoir, flushing for only 1 to 3 seconds.
◆ Clean the sampling site with an alcohol pad.
◆ Reactivate the monitor alarms.
◆ Use the blood transfer unit to transfer blood samples to specimen tubes.
◆ Send the labeled samples to the laboratory.

CHANGING ARTERIAL LINE TUBING

◆ Determine how much tubing length to change, according to facility policy.
◆ Inflate the pressure bag to 300 mm Hg, check it for air leaks, and release the pressure.
◆ Prepare the I.V. flush solution, prime the pressure tubing and transducer system, and add the drug and tubing labels.

⚡ **WARNING** *Priming tubing under pressure may cause microbubble formation.*

(continued)

- Apply 300 mm Hg of pressure to the system and hang the I.V. bag on an I.V. pole.
- Place the sheet protector under the affected extremity.
- Carefully remove the dressing from the catheter insertion site.
- Turn off or temporarily silence the monitor alarms, according to facility policy.
- Turn off the flow clamp of the tubing segment to be changed.
- Carefully disconnect the tubing from the catheter hub.
- Immediately insert new tubing into the catheter hub, secure the tubing, and activate the fast-flush release to clear it.
- Reactivate the monitor alarms.
- Apply an appropriate dressing.
- Level the zeroing stopcock of the transducer with the phlebostatic axis and zero the transducer system to atmospheric pressure.

REMOVING AN ARTERIAL CATHETER

- Determine if you're permitted to perform this procedure, according to facility policy.
- If permitted, record the patient's systolic, diastolic, and mean blood pressures.
- Obtain a manual blood pressure reading to establish a new baseline.
- Turn off the monitor alarms and the flow clamp to the flush solution.
- Carefully remove the dressing over the insertion site.
- Remove sutures using the suture removal kit.
- Withdraw the catheter using a gentle, steady motion, keeping the catheter parallel to the artery during withdrawal.
- Immediately apply pressure to the site with a sterile 4" × 4" gauze pad for at least 10 minutes (longer if bleeding or oozing persists) until hemostasis is obtained.
- If the patient has coagulopathy or is receiving anticoagulants, apply additional pressure to a femoral site.
- Cover the site with an appropriate dressing; secure the dressing with tape.

- Make a pressure dressing for a femoral site by folding four sterile 4" × 4" gauze pads in half. Place the dressing over the femoral site and cover with a tight adhesive bandage. Cover the bandage with a sandbag.
- Maintain the patient on bed rest for 6 hours with the sandbag in place.
- Observe the site for bleeding.
- Assess the extremity distal to the site by evaluating color, pulses, and sensation every 15 minutes for the first 4 hours, every 30 minutes for the next 2 hours, and hourly for the next 6 hours.

Catheter-tip culture

- If infection is suspected, obtain a culture of the catheter by cutting the tip so it falls into a sterile container. Label the specimen and send it to the laboratory.

SPECIAL CONSIDERATIONS

- Observe the pressure waveform on the monitor for abnormalities. (See *Recognizing abnormal waveforms*.)
- Change the pressure tubing every 2 to 3 days, according to facility policy.
- Change the catheter site dressing according to facility policy.
- Regularly assess the site for signs of infection, such as redness and swelling.

⚡ **WARNING** *Be aware that erroneous pressure readings may result from a catheter that's clotted or positional, loose connections, addition of extra stopcocks or extension tubing, inadvertent entry of air into the system, or improper calibration, leveling, or zeroing of the monitoring system.*

⚡ **WARNING** *A disparity of 5 to 20 mm Hg between direct and indirect arterial pressure measurements is a generally accepted range.*

- If the catheter lumen clots, check the flush system for proper pressure.
- Regularly assess the amount of flush solution in the I.V. bag and maintain 300 mm Hg pressure in the pressure bag.

COMPLICATIONS

- Nerve compression and injury
- Hemorrhage
- Infection
- Aneurysm
- Embolism
- Arterial spasm
- Necrosis of overlying skin
- Thrombosis
- Vasovagal reactions
- Hematoma
- Arteriovenous fistula
- Pseudoaneurysm

PATIENT TEACHING

- Explain why the procedure is performed.
- Describe how the arterial catheter is inserted.
- Tell the patient how to keep the affected limb still.
- State the anticipated duration of the catheter placement.
- Discuss discomfort at the insertion site.
- Explain monitoring and care performed while the arterial catheter is in place.
- Tell the patient when to notify the nurse — such as for bleeding.

Recognizing abnormal waveforms

Understanding a normal arterial waveform is relatively straightforward; however, an abnormal waveform is more difficult to decipher. Abnormal patterns and markings may provide important diagnostic clues to the patient's cardiovascular status, or they may simply signal trouble in the monitor. Use this table to help you recognize and resolve waveform abnormalities.

ABNORMALITY	POSSIBLE CAUSES	NURSING INTERVENTIONS
Alternating high and low waves in a regular pattern 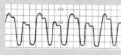	◆ Ventricular bigeminy	◆ Check the patient's electrocardiogram to confirm ventricular bigeminy. The tracing should reflect premature ventricular contractions every second beat.
Flattened waveform 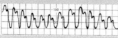	◆ Overdampened waveform or hypotensive patient	◆ Check the patient's blood pressure with a sphygmomanometer. If you obtain a reading, suspect overdampening. Correct the problem by trying to aspirate the arterial line. If you succeed, flush the line. If the reading is very low or absent, suspect hypotension.
Slightly rounded waveform with consistent variations in systolic height 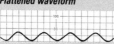	◆ Patient on ventilator with positive end-expiratory pressure	◆ Check the patient's systolic blood pressure regularly. The difference between the highest and lowest systolic pressure reading should be less than 10 mm Hg. If the difference exceeds that amount, suspect pulsus paradoxus, possibly from cardiac tamponade.
Slow upstroke 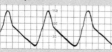	◆ Aortic stenosis	◆ Check the patient's heart sounds for signs of aortic stenosis. Also, notify the physician, who will document suspected aortic stenosis in his notes.
Diminished amplitude on inspiration 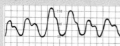	◆ Pulsus paradoxus, possibly from cardiac tamponade, constrictive pericarditis, or lung disease	◆ Note systolic pressure during inspiration and expiration. If inspiration pressure is at least 10 mm Hg less than expiratory pressure, call the physician. ◆ If you're also monitoring pulmonary artery pressure, observe for a diastolic plateau. This occurs when the mean central venous pressure (right arterial pressure), mean pulmonary artery pressure, and mean pulmonary artery wedge pressure are within 5 mm Hg of one another.

DOCUMENTATION

◆ Document the date and time of system setup, tubing or flush change, dressing change, and site care.
◆ Record the systolic, diastolic, and mean pressure.
◆ Report the neurovascular status of the extremity distal to the site.
◆ Note the amount of flush solution infused.
◆ Note the patient's position when the blood pressure reading is obtained.
◆ Describe the appearance of the waveform and include a monitor strip.
◆ Give a comparison with auscultated blood pressure.
◆ Note the insertion site appearance, including evidence of bleeding or infection.
◆ Document patient teaching.

SELECTED REFERENCES

Bourgoin, A., et al. "Increasing Mean Arterial Pressure in Patients with Septic Shock: Effects on Oxygen Variables and Renal Function," *Critical Care Medicine* 33(4):780-86, April 2005.

Eggen, M.A., and Brock-Utne, J.G. "Artifactual Increase in Arterial Pressure Waveform: Remember the Stopcock," *Anesthesia & Analgesia* 101(1):298-99, July 2005.

Garretson, S. "Haemodynamic Monitoring: Arterial Catheters," *Nursing Standard* 19(31):55-64, April 2005.

Michard, F. "Changes in Arterial Pressure during Mechanical Ventilation," *Anesthesiology* 103(2):419-28, August 2005.

Mukkamala, R., et al. "Continuous Cardiac Output Monitoring by Peripheral Blood Pressure Waveform Analysis," *IEEE Transactions on Bio-Medical Engineering* 53(3):459-67, March 2006.

Rose, J.C., et al. "Continuous Monitoring of the Microcirculation in Neurocritical Care: An Update on Brain Tissue Oxygenation," *Current Opinion in Critical Care* 12(2):97-102, April 2006.

Arterial puncture for blood gas analysis

DESCRIPTION

- The procedure requires percutaneous puncture of the brachial, radial, or femoral artery, or withdrawal of a sample from an arterial line.
- Arterial puncture is typically for patients with chronic obstructive pulmonary disease, pulmonary edema, acute respiratory distress syndrome, myocardial infarction, or pneumonia.
- A sample can be analyzed to determine arterial blood gas (ABG) values.
- ABG analysis tests ventilation by measuring blood pH and partial pressures of arterial oxygen (Pao_2) and carbon dioxide ($Paco_2$).
- Blood collection from the femoral artery is usually performed by a practitioner.
- Blood pH measurement reveals the blood's acid-base balance.
- Pao_2 indicates the amount of oxygen the lungs deliver to the blood.
- $Paco_2$ indicates the lungs' capacity to eliminate carbon dioxide.
- ABG values can be analyzed for oxygen content and saturation and for bicarbonate values.

CONTRAINDICATIONS

- Anticoagulant therapy
- History of clotting disorder (hemophilia)
- History of arterial spasms following previous punctures
- Severe peripheral vascular disease
- Abnormal or infectious skin processes at or near puncture sites
- Arterial grafts

EQUIPMENT

10-ml glass syringe or plastic Luer-lock syringe (specially made for drawing blood for ABG analysis) ◆ 1-ml ampule of aqueous heparin (1:1,000) ◆ 20G 1¼″ needle ◆ 22G 1″ needle ◆ gloves ◆ alcohol or povidone-iodine pad ◆ two 2″×2″ gauze pads ◆ rubber cap for syringe hub or rubber stopper for needle ◆ ice-filled plastic bag ◆ label ◆ laboratory request form ◆ adhesive bandage ◆ 1% lidocaine solution (optional)

⚫ **WARNING** *Many facilities use commercial ABG analysis kits that contain equipment listed above (except adhesive bandage and ice). If a kit isn't available, use a sterile syringe specially made for drawing blood for ABG values and use a clean emesis basin filled with ice instead of a plastic bag to transport the sample to the laboratory.*

PREPARATION

- Prepare collection equipment before entering the patient's room.
- Wash your hands.
- Open the ABG analysis kit (if using one) and remove the sample label and plastic bag.
- Record on the label the patient's name, room number, date, collection time, and practioner's name.
- Fill the plastic bag with ice and set it aside.
- If the syringe isn't heparinized, you'll have to do so.
- To heparinize the syringe, first attach the 20G needle to the syringe.
- Open the ampule of heparin and draw all of the heparin into the syringe to prevent the sample from clotting.

- Hold the syringe upright and pull the plunger back slowly to about the 7-ml mark.
- Rotate the barrel while pulling the plunger back to allow the heparin to coat the inside surface of the syringe.
- Slowly force the heparin toward the hub of the syringe and expel all but about 0.1 ml of heparin.
- To heparinize the needle, first replace the 20G needle with the 22G needle.
- Hold the syringe upright, tilt it slightly, and eject the remaining heparin.
- Excess heparin in the syringe alters blood pH and Pao_2 values.

- Confirm the patient's identity using two patient identifiers according to facility policy.
- Before attempting a radial puncture, Allen's test should be performed. (See *Performing Allen's test*.)
- Tell the patient you need to collect an arterial blood sample and explain the procedure to ease his anxiety and gain cooperation.
- Tell the patient that the needle stick will cause discomfort, but he must remain still during the procedure.
- After washing your hands and putting on gloves, place a rolled towel under the patient's wrist for support.
- Locate the artery and palpate for a strong pulse.
- Clean the puncture site with an alcohol or povidone-iodine pad.
- Don't wipe off the povidone-iodine with alcohol.
- Clean the area using a circular motion, starting at the center of the site and spiraling outward. If you use alcohol, apply it with friction for 30

seconds or until the final wipe comes away clean.
- Allow the skin to dry.
- Palpate the artery with the index and middle fingers of one hand while holding the syringe over the puncture site with the other hand.
- Hold the needle bevel up at a 30- to 45-degree angle. When puncturing the brachial artery, hold the needle at a 60-degree angle. (See *Arterial puncture technique*, page 18.)
- Puncture the skin and the arterial wall in one motion, following the path of the artery.
- Watch for blood backflow in the syringe.
- Don't pull back on the plunger because arterial blood should enter the syringe automatically.
- Fill the syringe to the 5-ml mark, and then remove the needle.
- After collecting the sample, press a gauze pad firmly over the puncture site until bleeding stops (at least 5 minutes).
- If the patient is receiving anticoagulant therapy or has a blood dyscrasia, apply pressure for 10 to 15 minutes; if

necessary, ask a coworker to hold the gauze pad in place while you prepare the sample for transport to the laboratory.
- Check the syringe for air bubbles. If any appear, remove them by holding the syringe upright and slowly ejecting some blood onto a $2'' \times 2''$ gauze pad.
- Insert the needle into a rubber stopper, or remove the needle and place a rubber cap directly on the syringe tip. This prevents the sample from leaking and keeps air out of the syringe.
- Put the labeled sample in an ice-filled plastic bag or emesis basin.
- Attach the completed laboratory request form and send the sample to the laboratory immediately.
- When the bleeding stops, apply a small adhesive bandage to the site.
- Monitor the patient's vital signs and watch for circulatory impairment, such as swelling, discoloration, pain, numbness, or tingling in the arm or leg.
- Watch for bleeding at the puncture site.

Performing Allen's test

Rest the patient's arm on the mattress or bedside stand, and support his wrist with a rolled towel. Have him clench his fist. Then, using your index and middle fingers, press on the radial and ulnar arteries. Hold this position for a few seconds.

Without removing your fingers from the patient's arteries, ask him to unclench his fist and hold his hand in a relaxed position. The palm will be blanched because pressure from your fingers has impaired the normal blood flow.

Release pressure on the patient's ulnar artery. If the hand becomes flushed, which indicates blood filling the vessels, you can safely proceed with the radial artery puncture. If the hand doesn't flush, perform the test on the other arm.

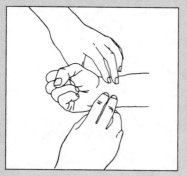
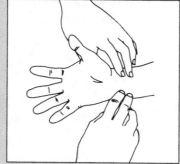
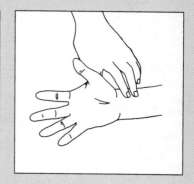

(continued)

◆ If the patient is receiving oxygen, make sure that therapy has been underway at least 15 minutes before collecting the arterial blood sample.

◆ Don't turn off the existing oxygen therapy before collecting arterial blood samples, unless ordered.

⚡ **WARNING** *If the patient has received a nebulizer treatment, wait 20 minutes before collecting the sample.*

◆ If necessary, anesthetize the puncture site with 1% lidocaine solution.

⚡ **WARNING** *Carefully consider the use of lidocaine because the patient may be allergic to the drug; resulting vasoconstriction may prevent successful puncture, and the use of lidocaine delays the procedure.*

◆ When filling out a laboratory request form for ABG analysis, be sure to include the necessary information to help laboratory staff calibrate equipment and correctly evaluate results.

– Record his current temperature.

– Note his most recent hemoglobin level.

– Give his current respiratory rate.

– Indicate if he's on a ventilator.

– Give fraction of inspired oxygen, tidal volume, and ventilatory frequency.

COMPLICATIONS

◆ Using too much force when puncturing the artery (causing the needle to touch the periosteum of the bone, producing pain)

◆ Advancing the needle through the opposite wall of the artery (If this happens, slowly pull the needle back a short distance and check for blood return.)

◆ Blood failing to enter the syringe (If this happens, withdraw the needle completely and start with a fresh heparinized needle.)

⚡ **WARNING** *Don't make more than two attempts to withdraw blood from the same site. Probing may injure the artery or radial nerve. Hemolysis will alter the test results.*

◆ If arterial spasm occurs, blood won't flow into the syringe and you won't be able to collect the sample. If this happens, replace the needle with a smaller one and puncture again.

◆ A smaller-bore needle is less likely to cause arterial spasm.

◆ Tell the patient to notify the nurse if bleeding occurs at the puncture site.

◆ Tell the patient to report paresthesia in the extremity where the procedure was done.

Arterial puncture technique

The angle of needle penetration in arterial blood gas sampling depends on which artery will be sampled. For the radial artery, which is used most commonly, the needle should enter bevel-up at a 30- to 45-degree angle over the artery.

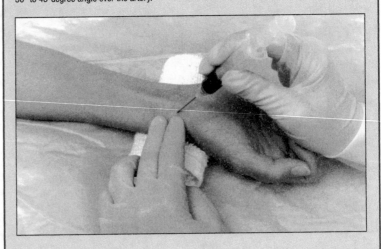

DOCUMENTATION

◆ Record the results of Allen's test.
◆ Note the time the sample was drawn.
◆ Note the patient's temperature.
◆ Indicate the site of the arterial puncture.
◆ Note the amount of time pressure was applied to the site to control bleeding.
◆ Note the type and amount of oxygen therapy the patient received.
◆ If the patient isn't receiving oxygen, indicate that he's breathing room air.
◆ Document patient teaching.

SELECTED REFERENCES

Crawford, A. "An Audit of the Patient's Experience of Arterial Blood Gas Testing," *British Journal of Nursing* 13(9):529-32, May 2004.

Dawson, D., and Hogg, K. "Topical Analgesia for Pain Reduction in Arterial Puncture," *Emergency Medicine Journal* 22(4):273-74, April 2005.

Diby, M., et al. "Harmonization of Practice among Different Groups of Caregivers: A Guideline on Arterial Blood Gas Utilization," *Journal of Nursing Care Quality* 20(4):327-34, October-December 2005.

Sado, D.M., and Deakin, C.D. "Local Anaesthesia for Venous Cannulation and Arterial Blood Gas Sampling: Are Doctors Using It?" *Journal of the Royal Society of Medicine* 98(4):158-60, April 2005.

Yildizdas, D., et al. "Correlation of Simultaneously Obtained Capillary, Venous, and Arterial Blood Gases of Patients in a Paediatric Intensive Care Unit," *Archives of Disease in Childhood* 89(2):176-80, February 2004.

Zavorsky, G.S., et al. "Comparison of Fingertip to Arterial Blood Samples at Rest and during Exercise," *Clinical Journal of Sports Medicine* 15(4):263-70, July 2005.

Arteriovenous hemofiltration, continuous

OVERVIEW

DESCRIPTION

- When patients have fluid overload but don't require or tolerate dialysis, continuous arteriovenous hemofiltration (CAVH) is used for treatment.
- CAVH filters fluid, solutes, and electrolytes from the patient's blood and infuses a replacement solution.
- CAVH carries a much lower risk of hypotension than conventional hemodialysis because it withdraws fluid more slowly — at about 200 ml/hour.
- CAVH can be performed in hypotensive patients who require fluid removal, who can't undergo peritoneal dialysis, or whose requirements for parenteral nutrition would make fluid volume control problematic.
- CAVH reduces the risk of other complications and makes maintaining a stable fluid volume and regulating fluid and electrolyte balance easier.
- A similar procedure, continuous arteriovenous filtration and hemodialysis combines hemodialysis with hemofiltration. Like CAVH, it can also be performed in patients with hypotension and fluid overload.
- Commonly used to treat patients in acute renal failure, CAVH is also used for treating fluid overload that doesn't respond to diuretics and for some electrolyte and acid-base disturbances.
- The hemofilter, composed of about 5,000 hollow fiber capillaries, filters blood at a rate of about 250 ml/minute and is driven by the patient's arterial blood pressure. (A systolic blood pressure of 60 mm Hg is adequate for the procedure.)
- Some of the ultrafiltrate collected during CAVH is replaced with a filter replacement fluid (FRF). This fluid can be lactated Ringer's solution or any solution that resembles plasma.
- Because the amount of fluid removed is greater than the amount replaced, the patient gradually loses fluid (12 to 15 L daily).

CONTRAINDICATIONS

- Active bleeding
- Recent cerebral hemorrhage

EQUIPMENT

CAVH equipment ◆ heparin flush solution ◆ occlusive dressings for catheter insertion sites ◆ sterile gloves ◆ sterile mask ◆ povidone-iodine solution ◆ sterile 4″ × 4″ gauze pads ◆ tape ◆ FRF, as ordered ◆ infusion pump

PREPARATION

- Prime the hemofilter and tubing according to the manufacturer's instructions.

KEY STEPS

- Wash your hands.
- Confirm the patient's identity using two patient identifiers according to facility policy.
- Assemble the equipment at the patient's bedside, and explain the procedure. (See *CAVH setup*.)
- Weigh the patient, take baseline vital signs, and make sure that all necessary laboratory studies have been done (usually electrolyte levels, coagulation factors, complete blood count, blood urea nitrogen, and creatinine studies).
- Monitor the patient's weight and vital signs hourly.
- Assess all pulses in the affected leg initially before access.
- Assess all pulses in the affected leg every hour for the first 4 hours and then every 2 hours afterward.
- If necessary, assist with inserting the catheters into the femoral artery and vein, using strict aseptic technique. (In some cases, an internal arteriovenous fistula or external arteriovenous shunt may be used instead of the femoral route.)
- If ordered, flush both catheters with the heparin flush solution to prevent clotting.
- Apply occlusive dressings to the insertion sites, and mark the dressings

with the date and time. Secure the tubing and connections with tape.
- Put on the sterile gloves and mask.
- Prepare the connection sites by cleaning them with gauze pads soaked in povidone-iodine solution, and then connect them to the exit port of each catheter.
- Connect the arterial and venous lines to the hemofilter. Use aseptic technique.
- Turn on the hemofilter and monitor the blood flow rate through the circuit. The flow rate is usually kept between 500 and 900 ml/hour.
- Inspect the ultrafiltrate during the procedure. It should remain clear yellow, with no gross blood. Pink-tinged or bloody ultrafiltrate may signal a membrane leak in the hemofilter, which permits bacterial contamination. If a leak occurs, follow facility policy. This may include physician notification, hemofilter replacement, or cessation of the procedure.
- Assess the affected leg for signs of obstructed blood flow, such as coolness, pallor, and weak pulse. Check the groin area on the affected side for signs of hematoma. Also, ask the patient if he has pain at the insertion sites.
- Calculate the amount of FRF every hour or as ordered, according to facility policy. Then infuse the prescribed amount and type of FRF through the infusion pump into the arterial side of the circuit.

SPECIAL CONSIDERATIONS

- Because blood flows through an extracorporeal circuit during CAVH, the blood in the hemofilter may need to be anticoagulated. To do this, infuse heparin in low doses (usually starting at 500 units/hour), according to the physician's order, into an infusion port on the arterial side of the setup. Then measure the thrombin clotting time or the activated clotting time (ACT). This ensures that the circuit, not the patient, is anticoagulated. A normal ACT is 100 seconds; during CAVH, keep it between 100 and 300 seconds, depending on the patient's clotting times. If the ACT is too high or too low, the physician will adjust the heparin dose accordingly.

◆ To prevent clotting in the hemofilter, don't infuse medications or blood through the venous line. Run infusions through another line if possible.

◆ Make sure that the patient doesn't bend the affected leg more than 30 degrees at the hip. This prevents catheter kinking and can prevent clot formation.

◆ To prevent infection, perform skin care at the catheter insertion sites every 48 hours, or per facility policy, using aseptic technique. Cover the sites with an occlusive dressing.

◆ If the ultrafiltrate flow rate decreases, raise the bed to increase the distance between the collection device and the hemofilter. Lower the bed to decrease the flow rate. (Clamping the ultrafiltrate line is contraindicated with some types of hemofilters because pressure may build up in the filter, clotting it and collapsing the blood compartment.)

COMPLICATIONS
◆ Bleeding
◆ Hemorrhage
◆ Hemofilter occlusion
◆ Infection
◆ Electrolyte imbalances
◆ Thrombosis

PATIENT TEACHING
◆ Explain the procedure to the patient and answer any of his questions.
◆ Instruct the patient to report pain at the insertion sites.
◆ Instruct the patient to not bend his leg at the hip anymore than 30 degrees to prevent kinking of the catheter and clot formation.

DOCUMENTATION
◆ Record the time the treatment began and ended, fluid balance information, times of dressing changes, complications, medications given, and the patient's tolerance.

SELECTED REFERENCES
de Francisco, A.L., and Pinera, C. "Challenges and Future of Renal Replacement Therapy," *Hemodialysis International* 10(suppl 1):S19-S23, January 2006.

Foland, J.A., et al. "Fluid Overload Before Continuous Hemofiltration and Survival in Critically Ill Children: A Retrospective Analysis," *Critical Care Medicine* 32(8):1771-776, August 2004.

Meyer, B., and Thalhammer, F. "Linezolid and Continuous Venovenous Hemofiltration," *Clinical Infectious Diseases* 42(3):435-36, February 2006.

Palsson, R., et al. "Choice of Replacement Solution and Anticoagulant in Continuous Venovenous Hemofiltration," *Clinical Nephrology* 65(1):34-42, January 2006.

CAVH setup

In continuous arteriovenous hemofiltration (CAVH), the physician inserts two large-bore, single-lumen catheters (as shown below). One catheter is inserted into an artery — most commonly, the femoral artery. The other catheter is inserted into a vein, usually the femoral, subclavian, or internal jugular vein. During CAVH, the patient's arterial blood pressure serves as a natural pump, driving blood through the arterial line. A hemofilter removes water and toxic solutes (ultrafiltrate) from the blood. Replacement fluid is infused into a port on the arterial side. The same port can be used to infuse heparin. The venous line carries the replacement fluid and purified blood to the patient.

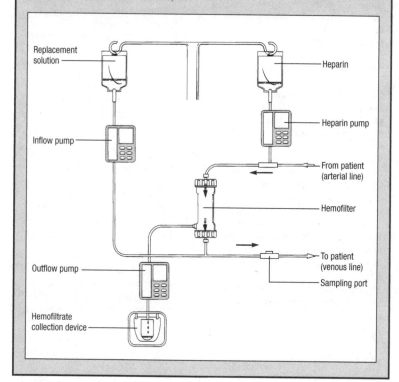

Arteriovenous shunt care

DESCRIPTION

- An arteriovenous (AV) shunt consists of two segments of tubing joined in a U-shape that divert blood from an artery to a vein.
- A shunt provides access to the circulatory system for hemodialysis.
- The device is usually inserted surgically in the forearm or (rarely) the ankle.
- After insertion, a shunt requires regular assessment for patency and examination of surrounding skin for infection.
- Device care also includes aseptically cleaning the arterial and venous exit sites, applying antiseptic ointment, and dressing the sites with sterile bandages.
- When done just before hemodialysis, care prolongs the life of a shunt, helps prevent infection, and allows early detection of clotting.
- Shunt site care is done more often if the dressing becomes wet or nonocclusive.

CONTRAINDICATIONS

- Absence of radial artery pulsation
- Signs of infection

EQUIPMENT

Drape ◆ stethoscope ◆ sterile gloves ◆ sterile 4″ × 4″ gauze pads ◆ sterile cotton-tipped applicators ◆ antiseptic (usually povidone-iodine solution) ◆ bulldog clamps ◆ plasticized or hypoallergenic tape ◆ swab specimen kit (optional) ◆ prescribed antimicrobial ointment (usually povidone-iodine) ◆ sterile elastic gauze bandage ◆ 2″ × 2″ gauze pads ◆ hydrogen peroxide ◆ prepackaged kits are available

KEY STEPS

- Confirm the patient's identity using two patient identifiers according to facility policy.
- Explain the procedure to the patient.
- Provide privacy and wash your hands.
- Place the drape on a stable surface, such as a bedside table, to reduce the risk of traumatic injury to the shunt site.
- Place the shunted extremity on the draped surface.
- Remove the two bulldog clamps from the elastic gauze bandage and unwrap the bandage from the shunt area.
- Carefully remove the gauze dressing covering the shunt and the 4″ × 4″ gauze pad under the shunt.
- Assess the arterial and venous exit sites for signs and symptoms of infection, such as erythema, swelling, excessive tenderness, or drainage.
- Obtain a swab specimen of purulent drainage and tell the practitioner immediately about signs of infection.
- Check the blood flow through the shunt by inspecting the color of the blood and comparing warmth of the shunt with that of the surrounding skin.
- The blood should be bright red and the shunt should feel as warm as the skin.

WARNING *If the blood is dark purple or black and temperature of the shunt is lower than the surrounding skin, clotting has occurred. Tell the practitioner immediately.*

- Use the stethoscope to auscultate the shunt between the arterial and venous exit sites. A bruit confirms normal blood flow.
- Don't use a Doppler device to auscultate because it will detect peripheral blood flow as well as shunt-related sounds.
- Palpate the shunt for a thrill (by lightly placing your fingertips over the access site and feeling for vibration), which also shows normal blood flow.
- Open a few 4″ × 4″ gauze pads and cotton-tipped applicators, and soak them with antiseptic.
- Put on sterile gloves.
- Clean the skin at one of the exit sites using a 4″ × 4″ gauze pad.
- Wipe away from the site to remove bacteria and prevent contamination of the shunt.
- Use the soaked cotton-tipped applicators to remove crusted material from the exit site; encrustations enable bacterial growth.
- Clean the other exit site using fresh, soaked 4″ × 4″ gauze pads and cotton-tipped applicators.
- Clean the rest of the skin that was covered by the gauze dressing with fresh, soaked 4″ × 4″ gauze pads.
- Apply antimicrobial ointment to the exit sites to prevent infection, if ordered.
- Place a dry, sterile 4″ × 4″ gauze pad under the shunt to prevent it from contacting the skin, which could cause irritation and breakdown.
- Cover the exit sites with dry, sterile 4″ × 4″ gauze pads; tape securely to keep the exit sites clean and protected.
- For daily care, wrap the shunt with an elastic gauze bandage.
- Leave a small part of the shunt cannula exposed so the patient can check for patency without removing the dressing.

- Place the bulldog clamps on the edge of the elastic gauze bandage so the patient can use them to stop hemorrhage in case the shunt separates.
- Follow facility procedure for shunt separation.
- For care before hemodialysis, don't re-dress the shunt, but keep the bulldog clamps accessible.

SPECIAL CONSIDERATIONS

WARNING *Make sure that the AV junction of the shunt is secured with plasticized or hypoallergenic tape to prevent separation of the two halves of the shunt and minimize the risk of hemorrhage.*

WARNING *To prevent shunt occlusion, avoid blood pressure measurement and venipuncture in the affected arm.*

- Handle the shunt and dressings carefully.
- Don't use sharp instruments or scissors to remove the dressing because you may cut the shunt.
- Never remove the tape securing the AV junction during dressing changes.
- Use each $4'' \times 4''$ gauze pad only once when cleaning shunt exit sites.
- Avoid wiping any area more than once to minimize the risk of contamination.
- Make sure that the tape doesn't kink or occlude the shunt when re-dressing the site.
- If the exit sites are heavily encrusted, place a $2'' \times 2''$ hydrogen peroxide-soaked gauze pad on the area for about 1 hour to loosen crust.
- Make sure that the patient isn't allergic to iodine before using povidone-iodine solution or ointment.

COMPLICATIONS
- Infection
- Hemorrhage (from shunt separation)

PATIENT TEACHING

- Teach the patient how to care for his shunt for proper home care. (See *Caring for an arteriovenous shunt at home*.)

Caring for an arteriovenous shunt at home

Before the patient leaves the health care facility, teach him how to care for his arteriovenous (AV) shunt. Be sure to cover:
- keeping the incision clean and dry to prevent infection
- cleaning the site daily until it heals completely and the sutures are removed (usually 10 to 14 days after surgery)
- notifying the practitioner about pain, swelling, redness, or drainage at the site
- using a stethoscope to auscultate for bruits and how to palpate a thrill
- using the arm freely after the site heals
- not allowing treatments or procedures on the arm with the AV shunt, including blood pressure monitoring or needle punctures
- avoiding excessive pressure on the arm
- avoiding lifting heavy objects, sleeping on the arm with the AV shunt, or wearing tight-sleeved shirts
- avoiding getting the hemodialysis access site wet for several hours after dialysis
- performing exercises for the affected arm to promote vascular dilation and blood flow, starting by squeezing a small rubber ball or other soft object for 15 minutes, when advised by the practitioner.

DOCUMENTATION

- Note that shunt care was given.
- Describe the condition of the shunt and surrounding skin.
- Note the ointment used.
- Report the instructions given to the patient.

SELECTED REFERENCES

Chen, H., et al. "Using an Anomalous Brachial Artery as an Alternative Choice of Arteriovenous Shunt Feeding Artery," *Nephrology Dialysis Transplantation* 20(11):2579-580, November 2005.

Huijbregts, H.J., and Blankestijn, P.J. "Dialysis Access-Guidelines for Current Practice," *European Journal of Vascular and Endovascular Surgery* 31(3):284-87, March 2006.

Mapes, D. "Nurses' Impact on the Choice and Longevity of Vascular Access," *Nephrology Nursing Journal* 32(6):670-74, November-December 2005.

McGill, R.L., et al. "Nurturing 'Fistula Culture' in a Hospital Environment," *Nephrology News & Issues* 19(6):53, 55, May 2005.

Saxena, A.K., and Panhotra, B.R. "Cardiovascular Mortality and Dialysis Access-Related Infections: Is There a Link?" *American Journal of Kidney Diseases* 46(6):1149-150, December 2005.

Arthroplasty care

DESCRIPTION

- Patient care after arthroplasty — surgical replacement of all or part of a joint — helps restore mobility and normal use of the affected limb.
- Care includes maintaining alignment of the affected joint, assisting with exercises, and providing routine postoperative care.
- Care also includes the responsibility of teaching safe mobility while performing activities of daily living.
- The two most commonly replaced joints are the hip and knee.

CONTRAINDICATIONS

- Active local or systemic infection
- Medical conditions that increase the risk of serious perioperative complications or death
- Severe peripheral vascular disease and some neurologic impairments

EQUIPMENT

Balkan frame with trapeze ◆ comfort device (such as static air mattress overlay, low-air-loss bed, or sheepskin) ◆ bed sheets ◆ incentive spirometer ◆ continuous passive motion (CPM) machine (total knee replacement) ◆ elastic stocking ◆ sterile dressings ◆ hypoallergenic tape ◆ ice bag ◆ skin lotion ◆ warm water ◆ crutches or walker ◆ analgesics ◆ closed-wound drainage system ◆ I.V. antibiotics ◆ pillow ◆ abduction splint and anticoagulants ◆ knee immobilizer (may be needed in the operating room)

PREPARATION

- After the patient goes to surgery, make a Balkan frame with a trapeze on the bed frame, so he can maintain limited mobility after surgery.
- Have the bed taken to the operating room to enable immediate patient placement after surgery and eliminate the need for an additional move from a recovery room bed.

KEY STEPS

- Confirm the patient's identity using two patient identifiers according to facility policy.
- Check the patient's vital signs every 30 minutes until stable, then every 2 to 4 hours, and routinely thereafter, according to facility policy.
- Report changes in vital signs because they may indicate infection and hemorrhage.
- Encourage the patient to perform deep-breathing and coughing exercises.
- Assist with incentive spirometry as ordered to prevent respiratory complications.
- Perform bilateral neurovascular assessment every 2 hours for the first 48 hours and then every 4 hours for signs of complications.
- Check the affected leg for color, temperature, toe movement, sensation, edema, capillary filling, and pedal pulse and compare to the unaffected extremity.
- Investigate complaints of pain, burning, numbness, or tingling.
- Apply elastic stockings or a sequential compression device, as ordered, to promote venous return and prevent phlebitis and pulmonary emboli.
- Once every 8 hours, remove the stocking, inspect the legs for pressure ulcers, and reapply it.
- Give analgesics as ordered.
- Give I.V. antibiotics as ordered.
- Give anticoagulant therapy as ordered.
- Check the leg for signs and symptoms of phlebitis, such as warmth, swelling, tenderness, redness, and a positive Homans' sign.
- Monitor laboratory results, such as complete blood count, prothrombin time, and partial thromboplastin time.
- Check dressings for excessive bleeding.
- Circle drainage on the dressing and mark it with your initials, date, and time.
- Apply additional sterile dressings, as needed, using hypoallergenic tape.
- Check the closed-wound drainage system for discharge color.
- Purulent discharge and fever may indicate infection.
- Empty and measure drainage, as ordered, using aseptic technique to prevent infection.
- Monitor fluid intake and output every shift; include wound drainage in output measurement.
- Apply an ice bag to the affected site for first 48 hours to reduce swelling, relieve pain, and control bleeding.
- Reposition the patient every 2 hours for comfort and prevention of pressure ulcers and respiratory complications.
- Help the patient use the trapeze to lift himself every 2 hours; provide skin care for the back and buttocks, using warm water and lotion.
- Before ambulation, give a mild analgesic, as ordered, because movement is painful.
- Encourage him during exercise.
- Help him with progressive ambulation as needed.

AFTER HIP ARTHROPLASTY

- Keep the affected leg in abduction and in neutral position to stabilize the hip and keep the cup and femur head in the acetabulum.
- Place a pillow between the patient's legs to maintain hip abduction.
- If desired, elevate the head of his bed 45 degrees for comfort. (Some physicians permit 60-degree elevation.)
- Limit elevation to 30 minutes at a time to prevent excessive hip flexion.

⚠ **WARNING** *Don't let the hip flex more than 90 degrees because the prosthesis may dislocate.*

- The day after surgery, have the patient begin plantar flexion and dorsiflexion exercises of the foot on the affected leg.
- Teach him to begin quadriceps exercises, when ordered.
- Progressive ambulation protocols vary. Most patients are permitted to begin transfer and progressive ambulation with assistive devices on the first day.

AFTER TOTAL KNEE REPLACEMENT

◆ Keep the knee immobilized in full extension immediately after surgery.
◆ Many health care facilities start CPM in the postanesthesia care unit.
◆ Elevate the affected leg to reduce swelling, as ordered.
◆ Instruct the patient to begin quadriceps and straight leg-raising exercises, when ordered (usually on the first postoperative day).
◆ Encourage flexion-extension exercises, when ordered (usually after the first dressing change).
◆ If the physician orders the use of a CPM machine, he'll adjust the machine daily to gradually increase the degree of flexion of the affected leg.
◆ The patient can usually dangle his feet the first day after surgery and begin ambulation with partial weight bearing as tolerated (cemented knee) or toe-touch ambulation only (uncemented knee) by the second day.
◆ He may need a knee immobilizer for support when walking; otherwise, he should be in CPM for most of the day and night or during waking hours only. Check facility protocol.

SPECIAL CONSIDERATIONS

◆ Before surgery, explain the procedure to the patient.
◆ Emphasize that frequent assessment — including monitoring the patient's vital signs, neurovascular integrity, and wound drainage — is normal after surgery.
◆ Inform him that he'll receive I.V. antibiotics for about 2 days.
◆ Make sure that the patient understands he'll receive drugs around the clock for pain control.
◆ Explain the need for immobilizing the affected leg and exercising the unaffected one.

COMPLICATIONS

◆ Pulmonary embolism
◆ Pneumonia
◆ Phlebitis
◆ Paralytic ileus
◆ Urine retention
◆ Bowel impaction
◆ Infection

> 🔲 **WARNING** *The presence of a deep wound or an infection at the prosthesis site is a serious complication that may require removal of the prosthesis.*

> 🔲 **WARNING** *Dislocation of a total hip prosthesis may occur after violent hip flexion or adduction or during internal rotation. Signs and symptoms include the inability to rotate the hip or bear weight, shortening of the leg, and increased pain.*

> 🔲 **WARNING** *Fat embolism, a potentially fatal complication resulting from the release of fat molecules in response to increased intermedullary canal pressure from the prosthesis, may develop within 72 hours after surgery. Watch for apprehension, diaphoresis, fever, dyspnea, pulmonary effusion, tachycardia, cyanosis, seizures, decreased level of consciousness, or petechial rash on the chest and shoulders.*

PATIENT TEACHING

◆ Teach the patient to perform muscle-strengthening exercises for the affected and unaffected extremities to maintain muscle strength and range of motion to prevent phlebitis.
◆ Before discharge, instruct the patient about home care and exercises.
◆ Tell the patient about drugs, including dosages and possible adverse effects.
◆ Advise the patient to avoid sexual intercourse for 4 to 8 weeks. Sexual activity can usually be resumed after the 2-month follow-up.
◆ Advise the patient he may return to work in 3 to 6 months or as instructed by the physician.
◆ Tell the patient not to drive a car until after the 2-month follow-up.
◆ Tell the patient to keep wearing elastic stockings until the 2-month follow-up.
◆ Advise the patient to not get the incision wet (no showers or tub baths) before staples are removed.

◆ Instruct the patient to inform dentists and other physicians of arthroplasty. He may require antibiotic prophylaxis for certain procedures.

DOCUMENTATION

◆ Record the patient's neurovascular status.
◆ Describe his position (especially the position of the affected leg).
◆ Note skin care and condition.
◆ Report respiratory care and condition.
◆ Document the use of elastic stockings.
◆ Document exercises performed and their effect.
◆ Record ambulatory efforts and the type of support used.
◆ Record the patient's vital signs and fluid intake and output on the flowchart.
◆ Record discharge instructions and the patient's understanding.

SELECTED REFERENCES

Altizer, L. "Patient Education for Total Hip or Knee Replacement," *Orthopaedic Nursing* 23(4):283-88, July-August 2004.

Best, J.T. "Revision Total Hip and Total Knee Arthroplasty," *Orthopaedic Nursing* 24(3):174-79, May-June 2005.

Hohler, S.E. "Looking into Minimally Invasive Total Hip Arthroplasty," *Nursing* 35(6):54-57, June 2005.

Pellino, T.A., et al. "Use of Nonpharmacologic Interventions for Pain and Anxiety after Total Hip and Total Knee Arthroplasty," *Orthopaedic Nursing* 24(3):182-90, May-June 2005.

Temple, J. "Total Hip Replacement," *Nursing Standard* 19(3):44-51, September-October 2004.

Timm, S. "Minimally Invasive Total Hip Arthroplasty: What Is It All About?" *Journal of Continuing Education in Nursing* 35(6):246-47, November-December 2004.

Autologous blood transfusion

OVERVIEW

DESCRIPTION

◆ Autologous transfusion (also called *autotransfusion*) is the collection, filtration, and reinfusion of the patient's own blood.

◆ Autologous transfusion has several advantages over transfusion of bank blood, including:
- lack of transfusion reactions
- prevention of disease transmission
- decreased need for anticoagulants (except in postoperative autotransfusion, when acid citrate dextrose [ACD] or citrate phosphate dextrose [CPD] is added)
- the blood supply isn't depleted.

◆ Autologous blood contains normal levels of 2,3-diphosphoglycerate, which increases in tissue oxygenation.

◆ Three techniques are preoperative blood donation, perioperative blood donation, and acute normovolemic hemodilution.

◆ Preoperative blood donation is recommended for patients scheduled for orthopedic surgery, which causes large blood loss.

◆ Donation begins 4 to 6 weeks before surgery.

◆ Perioperative blood may be collected during surgery or up to 12 hours afterward.

◆ Blood obtained postoperatively may be collected from chest tubes, mediastinal drains, or wound drains (placed in the surgical wound during surgery).

◆ Acute normovolemic hemodilution is used mainly in open-heart surgery.

◆ One or two units of blood are drawn immediately before or after anesthesia induction.

◆ The blood is replaced with a crystalloid or colloid solution, such as lactated Ringer's solution or dextran 40, to produce normovolemic anemia.

◆ The blood is reinfused after surgery.

◆ Acute normovolemic hemodilution is performed the same way as preoperative blood donation. Blood collected this way is reinfused the same way as with other transfusions.

CONTRAINDICATIONS

◆ Malignant neoplasms, coagulopathies, excessive hemolysis, and active infection

◆ Antibiotic use

◆ Blood that becomes contaminated by bowel contents

◆ Recent weight loss because of illness or malnutrition

◆ Cardiovascular disease with compromised hemodynamic reserves

◆ Anemia

◆ Conditions predisposing to bacteremia such as an indwelling urinary catheter

EQUIPMENT

Equipment listed here is for preoperative and perioperative blood donation only.

PREOPERATIVE BLOOD DONATION

Ferrous sulfate ◆ povidone-iodine solution ◆ alcohol ◆ tourniquet ◆ rubber ball ◆ large-bore needle for venipuncture ◆ collection bags ◆ I.V. line ◆ in-line filter for reinfusion

PERIOPERATIVE BLOOD DONATION

Autologous transfusion system (such as Davol or Pleur-evac systems) ◆ ACD or CPD collection bags ◆ vacuum source regulator ◆ suction tubing ◆ 18G needle ◆ blood administration set with in-line filter ◆ 500 ml of normal saline solution ◆ Hemovac and another autologous transfusion system (optional)

- Procedures presented are for preoperative and perioperative blood donation only.
- Steps depend on the circumstances of the autologous transfusion.

PREOPERATIVE BLOOD DONATION

- Explain autologous transfusion, including how and why it's performed, how often the patient can donate blood (every 7 days), and how much he can donate (1 unit every week until 3 to 7 days before surgery).
- Give him ferrous sulfate or another iron preparation to take three times per day at least 1 week before the first donation, or as ordered.
- To prevent hypovolemia, tell him to drink plenty of fluids before donating blood.
- Warn the patient that he may feel light-headed during the donation, but that it can easily be treated.
- Check his hemoglobin level, which must be 11 g/dl or higher to donate blood.
- Check the patient's vital signs before blood donation.
- Help him into a supine position.
- Clean the needle insertion site (usually the antecubital fossa) with alcohol or povidone-iodine solution.
- Apply a tourniquet.
- Insert the large-bore needle into the antecubital vein.
- Have him squeeze a rubber ball while you collect blood.
- Recheck the patient's vital signs after the collection.
- Provide replacement I.V. fluids immediately after the collection if ordered.
- Send a blood sample to the laboratory to be tested.

PERIOPERATIVE BLOOD DONATION

- Notify the patient if you know he'll leave surgery with a drain to the autologous transfusion device.

PERIOPERATIVE BLOOD DONATION USING A DAVOL SYSTEM

- Open the transfusion unit onto the sterile field.
- The physician inserts the drain tube (from the patient) to the connecting tube of the unit.
- The physician injects 25 to 35 ml of ACD or CPD into the injection port on top of the filter and wets the filter with anticoagulant to keep blood from clotting.
- Label the collection bag with the patient's name and time the transfusion was started so the reinfusion time is within guidelines.

AFTER PATIENT ARRIVAL IN POSTANESTHESIA CARE UNIT OR MEDICAL-SURGICAL UNIT

- Note on the bag and on the postoperative sheet the amount of blood in the bag.
- Attach the tube from the suction source to the port on the suction control module.
- Adjust the suction source to between 80 and 100 mm Hg on the wall regulator.
- Pinch the suction tube; if the regulator exceeds 100 mm Hg, turn the suction down. Suction set at more than 100 mm Hg may cause the collection bag to collapse, resulting in lysis of blood cells.
- If the collection bag collapses, change the entire collection setup.
- Start reinfusing blood when 500 ml has been collected or as ordered.

🔹 **WARNING** *Blood reinfusion must be completed within 4 hours of initiating collection in the operating room.*

- If less than 200 ml of blood is collected in 4 hours, record the amount on the intake and output sheet and the postoperative sheet.
- Discard drainage appropriately if the proportion of anticoagulant (inserted in the operating room) to blood is too great to infuse.
- If the blood can't be infused, switch from the collection container to a closed-wound suction unit.

- Remove the suction tube from the suction control unit.
- Clamp the connecting tubing above the filter.
- Detach the connecting tubing from the patient's tube and cap the patient's tube.
- Connect a closed-wound suction unit, such as a Hemovac, if you aren't going to collect more blood for reinfusion.
- If more than 500 ml of blood is collected in the first 4 hours, connect a new autologous transfusion unit to the patient.
- Reconnect the unit to suction, then monitor and record the drainage on the intake and output sheet.

BLOOD REINFUSION

- Prime the blood filter with 500 ml of normal saline solution.
- Twist the suction control module to remove it.
- Remove the hanger assembly from the collection bag.
- Pull the clear cap from the top of the bag, and discard the cap and filter.
- Insert a spike adapter into the large port on top of the bottle.
- Remove the protective seal to expose the filtered vent.
- Attach the blood to the Y-connector of the blood filter.
- Invert the bag and hang it.
- Obtain and document the patient's vital signs.
- Begin the infusion, following facility policy.
- Be sure to complete the infusion within 2 hours.

PERIOPERATIVE BLOOD DONATION USING THE PLEUR-EVAC SYSTEM CONNECTED TO A CHEST TUBE

- Establish underwater seal drainage.
- Connect the patient's chest tube, following steps printed on the Pleur-evac unit.
- Inspect the blood collection bag and tubing, making sure that all clamps are open and all connections are airtight.

(continued)

- If prescribed, add an anticoagulant, such as heparin or CPD, before collection.
- With CPD, add 1 part CPD to 7 parts blood.
- Inject anticoagulant through the red self-sealing port on the autologous transfusion connector using an 18G (or smaller) needle.
- After adding anticoagulant, the system is ready to use.
- You should see chest cavity blood begin to collect in the bag.
- To collect more than one bag of blood, open a replacement bag when the first is nearly full.
- Close the clamps on top of the second bag.
- Before removing the first collection bag from the drainage unit, reduce excess negativity by using the high-negativity relief valve.
- Depress the button.
- Watch the water seal manometer and release the relief valve button when negativity drops to the desired level.
- Close the white clamp on the patient tubing.
- Close the two white clamps on top of the collection bag.
- Disconnect all connectors on the first bag.
- Attach the red (female) and blue (male) connector sections on top of the autologous transfusion bag.
- Remove the protective cap from the collection tubing on the replacement bag.
- Using the red connectors, connect the collection tubing to the patient's chest drainage tube.
- Using the blue connectors, remove the protective cap from the replacement bag's suction tube and attach the tube to the Pleur-evac unit.
- Make sure that all connections are tight.
- Open all clamps and inspect the system for airtight connections.
- Spread the metal support arms and disconnect them.
- Remove the first bag from the drainage unit by disconnecting the foot hook.
- Use the foot hook and support arm to attach the replacement bag.

- Reinfuse blood from the original collection bag.
- Slide the bag off the support frame and invert it so the spike points upward.
- Remember to reinfuse blood within 4 hours of the start of collection.
- Never store the collected blood.
- Remove the protective cap from the spike port and insert a microaggregate filter into the port, using a twisting motion.
- Prime the filter by gently squeezing the inverted bag.
- Use a new filter with each bag.
- Continue squeezing until the filter is saturated and the drip chamber is one-half full.
- Close the clamp on the reinfusion line and remove residual air from the bag.
- Invert the bag and suspend it from an I.V. pole.
- After carefully flushing the I.V. line to remove all air, infuse the blood according to facility policy.

SPECIAL CONSIDERATIONS

PREOPERATIVE BLOOD DONATION
- Monitor the patient closely during and after donation and autologous transfusion.
- Vasovagal reactions are usually mild and easy to treat but can quickly progress to severe reactions, such as loss of consciousness and seizures.
- Make sure that the patient isn't bacteremic when he donates blood. Bacteria can proliferate in the collection bag and cause sepsis when reinfused.
- Clearly label the collection bag AUTOLOGOUS USE ONLY so the blood won't be subjected to rigorous blood bank testing or accidentally given to another patient.
- Before reinfusion, identify the patient and make sure that the collection bag is clearly marked with his name, identification number, and an autologous blood label.
- If signs of a hemolytic reaction occur, the patient may have received the wrong unit of blood.

ALL DONATION METHODS
- Check the patient's laboratory data (coagulation profile, hemoglobin and calcium levels, and hematocrit) after he donates blood and again after reinfusion.
- Before reinfusion, identify the patient and make sure that the collection bag is clearly marked with his name, identification number, and an autologous blood label.
- Be alert for signs and symptoms of a hemolytic reaction.
- If you observe pain at the I.V. site, fever, chills, back pain, hypotension, or anxiety, stop the transfusion and call the blood bank and physician. The patient may have received the wrong unit of blood.
- Check the patient's laboratory data again after reinfusion.

COMPLICATIONS
- Hemolysis
- Air and particulate emboli
- Coagulation
- Thrombocytopenia
- Vasovagal reactions (from transient hypotension and bradycardia)

AGE FACTOR *Hypovolemia can occur as a complication, especially in elderly patients. (See* Managing problems of autologous transfusion.*)*

- Have the patient lie down for at least 10 minutes after donating blood.
- Encourage the patient to drink more fluids than usual for a few hours after blood donation and to eat a large meal.
- Tell the patient to inspect the needle wound for a few hours after blood donation.
- If bleeding occurs, have the patient apply firm pressure for 5 to 10 minutes.
- Tell the patient that if bleeding doesn't stop, to notify the blood bank or his physician.
- If the patient feels light-headed or dizzy, advise him to sit and lower his head between his knees, or lie down with his head lower than the rest of his body until the feeling stops.
- Tell the patient he can resume normal activities after resting 15 minutes.

- Record the amount of blood the patient donated and had reinfused.
- Describe how the patient tolerated each procedure.

SELECTED REFERENCES

Dietrich, W., et al. "Autologous Blood Donation in Cardiac Surgery: Reduction of Allogenic Blood Transfusion and Cost-Effectiveness," *Journal of Cardiothoracic and Vascular Anesthesia* 19(5):589-96, October 2005.

Garvin, K.L., et al. "Blood Salvage and Allogenic Transfusion Needs in Revision Hip Arthroplasty," *Clinical Orthopaedics and Related Research* 441:205-209, December 2005.

Kirschman, R.A. "Finding Alternatives to Blood Transfusion," *Nursing* 34(6):58-62, June 2004.

Lewis, C.E., et al. "Autologous Blood Transfusion in Elective Cardiac Valve Operations," *Journal of Cardiac Surgery* 20(6):513-18, November-December 2005.

Rock, G., et al. "The Development of an Optimized Autologous Blood Donation Program," *Transfusion and Apheresis Science* 33(3):325-31, November 2005.

Managing problems of autologous transfusion

PROBLEM	POSSIBLE CAUSES	NURSING INTERVENTIONS
Citrate toxicity (rare, unpredictable)	• Chelating effect on calcium of citrate phosphate dextrose (CPD) • Predisposing factors, including hyperkalemia, hypocalcemia, acidosis, hypothermia, myocardial dysfunction, and liver or kidney problems	• Watch for hypotension, arrhythmias, and myocardial contractility. • Prophylactic calcium chloride may be given if more than 2,000 ml of CPD-anticoagulated blood is given over 20 minutes. • Stop infusing CPD and correct acidosis. Measure arterial blood gas values and serum calcium levels frequently to assess for toxicity.
Coagulation	• Not enough anticoagulant • Blood not defibrinated in mediastinum	• Add CPD or another regional anticoagulant at a ratio of 7 parts blood to 1 part anticoagulant. Keep blood and CPD mixed by shaking collection bottle regularly. • Check for anticoagulant reversal. Strip chest tubes as needed.
Coagulopathies	• Reduced platelet and fibrinogen levels • Platelets caught in filters • Enhanced levels of fibrin split products	• Patients receiving autologous transfusions of more than 4,000 ml of blood may also need transfusion of fresh frozen plasma or platelet concentrate.
Emboli	• Microaggregate debris • Air	• Don't use equipment with roller pumps or pressure infusion systems. Before reinfusion, remove air from blood bags. • Reinfuse with a 20- to 40-unit microaggregate filter.
Hemolysis	• Trauma to blood caused by turbulence or roller pumps	• Don't skim operative field or use equipment with roller pumps. When collecting blood from chest tubes, keep vacuum below 30 mm Hg; when aspirating from a surgical site, keep vacuum below 60 mm Hg.
Sepsis	• Lack of sterile technique • Contaminated blood	• Give broad-spectrum antibiotics. Use strict sterile technique. Reinfuse patient within 4 hours. • Don't infuse blood from infected areas or blood that contains feces, urine, or other contaminants.

Automated external defibrillation

DESCRIPTION

- Automated external defibrillation is used for early defibrillation, which is currently the most effective treatment for sudden cardiac arrest due to ventricular fibrillation.
- Some facilities require an automated external defibrillator (AED) in every noncritical care unit.
- AEDs are becoming common in public places, such as shopping malls, sports stadiums, health clubs, federal and state buildings, and airplanes.
- Instruction in using an AED is required in basic life support (BLS) and advanced cardiac life support (ACLS) training.
- AEDs are increasingly being used to provide early defibrillation — even when no health care professional is present.
- AEDs interpret the patient's cardiac rhythm and give the operator step-by-step directions if defibrillation is needed.
- Some AEDs have a "quick-look" feature that allows visualization of the rhythm using the paddles before the electrodes are connected.
- AEDs are equipped with a micro-computer that senses and analyzes a patient's heart rhythm at the push of a button.
- AEDs audibly, and sometimes visually, prompt you to deliver a shock.
- AED models all have the same basic function, but offer different operating options.
- AEDs communicate directions via voice commands and, sometimes, also on a display screen.
- Some AEDs simultaneously display a patient's heart rhythm.
- All devices record interactions with the patient during defibrillation, either on a cassette tape or in a solid-state memory module.
- Some AEDs have an integral printer for immediate event documentation.
- Facility policy determines who's responsible for reviewing AED interactions; the patient's practitioner always has that option.
- Local and state regulations govern who's responsible for collecting AED case data for reporting purposes.

CONTRAINDICATIONS

- Stable patient with a pulse
- Patient having a seizure
- In the patient who has made a legal documented request that he not be resuscitated
- If immediate danger to rescuers is evident because of environment, patient's location, or patient's condition

⚡ WARNING *Use with caution in a moving vehicle. If being used on a patient in transport, frequent stops for pulse and AED monitoring checks should be made.*

AED ◆ 2 prepackaged electrodes (pads)

- After determining that the patient is unresponsive, has no pulse, and is apneic, follow BLS and ACLS protocols.
- Ask a colleague to bring the AED into the patient's room and set it up before the code team arrives.
- Firmly press the AED's ON button and wait while the machine performs a brief self-test.
- Most AEDs signal readiness by a computerized voice that says, "Stand clear" or by emitting a series of loud beeps.
- If the AED is malfunctioning, it will convey the message "Do not use the AED. Remove and continue cardio-pulmonary resuscitation (CPR)." Report AED malfunctions in accordance with facility procedure.
- Open the foil packets containing two electrode pads. Attach the electrode cable to the AED.
- Expose the patients chest. Remove the plastic backing from the electrode pads and place the electrode pad on the right upper portion of the patient's chest, just beneath his clavicle. Place the second pad to the level of the heart's apex.
- At this point, the machine is ready to analyze the patient's heart rhythm.
- Ask everyone to stand clear.
- Press the ANALYZE button when the machine prompts you to.

WARNING *Be careful not to touch or move the patient while the AED is in analysis mode. (If you get the message "Check electrodes," make sure that the electrodes are correctly placed and the patient cable is securely attached; then press the ANALYZE button again.)*

♦ In 15 to 30 seconds, the AED will analyze the patient's rhythm.
♦ When the patient needs a shock, the AED will display a "Stand clear" message and emit a beep that changes into a steady tone as it's charging.
♦ When the AED is fully charged and ready to deliver a shock, it will prompt you to press the SHOCK button. (Some fully automatic AED models automatically deliver a shock within 15 seconds after analyzing the patient's rhythm.)
♦ If a shock isn't needed, the AED will display "No shock indicated," and you should then continue CPR.
♦ Make sure that no one is touching the patient or his bed, and call out "Stand clear."
♦ Press the SHOCK button on the AED.
♦ After the first shock at 360 joules (monophasic), the AED will automatically reanalyze the patient's rhythm.
♦ If no additional shock is needed, the machine will prompt you to check the patient. However, if he's still in ventricular fibrillation, perform CPR for 2 minutes and then press the ANALYZE button on the AED to identify the heart rhythm.
♦ If the patient is still in ventricular fibrillation, the AED will prompt you to press the SHOCK button. A second shock at 360 joules (monophasic) will be delivered.
♦ After five cycles of CPR (about 2 minutes), the AED should then analyze the cardiac rhythm and deliver another shock, if indicated.
♦ Repeat the steps performed earlier before delivering a shock to the patient.
♦ The energy level delivered may be different when using a defibrillator that delivers biphasic shocks (usually 120 to 200 joules) Follow facility policy.

WARNING *If the patient is still in ventricular fibrillation after three shocks, resume CPR.*

♦ Continue this sequence until the code team arrives.
♦ After the code, remove and transcribe the AED's computer memory module or tape, or prompt the AED to print a rhythm strip with code data.
♦ Follow facility policy for analyzing and storing code data.

WARNING *Don't remove the pads until directed to do so by the receiving practitioner or facility.*

SPECIAL CONSIDERATIONS

♦ AEDs vary by manufacturer. Familiarize yourself with your facility's equipment.
♦ AED operation should be checked at least every 8 hours and after each use.

COMPLICATIONS
♦ Accidental electric shock to care providers

PATIENT TEACHING

♦ Explain the procedure to the patient and answer his questions.

DOCUMENTATION

♦ Provide a summary of actions to the code team leader.
♦ Report the patient's name, age, and medical history.
♦ Note the time the patient was found in cardiac arrest.
♦ Note when you started CPR, when you applied the AED, and how many shocks he received.
♦ Note when the patient regained a pulse at any point.
♦ Note what postarrest care was given, if any.
♦ Document physical assessment findings.
♦ Later, document the code on the appropriate form.

SELECTED REFERENCES
Bar-Cohen, Y., et al. "First Appropriate Use of Automated External Defibrillator in an Infant," *Resuscitation* 67(1): 135-37, October 2005.
Craig, K. "Take Charge with an Automated External Defibrillator," *Nursing* 35(11): 50-52, November 2005.
Kyller, M., and Johnstone, D. "A 2-tiered Approach to In-hospital Defibrillation: Nurses Respond to a Trial of Using Automated External Defibrillators as Part of a Code-Team Protocol," *Critical Care Nurse* 25(4):25-33, August 2005.
Rea, T.D., et al. "Automated External Defibrillators: To What Extent Does the Algorithm Delay CPR?" *Annals of Emergency Medicine* 46(2):132-41, August 2005.
Riegel, B., et al. "How Well Are Cardiopulmonary Resuscitation and Automated External Defibrillator Skills Retained Over Time? Results from the Public Access Defibrillation (PAD) Trial," *Academic Emergency Medicine* 13(3):254-63, March 2006.
Weil, M.H., and Fries, M. "In-hospital Cardiac Arrest," *Critical Care Medicine* 33(12):2825-830, December 2005.

Balloon valvuloplasty

DESCRIPTION

- Surgery is the treatment of choice for valvular heart disease.
- For patients with critical stenoses, balloon valvuloplasty is an alternative to valve replacement.
- It enlarges the orifice of a heart valve that has been narrowed by a congenital defect, calcification, rheumatic fever, or aging.
- It's indicated for patients who face a high risk from surgery and for those who refuse surgery.

  AGE FACTOR *Balloon valvuloplasty is more tolerable than surgery for elderly patients, especially those older than age 80.*
- The procedure is done in the cardiac catheterization laboratory under local anesthesia and moderate sedation.
- The physician inserts a balloon-tipped catheter through the patient's femoral vein or artery, threads it into the heart, and repeatedly inflates it against the leaflets of the diseased valve.
- Inflation increases the size of the orifice, improving valvular function and helping prevent complications from decreased cardiac output.
- The nurse should teach the patient and his family about valvuloplasty and monitor the patient for potential complications.

CONTRAINDICATIONS

None known

EQUIPMENT

Povidone-iodine solution ◆ local anesthetic ◆ valvuloplasty or balloon-tipped catheter ◆ I.V. solution and tubing ◆ electrocardiogram (ECG) monitor and electrodes ◆ pulmonary artery (PA) catheter ◆ contrast medium ◆ oxygen ◆ sterile labels ◆ sterile marker ◆ nasal cannula ◆ sedative ◆ emergency medications ◆ scissors ◆ heparin for injection ◆ introducer kit for balloon catheter ◆ sterile gown, gloves, mask, cap, and drapes ◆ 5-lb (2.3-kg) sandbag ◆ nitroglycerin (optional)

KEY STEPS

BEFORE BALLOON VALVULOPLASTY

- Reinforce the physician's explanation of balloon valvuloplasty, including the risks and alternatives, to the patient and his family.
- Inform the patient that he'll be awake during the procedure, but will receive a sedative and a local anesthetic beforehand.
- Tell the patient that his groin area will be shaved and cleaned with an antiseptic.
- Tell the patient that he'll feel a brief sting when the local anesthetic is injected and may feel pressure as the catheter moves along the vessel.
- Describe the warm, flushed feeling the patient is likely to experience from injection of the contrast medium.
- Tell the patient that the procedure may last up to 4 hours and he may feel discomfort lying on a hard table that long.
- Make sure that the patient has no allergies to shellfish, iodine, or contrast media and that he or a family member has signed a consent form.
- Withhold food and fluids (except for drugs) for at least 6 hours before valvuloplasty or as ordered (usually after midnight the night before the procedure).
- Make sure that results of routine laboratory studies and blood typing and crossmatching are available.
- Insert an I.V. line to provide access for drugs.
- Take baseline peripheral pulses in all extremities.
- Clip hair from the insertion site, if needed.
- Clean the site with povidone-iodine solution.
- Give him a sedative as ordered.
- Have him void.
- When he arrives at the cardiac catheterization laboratory, apply ECG electrodes and ensure I.V. line patency.
- Label all medication syringes, medication containers, and solution containers on and off the sterile field.

DURING BALLOON VALVULOPLASTY

- Give oxygen by nasal cannula.
- The physician may insert a PA catheter if one isn't in place.
- The physician inserts a large guide catheter into the site through an introducer sheath and threads a valvuloplasty or balloon-tipped catheter up into the heart.
- The physician injects a contrast medium to visualize the heart valves and assess the stenosis.
- The physician injects heparin to prevent the catheter from clotting.
- Using low pressure, he inflates the balloon on the valvuloplasty catheter for a short time, usually 15 to 30 seconds, gradually increasing the time and pressure.
- If the stenosis isn't reduced, a larger balloon may be used.
- After completion of valvuloplasty, a series of angiograms are taken to evaluate the effectiveness of treatment.
- The physician sutures the guide catheter in place.
- The physician removes the guide catheter after the effects of the heparin have worn off.

AFTER BALLOON VALVULOPLASTY

- When the patient returns to the cardiac intensive care unit, he may be receiving I.V. heparin or nitroglycerin.
- He may also have a sandbag on the insertion site as a reminder to maintain limb position.
- Monitor ECG rhythm and arterial pressures.

  AGE FACTOR *Monitor the insertion site frequently for signs of hemorrhage because exsanguination can occur rapidly.*
- Keep the affected leg straight and elevate the head of the bed no more than 15 degrees to prevent excessive

hip flexion and migration of the catheter.

◆ Use a soft restraint, if necessary.

◆ Monitor the patient's vital signs every 15 minutes for the first hour, every 30 minutes for the next 2 hours, and then hourly for the next 5 hours.

⚫ **WARNING** *If the patient's vital signs are unstable, notify the physician and continue to check them every 5 minutes.*

◆ When you take vital signs, assess peripheral pulses distal to the catheter insertion site as well as the color, sensation, temperature, and capillary refill of the affected extremity.

◆ Assess the catheter site for hematoma, ecchymosis, and hemorrhage.

⚫ **WARNING** *If a hematoma expands, mark the site and alert the physician.*

◆ Auscultate regularly for murmurs, which may indicate worsening valvular insufficiency.

◆ Notify the physician if you detect a new or worsening murmur.

◆ Provide I.V. fluids at a rate of at least 100 ml/hour to help the kidneys excrete the contrast medium.

⚫ **WARNING** *Assess the patient for signs of fluid overload, including distended jugular veins, atrial and ventricular gallop, dyspnea, pulmonary congestion, tachycardia, hypertension, and hypoxemia.*

◆ Monitor intake and output closely.

◆ Encourage the patient to perform deep-breathing exercises to prevent atelectasis.

◆ After the guide catheter is removed (usually 6 to 12 hours after valvuloplasty), apply direct pressure for at least 10 minutes, and monitor the site frequently.

SPECIAL CONSIDERATIONS

◆ Assess the patient's vital signs constantly during the procedure, especially if it's an aortic valvuloplasty.

◆ During balloon inflation, the aortic outflow tract is completely obstructed, causing blood pressure to fall dangerously low.

◆ Ventricular ectopy is common during balloon positioning and inflation.

◆ Start treatment for ectopy when symptoms develop or when ventricular tachycardia is sustained.

◆ Assess for embolism, hemorrhage, chest pain, and cardiac tamponade.

⚫ **WARNING** *Using heparin and a large-bore catheter can lead to arterial hemorrhage. This can be reversed with protamine sulfate when the sheath is removed, or the sheath can be left in place and removed 6 to 8 hours after heparin is discontinued.*

⚫ **WARNING** *Carefully assess the patient's respiratory status — changes in rate and pattern can be the first sign of a complication such as embolism.*

◆ Assess pedal pulses with a Doppler stethoscope. Pedal pulses will be difficult to detect, especially if the catheter sheath remains in place.

◆ Assess for symptoms of myocardial ischemia because chest pain can result from obstruction of blood flow during aortic valvuloplasty.

⚫ **WARNING** *Stay alert for symptoms of cardiac tamponade (decreased or absent peripheral pulses, pale or cyanotic skin, hypotension, and paradoxical pulse), which requires emergency surgery.*

COMPLICATIONS

◆ Bleeding or hematoma at the insertion site

◆ Arrhythmias

◆ Circulatory disorders distal to the insertion site

◆ Guide wire perforation of the ventricle leading to tamponade

◆ Disruption of the valve ring

◆ Restenosis of the valve

◆ Valvular insufficiency, which can contribute to heart failure and reduced cardiac output

◆ Infection

◆ Allergic reaction to the contrast medium

PATIENT TEACHING

◆ Instruct the patient to report chest pain or bleeding from the insertion sites.

◆ Teach the patient deep-breathing exercises.

◆ Instruct the patient to keep the leg with the insertion site straight after the procedure, as ordered by the physician.

DOCUMENTATION

◆ Document complications and interventions.

◆ Note the patient's tolerance of the procedure and his condition afterward.

SELECTED REFERENCES

Chlan, L.L., et al. "Effects of Three Groin Compression Methods on Patient Discomfort, Distress, and Vascular Complications Following a Percutaneous Coronary Intervention Procedure," *Nursing Research* 54(6):391-98, November-December 2005.

Liu, T., et al. "Prevention of Ischemic Cerebral Stroke by Percutaneous Balloon Valvuloplasty in Patients with Symptomatic Rheumatic Mitral Stenosis," *Stroke* 37(2):714, February 2006.

McElhinney, D.B., et al. "Left Heart Growth, Function, and Reintervention after Balloon Aortic Valvuloplasty for Neonatal Aortic Stenosis," *Circulation* 111(4):451-58, February 2005.

Tagney, J., and Lackie, D. "Bed-rest Postfemoral Arterial Sheath Removal — What Is Safe Practice? A Clinical Audit," *Nursing in Critical Care* 10(4):167-73, July-August 2005.

Bed equipment, supplemental

DESCRIPTION

◆ Certain equipment can promote a bedridden patient's comfort and help prevent pressure ulcers and other complications of immobility.

◆ A wood or hard plastic footboard prevents footdrop by maintaining proper alignment.

◆ A footboard raises bed linens off the patient's feet.

◆ A foot cradle, a footboard bar over the end of the bed, also keeps bed linens off of the patient's feet, preventing skin irritation and breakdown, especially in the patient with peripheral vascular disease or neuropathy.

◆ A bed board, made of wood or wood covered with canvas, firms the mattress and is especially useful for a patient with spinal injuries.

◆ The metal basic frame and metal trapeze (a triangular piece attached to the frame) allow the patient with arm mobility and strength to lift himself off the bed, facilitating bed making and bedpan positioning.

◆ The metal overbed cradle, a cagelike frame positioned on top of the mattress, keeps linens off a patient with burns, open wounds, or a wet cast.

◆ A vinyl water mattress used to prevent or treat pressure ulcers exerts less pressure on the skin than a standard hospital mattress.

◆ An alternating pressure pad (a vinyl pad divided into chambers filled with air or water and attached to an electric pump) serves the same purpose as a vinyl mattress, but also stimulates circulation by alternately inflating and deflating its chambers.

◆ The reusable water mattress replaces the standard hospital mattress and rests on a sheet of heavy cardboard placed over the bedsprings.

◆ The smaller, less bulky disposable mattress rests on top of the standard hospital mattress.

CONTRAINDICATIONS

None known

EQUIPMENT

Footboard and cover ◆ drawsheet ◆ bath blanket ◆ foot cradle ◆ bed board ◆ basic frame with trapeze ◆ overbed cradle ◆ roller gauze ◆ water mattress ◆ stretcher ◆ alternating pressure pad ◆ pump and tubing ◆ footstool ◆ linen-saver pad

PREPARATION
Footboard

◆ When preparing a footboard, place a cover over it to provide padding, or pad it with a folded drawsheet or bath blanket.

◆ Bring the top and side edges of the sheet or blanket to the back of the footboard, miter the corners, and secure them at the center with safety pins.

◆ Padding cushions the patient's feet against pressure from the hard footboard, helping to prevent skin irritation and breakdown.

◆ To prevent skin irritation, avoid wrinkles.

KEY STEPS

◆ Confirm the patient's identity using two patient identifiers according to facility policy.

◆ Explain to the patient what you're going to do and describe the equipment.

◆ Wash your hands.

USING A FOOTBOARD

◆ Move the patient up in bed to allow room for the footboard.

◆ Loosen the top linens at the foot of the bed and fold them back over the patient to expose his feet.

◆ Lift the mattress at the foot of the bed and place the lip of the footboard between the mattress and the bedsprings, or secure the footboard under both sides of the mattress.

◆ Adjust the footboard so the patient's feet rest comfortably against it.

◆ If the footboard isn't adjustable, tuck a folded bath blanket between the board and his feet.

◆ Unless the footboard has side supports, place a sandbag, a folded bath blanket, or a pillow along each foot to maintain 90-degree foot alignment.

◆ Fold the top linens over the footboard, tuck them under the mattress, and miter the corners.

USING A FOOT CRADLE

◆ Loosen the top linens at the foot of the bed and fold them over the patient or to one side.

◆ When using a one-piece cradle, place one side arm under the mattress, extend the arch over the bed, and place the other side arm under the mattress on the opposite side. Adjust the tension rods so they rest securely over the edge of the mattress.

◆ When using a sectional cradle with two side arms, place the side arms under the mattress. Secure the tension rods over the edge of the mattress. Place the arch over the bed and connect it to the side arms.

◆ When using a sectional cradle with one side arm, connect the side arm and horizontal cradle bar before placement. Place the side arm under the mattress on one side of the bed.

◆ Cover the cradle with the top linens, tuck them under the mattress at the foot of the bed, and miter the corners.

USING A BED BOARD

◆ Transfer the patient from his bed to a stretcher or chair.

◆ Strip the linens from the bed.

◆ If the bed board consists of wooden slats encased in canvas, lift the mattress at the head of the bed and center the board over the bedsprings to prevent it from jutting out and causing injury.

◆ Unroll the slats to cover the bedsprings at the head of the bed.

◆ Lift the mattress at the foot of the bed and unroll the remaining slats.

◆ If the bed board consists of one solid or two hinged pieces of wood, lift the mattress on one side of the bed and center the board over the bedsprings.

◆ After positioning the bed board, replace the linens.

◆ Return the patient to the bed.

USING A BASIC FRAME WITH A TRAPEZE

◆ If an orthopedic technician isn't available to secure the frame and trapeze, get assistance to attach these devices to the bed, as necessary.

◆ Be sure to hang the trapeze within easy reach.

USING AN OVERBED CRADLE

◆ Loosen and remove the top linens.

◆ Carefully lower the cradle onto the patient's bed and secure.

◆ Wrap roller gauze around both sides of the cradle.

◆ Pull the gauze taut and attach it to the bedsprings.

◆ Cover the cradle with the top linens, tuck them under the mattress at the foot of the bed, and miter the corners.

USING A PORTABLE WATER MATTRESS

◆ A portable water mattress is heavy and bulky. Enlist several coworkers to help transfer it from the stretcher to the patient's bed.

⚡ **WARNING** *Check with the maintenance department before transferring the mattress because its weight may rule out use on some electric beds.*

◆ Make sure that the patient isn't prone to motion sickness; movement of the water may cause nausea.

◆ Position the mattress on the bed and place the protective cover over it.

◆ Place a bottom sheet over the cover and tuck it in loosely.

◆ Place a sheepskin, linen-saver pad, or drawsheet over the bottom sheet, as needed.

◆ Position the patient comfortably on the mattress.

◆ Cover him with the top linens and tuck them in loosely.

◆ Check the water mattress daily to ensure adequate flotation.

◆ To check a water mattress, place your hand under the patient's thighs. Arrange to have water added if you feel the bottom of the mattress.

USING AN ALTERNATING PRESSURE PAD

◆ Transfer the patient from his bed to a chair or stretcher. Get help, if necessary.

◆ Strip the linens from the bed.

◆ Inspect the plug and electrical cord of the alternating pressure pad for defects. Don't use the unit if it appears damaged.

◆ Unfold the pad on top of the mattress with the appropriate side facing up.

◆ Place the motor on a linen-saver pad on the floor or on a footstool near the mattress outlets.

◆ Connect the tubing securely to the motor and mattress outlets, and plug the cord into an electrical outlet.

◆ Turn the motor on.

◆ After several minutes, observe the emptying and filling of the pad's chambers and check the tubing for kinks because they could interfere with the pad's function.

◆ Place a bottom sheet over the pad and tuck it in loosely.

◆ To avoid tube constriction, don't miter the corner where the tubing is attached.

◆ Position the patient comfortably on the pad, cover him with the top linens, and tuck them in loosely.

◆ If the pad becomes soiled, clean it with a damp cloth and mild soap and then dry it well. To avoid damaging the pad's surface, don't use alcohol.

◆ Fold and store or discard the pad, or give the pad to the patient to take home, if applicable.

SPECIAL CONSIDERATIONS

◆ Place the patient in bed before positioning and securing an overbed or foot cradle to ensure its proper placement and prevent injury.

◆ Remove the cradle before he gets out of bed.

◆ When turning or positioning him on his side, make sure that the foot cradle's tension rod doesn't rest against his skin because this may cause pressure and predispose him to skin breakdown.

◆ Use caution when turning an obese patient on a water mattress because turning displaces a large volume of water. Be sure to keep the side rails raised when turning to prevent falls.

◆ Avoid placing excessive layers of drawsheets or linen-saver pads between the alternating pressure pad and the patient because they decrease the pad's effectiveness.

◆ Avoid using pins or sharp instruments near an alternating pressure pad or water mattress to prevent accidental puncture.

⚡ **WARNING** *Make sure that a coworker is standing on the opposite side of the bed when you're transferring the patient from the stretcher to the bed because a plastic-covered mattress slides off a bed board easily.*

COMPLICATIONS

None known

PATIENT TEACHING

◆ Explain to the patient how to use each piece of the bed equipment.

◆ Before discharge, advise the patient where to obtain, or how to improvise, bed equipment for home use.

DOCUMENTATION

◆ Record the type of supplemental bed equipment used.

◆ Document the time and date of use.

◆ Describe the patient's response to treatment.

SELECTED REFERENCES

Compton, G.A., et al. "Use of a Heel Pressure Relief Mattress Replacement System in a Large Post Acute Rehabilitation Program," *Journal of the American Geriatrics Society* 53(Suppl 1):S214-215, April 2005.

van Schie, C.H.M., et al. "Heel Blood Flow Studies Using Alternating Pressure Air Mattress Systems in Diabetic Patients," *Diabetic Medicine Supplement* 21(Suppl 2):95, April 2004.

Bedside spirometry

OVERVIEW

DESCRIPTION

◆ Spirometry measures forced vital capacity (FVC) and forced expiratory volume (FEV), allowing calculation of other pulmonary function indices such as timed forced expiratory flow rate.

◆ Depending on the type of spirometer used, it can also allow direct measurement of vital capacity and tidal volume. (See *Digital bedside spirometer.*)

◆ Spirometry aids in diagnosing obstructive or restrictive pulmonary dysfunction, evaluating its severity, and determining the patient's response to therapy.

◆ Assessment of the relationship of flow rate to vital capacity helps distinguish between obstructive and restrictive pulmonary disease.

◆ Spirometry is useful for evaluating preoperative anesthesia risk.

◆ Required breathing patterns can aggravate such conditions as bronchospasm; use requires review of the patient's history and close observation during the test.

CONTRAINDICATIONS

None known

EQUIPMENT

Spirometer ◆ disposable mouthpiece ◆ breathing tube, if required ◆ spirographic chart, if required ◆ chart and pen, if required ◆ vital capacity predicted-values table and noseclips (optional)

PREPARATION

◆ Review the manufacturer's instructions for the assembly and use of the spirometer.

◆ Firmly insert the breathing tube, if necessary, to ensure a tight connection.

◆ If the tube comes preconnected, check the seals for tightness and the tubing for leaks.

◆ Check the operation of the recording mechanism and insert a chart and pen, if necessary.

◆ Insert the disposable mouthpiece and make sure that it's tightly sealed.

Digital bedside spirometer

Various models of bedside spirometers are available. The instrument shown here has a digital readout. Other models display results on an individual chart record or on a roll of chart paper.

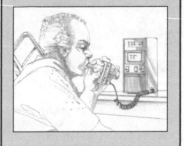

KEY STEPS

◆ Confirm the patient's identity using two patient identifiers according to facility policy.

◆ Explain the procedure to the patient.

◆ Emphasize that cooperation is essential to ensure accurate results.

◆ Tell the patient to remove or loosen constricting clothing to prevent alteration of the test results from restricted thoracic expansion and abdominal mobility.

◆ Before the procedure, have the patient void to prevent abdominal discomfort.

◆ Don't perform pulmonary function tests immediately after a large meal because the patient may experience abdominal discomfort.

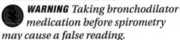 **WARNING** *Taking bronchodilator medication before spirometry may cause a false reading.*

◆ If the patient wears dentures that fit poorly, remove them to prevent incomplete closure of his mouth, which could allow air to leak around the mouthpiece. If the dentures fit well, leave them in place to promote a tight seal.

◆ Plug in the spirometer and set the baseline time.

◆ Allow him to practice required breathing with the breathing tube unhooked, if desired.

◆ After practice, replace the tube and check the seal.

◆ Tell him not to breathe through his nose; if he has difficulty, apply a noseclip.

◆ To measure vital capacity, tell the patient to inhale as deeply as possible, and then insert the mouthpiece so his lips are sealed tightly around it to prevent air leakage and ensure an accurate digital readout or spirogram recording.

◆ Tell him to exhale completely.

◆ Remove the mouthpiece to prevent recording his next inspiration.

◆ Allow him to rest; repeat the procedure twice.

- To measure FEV and FVC, repeat the procedure with the chart or timer on, but instruct him to exhale as quickly and completely as possible.
- Tell him when to start and turn on the recorder or timer.
- Allow him to rest; repeat the procedure twice.
- After completing the procedure, discard the mouthpiece, remove the spirographic chart, and follow the manufacturer's instructions for cleaning and sterilizing.

SPECIAL CONSIDERATIONS

- Encourage the patient during the test to help him exhale more forcefully, which is needed for best results.
- If he coughs during expiration, wait until coughing subsides before repeating the measurement.
- Read the vital capacity directly from the readout or spirogram chart.
- The FVC is the highest volume recorded on the curve.
- Of the 3 trials, accept the highest recorded exhalation as the vital capacity result.
- To determine the percentage of predicted vital capacity, locate the patient's predicted value on the vital capacity predicted-values table.
- Calculate the percentage using this formula: (observed vital capacity divided by predicted vital capacity) $\times$ 100 = % predicted vital capacity.
- To determine FEV for a specified time, mark the point on the spirogram where it crosses the desired time and draw a straight line from this point to the side of the chart, which indicates volume in liters.
- This measurement is usually calculated for 1, 2, and 3 seconds and reported as a percentage of vital capacity.
- A healthy patient will have exhaled 75%, 85%, and 95%, respectively, of his FVC. Calculate this percentage using this formula: (observed forced expiratory volume divided by predicted vital capacity) $\times$ 100 = % vital capacity.

COMPLICATIONS

- Dizziness or light-headedness
- Bronchospasm
- Increased exhaustion (possibly to where the patient will require mechanical support)
- Increased air trapping in the patient with emphysema

PATIENT TEACHING

- Explain the procedure to the patient and answer any of his questions.
- Demonstrate how the patient should inhale and exhale and encourage him during his practice time and during the test.

DOCUMENTATION

- Document the date and time of the procedure.
- Record the observed and calculated values, including FEV at 1, 2, and 3 seconds.
- Note the complications and nursing actions taken.
- Describe the patient's tolerance of the procedure.

SELECTED REFERENCES

Dindas, I., and Mcendzie, S. "Spirometry in the Diagnosis of Asthma in Children," *Current Opinion in Pulmonary Medicine* 12(1):28-33, January 2006.

Gibbons, D. "A Comprehensive Guide to the Accurate Performance of Spirometry Tests," *Professional Nurse* 19(11):39-40, 42, July 2004.

Petty, T.L. "Benefits of and Barriers to the Widespread Use of Spirometry," *Current Opinion in Internal Medicine* 4(3):297-302, June 2005.

Pullen, R.L. Jr. "Teaching Bedside Incentive Spirometry," *Nursing* 33(8):24, August 2003.

Yin, X., et al. "The Clinical Application of Portable Spirometry in Asthma," *Respirology* 10(Suppl):A110, November 2005.

Binders

DESCRIPTION

- Binders, also known as *self-closures*, are lengths of cloth or elasticized material that encircle the chest, abdomen, or groin.
- Typically, cloth binders are fastened with safety pins and elasticized binders are fastened with Velcro.
- Binders are used to:
- provide support
- keep dressings in place (especially for patients allergic to tape)
- reduce tension on wounds and suture lines
- reduce breast engorgement in the non–breast-feeding mother (although a snug-fitting support bra is usually recommended).

CONTRAINDICATIONS

None known

EQUIPMENT

Tape measure ◆ binder of appropriate size and type ◆ safety pins ◆ gloves (if necessary)

TYPES OF BINDERS

- Commercial elastic binders with Velcro closings are now commonly used instead of standard cotton straight and scultetus binders, which require pins.
- Disposable T-binders are available, and scrotal supports typically replace binders for male patients, except after abdominal-perineal resection.

PREPARATION

- Measure the area the binder must fit.
- Obtain the proper size and type of binder.

KEY STEPS

- Confirm the patient's identity using two patient identifiers according to facility policy.
- Check the practitioner's order and assess the patient's condition.
- Explain the procedure, provide privacy, wash your hands thoroughly, and put on gloves, if necessary.
- Raise the patient's bed to its highest position to avoid muscle strain when applying the binder.
- Change the dressing and inspect the wound or suture line, if appropriate.

APPLYING A STRAIGHT ABDOMINAL BINDER

- Accordion-fold half of the binder, slip it under the patient, and pull it through from the other side.
- Make sure that the binder is straight, wrinkle-free, and evenly distributed under the patient.
- The binder's lower edge should extend well below his hips.
- Overlap one side of the binder snugly onto the other.
- Insert one finger under the binder's edge to ensure a snug fit that's still loose enough to avoid impaired circulation and discomfort.
- Close the Velcro closure, starting at the lower edge.
- Make darts in the binder as needed.
- ⚡ **WARNING** *Avoid making the binder too tight around the diaphragm because it may interfere with breathing.*

APPLYING A SCULTETUS BINDER

- A scultetus binder is placed under the patient's hips and buttocks. (See *Applying a scultetus binder.*)

APPLYING A T-BINDER

- Slip the T-binder under the patient's waist, with its tails extending below the buttocks.
- Smooth the waistband and tails to remove twists, which can chafe and create pressure on the patient's skin.
- Pull the waistband snugly into position at the patient's waistline or lower the waistband across the abdomen.

- Fasten the Velcro closure.
- Bring the free tail up between the patient's legs over the dressing or perineal pad.
- For a female patient, bring the single tail up to the center of the waist, loop it behind and over the waistband, and secure it to the waistband with the Velcro closures.
- For a male patient, bring the two tails up on either side of the penis to provide even support for the testes.
- Loop the ends behind and over the waistband on either side of the midline, and fasten them to the waistband with the Velcro closures.
- Pinning through multiple layers keeps the straps from slipping sideways as the patient moves.
- Tell the patient to call you when he needs to void or defecate, to unfasten and reapply the binder.

APPLYING A BREAST BINDER

- Slip the binder under the patient's chest so its lower edge aligns with the waist.
- Straighten the binder to distribute evenly on either side.
- Place the binder so her nipples are centered in the breast tissue. This ensures proper breast alignment and support and produces faster tissue involution.
- Pull the binder's edges snugly together and begin closing the Velcro closures upward from the waist.
- Adjust the shoulder straps to fit properly and secure with the Velcro fasteners.

APPLYING ANY BINDER

- Ask the patient if the binder feels comfortable.
- Tell the patient it may feel tight at first but should soon feel comfortable.
- Tell the patient to notify you immediately if the binder feels too tight, too loose, or comes apart.
- Ask the patient to ambulate, if he can, to evaluate the fit of the binder.

- For maximum support, wrap the binder so it applies even pressure across the body section.
- Eliminate all wrinkles and avoid placing pressure over bony prominences.
- In surgical applications, fasten straight and scultetus binders from the bottom upward to relieve gravitational pull on the wound.
- In obstetric applications, fasten from the top downward to direct the uterus into the pelvis.

⚡ **WARNING** *Be careful not to compress tubes, drains, or catheters and be sure to position them properly so they're working with gravity.*

- Don't allow binder placement to interfere with elimination.
- Use a double T-binder on a female patient after extensive surgery that requires a large dressing.
- Use a straight or scultetus binder as a breast binder, if necessary.
- Observe the patient and check binder placement every 8 hours.

- Check the skin for color, palpate it for warmth, check pulses, and assess for tingling or numbness.
- Reapply the binder when a dressing needs changing, when the binder becomes loose or too tight, and per physician's orders.
- When changing the binder, observe the skin for signs of irritation.
- Provide appropriate skin care before reapplying the binder.

COMPLICATIONS
- Irritation of the underlying skin resulting from perspiration or friction

- If the patient needs a binder after discharge, teach him and a family member how to remove it, inspect the skin, bathe the area, and reapply the binder.
- Tell the patient and his family where binders can be purchased and how to care for them.
- Advise the patient and his family that a clean towel can be used if commercially manufactured binders are unavailable.

DOCUMENTATION

- Record the dates and times of binder application, reapplication, and removal.
- Record the binder type and location.
- Note the purpose of application.
- Describe the skin condition before and after application.
- Note dressing changes or skin care.
- Report complications.
- Describe the patient's tolerance of the treatment.

SELECTED REFERENCES

Bodin, P., et al. "Effects of Abdominal Binding on Breathing Patterns during Breathing Exercises in Persons with Tetraplegia," *Spinal Cord* 43(2):117-22, February 2005.

Carr, C.A. "Use of a Maternity Support Binder for Relief of Pregnancy-Related Back Pain," *Journal of Obstetric, Gynecologic, and Neonatal Nursing* 32(4): 495-502, July-August 2003.

Laura, S., et al. "Patient Preference for Bra or Binder after Breast Surgery," *ANZ Journal of Surgery* 74(6):463-64, June 2004.

Swift, K., and Janke, J. "Breast Binding…Is It All that It's Wrapped Up to Be?" *Journal of Obstetric, Gynecologic, and Neonatal Nursing* 32(3):332-39, May-June 2003.

Applying a scultetus binder

After centering the binder's solid portion under the patient, with tails distributed evenly on each side, bring the lowest tail straight across the patient's abdomen, hold it snugly, and bring the next higher tail across to overlap it. Alternate tails in this manner, with the next higher tail overlapping the one below it by about one-half its width.

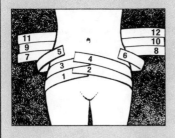

Bispectral index monitoring

DESCRIPTION

- Bispectral index monitoring involves the use of an electronic device that converts EEG waves into a statistically derived number that indicates the depth of a patient's sedation, providing a measure of sedative and anesthetic effects on the brain.
- The procedure provides objective, reliable data on which to base care, thus lessening the risks of oversedation and undersedation.
- The bispectral index monitor is attached to a sensor applied to the patient's forehead.
- The sensor obtains information about the patient's electrical brain activity and translates it into a number from 0 (indicating no brain activity) to 100 (indicating a patient who is awake and alert).
- Bispectral index monitoring is used to assess sedation when the patient is receiving mechanical ventilation or neuromuscular blockers or during barbiturate coma or bedside procedures.

CONTRAINDICATIONS

None known

EQUIPMENT

Bispectral index monitor and cable ◆ bispectral index sensor ◆ alcohol swabs ◆ soap and water

PREPARATION

- Place the bispectral index monitor close to the patient's bed.
- Plug the power cord into the wall outlet.

KEY STEPS

- Confirm the patient's identity using two patient identifiers according to facility policy.
- Gather the necessary equipment and explain the procedure and rationale to the patient and her family. (See *Bispectral index monitoring.*)
- Provide privacy, wash your hands, and follow standard precautions.
- Clean the patient's forehead with soap and water and allow it to dry.
- If necessary, wipe her forehead with an alcohol swab to ensure the skin is oil-free; allow the alcohol to dry.
- Open the sensor package and apply the sensor to her forehead.
- Position the circle labeled "1" midline about 1½" (4 cm) above the bridge of the nose.

Bispectral index monitoring

Bispectral index monitoring consists of a monitor and cable connected to a sensor that's applied to the patient's forehead (as shown here).

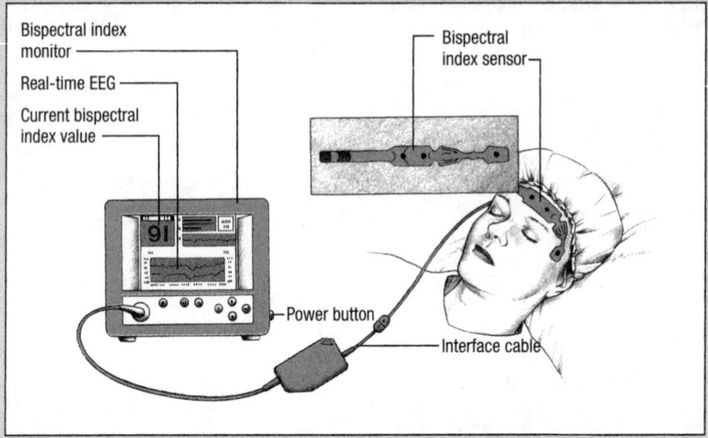

TROUBLESHOOTER

Sensor problems

When initiating bispectral index monitoring, be aware that the monitor may display messages that indicate a problem. This chart highlights these messages and offers possible solutions.

MESSAGE	POSSIBLE SOLUTIONS
High impedance	Check sensor adhesion; reapply firm pressure to each of the numbered circles on the sensor for 5 seconds; if the message continues, check the connection between the sensor and the monitor; if necessary, apply a new sensor.
Noise	Remove possible pressure on the sensor; investigate possible electrical interference from equipment.
Lead-off	Check sensor for electrode displacement or lifting; reapply with firm pressure or, if necessary, apply a new sensor.

- Position the circle labeled "3" on the right or left temple — level with the outer canthus of the eye — between the corner of her eye and her hairline.
- Make sure that the circle labeled "4" and the line below it are parallel to the eye on the appropriate side.
- Apply gentle, firm pressure around the edges of the sensor, including areas between the numbered circles, to ensure proper adhesion.
- Press firmly on the numbered circles for about 5 seconds each to make sure that the electrodes stick to the skin.
- Connect the sensor to the interface cable and monitor.
- Turn on the monitor and watch it for information related to impedance (electrical resistance) testing.

⚡ *WARNING For the monitor to display a reading, impedance values must be below a specified threshold. If they aren't, be prepared to troubleshoot sensor problems. (See Sensor problems.)*

- Select a smoothing rate (the time it takes to analyze data for calculation of the bispectral index; usually 15 to 30 seconds) using the ADVANCE SETUP button, based on facility policy.
- Read and record the bispectral index value.

Interpreting bispectral index values

Use these guidelines to interpret your patient's bispectral index value.

BISPECTRAL INDEX

100	Awake
80	Light/moderate sedation
70	Deep sedation (low probability of explicit recall)
60	General anesthesia (low probability of consciousness)
40	Deep hypnotic state
0	Flat-line EEG

Light hypnotic state

Moderate hypnotic state

SPECIAL CONSIDERATIONS

- Evaluate the bispectral index value in relation to other assessments. (See *Interpreting bispectral index values.*)
- Don't rely on the bispectral index value alone.
- Keep in mind that movement may occur with low bispectral index values.
- Stay alert for artifacts that could falsely elevate bispectral index values.

⚡ *WARNING Bispectral index values may be elevated because of muscle shivering, tightening, or twitching or with the use of mechanical devices either with the patient or close to the patient, the bispectral index monitor, or the sensor. Interpret the bispectral index value cautiously in these situations.*

- Anticipate the need to adjust the dosage of sedation based on the patient's bispectral index value.

⚡ *WARNING A decrease in stimulation, increased sedation, recent administration of a neuromuscular blocking agent or analgesia, or hypothermia may decrease the bispectral index and indicate the need for a decrease in sedative agents. Pain may cause an elevated bispectral index, indicating a need for an increase in sedation.*

- Check the sensor site according to facility policy.
- Change the sensor every 24 hours.

COMPLICATIONS
None known

PATIENT TEACHING

- Explain the procedure to the patient and family and answer any of their questions.

DOCUMENTATION

- Note the initiation of bispectral index monitoring, including the baseline bispectral index value and location of the sensor.
- Record assessment findings with the bispectral index value to indicate the patient's condition.
- Report increases or decreases in the bispectral index value, along with actions taken based on values and changes in sedative agents given.

SELECTED REFERENCES

Bader, M.K., et al. "Refractory Increased Intracranial Pressure in Severe Traumatic Brain Injury: Barbiturate Coma and Bispectral Index Monitoring," *AACN Clinical Issues* 16(4):526-41, October-December 2005.

Gambrell, M. "Using the BIS Monitor in Palliative Care: A Case Study," *Journal of Neuroscience Nursing* 37(3):140-43, June 2005.

Leblanc, J.M., et al. "Role of the Bispectral Index in Sedation Monitoring in the ICU," *Annals of Pharmacotherapy* 40(3):490-500, March 2006.

Luebbehusen, M. "Technology Today: Bispectral Index Monitoring," *RN* 68(9):50-54, September 2005.

Olson, D.M., et al. "The Impact of Bispectral Index Monitoring on Rates of Propofol Administration," *AACN Clinical Issues* 15(1):63-73, January-March 2004.

Olson, D.M., and Krebbs, L.M. "Use Bispectral Index to Gauge Consciousness," *Nursing* 34(7):53, July 2004.

Bladder irrigation, continuous

DESCRIPTION

- Continuous bladder irrigation helps prevent urinary tract obstruction by flushing out small blood clots that form after prostate or bladder surgery.
- It can be used to treat an irritated, inflamed, or infected bladder lining.
- Continuous flow of irrigating solution through the bladder creates a mild tamponade that may help prevent venous hemorrhage. (See *Setup for continuous bladder irrigation.*)
- The catheter is usually inserted during prostate or bladder surgery, but may be inserted at the bedside for a nonsurgical patient.

CONTRAINDICATIONS

None known

EQUIPMENT

One 4,000-ml container or two 2,000-ml containers of irrigating solution (usually normal saline solution) or prescribed amount of medicated solution ◆ Y-type tubing made specifically for bladder irrigation ◆ alcohol or chlorhexidine pad

PREPARATION

- Use Y-type tubing to allow immediate irrigation with reserve solution.
- Large volumes of irrigating solution are usually required during the first 24 to 48 hours after surgery.
- Before starting, double-check the irrigating solution against the practitioner's order.
- If the solution contains an antibiotic, check the patient's chart to make sure that he isn't allergic to the drug.
- The patient should remain on bed rest throughout continuous bladder irrigation, unless specified otherwise.

KEY STEPS

- Confirm the patient's identity using two patient identifiers according to facility policy.
- Wash your hands and put on gloves.
- Assemble all equipment at the patient's bedside.
- Explain the procedure and provide privacy.
- Insert the spike of the Y-type tubing into the container of irrigating solution.
- If you have a two-container system, insert one spike into each container.
- Squeeze the drip chamber on the spike of the tubing.
- Open the flow clamp and flush the tubing to remove air that could cause bladder distention.
- Close the clamp.

- Hang the bag of irrigating solution on the I.V. pole.
- Clean the opening to the inflow lumen of the catheter with the alcohol or chlorhexidine pad.
- Insert the distal end of the Y-type tubing securely into the inflow lumen (third port) of the catheter using sterile technique.
- Make sure that the catheter's outflow lumen is securely attached to the drainage bag tubing.
- Open the flow clamp under the container of the irrigating solution and set the drip rate as ordered.
- To prevent air from entering the system, don't allow the primary container to empty completely before replacing it.
- If you have a two-container system, simultaneously close the flow clamp under the nearly empty container

Setup for continuous bladder irrigation

In continuous bladder irrigation, a triple-lumen catheter allows irrigating solution to flow into the bladder through one lumen and flow out through another, as shown in the inset. The third lumen is used to inflate the balloon that holds the catheter in place.

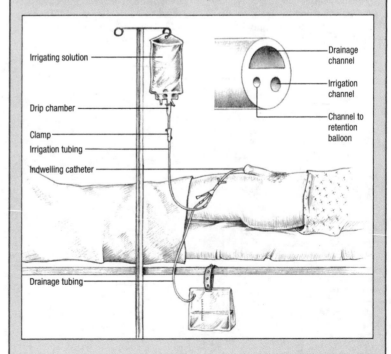

Irrigating solution

Drip chamber

Clamp

Irrigation tubing

Indwelling catheter

Drainage tubing

Drainage channel

Irrigation channel

Channel to retention balloon

and open the flow clamp under the reserve container. This prevents reflux of irrigating solution from the reserve container into the nearly empty one.

◆ Hang a new reserve container on the I.V. pole and insert the tubing, maintaining asepsis.

◆ Empty the drainage bag about every 4 hours or as often as needed.

◆ Use sterile technique to avoid the risk of contamination.

◆ Monitor the patient's vital signs at least every 4 hours during irrigation, increasing the frequency if the patient becomes unstable.

SPECIAL CONSIDERATIONS

◆ Check inflow and outflow lines periodically for kinks to make sure that the solution is running freely.

◆ If the solution flows rapidly, check the lines frequently.

◆ Measure the outflow volume accurately.

◆ The outflow should be the same or slightly more than the inflow volume, allowing for urine production.

⚡ **WARNING** *Postoperative inflow volume exceeding outflow volume may indicate bladder rupture at the suture lines or renal damage; notify the practitioner immediately.*

◆ Assess outflow for changes in appearance and for blood clots, especially if irrigation is being done postoperatively to control bleeding.

⚡ **WARNING** *If the drainage is bright red, the irrigating solution should be infused rapidly with the clamp wide open until drainage clears. Notify the practitioner immediately if you suspect hemorrhage.*

◆ If the drainage is clear, the solution is usually given at a rate of 40 to 60 drops/minute.

◆ The practitioner usually specifies the rate for antibiotic solutions.

◆ Encourage oral fluid intake of 2 to 3 qt (2 to 3 L)/day unless contraindicated.

COMPLICATIONS

◆ Infection that's caused by interruptions in a continuous irrigation system

◆ Bladder distention that's caused by obstruction in the catheter's outflow lumen

PATIENT TEACHING

◆ Instruct the patient to notify the nurse if he experiences abdominal discomfort.

◆ Instruct the patient to remain on bed rest (unless otherwise specified).

DOCUMENTATION

◆ Each time a container of solution is finished, record the date, time, and amount of fluids on the intake and output record.

◆ Record the time and amount of fluid each time you empty the drainage bag.

◆ Note the appearance of the drainage and patient complaints.

SELECTED REFERENCES

Braasch, M., et al. "Irrigation and Drainage Properties of Three-way Urethral Catheters," *Urology* 67(1):40-44, January 2006.

Chan, P.T., et al. "A Modified Bladder Irrigation System after Transurethral Resection of Prostate," *International Journal of Urology* 11(Suppl 1):A72, October 2004.

Cutts, B. "Developing and Implementing a New Bladder Irrigation Chart," *Nursing Standard* 20(8):48-52, November 2005.

Bladder ultrasonography

OVERVIEW

DESCRIPTION

◆ Urine retention, a potentially life-threatening condition, may result from neurologic or psychological disorders or obstruction of urine flow.
◆ Medications, such as anticholinergics, antihistamines, and antidepressants, may also cause urine retention.
◆ Traditionally, the amount of urine retained in the bladder was measured by urinary catheterization, placing the patient at risk for infection.
◆ Noninvasive bladder ultrasonography provides an assessment of bladder volume while lowering the risk of urinary tract infection.

CONTRAINDICATIONS

None known

EQUIPMENT

BladderScan unit with scanhead ◆ ultrasonic transmission gel ◆ alcohol pad ◆ washcloth ◆ gloves

KEY STEPS

◆ Bring the BladderScan unit to the bedside.
◆ Confirm the patient's identity using two patient identifiers according to facility policy.
◆ Explain the procedure to the patient to help reduce his anxiety.
◆ Provide privacy, wash your hands, and put on gloves.
◆ If this is a postvoiding scan, ask the patient to void and assist him with this, if necessary.
◆ Position the patient in a supine position.
◆ Clean the rounded end of the scanhead with an alcohol pad.
◆ Expose the patient's suprapubic area.
◆ Turn on the BladderScan by pressing the button (designated by a dot within a circle) on the far left and then press SCAN.
◆ Place ultrasonic gel on the scanhead to promote an airtight seal for optimal sound-wave transmission.
◆ Tell the patient that the gel will feel cold when placed on the abdomen.
◆ Locate the symphysis pubis, and place the scanhead about 1″ (2.5 cm) superior to the symphysis pubis.
◆ Locate the icon (a rough figure of a patient) on the probe and make sure that the head of the icon points toward the head of the patient.
◆ Press the scanhead button marked with a soundwave pattern to activate the scan.
◆ Hold the scanhead steady until you hear the beep.
◆ Look at the aiming icon and screen, which displays the bladder position and volume. Reposition the probe and scan until the bladder is centered in the aiming screen.
◆ The largest measurement will be saved.
◆ Press DONE when finished.
◆ The BladderScan will display the measured urine volume and the longitudinal and horizontal axis scans.
◆ Press PRINT to obtain a hard copy of your results.
◆ Turn off the BladderScan.

- Use an alcohol pad to clean the gel off the scanhead.
- Using a washcloth, remove the gel from the patient's skin.
- Remove your gloves and wash your hands.

SPECIAL CONSIDERATIONS

None

COMPLICATIONS
None known

PATIENT TEACHING

- Explain the procedure to the patient and answer any of his questions.

DOCUMENTATION

- Write the patient's name, date, and time on the printout and attach it to the patient's medical record.
- Document the procedure and urine volume as well as any treatment in the patient's medical record.
- Describe the patient's tolerance of the procedure.

SELECTED REFERENCES

Hirahara, N., et al. "Four-dimensional Ultrasonography for Dynamic Bladder Shape Visualization and Analysis during Voiding," *Journal of Ultrasound in Medicine* 25(3):307-13, March 2006.

Ozden, E., et al. "Is Fluid Ingestion Really Necessary during Ultrasonography for Detecting Ureteral Stones? A Prospective Randomized Study," *Journal of Ultrasound in Medicine* 24(12):1651-657, December 2005.

Porpiglia, F., et al. "Real Time Ultrasound in Laparoscopic Bladder Diverticulectomy," *International Journal of Urology* 12(10):933-35, October 2005.

Rafique, M. "Value of Routine Renal and Abdominal Ultrasonography in Patients Undergoing Prostatectomy," *International Urology and Nephrology* 38(1):153-56, 2006.

Ransley, P.G., et al. "Bladder Ultrasonography in the Evaluation of the Efficacy of Dextranomer/Myaluronic Acid Injection for Treating VUR," *BJU International Supplement* 93(Suppl 2):2, April 2004.

Blood culture

DESCRIPTION

- Bacteria-free blood is susceptible to infection through infusion lines as well as from thrombophlebitis, infected shunts, or bacterial endocarditis caused by prosthetic heart valve replacements.
- Bacteria may also invade the vascular system from local tissue infections through the lymphatic system and thoracic duct.
- Blood cultures are performed to detect bacterial invasion (bacteremia) and the systemic spread of infection (septicemia) through the bloodstream.
- To determine bacteremia, a venous blood sample is collected by venipuncture and transferred into two bottles, one containing an anaerobic medium and the other, an aerobic medium.
- The bottles are incubated to encourage organisms present in the sample to grow in the media.
- Blood cultures allow identification of about 67% of pathogens within 24 hours and up to 90% within 72 hours. (See *Isolator blood-culturing system,* for a description of another type of culturing procedure.)
- The importance of the timing of culture collections isn't clear; some authorities recommend drawing three blood samples at least 1 hour apart.
- The first of these samples should be collected at the earliest sign of suspected bacteremia or septicemia.
- To check for suspected bacterial endocarditis, three or four samples may be collected at 5- to 30-minute intervals before starting antibiotic therapy.

CONTRAINDICATIONS

None known

Tourniquet ◆ gloves ◆ alcohol or povidone-iodine pads (check facility policy for specific antiseptic solution) ◆ 10-ml syringe for an adult; 6-ml syringe for a child ◆ three or four 20G 1½″ needles ◆ two or three blood culture bottles (50-ml bottles for adults, 20-ml bottles for infants and children) with sodium polyethanol sulfonate added (one aerobic bottle containing a suitable medium, such as Trypticase soy broth with 10% carbon dioxide atmosphere; one anaerobic bottle with prereduced medium; and, possibly, one hyperosmotic bottle with 10% sucrose medium) ◆ laboratory request form ◆ 2″×2″ gauze pads ◆ small adhesive bandages ◆ labels

PREPARATION

- Check the expiration dates on the culture bottles and replace outdated bottles.

- Confirm the patient's identity using two patient identifiers according to facility policy.
- Tell the patient you need to collect a series of blood samples to check for infection.
- Explain the procedure to ease his anxiety and promote cooperation.
- Explain that the procedure usually requires three blood samples collected at different times.
- Wash your hands and put on gloves.
- Tie a tourniquet 2″ (5 cm) proximal to the area chosen.
- Clean the venipuncture site with an alcohol or povidone-iodine pad. Start at the site and work outward.
- Wait 30 to 60 seconds for the skin to dry.

  WARNING *Don't wipe off the povidone-iodine with alcohol because alcohol cancels the effect of povidone-iodine.*
- Perform a venipuncture, drawing 10 ml of blood from an adult.

  WARNING *Observe the needle for defects, such as burrs, which could cause increased discomfort and damage to the patient's vein.*

  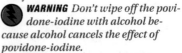 **AGE FACTOR** *Draw 2 to 6 ml of blood from a child.*
- Remove the tourniquet.
- Apply pressure to the venipuncture site using a 2″×2″ gauze pad.
- Cover the site with a small adhesive bandage.
- Wipe the diaphragm tops of the culture bottles with a povidone-iodine pad and replace the needle on the syringe used to draw the blood with a sterile needle before injecting the specimen into the culture bottle.
- Inject 5 ml of blood into each 50-ml bottle or 2 ml into a 20-ml pediatric culture bottle.
- Bottle size may vary with your facility's protocol, but the sample dilution should always be 1:10.
- Label the culture bottles with the patient's name, room number, physician's name, and date and time of collection.

- Indicate the suspected diagnosis and the patient's temperature, and note on the laboratory request any recent antibiotic therapy.
- Send the samples to the laboratory immediately.
- Discard syringes, needles, and gloves in appropriate containers.

SPECIAL CONSIDERATIONS

- Obtain each set of cultures from a different site.
- Avoid using existing blood lines for cultures unless the sample is drawn when the line is inserted or catheter sepsis is suspected.

COMPLICATIONS

- Hematoma (most common; apply pressure to site)

PATIENT TEACHING

- Instruct the patient to briefly apply pressure to the venipuncture site.
- Instruct the patient to notify the nurse or physician if persistent or recurrent bleeding or an expanding hematoma occurs at the venipuncture site.

DOCUMENTATION

- Document the date and time of the blood sample collection.
- Record the name of the test.
- Report the amount of blood collected.
- Note the number of bottles used.
- Record the patient's temperature.
- Report adverse reactions to the procedure.

SELECTED REFERENCES

Berild, D., et al. "Adjustment of Antibiotic Treatment According to the Results of Blood Cultures Leads to Decreased Antibiotic Use and Costs," *Journal of Antimicrobial Chemotherapy* 57(2):326-30, February 2006.

Freedman, S.B., and Roosevelt, G.E. "Utility of Anaerobic Blood Cultures in a Pediatric Emergency Department," *Pediatric Emergency Care* 20(7):433-36, July 2004.

Madeo, M., et al. "Simple Measures to Reduce the Rate of Contamination of Blood Cultures in Accident and Emergency," *Emergency Medicine Journal* 22(11):810-11, November 2005.

Mountain, D., et al. "Blood Cultures Ordered in the Adult Emergency Department Are Rarely Useful," *European Journal of Emergency Medicine* 13(2): 76-78, April 2006.

Rushing, J. "Drawing Blood Culture Specimens for Reliable Results," *Nursing* 34(12):20, December 2004.

Weinstein, M.P. "Blood Culture Contamination: Persisting Problems and Partial Progress," *Journal of Clinical Microbiology* 41(6):2275-278, June 2003.

Isolator blood-culturing system

A single-tube blood-culturing system, the Isolator uses lysis and centrifugation to help detect septicemia and monitor the effectiveness of antibacterial drug therapy.

The Isolator evacuated tube, used to collect the blood sample, contains a substance that lyses red blood cells. Then, centrifugation concentrates bacteria and other organisms in the sample onto an inert cushioning pad; the concentrate can then be applied onto four agar plates.

The Isolator has several advantages over conventional blood-culturing methods. This system:
- provides faster results
- improves bacterial survival
- results in more valid positive results through direct application onto agar plates, which more effectively dilutes any antibiotic present in the sample
- detects more yeast and polymicrobial infections
- improves the laboratory's ability to detect difficult to grow organisms
- is easier to use at the patient's bedside and to transport because blood is drawn directly into the Isolator tube.

Blood glucose tests

OVERVIEW

DESCRIPTION

◆ Rapid, easy-to-perform reagent strip tests (such as Glucostix, Trendstrips, Chemstrip bG, and Multistix) use a drop of capillary blood obtained by fingerstick, heelstick, or earlobe puncture as a sample.

◆ Reagent strip tests can detect or monitor elevated blood glucose levels in the patient with diabetes, screen for diabetes mellitus and neonatal hypoglycemia, and help distinguish diabetic coma from non-diabetic coma.

◆ Blood glucose tests can be performed in the hospital, physician's office, or patient's home.

◆ A blood glucose test strip consists of a reagent patch on the tip of a hand-held plastic strip, which changes color in response to the amount of glucose in the blood sample.

◆ Comparing the color change with a standardized color chart provides a semiquantitative measurement of blood glucose levels.

◆ Inserting the test strip in a portable blood glucose meter (such as Glucometer II, Accu-Chek II, and One Touch) provides quantitative measurements that are as accurate as other laboratory tests.

◆ Some meters store successive test results electronically to help determine glucose patterns.

CONTRAINDICATIONS

None known

EQUIPMENT

Reagent strips ◆ portable blood glucose meter, if available ◆ alcohol pads ◆ gauze pads ◆ disposable lancets or mechanical blood-letting devices ◆ small adhesive bandage ◆ watch or clock with a second hand ◆ sharps container

KEY STEPS

◆ Confirm the patient's identity using two patient identifiers according to facility policy.

◆ Explain the procedure to the patient or to the child's parents.

◆ Select the puncture site — usually the fingertip or earlobe for an adult or a child.

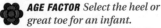 **AGE FACTOR** *Select the heel or great toe for an infant.*

◆ Wash your hands and put on gloves.

◆ If necessary, dilate the capillaries by applying a warm, moist compress to the area for about 10 minutes.

◆ Wipe the puncture site with an alcohol pad, and dry it thoroughly with a gauze pad.

Oral and I.V. glucose tolerance tests

For monitoring trends in glucose metabolism, two tests may offer benefits over testing blood with reagent strips.

ORAL GLUCOSE TOLERANCE TEST

The most sensitive test for detecting borderline diabetes mellitus, the oral glucose tolerance test (OGTT) measures carbohydrate metabolism after ingestion of a challenge dose of glucose. The body absorbs this dose rapidly, causing plasma glucose levels to rise and peak within 30 minutes to 1 hour. The pancreas responds by secreting insulin, causing glucose levels to return to normal within 2 to 3 hours. During this period, plasma and urine glucose levels are monitored to assess insulin secretion and the body's ability to metabolize glucose.

Although you may not collect the blood and urine specimens (usually five of each) required for this test, you'll be responsible for preparing the patient and monitoring his physical condition during the test.

Explain the OGTT to the patient. Then tell him to maintain a high-carbohydrate diet for 3 days and to fast for 10 to 16 hours before the test, as ordered. The patient must not smoke, drink coffee or alcohol, or exercise strenuously for 8 hours before or during the test. Inform him that he'll then receive a challenge dose of 100 g of carbohydrate (usually a sweetened carbonated beverage or gelatin).

Tell the patient who will perform the venipunctures, when they'll be done, and that he may feel slight discomfort from the needle punctures and the pressure of the tourniquet. Reassure him that collecting each blood sample usually takes less than 3 minutes. As ordered, withhold drugs that may affect test results. Remind him not to discard the first urine specimen voided after waking.

During the test period, watch for signs and symptoms of hypoglycemia — weakness, restlessness, nervousness, hunger, and sweating — and report these to the practitioner immediately. Encourage the patient to drink plenty of water to promote adequate urine excretion. Provide a bedpan, urinal, or specimen container when necessary.

I.V. GLUCOSE TOLERANCE TEST

The I.V. glucose tolerance test may be chosen for patients who can't absorb an oral dose of glucose — for example, those with malabsorption disorders or short-bowel syndrome or those who have had a gastrectomy. This test measures blood glucose after an I.V. infusion of 50% glucose over 3 or 4 minutes. Blood samples are then drawn after 30 minutes, 1 hour, 2 hours, and 3 hours. After an immediate glucose peak of 300 to 400 mg/dl (accompanied by glycosuria), the normal glucose curve falls steadily, reaching fasting levels within 1 to 1¼ hours. Failure to achieve fasting glucose levels within 2 to 3 hours typically confirms diabetes.

- To collect a sample from the fingertip with a disposable lancet (smaller than 2 mm), position the lancet on the side of the patient's fingertip perpendicular to the lines of the fingerprints.
- Pierce the skin sharply and quickly to minimize anxiety and pain and to increase blood flow.
- Alternatively, you can use a mechanical bloodletting device, such as an Autolet, which uses a spring-loaded lancet.
- After puncturing the finger, don't squeeze the puncture site; this can dilute the sample with tissue fluid.
- Touch a drop of blood to the reagent patch on the strip, making sure that you cover the entire patch.
- After collecting the blood sample, briefly apply pressure to the puncture site to prevent painful extravasation of blood into subcutaneous tissues.
- Ask the adult patient to hold a gauze pad firmly over the puncture site until the bleeding stops.
- Make sure that you leave the blood on the strip for exactly 60 seconds.
- Compare the color change on the strip with the standardized color chart on the product container.
- If you're using a blood glucose meter, follow the manufacturer's instructions.
- Designs vary, but all meters analyze glucose levels from a single drop of blood that's placed on a machine-specific reagent strip and provide a digital display of the result.
- After the bleeding has stopped, apply a small adhesive bandage to the puncture site.

SPECIAL CONSIDERATIONS

- Before using reagent strips, check the expiration date on the package and replace outdated strips.
- Check for special instructions related to the specific reagent.
- The reagent area of a fresh strip should match the color of the "0" block on the color chart.
- **WARNING** *Protect the strips from light, heat, and moisture.*
- Before using a blood glucose meter, calibrate it and run it with a control sample to ensure accurate test results. Follow the manufacturer's instructions for calibration.
- Follow facility policy and procedure for bedside point-of-care testing.
- To ensure an adequate sample, avoid selecting cold, cyanotic, or swollen puncture sites.
- If you can't obtain a capillary sample, perform venipuncture and place a large drop of venous blood on the reagent strip.
- If you want to test blood from a refrigerated sample, allow the blood to return to room temperature before testing it.
- To help detect abnormal glucose metabolism and diagnose diabetes mellitus, the practitioner may order other blood glucose tests. (See *Oral and I.V. glucose tolerance tests.*)
- Newer blood glucose meters (such as One Touch Ultra) require smaller amounts of blood; the puncture may be done on the patient's arm.

COMPLICATIONS

None known

PATIENT TEACHING

- If the patient will use the reagent strip system at home, teach him the proper use of the lancet or Autolet, reagent strips, and portable blood glucose meter.
- Ensure the patient's ability to obtain all necessary supplies, which may not be covered by his health insurance.
- Instruct the patient how to record blood glucose levels and when to notify his health care provider.
- Provide the patient with written guidelines.

DOCUMENTATION

- Record the reading from the reagent strip (using a portable blood glucose meter or a color chart) in your notes or in a special flowchart, if available.
- Document the time and date of the test.

SELECTED REFERENCES

Dale, L. "Make a Point about Alternate Site Blood Glucose Sampling," *Nursing* 36(2):52-53, February 2006.

Fain, J.A. "Blood Glucose Meters: Different Strokes for Different Folks," *Nursing* 34(11):48-51, November 2004.

Mensing, C. "Helping Patients Choose the Right Blood Glucose Meter," *The Nurse Practitioner* 29(5):43-45, May 2004.

Moore, S., and Avery, L. "Enabling Effective Blood Glucose Monitoring," *Diabetic Medicine* 23(Suppl 2):113, March 2006.

Traynor, K. "Experts Call for Better Management of Blood Glucose in Hospitalized Patients," *American Journal of Health-System Pharmacy* 63(6):488, 491, March 2006.

Blood pressure assessment

DESCRIPTION

◆ Blood pressure is the lateral force exerted by blood on the arterial walls. It depends on the force of ventricular contractions, arterial wall elasticity, peripheral vascular resistance, and blood volume and viscosity.

◆ Systolic, or maximum pressure, occurs during left ventricular contraction and indicates the integrity of the heart, arteries, and arterioles.

◆ Diastolic, or minimum pressure, occurs during left ventricular relaxation and indicates blood vessel resistance.

◆ Pulse pressure, the difference between systolic and diastolic pressures, varies inversely with arterial elasticity.

◆ Rigid vessels, incapable of distention and recoil, produce high systolic pressure and low diastolic pressure.

◆ Systolic pressure normally exceeds diastolic pressure by about 40 mm Hg.

◆ Narrowed pulse pressure — a difference less than 30 mm Hg — occurs when systolic pressure falls and diastolic pressure rises. These changes reflect reduced stroke volume, increased peripheral resistance, or both.

◆ Widened pulse pressure — a difference of more than 50 mm Hg between systolic and diastolic pressures — occurs when systolic pressure rises and diastolic pressure remains constant, or when systolic pressure rises and diastolic pressure falls. These changes reflect increased stroke volume, decreased peripheral resistance, or both.

◆ Blood pressure is measured in millimeters of mercury with a sphygmomanometer and a stethoscope, usually at the brachial artery (less commonly at the popliteal or radial artery).

AGE FACTOR *Blood pressure is lowest in the neonate and increases with age, weight gain, prolonged stress, and anxiety.*

◆ Frequent blood pressure measurement is critical after serious injury, surgery, or anesthesia and during an illness or condition that threatens cardiovascular stability.

◆ Frequent measurement may be done with an automated vital signs monitor.

◆ Regular measurement is indicated for the patient with a history of hypertension or hypotension; yearly screening is recommended for adults.

CONTRAINDICATIONS

◆ Mastectomy (Don't take blood pressure in the arm on the affected side; it may decrease already compromised lymphatic circulation, worsen edema, and damage the arm.)

◆ Arteriovenous fistula or hemodialysis shunt (Don't take blood pressure on these areas of the arm; blood flow through the vascular device may be compromised.)

Mercury or aneroid sphygmomanometer ◆ stethoscope ◆ alcohol pad ◆ automated vital signs monitor (if available)

PREPARATION

◆ The sphygmomanometer consists of an inflatable compression cuff linked to a manual air pump and a mercury manometer or an aneroid gauge.

◆ The mercury sphygmomanometer is more accurate and requires calibration less frequently than the aneroid model, but is larger and heavier.

◆ Hook, bandage, snap, or Velcro cuffs come in six standard sizes ranging from neonate to extra-large adult. Disposable cuffs are available.

◆ The automated vital signs monitor is a noninvasive device that measures pulse rate, systolic and diastolic pressures, and mean arterial pressure at preset intervals.

◆ Carefully choose a cuff of appropriate size for the patient.

◆ To obtain an accurate reading, rest the gauge on a level surface and view the meniscus at eye level.

◆ You can rest an aneroid gauge in any position, but you must view it directly from the front.

WARNING *An excessively narrow cuff may cause a false-high pressure reading; an excessively wide one, a false-low reading.*

◆ To use an automated vital signs monitor, collect the monitor, dual air hose, and pressure cuff.

◆ Confirm the patient's identity using two patient identifiers according to facility policy.

◆ Tell the patient that you're going to take his blood pressure.

◆ Have the patient lie in a supine position or sit erect during blood pressure measurement.

◆ His arm should be extended at heart level and be well supported.

◆ If the artery is below heart level, you may get a false-high blood pressure reading.

◆ Make sure that the patient is relaxed and comfortable so his blood pressure stays at its normal level.

◆ Wrap the deflated cuff snugly around the upper arm.

◆ Connect the appropriate tube to the rubber bulb of the air pump and the other tube to the manometer, if necessary.

◆ To determine how high to pump the blood pressure cuff, estimate the systolic blood pressure by palpation.

◆ As you feel the radial artery with your fingers of one hand, inflate the cuff until the radial pulse disappears.

◆ Read this pressure on the manometer and add 30 mm Hg.

◆ Use the sum as the target inflation to prevent discomfort from overinflation.

◆ Deflate the cuff.

◆ Pump up the cuff to the predetermined level.

◆ Locate the brachial artery by palpation.

◆ Center the bell of the stethoscope over the part of the artery where you detect the strongest beats, holding the bell of the stethoscope in place with one hand.

- The bell of the stethoscope transmits low-pitched arterial blood sounds more effectively than the diaphragm.
- Turn the thumbscrew on the rubber bulb of the air pump clockwise, using the thumb and index finger of your other hand, to close the valve.
- Carefully open the valve of the air pump and slowly deflate the cuff — no faster than 5 mm Hg/second.
- While releasing air, watch the mercury column or aneroid gauge and auscultate for the sound over the artery.
- When you hear the first beat or clear tapping sound, note the pressure on the column or gauge. This is the systolic pressure.
- The beat or tapping sound is the first of five Korotkoff sounds:
  - the second sound resembles a murmur or swish
  - the third sound is a crisp tapping
  - the fourth sound is a soft, muffled tone
  - the fifth sound is the last sound heard.
- Continue to release air gradually while auscultating for the sound over the artery.
- Note the diastolic pressure — the fourth Korotkoff sound.
- If you continue to hear sounds as the column or gauge falls to zero (common in children), record the pressure at the beginning of the fourth sound. This is important because, in some patients, a distinct fifth sound is absent.
- Rapidly deflate the cuff.
- Record the pressure, wait 15 to 30 seconds, and then repeat the procedure to confirm your original findings.
- Remove and fold the cuff, and return it to storage.

SPECIAL CONSIDERATIONS

- If you can't auscultate blood pressure, you may estimate systolic pressure.
- To estimate systolic pressure, palpate the brachial or radial pulse.
- Inflate the cuff until you no longer detect the pulse.

- Slowly deflate the cuff and when you detect the pulse again, record the pressure as the palpated systolic pressure.
- When measuring blood pressure in the popliteal artery, position the patient on his abdomen, wrap a cuff around the middle of the thigh, and proceed with blood pressure measurement.
- Palpation of systolic blood pressure may also be important to avoid underestimating blood pressure in patients with an auscultatory gap, which is a loss of sound between the first and second Korotkoff sounds that may be as great as 40 mm Hg.
- Auscultatory gaps may occur in patients with venous congestion or hypotension.
- If your facility considers the fourth and fifth Korotkoff sounds as the first and second diastolic pressures, record both pressures.
- Malfunction in an aneroid sphygmomanometer can be identified by checking it against a mercury manometer of known accuracy.
- Be sure to periodically check your aneroid manometer.
- Malfunction in a mercury manometer is evident in abnormal actions of the mercury column.
- Don't attempt to repair either type yourself.
- Blood pressure must sometimes be measured in both arms or with the patient in two positions (such as lying and standing or sitting and standing).
- Observe and record significant differences between the two readings and record the blood pressure and extremities and positions used.
- Measure the blood pressure of patients taking antihypertensive drugs in a sitting position to ensure accurate measurements.

COMPLICATIONS
None known

PATIENT TEACHING

- If the patient will be monitoring his blood pressure at home, teach him how to do so and have him do a return demonstration.
- Teach him how to record his blood pressure reading and how often he should take his blood pressure, as ordered by his practitioner.

DOCUMENTATION

- Record blood pressure as systolic over diastolic pressures such as 120/78 mm Hg.
- Record systolic pressure over the two diastolic pressures, such as 120/78/20 mm Hg, if necessary.
- Chart an auscultatory gap if present.
- If required by your facility, chart blood pressures on a graph, using dots or checkmarks.
- Document the extremity used and the patient's position.

SELECTED REFERENCES
Bursztyn, M. "Out-of-office Blood Pressure Measurement: A New Era," *Hypertension* 45(6):1070-71, June 2005.
Houweling, S.T., et al. "Pitfalls in Blood Pressure Measurement in Daily Practice," *Family Practice* 23(1):20-27, February 2006.
Karagiannis, A., et al. "The Unilateral Measurement of Blood Pressure May Mask the Diagnosis or Delay the Effective Treatment of Hypertension," *Angiology* 56(5):565-69, September-October 2005.
Myers, M.G. "Automated Blood Pressure Measurement in Routine Clinical Practice," *Blood Pressure Monitoring* 11(2): 59-62, April 2006.
Parati, G., and Mancia, G. "Assessing the White-coat Effect: Which Blood Pressure Measurement Should Be Considered?" *Journal of Hypertension* 24(1): 29-31, January 2006.

Bone growth stimulation, electrical

DESCRIPTION

- ◆ Electrical bone growth stimulation initiates or accelerates the healing process in a fractured bone that fails to heal by imitating the body's natural electrical forces.
- ◆ About 1 in 20 fractures may fail to heal properly, possibly as a result of infection, insufficient reduction or fixation, pseudarthrosis, or severe tissue trauma around the fracture.
- ◆ The stimulating effects of electrical currents on osteogenesis have led to using electrical bone growth stimulation to promote healing.
- ◆ Electrical stimulation may also be used for treating spinal fusions.
- ◆ The three electrical stimulation techniques include:
- – fully implantable direct current stimulation
- – semi-invasive percutaneous stimulation

- – noninvasive electromagnetic coil stimulation. (See *Methods of electrical bone growth stimulation* for explanations of invasive and noninvasive systems.)
- ◆ Choice of technique depends on:
- – fracture type and location
- – physician's preference
- – patient's ability and willingness to comply.
- ◆ The fully implantable device requires little or no patient management.
- ◆ The semi-invasive and noninvasive techniques require the patient to manage his treatment schedule and maintain the equipment.
- ◆ Treatment time averages from 3 to 6 months.

CONTRAINDICATIONS

- ◆ The pregnant patient, the patient with a tumor, and the patient with an arm fracture, who also has pacemaker, due to electromagnetic coils
- ◆ Any kind of inflammatory process (with percutaneous electrical bone growth stimulation)

⚡ **WARNING** *Use caution in the patient who's sensitive to nickel or chromium because both are present in the electrical bone growth stimulation system.*

DIRECT CURRENT STIMULATION
Small generator with lead wires connecting to surgically implanted titanium cathode wire into nonunited bone site

PERCUTANEOUS STIMULATION
External anode skin pad with a lead wire ◆ lithium battery pack ◆ 1 to 4 surgically implanted Teflon-coated stainless steel cathode wires

ELECTROMAGNETIC STIMULATION
Generator that plugs into a standard 110 V outlet ◆ 2 strong electromagnetic coils (placed on either side of injured area; they can be incorporated into a cast, cuff, or orthotic device)

PREPARATION
- ◆ All equipment comes with instructions provided by the manufacturer. Follow the instructions carefully.
- ◆ Make sure that all parts are included and sterilized according to facility policy and procedure.

Methods of electrical bone growth stimulation

Electrical bone growth stimulation may be invasive or noninvasive.

INVASIVE SYSTEM
An invasive system involves placing a spiral cathode inside the bone at the fracture site. A wire leads from the cathode to a battery-powered generator, also implanted in local tissues. The patient's body completes the circuit.

NONINVASIVE SYSTEM
A noninvasive system may include a cufflike transducer or fitted ring that wraps around the patient's limb at the level of the injury. Electric current penetrates the limb.

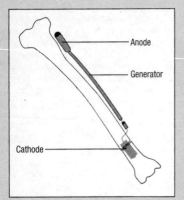

- Anode
- Generator
- Cathode

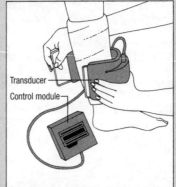

- Transducer
- Control module

KEY STEPS

- Discuss with the patient the use of anesthetics.

DIRECT CURRENT STIMULATION

- Implantation is performed with the patient under general anesthesia.
- The practitioner may apply a cast or external fixator to immobilize the limb.
- The patient is usually hospitalized for 2 to 3 days after implantation.
- Weight bearing may be ordered as tolerated.
- After the bone fragments join, the generator and lead wire can be removed under local anesthesia.
- The titanium cathode remains implanted.

PERCUTANEOUS STIMULATION

- Remove excessive hair from the injury site before applying the anode pad.
- Avoid stressing or pulling on the anode wire.
- Tell the patient to change the anode pad every 48 hours.
- Tell him to report local pain to the physician and to follow weight-bearing status as prescribed by the physician.

ELECTROMAGNETIC STIMULATION

- Show the patient where to place the coils and tell him to apply them for 3 to 10 hours each day, or as ordered.
- Many patients find it most convenient to perform the procedure at night.
- Advise the patient to not interrupt the treatments for more than 10 minutes at a time.
- Teach the patient how to use and care for the generator.
- Restate the physician's instructions for weight bearing. The physician usually will advise against bearing weight until evidence of healing appears on X-rays.

SPECIAL CONSIDERATIONS

- A patient with direct current electrical bone growth stimulation shouldn't undergo electrocauterization, diathermy, or magnetic resonance imaging (MRI).
- Electrocautery may "short" the system.
- Diathermy may potentiate the electrical current, possibly causing tissue damage.
- MRI interferes with or stops the current.

COMPLICATIONS

- Infection with direct current electrical bone growth stimulation equipment
- Local irritation or skin ulceration around cathode pin sites with percutaneous devices
- None known with electromagnetic coils

PATIENT TEACHING

- Teach the patient how to care for his cast or external fixation devices.
- Tell the patient how to care for the electrical generator.
- Urge the patient to follow treatment instructions.

DOCUMENTATION

- Note the type of electrical bone growth stimulation equipment provided.
- Note the date, time, and location of stimulation, as appropriate.
- Record the patient's skin condition and tolerance of the procedure.
- Document the instructions given to the patient and his family.

SELECTED REFERENCES

Hannay, G., et al. "Timing of Pulsed Electromagnetic Field Stimulation Does not Affect the Promotion of Bone Cell Development," *Bioelectromagnetics* 26(8):670-76, December 2005.

Huang, A.J., et al. "Health Plans' Coverage Determinations for Technology-Based Interventions: The Case of Electrical Bone Growth Stimulation," *American Journal of Managed Care* 10(12):957-62, December 2004.

Park, S.H., and Silva, M. "Neuromuscular Electrical Stimulation Enhances Fracture Healing: Results of an Animal Model," *Journal of Orthopaedic Research* 22(2):382-87, March 2004.

Resnick, D.K., et al. "Guidelines for the Performance of Fusion Procedures for Degenerative Disease of the Lumbar Spine. Part 17: Bone Growth Stimulators and Lumbar Fusion," *Journal of Neurosurgery-Spine* 2(6):737-40, June 2005.

Weinraub, G.M. "Orthobiologics: A Survey of Materials and Techniques," *Clinics in Podiatric Medicine and Surgery of North America* 22(4):509-19, v., October 2005.

Bone marrow aspiration and biopsy

DESCRIPTION

- A specimen of bone marrow — the major site of blood cell formation — may be obtained by aspiration or needle biopsy.
- The procedure allows evaluation of overall blood composition by studying blood elements and precursor cells as well as abnormal or malignant cells.
- Aspiration removes cells through a needle inserted into the marrow cavity of the bone; a biopsy removes a small, solid core of marrow tissue through the needle.
- Both procedures are usually performed by a physician, but some trained chemotherapy nurses or nurse clinicians perform them with assistance.
- Aspirates aid in diagnosing various disorders and cancers, such as oat cell carcinoma, leukemia, and lymphomas such as Hodgkin's disease.
- Biopsies are commonly performed simultaneously to stage the disease and monitor response to treatment.

CONTRAINDICATIONS

None known

EQUIPMENT

ASPIRATION

Prepackaged bone marrow set, which includes: povidone-iodine pads ◆ two sterile drapes (one fenestrated, one plain) ◆ ten 4″ × 4″ gauze pads ◆ ten 2″ × 2″ gauze pads ◆ two 12-ml syringes ◆ 22G 1″ or 2″ needle ◆ scalpel ◆ sedative ◆ specimen containers ◆ bone marrow needle ◆ 70% isopropyl alcohol ◆ 1% lidocaine (unopened bottle) ◆ 26G or 27G ½″ to ⅝″ needle ◆ adhesive tape ◆ sterile gloves ◆ glass slides and cover glass labels ◆ sterile labels ◆ sterile marker

BIOPSY

All equipment listed above ◆ Vim-Silverman, Jamshidi, Illinois sternal, or Westerman-Jensen needle ◆ Zenker's fixative

---

KEY STEPS

- Confirm the patient's identity using two patient identifiers according to facility policy.
- Check the patient's history for hypersensitivity to the local anesthetic.
- Provide a sedative before the test as ordered.

- Obtain the patient's baseline vital signs.
- Position the patient according to the selected puncture site. (See *Common sites for bone marrow aspiration and biopsy.*)
- Clean the puncture site with povidone-iodine solution, using sterile technique.
- Allow the site to dry, and drape the area.
- Label all medication syringes, medication containers, and solution containers on and off the sterile field.
- To anesthetize the site, the physician infiltrates it with 1% lidocaine, using a 26G or 27G ½″ to ⅝″ needle to inject a small amount intradermally and then a larger 22G 1″ or 2″ needle to anesthetize the tissue down to the bone.
- When the needle tip reaches the bone, the physician anesthetizes the periosteum by injecting a small amount of lidocaine in a circular area about ¾″ (2 cm) in diameter.
- The needle should be withdrawn from the periosteum after each injection.
- After allowing about 1 minute for the lidocaine to take effect, a scalpel may be used to make a small stab incision in the patient's skin to accommodate the bone marrow needle. This technique avoids pushing skin into the

---

Common sites for bone marrow aspiration and biopsy

The posterior superior iliac crest is the preferred site for aspiration because no vital organs or vessels are nearby. The patient is placed in either a lateral position with one leg flexed or in a prone position.

For aspiration or biopsy from the anterior iliac crest, the patient is placed in the supine or side-lying position. This site is used with a patient who can't lie prone because of severe abdominal distention.

Aspiration from the sternum involves the greatest risk but may be chosen because the site is near the surface, the cortical bone is thin, and the marrow cavity contains numerous cells and relatively little fat or supporting bone. The sternum is seldom used for biopsy.

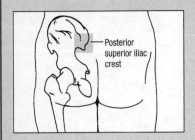

Posterior superior iliac crest

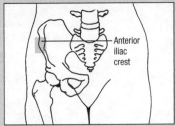

Anterior iliac crest

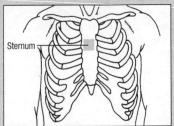

Sternum

bone marrow and also helps avoid unnecessary skin tearing and reduces the risk of infection.

◆ Explain the procedure to the patient to ease his anxiety and ensure cooperation.

◆ Make sure that the patient or a responsible family member understands the procedure and signs a consent form.

◆ Tell the patient the procedure usually takes 5 to 10 minutes, that test results are usually available in 1 day, and that more than one marrow specimen may be required.

◆ Tell the patient which bone will be sampled.

◆ Tell the patient that he'll receive a local anesthetic.

◆ Explain to the patient that he'll feel heavy pressure from insertion of the biopsy or aspiration needle as well as a brief, pulling sensation.

◆ Tell the patient that the physician may make a small incision to avoid tearing the skin.

◆ If the patient has osteoporosis, explain that the needle pressure may be minimal and that a drill may be needed.

◆ Explain to the patient that a pressure dressing may be applied and, if so, the patient shouldn't remove it.

ASPIRATION

◆ The physician inserts the bone marrow needle and lodges it firmly in the bone cortex.

◆ If the patient feels sharp pain instead of pressure when the needle first touches the bone, the needle was probably inserted outside the anesthetized area.

◆ To correct the needle insertion, withdraw slightly and move it toward the anesthetized area.

◆ The needle is advanced by applying an even, downward force with the heel of the hand or the palm, while twisting it back and forth slightly.

◆ A crackling sensation means the needle has entered the marrow cavity.

◆ Next, the physician removes the inner cannula, attaches the syringe to the needle, aspirates the required specimen, and withdraws the needle.

◆ The specimen is placed on glass slides and covered with the coverglass.

◆ Label the specimen with the patient's name and the date.

◆ Put on gloves and apply pressure to the aspiration site with a gauze pad for 5 minutes to control bleeding, while an assistant prepares the marrow slides.

◆ Clean the area with alcohol to remove the povidone-iodine.

◆ Dry the skin thoroughly with a $4'' \times 4''$ gauze pad, and apply a sterile pressure dressing.

BIOPSY

◆ The physician inserts the biopsy needle into the periosteum and advances it steadily until the outer needle passes into the marrow cavity.

◆ The biopsy needle is directed into the marrow cavity by alternately rotating the inner needle clockwise and counterclockwise.

◆ A plug of tissue is removed, the needle assembly is withdrawn, and the marrow specimen is expelled into a properly labeled specimen bottle containing Zenker's fixative or formaldehyde.

◆ Put on gloves.

◆ Clean the area around the biopsy site with alcohol to remove the povidone-iodine solution.

◆ Firmly press a sterile $2'' \times 2''$ gauze pad against the incision to control bleeding, and apply a sterile pressure dressing.

SPECIAL CONSIDERATIONS

◆ Faulty needle placement may yield too little aspirate.

◆ If no specimen is produced, the needle must be withdrawn from the bone (but not from the overlying soft tissue), the stylet replaced, and the needle inserted into a second site within the anesthetized field.

◆ Bone marrow specimens shouldn't be collected from irradiated areas because radiation may have altered or destroyed the marrow.

COMPLICATIONS

⬤ **WARNING** *Bleeding and infection are potentially life-threatening complications of aspiration or biopsy at any site.*

◆ Potential complications include:

– puncturing the heart and major vessels, causing severe hemorrhage

– puncturing the mediastinum, causing mediastinitis or pneumomediastinum

– puncturing the lung, causing pneumothorax

◆ Hematoma that occurs around the puncture site (Apply pressure and give analgesics for site pain or tenderness.)

PATIENT TEACHING

◆ Instruct the patient to contact the nurse or physician if signs of infection appear at the puncture site.

DOCUMENTATION

◆ Document the time, date, location, and patient's tolerance of the procedure and what specimen was obtained.

SELECTED REFERENCES

Antmen, B., et al. "Safe and Effective Sedation and Analgesia for Bone Marrow Aspiration Procedures in Children with Alfentanil, Remifentanil and Combinations with Midazolam," *Pediatric Anesthesia* 15(3):214-19, March 2005.

Bain, B.J. "Bone Marrow Biopsy Morbidity: Review of 2003," *Journal of Clinical Pathology* 58(4):406-408, April 2005.

Eikelboom, J.W. "Bone Marrow Biopsy in Thrombocytopenic or Anticoagulated Patients," *British Journal of Haematology* 129(4):562-63, May 2005.

Marti, J., et al. "Complications of Bone Marrow Biopsy," *British Journal of Haematology* 124(4):557-58, February 2004.

Rushing, J. "Assisting with Bone Marrow Aspiration and Biopsy," *Nursing* 36(3): 68, March 2006.

Bryant's traction

OVERVIEW

DESCRIPTION

- Also called *vertical suspension,* Bryant's traction is used primarily to reduce congenital hip dislocations in children.
- With the patient lying supine in a bed or crib, the traction extends the legs vertically at a 90-degree angle to the body.
- Even if the disorder affects only one leg, the patient has traction applied to both legs to prevent hip rotation and to ensure equal stress on the legs and even, bilateral bone growth.
- Bryant's traction continues for about 2 to 4 weeks. Afterward, the patient may be immobilized in a hip-spica cast.
- Bryant's traction is usually chosen for children younger than age 2 who weigh 25 to 30 lb (11.5 to 13.5 kg).

CONTRAINDICATIONS

- Children heavier than 30 lb because the risk of positional hypertension rises with increased weight

EQUIPMENT

Traction setup (supplied by the orthopedic department) ◆ moleskin traction straps ◆ elastic bandages ◆ foam rubber padding ◆ cotton balls ◆ compound benzoin tincture ◆ adhesive tape ◆ jacket restraint ◆ optional: safety razor, cotton batting, convoluted foam mattress, and sheepskin pad

PREPARATION

- Assist the physician and orthopedic technician with measuring and cutting the moleskin straps and with assembling the traction equipment.

KEY STEPS

- Confirm the patient's identity using two patient identifiers according to facility policy.
- Thoroughly explain the purpose and function of the traction to enhance learning and alleviate patient and family anxiety. If possible, use visual aids to illustrate your teaching. Keep a diagram handy for the parents and a doll in traction for the patient.
- Ask the parents whether their child is sensitive or allergic to rubber or to adhesive tape.
- If the patient has hairy legs, shave or clip the hair with a safety razor to ensure good contact between the moleskin traction straps and the skin. Use soap, warm water, and long, downward strokes to minimize nicking.
- Use cotton balls to apply the compound benzoin tincture, if ordered, to the patient's legs to protect the skin.
- Assist the physician or orthopedic technician with placing foam rubber padding and moleskin traction straps against the patient's legs and securing the straps with elastic bandages from foot to thigh. Secure the elastic bandages with adhesive tape. If the patient is allergic to rubber or to adhesive tape, wrap the legs in cotton batting before applying the straps.
- If necessary to keep the patient positioned properly, apply a jacket restraint to keep the weights from pulling the patient forward and altering the tractional force.
- Carefully monitor the circulatory status of the patient's legs 15 minutes and 30 minutes after applying initial traction. Then check circulatory status every 4 hours to detect impairment caused by the traction. Assess capillary refill, skin color, sensation, movement, temperature, peripheral pulses, and bandage tightness. If you detect circulatory compromise, loosen the elastic bandages and notify the physician.
- Take care to position the elastic bandages precisely. Unless contraindicated, periodically remove the bandages from the unaffected leg to assess circulation and provide skin care. When doing so, have another person hold the traction straps in place to prevent slipping. Don't unwrap the affected leg unless ordered to do so by the physician.
- Check the patient's position regularly to ensure optimum traction. Be sure to raise the patient's buttocks high enough off the mattress to allow one hand to slide between the skin and the mattress. Avoid raising the buttocks too high, however, because this may reduce the effectiveness of the traction.
- Try marking the bed sheet with an "X" at the correct shoulder position as a guide to correct body alignment. Near the patient's bed, post an illustration of the correct alignment to guide other nurses and caregivers. (See *Maintaining body alignment and traction.*)
- Provide skin care every 4 hours, focusing especially on the back, buttocks, and elbows — the areas most prone to breakdown. Place a convoluted foam mattress or a sheepskin pad — or both — beneath the patient to help prevent or alleviate skin problems.
- Inspect the traction apparatus at least every 2 hours to ensure the correct weight. Make sure that the weights hang freely, the pulleys glide easily, the ropes aren't frayed, and the knots remain snugly tied and taped.
- Encourage the patient to take deep breaths at least every 2 hours to minimize the risk of developing hypostatic pneumonia.
- Review the patient's diet to make sure that he consumes enough fiber and fluid to prevent constipation and urinary stasis. (Infants should consume about 130 ml of fluid for each kilogram of body weight every 24 hours; toddlers should consume about 115 ml/kg.)
- Promote safety by keeping the side rails raised on the patient's bed whenever you aren't at the bedside.

SPECIAL CONSIDERATIONS

◆ To promote regular deep breathing and guard against pneumonia, allow the patient to blow a horn, a whistle, a pinwheel, or bubbles heartily or encourage him to sing. This promotes lung expansion and enjoyment at the same time.

◆ Because a child can't always tell you that he's in pain, carefully observe his behavior, facial expression, and cry to judge discomfort levels. Besides needing an analgesic or sedative, the patient may need an antispasmodic medication to relieve irritable muscles and prevent muscle spasms.

◆ To foster development, diversion, and mobility, provide age-appropriate games and activities as permitted within the confines of traction. For infants, this can include mobiles, music boxes, and rattles. Toddlers may enjoy puppets, large-pieced puzzles, and dolls. Involve the family in their child's care and recreational activities to increase the patient's sense of security and to minimize the family's sense of anxiety. If facility policy permits, consider moving the infant's crib to the playroom so that he can be around other children.

◆ Eating and drinking are difficult and inconvenient for the patient in Bryant's traction because of the head-down position. To facilitate digestion and encourage eating — especially if the patient refuses food — place a small pillow under his head at mealtime. If possible, allow him to choose his own foods, and encourage his family to bring food from home.

◆ To minimize patient movement, change bed linens every other day unless the linens get wet or soiled. Keep sheets taut and wrinkle-free to help prevent skin breakdown.

COMPLICATIONS

◆ Pneumonia
◆ Skin necrosis
◆ Urinary stasis
◆ Constipation

PATIENT TEACHING

◆ Instruct the parents how to help the child maintain proper body alignment to prevent disalignment.
◆ Teach the parents how to check the child's skin for possible breakdown to prevent tissue damage and infection.

DOCUMENTATION

◆ Record the date and time that traction was applied, the amount of weight applied, and the patient's circulatory status, skin condition, and position.
◆ Note whether the weights hang freely.
◆ Note changes in the patient's status.
◆ Describe the patient's and family's response to the traction.
◆ Note the patient's and family's response to patient teaching.

SELECTED REFERENCES

Cassinelli, E.H., et al. "Spica Cast Application in the Emergency Room for Select Pediatric Femur Fractures," *Journal of Orthopaedic Trauma* 19(10):709-16, November-December 2005.

Song, K.S., and Kim, H.K. "Femoral Neck Fracture in a Child with Autosomal-Dominant Osteopetrosis: Failure of Spica Cast Treatment and Successful Outcome by Internal Fixation," *Journal of Orthopaedic Trauma* 19(7):494-97, August 2005.

Yamada, N., et al. "Closed Reduction of Developmental Dislocation of the Hip by Prolonged Traction," *Journal of Bone and Joint Surgery* (British volume) 85(8):1173-177, November 2003.

Maintaining body alignment and traction

Keeping the child's body in the correct position with Bryant's traction requires precision as well as continual supervision and adjustment.

At the same time that the traction apparatus holds the patient's legs perpendicular to the mattress, you need to make sure that his buttocks stay slightly elevated to provide countertraction and that his shoulders stay flat and in the same position on the mattress to maintain body alignment.

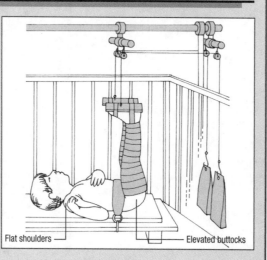

Flat shoulders —— —— Elevated buttocks

Buccal, sublingual, and translingual drug administration

OVERVIEW

DESCRIPTION

- Certain drugs are given buccally, sublingually, or translingually for rapid absorption and to prevent their destruction or transformation in the stomach or small intestine.
- These drugs act quickly because the oral mucosa's thin epithelium and abundant vasculature allow direct absorption into the bloodstream.
- Drugs given buccally include nitroglycerin and methyltestosterone.
- Drugs given sublingually include ergotamine tartrate, isosorbide dinitrate, and nitroglycerin.
- Translingual drugs, which are sprayed onto the tongue, include nitrate preparations for patients with chronic angina.

CONTRAINDICATIONS

None known

EQUIPMENT

Patient's drug record and chart ◆ prescribed drug ◆ drug cup

KEY STEPS

- Confirm the patient's identity using two patient identifiers according to facility policy.
- Verify the order on the patient's drug record by checking it against the practitioner's order on his chart.
- Wash your hands thoroughly.
- Explain the procedure to the patient if he has never taken a drug buccally, sublingually, or translingually.
- Check the label on the drug before giving it to make sure that you'll be giving the prescribed drug.
- Verify the expiration date of all drugs, especially nitroglycerin.
- Confirm the patient's identity by asking his name and checking the name, room, and bed number on his wristband.

Placing drugs in the oral mucosa

Buccal and sublingual administration routes allow some drugs, such as nitroglycerin or methyltestosterone, to enter the bloodstream rapidly without being degraded in the GI tract.

To give a drug buccally, insert it between the patient's cheek and teeth (as shown here). Ask him to close his mouth and hold the tablet against his cheek until it's absorbed.

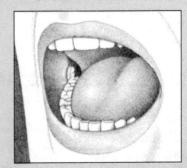

To give a drug sublingually, place it under the patient's tongue (as shown here), and ask him to leave it there until it's dissolved.

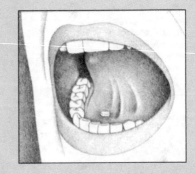

BUCCAL AND SUBLINGUAL ADMINISTRATION

- To give a drug buccally, place the tablet in the buccal pouch, between the cheek and gum.
- To give a drug sublingually, place the tablet under the patient's tongue. (See *Placing drugs in the oral mucosa.*)
- Tell the patient to keep the drug in place until it dissolves completely to ensure absorption.
- Tell the patient not to rinse his mouth until the tablet has been absorbed.
- Tell the patient with angina to wet the nitroglycerin tablet with saliva and to keep it under his tongue until fully absorbed.

  WARNING *Caution the patient against chewing the tablet or touching it with his tongue to prevent accidental swallowing.*

  WARNING *Tell the patient not to smoke before the drug has dissolved because nicotine's vasoconstrictive effects slow absorption.*

TRANSLINGUAL ADMINISTRATION

- To give a drug translingually, tell the patient to hold the drug canister vertically with the valve head at the top and the spray orifice as close to his mouth as possible.
- Tell the patient to spray the dose onto his tongue by pressing the button firmly.
- Remind the patient using a translingual aerosol form that he shouldn't inhale the spray but should release it under his tongue.
- Tell the patient to wait about 10 seconds before swallowing.

SPECIAL CONSIDERATIONS

- Don't give liquids to a patient who's receiving a buccal drug because some buccal tablets can take up to 1 hour to be absorbed.

COMPLICATIONS

- Some buccal drugs that irritate the mucosa
- Irritation of the same site (use alternate sides of the mouth for repeat doses)
- Sublingual drugs, such as nitroglycerin, which may cause a tingling sensation under the tongue (to avoid, place the drug in the buccal pouch)

PATIENT TEACHING

- Explain the procedure to the patient and answer any of his questions.
- Review his medications with him, including any possible adverse reactions.
- Review with the patient that he shouldn't rinse his mouth until the tablet has absorbed.

DOCUMENTATION

- Record the drug given.
- Document the dose, date, and time.
- Describe the patient's reaction.

SELECTED REFERENCES

Ferguson, A. "Administration of Oral Medication," *Nursing Times* 101(45):24-25, November 2005.

Finn, A., et al. "Bioavailability and Metabolism of Prochlorperazine Administered via the Buccal and Oral Delivery Route," *Journal of Clinical Pharmacology* 45(12):1383-390, December 2005.

Lee, M.C., and Menon, D.K. "Sublingual Drug Delivery during Functional Magnetic Resonance Imaging," *Anaesthesia* 60(8):821-22, August 2005.

Smart, J.D. "Buccal Drug Delivery," *Expert Opinion on Drug Delivery* 2(3):507-17, May 2005.

Burn care

DESCRIPTION

- The goals of burn care are to maintain the patient's physiologic stability, repair skin integrity, prevent infection, and maximize functionality and psychosocial health.
- Competent care immediately after a burn occurs can dramatically improve the success of overall treatment.
- Burn severity is determined by the depth and extent of the burn and the presence of other factors, such as age, complications, and coexisting illnesses. (See *Evaluating burn severity*.)
- To promote stability, carefully monitor your patient's respiratory status, especially if he suffered smoke inhalation.

- A patient with burns involving more than 20% of his total body surface area usually needs fluid resuscitation to support his body's compensatory mechanisms without overwhelming them.
- Give fluids (such as lactated Ringer's solution) to keep the patient's urine output to at least 30 to 50 ml/hour; monitor blood pressure and heart rate.
- Control the patient's body temperature because skin loss interferes with temperature regulation.
- Use warm fluids, heat lamps, and hyperthermia blankets, as appropriate, to keep the patient's temperature above 97° F (36.1° C), if possible.
- Frequently review laboratory values, such as serum electrolyte levels, to detect early changes in the patient's condition.
- Infection can increase wound depth, cause rejection of skin grafts, slow healing, worsen pain, prolong hospitalization, and lead to death. For prevention, use strict aseptic technique during care, dress the burn site as ordered, monitor and rotate I.V. lines regularly, and carefully assess the burn extent, body system function, and patient's emotional status.
- Other interventions, such as careful positioning and regular exercise for burned extremities, help maintain joint function, prevent contractures, and minimize deformity. (See *Positioning the burn patient to prevent deformity*.)
- Skin integrity is repaired through aggressive wound debridement, followed by maintenance of a clean wound bed until the wound heals or is covered with a skin graft.
- Full-thickness burns and some deep partial-thickness burns must be debrided and grafted in the operating room. Surgery takes place as soon as possible after fluid resuscitation.
- Most wounds are managed with twice-daily dressing changes using topical antibiotics.
- Burn dressings encourage healing by barring germ entry and removing exudate, eschar, and other debris that host infection.
- After thorough wound cleaning, topical antibacterial agents are applied, and the wound is covered with absorptive, coarse mesh gauze.
- Roller gauze typically tops the dressing and is secured with elastic netting or tape.

CONTRAINDICATIONS
None known

Evaluating burn severity

To judge a burn's severity, assess its depth and extent as well as the presence of other factors.

SUPERFICIAL PARTIAL-THICKNESS (FIRST-DEGREE) BURN

Does the burned area appear pink or red with minimal edema? Is the area sensitive to touch and temperature changes? If so, your patient probably has a superficial partial-thickness, or first-degree, burn (shown at right) affecting only the epidermal skin layer.

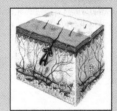

DEEP PARTIAL-THICKNESS (SECOND-DEGREE) BURN

Does the burned area look pink or red and have a mottled appearance? Do red areas blanch when you touch them? Does the skin have large, thick-walled blisters with subcutaneous edema? Does touching the burn cause severe pain? Is hair still present? If so, your patient probably has a deep partial-thickness, or second-degree, burn (shown at right) affecting the epidermal and dermal layers.

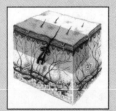

FULL-THICKNESS (THIRD-DEGREE) BURN

Does the burned area appear red, waxy white, brown, or black? Does red skin remain red with no blanching when you touch it? Is the skin leathery with extensive subcutaneous edema? Is the skin insensitive to touch? Does the hair fall out easily? If so, your patient probably has a full-thickness, or third-degree, burn that affects all skin layers.

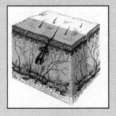

EQUIPMENT

Normal saline solution ◆ sterile bowl ◆ scissors ◆ tissue forceps ◆ ordered topical medication ◆ burn gauze ◆ roller gauze ◆ elastic netting or tape ◆ fine-mesh gauze ◆ elastic gauze ◆ cotton-tipped applicators or sterile tongue depressor ◆ ordered pain medication ◆ three pairs of sterile gloves ◆ sterile gown ◆ mask ◆ surgical cap ◆ heat lamps ◆ impervious plastic trash bag ◆ cotton bath blanket ◆ 4″ × 4″ gauze pad

PREPARATION
◆ A sterile field is required and all equipment and supplies used in the dressing should be sterile.
◆ Open equipment packages using aseptic technique.
◆ Arrange supplies on a sterile field in the order of their use.
◆ Dress the cleanest areas first and the dirtiest or most contaminated areas last to prevent cross-contamination.
◆ You may need to dress in stages to avoid exposing all wounds at the same time to help prevent excessive pain or cross-contamination.

KEY STEPS
◆ Confirm the patient's identity using two patient identifiers according to facility policy.
◆ Give the ordered analgesic about 20 minutes before beginning wound care to maximize patient comfort and cooperation.
◆ Explain the procedure and provide privacy.
◆ Turn on overhead heat lamps to keep him warm. Make sure that they don't overheat him.
◆ Pour warmed normal saline solution into the sterile bowl in the sterile field.
◆ Wash your hands.

REMOVING A DRESSING WITHOUT HYDROTHERAPY
◆ Put on a gown, a mask, and sterile gloves.

Positioning the burn patient to prevent deformity

For each of the potential deformities listed here, you can use the corresponding positioning and interventions to help prevent the deformity.

BURNED AREA	POTENTIAL DEFORMITY	PREVENTIVE POSITIONING	NURSING INTERVENTIONS
Neck	◆ Flexion contraction of neck ◆ Extensor contraction of neck	◆ Extension ◆ Prone with head slightly raised	◆ Remove pillow from bed. ◆ Place pillow or rolled towel under upper chest to flex cervical spine, or apply cervical collar.
Axilla	◆ Adduction and internal rotation ◆ Adduction and external rotation	◆ Shoulder joint in external rotation and 100- to 130-degree abduction ◆ Shoulder joint in forward flexion and 100- to 130-degree abduction	◆ Use an I.V. pole, bedside table, or sling to suspend arm. ◆ Use an I.V. pole, bedside table, or sling to suspend arm.
Pectoral region	◆ Shoulder protraction	◆ Shoulders abducted and externally rotated	◆ Remove pillow from bed.
Chest or abdomen	◆ Kyphosis	◆ Same as for pectoral region, with hips neutral (not flexed)	◆ Use no pillow under head or legs.
Lateral trunk	◆ Scoliosis	◆ Supine; affected arm abducted	◆ Put pillows or blanket rolls at sides.
Elbow	◆ Flexion and pronation	◆ Arm extended and supinated	◆ Use elbow splint, arm board, or bedside table.
Wrist	◆ Flexion ◆ Extension	◆ Splint in 15-degree extension ◆ Splint in 15-degree flexion	◆ Apply a hand splint. ◆ Apply a hand splint.
Fingers	◆ Adhesions of the extensor tendons; loss of palmar grip	◆ Metacarpophalangeal joints in maximum flexion; interphalangeal joints in slight flexion; thumb in maximum abduction	◆ Apply hand splint; wrap fingers separately.
Hip	◆ Internal rotation, flexion, and adduction; possibly, joint subluxation if contracture is severe	◆ Neutral rotation and abduction; maintain extension by prone position	◆ Put pillow under buttocks (if supine) or use trochanter rolls or knee or long leg splints.
Knee	◆ Flexion	◆ Maintain extension	◆ Use knee splint with no pillows under legs.
Ankle	◆ Plantar flexion if foot muscles are weak or their tendons are divided	◆ 90-degree dorsiflexion	◆ Use footboard or ankle splint.

(continued)

- Remove dressing layers down to the innermost layer by cutting the outer dressings with sterile blunt scissors.
- Lay open these dressings.
- If the inner layer appears dry, soak it with warm normal saline solution to ease removal.
- Remove the inner dressing with sterile tissue forceps or your sterile gloved hand.
- Dispose of soiled dressings carefully in an impervious plastic trash bag according to facility policy because these dressings harbor infection.
- Dispose of your gloves and wash your hands.
- Put on a new pair of sterile gloves.
- Using gauze pads moistened with normal saline solution, gently remove exudate and old topical drug.
- Carefully remove all loose eschar with sterile forceps and scissors, if ordered.
- Assess the wound's condition. It should appear clean, with no debris, loose tissue, purulence, inflammation, or darkened margins.
- Before applying a new dressing, remove your gown, gloves, and mask.
- Discard them properly; put on a clean mask, surgical cap, gown, and sterile gloves.

APPLYING A WET DRESSING
- Soak fine-mesh gauze and the elastic gauze dressing in a large sterile basin containing the ordered solution.
- Wring out the fine-mesh gauze until it's moist but not dripping, and apply it to the wound.
- Warn the patient that he may feel transient pain when you apply the dressing.
- Wring out the elastic gauze dressing and position it to hold the fine-mesh gauze in place.
- Roll elastic gauze dressing over the fine-mesh dressing to keep it intact.
- Cover the patient with a cotton bath blanket to prevent chills.
- Change the blanket if it becomes damp.
- Use an overhead heat lamp, if necessary.

- Change the dressings frequently, as ordered, to keep the wound moist, especially if you're using silver nitrate.
- If the dressings become dry, silver nitrate becomes ineffective and the silver ions may damage tissue.
- To maintain moist dressings, some protocols call for irrigating the dressing with solution at least every 4 hours through small slits cut into the outer dressing.

APPLYING A DRY DRESSING WITH A TOPICAL DRUG
- Remove old dressings and clean the wound (as described previously).
- Apply the drug to the wound in a thin layer — about 2 to 4 mm thick — with your sterile gloved hand or a sterile tongue blade.
- Apply several layers of burn gauze over the wound to contain the drug but allow exudate to escape.
- Cut the dressing to fit only the wound areas.
- Don't cover unburned areas.
- Cover the entire dressing with roller gauze and secure it with elastic netting or tape.

PROVIDING ARM AND LEG CARE
- Apply the dressings from the distal to the proximal area to stimulate circulation and prevent constriction.
- Wrap the burn gauze once around the arm or leg so the edges overlap slightly.
- Continue wrapping until the gauze covers the wound.
- Apply a dry roller gauze dressing to hold bottom layers in place.
- Secure with elastic netting or tape.

PROVIDING HAND AND FOOT CARE
- Wrap each finger separately with a single 4″ × 4″ gauze pad to allow the patient to use his hands and to prevent webbing contractures.
- Place the hand in a functional position, and secure using a dressing.
- Apply splints if ordered.

- Put gauze between each toe, as appropriate, to prevent webbing contractures.

PROVIDING CHEST, ABDOMEN, AND BACK CARE
- Apply the ordered drug to the wound in a thin layer.
- Cover the entire burned area with sheets of burn gauze.
- Wrap with roller gauze or apply a specialty vest dressing to hold the burn gauze in place.
- Secure the dressing with elastic netting or tape.
- Make sure that the dressing doesn't restrict respiratory motion, especially in very young or elderly patients, or in those with circumferential injuries.

PROVIDING SCALP AND FACIAL CARE
- If the patient has scalp burns, clip or shave the hair around the burn as ordered.
- Clip other hair until it's about 2″ (5 cm) long to prevent contamination of burned scalp areas.
- Shave facial hair if it comes in contact with burned areas.
- Typically, facial burns are managed with milder topical agents (such as triple antibiotic ointment) and are left open to air.
- If dressings are required, make sure that they don't cover the eyes, nostrils, or mouth.

PROVIDING EAR CARE
- Clip or shave hair around the affected ear.
- Remove exudate and crusts with cotton-tipped applicators dipped in normal saline solution.
- Place a layer of 4″ × 4″ gauze behind the auricle to prevent webbing.
- Apply the ordered topical drug to 4″ × 4″ gauze pads and place them over the burned area.
- Before securing the dressing with a roller bandage, position the patient's ears normally to avoid damaging the auricular cartilage.
- Assess the patient's hearing ability.

PROVIDING EYE CARE

- Clean the area around his eyes and eyelids with a cotton-tipped applicator and normal saline solution every 4 to 6 hours, or as needed, to remove crust and drainage.
- Give ordered eye ointments or drops.
- If his eyes can't be closed, apply lubricating ointments or drops as ordered.
- Be sure to close his eyes before applying eye pads to prevent corneal abrasion.
- Don't apply topical ointments near his eyes without a practitioner's order.

PROVIDING NASAL CARE

- Check the patient's nostrils for inhalation injury, such as the presence of inflamed mucosa, singed vibrissae, and soot.
- Clean his nostrils with cotton-tipped applicators dipped in normal saline solution.
- Remove crust.
- Apply the ordered ointments.
- If he has a nasogastric tube, use tracheostomy ties to secure the tube.
- Be sure to check tracheostomy ties frequently for tightness caused by swelling facial tissue.
- Clean the area around the tube every 4 to 6 hours.

SPECIAL CONSIDERATIONS

- Thorough assessment and documentation of the wound's appearance are essential to detect infection and other complications.

⚡ **WARNING** *A purulent wound or green-gray exudate indicates infection, an overly dry wound suggests dehydration, and a wound with a swollen, red edge suggests cellulitis. Suspect a fungal infection if the wound is white and powdery.*

- Healthy granulation tissue appears clean, pinkish, faintly shiny, and free from exudate.
- Blisters protect underlying tissue; leave them intact unless they impede joint motion, become infected, or cause discomfort.
- Be sure to meet the increased nutritional needs of the patient with healing burns; extra protein and carbohydrates are required to accommodate an almost doubled basal metabolism.
- If you must manage a burn with topical drugs, exposure to air, and no dressing, watch for such problems as wound adherence to bed linens, poor drainage control, and partial loss of topical drugs.

COMPLICATIONS

- Infection (most common)
- Sepsis
- Allergic reaction to ointments or dressings
- Renal failure
- Multisystem organ dysfunction

PATIENT TEACHING

- Begin discharge planning as soon as the patient enters the facility to help him (and his family) transition from facility to home.
- To encourage therapeutic compliance, prepare the patient to expect scarring, but advise him that proper therapy can minimize scarring.
- Teach the patient wound management and pain control, and urge him to do the prescribed exercises.

- Provide encouragement and emotional support, and urge the patient to join a burn survivor support group.
- Teach the family or caregivers how to encourage, support, and provide care for the patient.

DOCUMENTATION

- Record the dates and times for all care provided.
- Describe the wound's condition.
- Report special dressing-change techniques.
- List topical drugs given.
- Note the positioning of the burned area.
- Describe the patient's tolerance of the procedure.

SELECTED REFERENCES

Gilbride, J. "Not Just Skin Deep: A History of Pediatric Burn Trauma," *Pediatric Nursing* 31(5):412-13, September-October 2005.

Hall, B. "Wound Care for Burn Patients in Acute Rehabilitation Settings," *Rehabilitation Nursing* 30(3):114-19, May-June 2005.

Kavanagh, S., et al. "Care of Burn Patients in the Hospital," *Burns* 30(8):A2-6, December 2004.

Laskowski-Jones, L. "First Aid for Burns," *Nursing* 36(1):41-43, January 2006.

Mendez-Eastman, S. "Burn Injuries," *Plastic Surgical Nursing* 25(3):133-39, July-September 2005.

Nowlin, A. "The Delicate Business of Burn Care," *RN* 69(1):52, 56-57, January 2006.

Supple, K.G. "Handle with Care. An Overview of Burn Injury," *Advance for Nurse Practitioners* 13(7):24-29, July 2005.

Burn dressings, biological

DESCRIPTION

◆ Biological dressings provide a temporary protective covering for burn wounds and for clean granulation tissue.

◆ Biological dressings temporarily secure fresh skin grafts and protect graft donor sites.

◆ Common organic materials for burn dressings include pigskin, cadaver skin, and amniotic membrane.

◆ Biobrane is a synthetic material used for burn dressings. (See *Comparing biological dressings*.)

◆ Besides stimulating new skin growth, these dressings act like normal skin to reduce heat loss, block infection, and minimize fluid, electrolyte, and protein losses.

◆ Amniotic membrane or fresh cadaver skin is usually applied to the patient in the operating room, although it may be applied in a treatment room.

◆ Pigskin or Biobrane may be applied in either the operating room or a treatment room.

◆ Before applying a biological dressing, the practitioner must clean and debride the wound.

◆ The frequency of dressing changes depends on the type of wound and the dressing's specific function.

CONTRAINDICATIONS

None known

EQUIPMENT

Ordered analgesic ◆ cap ◆ mask ◆ two pairs sterile gloves ◆ sterile or clean gown ◆ shoe covers ◆ biological dressing ◆ normal saline solution ◆ sterile basin ◆ Xeroflo gauze ◆ sterile forceps ◆ sterile scissors ◆ sterile hemostats ◆ elastic netting

PREPARATION

◆ Place the biological dressing in the sterile basin containing sterile normal saline solution (or open the Biobrane package).

◆ Using aseptic technique, open the sterile dressing packages.

◆ Arrange the equipment on the dressing cart and keep the cart accessible.

◆ Make sure the treatment area has adequate light to allow accurate wound assessment and dressing placement.

Comparing biological dressings

TYPE	DESCRIPTION AND USES	NURSING CONSIDERATIONS
Cadaver (homograft)	◆ Applied in the operating room or at the bedside to debrided, untidy wounds ◆ Available as fresh cryopreserved homografts in tissue banks nationwide ◆ Provides protection, especially to granulation tissue after escharotomy ◆ May be used in some patients as a test graft for autografting ◆ Obtained at autopsy up to 24 hours after death ◆ Covers excised wounds immediately	◆ Observe for exudate. ◆ Watch for signs of rejection. ◆ Keep in mind that the gauze dressing may be removed every 8 hours to observe the graft.
Pigskin (heterograft or xenograft)	◆ Applied in the operating room or at the bedside ◆ Comes fresh or frozen in rolls or sheets ◆ Can cover and protect debrided, untidy wounds, mesh autografts, clean (eschar-free) partial-thickness burns, and exposed tendons	◆ Reconstitute frozen form with normal saline solution 30 minutes before use. ◆ Watch for signs of rejection. ◆ Cover with gauze dressing or leave exposed to air, as ordered.
Amniotic membrane (homograft)	◆ Available from the obstetric department ◆ Must be sterile and come from an uncomplicated birth; serologic tests must be done ◆ Bacteriostatic condition doesn't require antimicrobials ◆ May be used to protect partial-thickness burns or (temporarily) granulation tissue before autografting ◆ Applied by the practitioner to clean wounds only	◆ Change the membrane every 48 hours. ◆ Cover the membrane with a gauze dressing or leave it exposed as ordered. ◆ If you apply a gauze dressing, change it every 48 hours.
Biobrane (biosynthetic membrane)	◆ Comes in sterile, prepackaged sheets in various sizes and in glove form for hand burns ◆ Used to cover donor graft sites, superficial partial-thickness burns, debrided wounds awaiting autograft, and meshed autografts ◆ Provides significant pain relief ◆ Applied by the nurse	◆ Leave the membrane in place for 3 to 14 days, possibly longer. ◆ Don't use this dressing for preparing a granulation bed for subsequent autografting.

- Confirm the patient's identity using two patient identifiers according to facility policy.
- If this is the patient's first treatment, explain the procedure to allay his fears and promote cooperation.
- Provide privacy.
- If ordered, give an analgesic to the patient 20 minutes before beginning the procedure, or give an analgesic I.V. immediately before the procedure to increase the patient's comfort and tolerance.
- Wash your hands and put on a cap, mask, gown, shoe covers, and sterile gloves.
- Clean and debride the wound to reduce bacteria.
- Remove and dispose of your gloves.
- Wash your hands and put on a fresh pair of sterile gloves.
- Place the dressing directly on the wound surface.
- Apply pigskin dermal (shiny) side down.
- Apply Biobrane nylon-backed (dull) side down.
- Roll the dressing directly onto the skin, if applicable.
- Place the dressing strips so that the edges touch but don't overlap.
- Use sterile forceps, if necessary.
- Smooth the dressing.
- Eliminate folds and wrinkles by rolling out the dressing with the hemostat handle, the forceps handle, or your sterile-gloved hand to cover the wound completely and ensure adherence.
- Use the scissors to trim the dressing around the wound so the dressing fits the wound without overlapping adjacent areas.
- Place Xeroflo gauze directly over an allograft, pigskin graft, or amniotic membrane.
- Place a few layers of gauze on top to absorb exudate, and wrap with roller gauze dressing.
- Secure the dressing with tape or elastic netting.

- During daily dressing changes, the dressing will be removed down to the Xeroflo gauze, and the gauze will be replaced after the Xeroflo is inspected for drainage, adherence, and signs of infection.
- Place a nonadhesive dressing (such as Exu-dry) over the Biobrane to absorb drainage and provide stability.
- Wrap the dressing with roller gauze dressing and secure it with tape or elastic netting.
- During daily dressing changes, remove the dressing down to the Biobrane and inspect the site for signs of infection.
- After the Biobrane adheres (usually in 2 to 3 days), it doesn't need to be covered with a dressing.
- Position the patient comfortably, elevating the area if possible, to reduce edema, which may prevent the biological dressing from adhering.

SPECIAL CONSIDERATIONS

- Handle the biological dressing as little as possible.

COMPLICATIONS
- Infection that may develop under a biological dressing

  WARNING *Observe the wound carefully during dressing changes for signs of infection. If wound drainage appears purulent, remove the dressing, clean the area with normal saline solution or another prescribed cleaning solution, as ordered, and apply a fresh biological dressing.*

PATIENT TEACHING

- Tell the patient or caregiver to assess the site daily for signs of infection, swelling, blisters, drainage, and separation.
- Make sure that the patient knows who to contact if complications develop.

DOCUMENTATION

- Document the times and dates of dressing changes.
- List the areas of application.
- Note the quality of adherence.
- Report purulent drainage or other signs of infection.
- Describe the patient's tolerance of the procedure.

SELECTED REFERENCES
Chiu, T., and Burd, A. "'Xenograft Dressing in the Treatment of Burns," *Clinics in Dermatology* 23(4):419-23, July-August 2005.

Chiu, T., et al. "Porcine Skin: Friend or Foe?" *Burns* 30(7):739-41, November 2004.

Gajiwala, K., and Gajiwala, A.L. "Evaluation of Lyophilized, Gamma-irradiated Amnion as a Biological Dressing," *Cell and Tissue Banking* 5(2):73-80, 2004.

Hassan, Z., and Shah, M. "Porcine Xenograft Dressing for Facial Burns: Meshed Versus Non-meshed," *Burns* 30(7):753, November 2004.

Hassan, Z., and Shah, M. "Punctate Scarring from Use of Porous Biobrane," *Burns* 32(2):258-60, March 2006.

Lang, E.M., et al. "Biobrane in the Treatment of Burn and Scald Injuries in Children," *Annals of Plastic Surgery* 55(5):485-89, November 2005.

Canes

DESCRIPTION

- Canes are indicated for the patient with one-sided weakness or injury, occasional loss of balance, or increased joint pressure.
- They provide balance and support for walking and reduce fatigue and strain on weight-bearing joints.
- Canes are available in various sizes to ensure proper fit. The cane should extend from the greater trochanter to the floor and have a rubber tip to prevent slipping.

CONTRAINDICATIONS

- Bilateral weakness (should use crutches or a walker)

WARNING *A poorly fitted cane can cause the patient to lose balance and fall.*

Rubber-tipped cane ◆ walking belt (optional)

PREPARATION

- Ask the patient to hold the cane on the uninvolved side 4″ to 6″ (10 to 15 cm) from the base of his little toe.

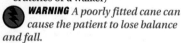 **TROUBLESHOOTER** *If using an adjustable aluminum cane, adjust height by pushing in the metal button on the shaft and raising or lowering the shaft. To shorten a wood cane, remove the rubber tip and saw off excess length.*

- At the correct height, the handle of the cane is level with the greater trochanter and allows about 15 degrees of flexion at the elbow.
- If the cane is too short, he'll need to drop his shoulder to lean on the cane.
- If it's too long, he'll need to raise his shoulder, making it difficult to support his weight.

- Confirm the patient's identity using two patient identifiers according to facility policy.
- Explain the mechanics of cane walking to the patient.
- Demonstrate the technique and ask him to repeat it.
- Coordinate practice sessions in the physical therapy department, if necessary.

NEGOTIATING STAIRS

- Tell the patient to use railings whenever possible.
- To go up stairs, the patient should lead with the uninvolved leg and follow with the involved leg.
- To go down stairs, the patient should lead with the involved leg and follow with the uninvolved one.
- Teach him the mnemonic device "The good goes up; the bad goes down" to help remember which leg to lead with on stairs.
- To negotiate stairs without a railing, he should use the walking technique to go up and down stairs but should move the cane just before the involved leg.
- To go up stairs, he should hold the cane on the uninvolved side, step with the uninvolved leg, advance the cane, and follow with the involved leg.
- To go down stairs, he should hold the cane on the uninvolved side, lead with the cane, advance the involved leg, and follow with the uninvolved leg.

USING A CHAIR

- To teach him to sit, stand by his affected side and tell him to place the backs of his legs against the edge of the chair seat.
- Tell him to move the cane out from his side and reach back with both hands to grasp the chair's armrests.
- Supporting his weight on the armrests, he can lower himself onto the seat.
- While he's seated, he should keep the cane hooked on the armrest or chair

back, or keep it within easy reach if he's using a quad or straight-handled cane.

- ◆ To teach him to get up, stand by his affected side, and tell him to hold the cane in his stronger hand as he grasps the armrests.
- ◆ Tell him to move his uninvolved foot slightly forward and lean slightly forward, then push against the armrests to raise himself.
- ◆ To prevent falls, tell him not to lean on the cane when sitting or rising from the chair.
- ◆ Supervise him each time he gets in or out of a chair until you're both certain he can do it alone.

SPECIAL CONSIDERATIONS

- ◆ Three types of aluminum canes are used most commonly; wooden canes can also be used.
- ◆ A standard aluminum cane (used by the patient who needs only slight assistance walking) provides least support.
- ◆ The half-circle handle of a standard aluminum cane allows it to be hooked on chairs.
- ◆ A T-handle cane (used by the patient with hand weakness) has a straight-shaped handle with grips and a bent shaft.
- ◆ A T-handle cane provides greater stability than a standard cane.
- ◆ Three- or four-pronged (quad) canes are used by patients with poor balance or one-sided weakness and inability to hold onto a walker with both hands.
- ◆ The base of quad canes splits into three or four short, splayed legs; it provides greater stability than a standard cane but provides considerably less stability than a walker.
- ◆ To prevent falls during the learning period, guard the patient carefully by standing behind him slightly to his stronger side and putting one foot between his feet and your other foot to the outside of the uninvolved leg.
- ◆ Use a walking belt, if necessary.

COMPLICATIONS
None known

PATIENT TEACHING

- ◆ Tell the patient to hold the cane on the uninvolved side to promote a reciprocal gait pattern and distribute weight away from involved side.
- ◆ Tell the patient to hold the cane close to his body to prevent leaning and to move the cane and involved leg simultaneously, followed by the uninvolved leg.
- ◆ Encourage the patient to make the stride length of each leg and the timing of each step (cadence) equal.

DOCUMENTATION

- ◆ Record type of cane used.
- ◆ Log distance walked.
- ◆ Describe the patient's understanding and tolerance of cane walking.

SELECTED REFERENCES
Chan, G.N., et al. "Changes in Knee Moments With Contralateral Versus Ipsilateral Cane Usage in Females With Knee Osteoarthritis," *Clinical Biomechanics* 20(4):396-404, May 2005.

Ivanoff, S.D., and Sonn, U. "Changes in the Use of Assistive Devices Among 90-year-old Persons," *Aging Clinical and Experimental Research* 17(3): 246-51, June 2005.

Ray, W.A., et al. "Prevention of Fall-Related Injuries in Long-Term Care: A Randomized Controlled Trial of Staff Education," *Archives of Internal Medicine* 165(19):2293-98, October 2005.

"Stepping Out: How to Select a Walking Device," *Johns Hopkins Medical Letter Health After 50* 17(9):6-7, November 2005.

Youdas, J.W., et al. "Partial Weight-Bearing Gait Using Conventional Assistive Devices," *Archives of Physical Medicine and Rehabilitation* 86(3):394-98, March 2005.

Cardiac monitoring

DESCRIPTION

◆ Cardiac monitoring is used in patients with conduction disturbances or those at risk for life-threatening arrhythmias; it allows for continuous observation of the heart's electrical activity.
◆ Electrodes are placed on the patient's chest to transmit electrical signals that are converted into tracing of cardiac rhythm on an oscilloscope.
◆ Two types of monitoring are used: hardwire or telemetry.
◆ With hardwire, the patient is connected to a monitor at the bedside, where cardiac rhythm is displayed. It can also be transmitted to a remote console.
◆ Telemetry uses a small transmitter connected to the ambulatory patient to send electrical signals to a display monitor at another location.
◆ Telemetry is useful for monitoring arrhythmias that occur during sleep, rest, exercise, or stress.
◆ Unlike hardwire monitoring, telemetry monitors only heart rate and rhythm.
◆ Cardiac monitors display the patient's heart rate and rhythm, produce a printed record of cardiac rhythm, and sound an alarm if the patient's heart rate goes above or below specified limits, regardless of monitor type.
◆ Monitors also recognize and count abnormal heartbeats and changes.

⚡ **WARNING** *The ST segment represents early ventricular repolarization; changes in this waveform component reflect alterations in myocardial oxygenation. A monitoring lead that views an ischemic heart region will reveal ST-segment changes.*

◆ The monitor's software creates a template of the patient's normal QRST pattern from selected leads; then the monitor displays ST-segment changes.
◆ Some monitors display changes continuously; others only on command.

CONTRAINDICATIONS

None known

Cardiac monitor ◆ leadwires ◆ patient cable ◆ disposable pre-gelled electrodes (number of electrodes varies from 3 to 5, depending on facility's type of monitor) ◆ washcloth ◆ 4″ × 4″ gauze pads ◆ hair clipping supplies and alcohol pads (optional)

Telemetry monitoring requires additional use of: transmitter ◆ transmitter pouch ◆ telemetry battery pack ◆ leads ◆ electrodes

PREPARATION

◆ Plug the cardiac monitor into the electrical outlet and turn it on.
◆ Insert the cable into the appropriate socket in the monitor.
◆ Connect the leadwires to the cable. In some systems, leadwires are permanently secured to the cable.
◆ Each leadwire should indicate the location for attachment to the patient: right arm (RA), left arm (LA), right leg (RL), left leg (LL), and chest (C). The indication should appear on the leadwire — if it's permanently connected — or at the connection of the leadwires and cable to the patient.
◆ Connect an electrode to each leadwire, carefully checking that each leadwire is in its correct outlet.
◆ For telemetry, put a new battery in the transmitter.
◆ Be sure to match the poles on the battery with polar markings on the transmitter case.
◆ If leadwires aren't permanently affixed to the telemetry unit, attach them securely.
◆ If the leadwires must be attached individually, be sure to connect each one to the correct outlet.

HARDWIRE MONITORING

◆ Wash your hands.
◆ Confirm the patient's identity using two patient identifiers according to facility policy.
◆ Explain the procedure to patient, provide privacy, and expose his chest.
◆ Determine the electrode positions on the patient's chest, based on the system and lead you're using. (See *Positioning monitoring leads*.)
◆ If the leadwires and patient cables aren't permanently attached, verify that the electrode placement corresponds to the label on the patient cable.
◆ Clip the patient's hair in an area about 4″ (10 cm) in diameter around each electrode site, if necessary.
◆ Clean the area with soap and water and dry completely to remove skin secretions that may interfere with electrode function. You may use an alcohol pad to clean the area if the skin is diaphoretic or oily.
◆ Gently abrade the dried area by rubbing it briskly with a dry washcloth or gauze until it reddens to promote better electrical contact.
◆ Remove the backing from the pre-gelled electrode.
◆ Apply the electrode to the site and press firmly to ensure a tight seal.
◆ Repeat the process with the remaining electrodes and attach the leadwires and cable.
◆ When all electrodes are in place, check for a tracing on the cardiac monitor.
◆ Assess the quality of the electrocardiogram (ECG). (See *Identifying cardiac monitor problems*, page 71.)
◆ To verify that the monitor is detecting each beat, compare the digital heart rate display with your count of the patient's heart rate.

■ **TROUBLESHOOTER** *If necessary, use "gain control" to adjust the size of the rhythm tracing, and "position control" to adjust the waveform position on the recording paper.*

- Set the upper and lower limits of the heart rate alarm, based on unit policy, and make sure the alarm is turned on.

TELEMETRY MONITORING

- Wash your hands.
- Explain the procedure to the patient, provide privacy, and expose his chest.
- Select the lead arrangement.
- Remove the backing from one of the gelled electrodes.
- Apply the electrode to the appropriate site by pressing one side of the electrode against the patient's skin, pulling gently, and then pressing the other side against the skin.
- Press your fingers in a circular motion around the electrode to fix the gel and stabilize the electrode.
- Repeat for each electrode.
- Attach the appropriate leadwire to each electrode.
- Place the transmitter in the pouch.
- Tie the pouch strings around the patient's neck and waist, making sure the pouch fits snugly without causing discomfort.
- If no pouch is available, place the transmitter in the patient's bathrobe pocket.
- Check the patient's waveform for clarity, position, and size.
- Adjust the gain and baseline as needed.
- If necessary, ask him to remain resting or sitting in his room while you locate his telemetry monitor at the central station.
- To obtain a rhythm strip, press the RECORD key at the central station.
- Label the strip with patient's name, room number, date, and time; measure the intervals, and identify the rhythm.
- Place the rhythm strip in the appropriate location in the patient's chart.

Positioning monitoring leads

This chart shows the correct electrode positions for some of the monitoring leads you'll use most often. For each lead, you'll see electrode placement for two hardwire systems (the five- and the three-leadwire systems) and a telemetry system.

In the two hardwire systems, the electrode positions for one lead may be identical to the electrode positions for another lead. In this case, you simply change the lead selector switch to the setting that corresponds to the lead you want. In some cases, you'll need to reposition the electrodes.

In the telemetry system, you can create the same lead with two electrodes that you do with three, simply by eliminating the ground electrode.

The illustrations below use these abbreviations: RA, right arm; LA, left arm; RL, right leg; LL, left leg; C, chest; and G, ground.

FIVE-LEADWIRE SYSTEM	THREE-LEADWIRE SYSTEM	TELEMETRY SYSTEM

Lead I

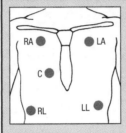 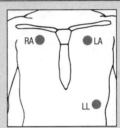 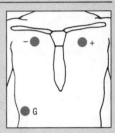

Lead II

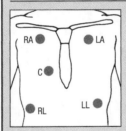 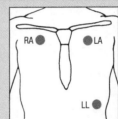 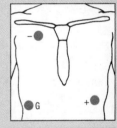

Lead III

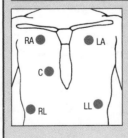 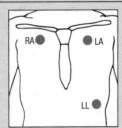 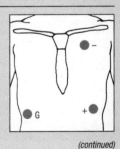

(continued)

(continued)

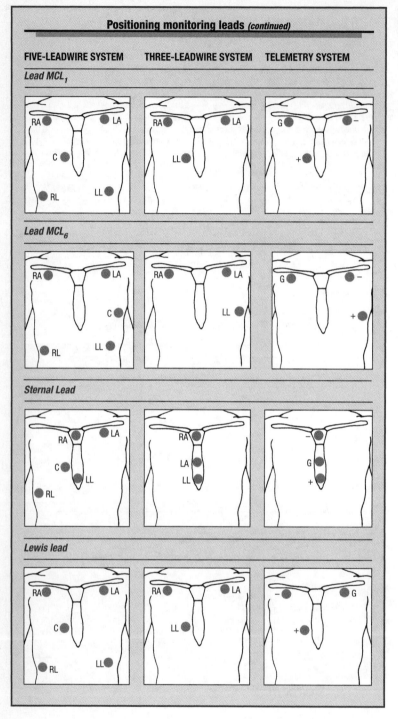

FIVE-LEADWIRE SYSTEM   THREE-LEADWIRE SYSTEM   TELEMETRY SYSTEM

Lead MCL₁

Lead MCL₆

Sternal Lead

Lewis lead

SPECIAL CONSIDERATIONS

TROUBLESHOOTER Make sure all electrical equipment and outlets are grounded to avoid electric shock and interference (artifacts).

◆ Avoid placing electrodes on bony prominences, hairy areas, areas where defibrillator pads will be placed, or areas for chest compression.

◆ If the patient's skin is exceptionally oily, scaly, or diaphoretic, rub the electrode site with a dry 4″×4″ gauze pad before applying the electrode to reduce interference in tracing.

◆ If the patient's respirations distort recording, ask him to hold his breath briefly to reduce baseline wander in the tracing.

◆ Assess skin integrity, and reposition electrodes every 24 hours or as necessary.

COMPLICATIONS
None known

- If the patient is being monitored by telemetry, show him how the transmitter works.
- If applicable, show the patient the button that will produce a recording of his ECG at the central station.
- Tell the patient to push the button whenever he has symptoms. This causes the central console to print a rhythm strip.
- Tell the patient to remove the transmitter if he takes a shower or bath.
- Tell the patient to alert the nurse before removing the unit.

DOCUMENTATION

- Record date and time monitoring begins and which monitoring lead is used.
- Document a rhythm strip at least every 8 hours with changes in the patient's condition or by facility policy.
- Label the rhythm strip with the patient's name, room number, date, and time.

SELECTED REFERENCES

Helms, S. "Telemetry Heightens Nurses' Vigilance, Patients' Mobility," *Nursing Management* 34(12):29-30, December 2003.

Lapensky, J. "Integrated Technologies Transform Telemetry," *Nursing Management* 36(12):23-26, December 2005.

Schneck, M.J., et al. "Utility of Routine Telemetry in Patients with Acute Stroke or Transient Ischemic Attacks," *Stroke* 37(2):702, February 2006.

Singer, A.J., et al. "Telemetry Monitoring During Transport Of Low-Risk Chest Pain Patients From The Emergency Department: Is It Necessary?" *Academic Emergency Medicine* 12(10):965-69, October 2005.

Identifying cardiac monitor problems

PROBLEM	POSSIBLE CAUSES	NURSING INTERVENTIONS
False-high-rate alarm	- Monitor interpreting large T waves as QRS complexes, which doubles the rate - Skeletal muscle activity	- Reposition electrodes to lead where QRS complexes are taller than T waves. - Place electrodes away from major muscle masses.
False-low-rate alarm	- Shift in electrical axis from patient movement, making QRS complexes too small to register - Low amplitude of QRS - Poor contact between electrode and skin	- Reapply electrodes. Set gain so height of complex is greater than 1 millivolt. - Increase gain. - Reapply electrodes.
Low amplitude	- Gain dial set too low - Poor contact between skin and electrodes; dried gel; broken or loose leadwires; poor connection between patient and monitor; malfunctioning monitor; physiologic loss of QRS amplitude	- Increase gain. - Check connections on all leadwires and monitoring cable. Replace electrodes as necessary. Reapply electrodes, if required.
Wandering baseline	- Poor position or contact between electrodes and skin - Thoracic movement with respirations	- Reposition or replace electrodes. - Reposition electrodes.
Artifact (waveform interference)	- Patient having seizures, chills, or anxiety - Patient movement - Electrodes applied improperly - Static electricity - Electrical short circuit in leadwires or cable - Interference from decreased room humidity	- Notify physician and treat patient as ordered. Keep patient warm and reassure him. - Help patient relax. - Check electrodes and reapply, if necessary. - Make sure cables don't have exposed connectors. Change patient's static-causing gown or pajamas. - Replace broken equipment. Use stress loops when applying leadwires. - Regulate humidity to 40%.
Broken leadwires or cable	- Stress loops not used on leadwires - Cables and leadwires cleaned with alcohol or acetone, causing brittleness	- Replace leadwires and retape them, using stress loops. - Clean cable and leadwires with soapy water. *Do not allow cable ends to become wet.* Replace cable as necessary.
60-cycle interference (fuzzy baseline)	- Electrical interference from other equipment in room - Patient's bed improperly grounded	- Attach all electrical equipment to common ground. Check plugs to make sure prongs aren't loose. - Attach bed ground to the room's common ground.
Skin excoriation under electrode	- Patient allergic to electrode adhesive - Electrode on skin too long	- Remove electrodes and apply nonallergenic electrodes and nonallergenic tape. - Remove electrode, clean site, and reapply electrode at new site.

Cardiac output measurement

DESCRIPTION

- Cardiac output (amount of blood ejected by the heart) helps evaluate cardiac function.
- The bolus thermodilution technique is the most widely used method of calculating cardiac output.
- The technique is performed at the patient's bedside.
- Thermodilution is the most practical method for evaluating the cardiac status of critically ill patients and those suspected to have cardiac disease.
- Other methods include the Fick method and the dye dilution test.
- To measure cardiac output, a quantity of solution colder than the patient's blood is injected into the right atrium via a pulmonary artery (PA) catheter port.
- Indicator solution mixes with the blood as it travels through the right ventricle into the pulmonary artery, and a thermistor on the catheter registers the temperature change of flowing blood.
- A computer plots the temperature change over time as a curve and calculates flow based on the area under the curve.
- Accuracy of bolus thermodilution depends on the computer's ability to differentiate temperature change caused by the injectate in the pulmonary artery and temperature changes in the pulmonary artery.
- Accuracy of measurement also depends on injection time. Prolonged or irregular injection technique (should be less than 4 seconds) may produce inaccurately high measurements.

CONTRAINDICATIONS

None known

Thermodilution PA catheter in position ◆ output computer and cables (or a module for the bedside cardiac monitor) ◆ closed or open injectant delivery system ◆ 10-ml syringe ◆ 500-ml bag of dextrose 5% in water or normal saline solution

PREPARATION

- Confirm the patient's identity using two patient identifiers according to facility policy.
- Wash your hands and assemble the equipment at the bedside.
- Insert the closed injectant system tubing into a 500-ml bag of I.V. solution.
- Connect the 10-ml syringe to the system tubing and prime the tubing with I.V. solution until it's free from air.
- Clamp the tubing.
- After clamping the tubing, connect the primed system to the stopcock of the proximal injectant lumen of the PA catheter.
- Connect the temperature probe from the cardiac output computer to the closed injectant system's flow-through housing device.
- Connect the cardiac output computer cable to the thermistor connector on the PA catheter and verify blood temperature reading.
- Turn on the cardiac output computer and enter the correct computation constant, as provided by the catheter's manufacturer.
- The constant is determined by the volume and temperature of the injectant and size and type of catheter.

AGE FACTOR *For children, adjust the computation constant to reflect a smaller volume and a smaller catheter size.*

- Make sure the patient is comfortable.

WARNING *Maintain consistency of technique and patient body positioning for serial cardiac output measurements.*

- Tell him not to move during the procedure because movement can cause measurement errors.
- Explain that the procedure will help determine how well his heart is pumping and that he'll feel no discomfort.
- Verify the presence of a pulmonary artery waveform on the cardiac monitor.
- Unclamp the I.V. tubing and withdraw exactly 10 ml of solution.
- Reclamp the tubing.
- Turn the stopcock at the catheter injectant hub to open a fluid path between the injectant lumen of the PA catheter and the syringe.
- Press the START button on the cardiac output computer or wait for the "Inject" message to flash.
- Inject solution smoothly within 4 seconds, making sure it doesn't leak at the connectors.
- If available, analyze the contour of the thermodilution washout curve on a strip chart recorder for a rapid upstroke and a gradual, smooth return to baseline.
- Repeat steps until three values are within 10% to 15% of the median value.
- Compute the average of three values and record the patient's cardiac output.
- Return the stopcock to the original position and make sure the injectant delivery system tubing is clamped.
- Verify the presence of a pulmonary artery waveform on the cardiac monitor.
- Discontinue cardiac output measurements when patient is hemodynamically stable and weaned from vasoactive and inotropic drugs.

- Leave the PA catheter inserted for pressure measurements.
- Disconnect and discard the injectant delivery system and I.V. bag.
- Cover exposed stopcocks with air-occlusive caps.

⚡ **WARNING** *Monitor the patient for signs or symptoms of inadequate perfusion, including restlessness, fatigue, changes in level of consciousness, decreased capillary refill time, diminished peripheral pulses, oliguria, and pale, cool skin.*

SPECIAL CONSIDERATIONS

- Newer bedside cardiac monitors measure cardiac output continuously using either an invasive or a noninvasive method.
- If the bedside monitor doesn't have continuous output capability, you'll need a freestanding cardiac output computer.
- Normal range for cardiac output is 4 to 8 L/minute.
- Adequacy of the patient's cardiac output is better assessed by calculating his cardiac index (CI), adjusted for his body size.
- To calculate the patient's CI, divide his cardiac output by his body surface area (BSA), a function of height and weight. For example, a cardiac output of 4 L/minute might be adequate for a 65″, 120-lb (165.1-cm, 54.4-kg) patient (normally a BSA of 1.59 and a CI of 2.5) but would be inadequate for a 74″, 230-lb (188-cm, 104.3-kg) patient (normally a BSA of 2.26 and a CI of 1.8).
- Normal CI for adults ranges from 2.5 to 4.2 L/minute/m^2 and 3.5 to 6.5 L/minute/m^2 for pregnant women.

✿ **AGE FACTOR** *Normal CI for infants and children is 3.5 to 4.5 L/minute/m^2.*

✿ **AGE FACTOR** *Normal CI for elderly adults is 2 to 2.5 L/minute/m^2.*

- Add the fluid volume injected for cardiac output determinations to the patient's total intake.
- Injectant delivery of 30 ml/hour will contribute 720 ml to the patient's 24-hour intake.
- After cardiac output measurement, make sure the clamp on the injectant bag is secured to prevent inadvertent delivery of injectant to the patient.

COMPLICATIONS
None known

PATIENT TEACHING

- Explain the procedure to the patient and answer any questions.

DOCUMENTATION

- Record cardiac output, CI, and other hemodynamic values and vital signs at the time of measurement.
- Note the patient's position during measurement and unusual occurrences, such as bradycardia or neurologic changes.

SELECTED REFERENCES
Baulig, W., et al. "Cardiac Output Measurement by Pulse Dye Densitometry in Cardiac Surgery," *Anaesthesia* 60(10):968-73, October 2005.

Pittman, J., et al. "Continuous Cardiac Output Monitoring With Pulse Contour Analysis: A Comparison With Lithium Indicator Dilution Cardiac Output Measurement," *Critical Care Medicine* 33(9):2015-021, September 2005.

Taguchi, N., et al. "Cardiac Output Measurement by Pulse Dye Densitometry Using Three Wavelengths," *Pediatric Critical Care Medicine* 5(4):343-50, July 2004.

Cardiopulmonary resuscitation, adult

OVERVIEW

DESCRIPTION

- Cardiopulmonary resuscitation (CPR) is used to restore and maintain the patient's respiration and circulation after a heartbeat and breathing have stopped.
- CPR is a basic life support (BLS) procedure performed on patients in cardiac arrest.
- Another BLS procedure is clearing the obstructed airway.
- Most adults in sudden cardiac arrest develop ventricular fibrillation and require defibrillation.
- CPR alone doesn't improve the chances of survival in adults requiring defibrillation.
- Assess the patient, then contact emergency medical services (EMS) or call a code before starting CPR. Timing is critical.
- Early access to EMS, early CPR, and early defibrillation greatly improve survival chances.
- It's generally performed to keep the patient alive until advanced cardiac life support (ACLS) can begin.
- Basic CPR procedure consists of assessing the patient, calling for help, then following the ABC protocol:
  - opening Airway
  - restoring Breathing
  - restoring Circulation.
- After the airway has been opened and breathing and circulation are restored, drug therapy, diagnosis by electrocardiogram, or defibrillation may follow.

CONTRAINDICATIONS

- A do-not-resuscitate (DNR) order

EQUIPMENT

Hard surface (to place patient on) ◆ protective equipment such as disposable airway device (optional)

KEY STEPS

- These instructions provide a step-by-step guide for CPR as currently recommended by the American Heart Association (AHA).

ONE-PERSON RESCUE

- If you're the sole rescuer, determine unresponsiveness, call for help, open the patient's airway, check for breathing, give rescue breaths, assess for circulation, and begin compressions.
- Assess the patient to determine if he's unconscious (as shown below).

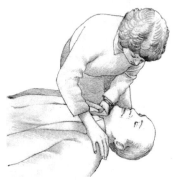

- To ensure you don't start CPR on a person who's conscious, gently shake his shoulders and shout, "Are you okay?"
- If there's no response, check whether the patient has an injury, particularly to the head or neck.
  - **WARNING** *If you suspect a head or neck injury, move the patient as little as possible to reduce risk of paralysis.*
- Call out for help.
- Send someone to contact EMS or call a code, as appropriate.
- Put the patient in the supine position on a hard, flat surface.
- When moving the patient, roll his head and torso as a unit. Avoid twisting or pulling his neck, shoulders, or hips.
- Kneel near the patient's shoulders to gain easy access to his head and chest.
- Usually, the muscles controlling the patient's tongue will be relaxed, causing the tongue to obstruct the airway.

Open the airway: head-tilt, chin-lift maneuver

- If the patient doesn't appear to have a neck injury, use the head-tilt, chin-lift maneuver to open his airway.
- To open the patient's airway, place one hand on his forehead and apply pressure to tilt his head back.
- Place the fingertips of your other hand under the bony part of his lower jaw near his chin.
- Lift his chin while keeping his mouth partially open (as shown below).

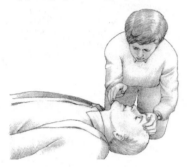

- Avoid placing your fingertips on the soft tissue under his chin because this maneuver may obstruct the airway.

Open the airway: jaw-thrust maneuver

- If you suspect a neck injury, use the jaw-thrust maneuver instead of the head-tilt, chin-lift maneuver.
- Kneel at the patient's head with your elbows on the ground.
- Rest your thumbs on the patient's lower jaw near the corners of the mouth, pointing your thumbs toward his feet.
- Place your fingertips around the lower jaw.
- To open the airway, lift the lower jaw with your fingertips (as shown below).

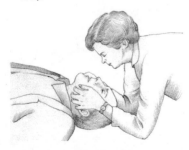

Check for breathing

- While maintaining the open airway, place your ear over his mouth and nose.
- Listen for air moving and note whether his chest rises and falls.
- You may also feel for airflow on your cheek.
- If he starts to breathe, keep the airway open and continue checking breathing until help arrives (as shown below).

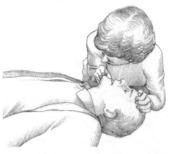

- If he doesn't start breathing after you open his airway, begin rescue breathing.
- Pinch his nostrils shut using the hand you had on his forehead (as shown below).

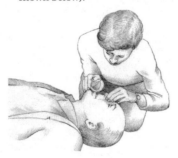

- Take a regular (not deep) breath and place your mouth over his, creating a tight seal (as shown below).

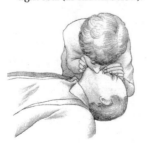

- Give two full breaths that make his chest rise.
- Each ventilation should last over 1 second.
- If the ventilation isn't successful, reposition his head and try again.
- If you aren't successful, check for dentures or another foreign-body airway obstruction and follow the procedure for clearing obstruction.

Assess circulation

- Keep your hand on his forehead so the airway remains open.
- Palpate the carotid artery closer to you with your other hand.
- Place your index and middle fingers in the groove between the trachea and the sternocleidomastoid muscle.
- Palpate for 10 seconds (as shown below) and observe for signs of circulation (skin color and warmth).

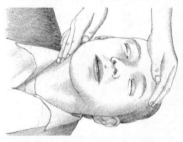

⬤ **WARNING** *If you detect a pulse, don't start chest compressions. Instead, do rescue breathing, giving 10 to 12 breaths (one for every 5 to 6 seconds.) After 2 minutes, recheck pulse. Each breath should be given over 1 second and cause a visible chest rise. After 2 minutes, recheck his pulse but spend only 10 seconds doing so.*

- If there's no pulse, start giving chest compressions.
- Make sure the patient is lying on a hard surface.
- Make sure your knees are apart for a wide base of support.
- Put the heel of your other hand on the center of his chest at the nipple line.

(continued)

- Place the other hand directly on top of the first hand, making sure your fingers aren't on his chest (as shown below). This position will keep the compression force on the sternum and reduce the risk of rib fracture, lung puncture, or liver laceration.

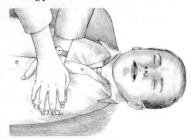

- With elbows locked, arms straight, and shoulders directly over your hands (as shown below), you're ready to give chest compressions.

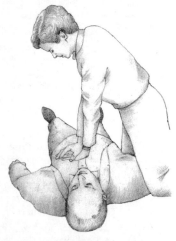

- Compress the patient's sternum 1½" to 2" (4 to 5 cm) using your upper body weight; deliver pressure through the heels of your hands.
- After each compression, release pressure completely and allow the chest to return to a normal position so the heart can fill with blood.
- **WARNING** *Don't change hand position during compressions — you might injure the patient.*
- Give 30 chest compressions at a rate of about 100 per minute. Push hard and fast.
- Open the airway and give two ventilations.

- Find the proper hand position again and give 30 more compressions.
- Continue chest compressions until EMS arrives or another rescuer arrives with the automated external defibrillator (AED).
- Health care professionals should interrupt chest compressions as infrequently as possible. Interruptions should last no longer than 10 seconds except for special interventions, such as use of an AED or insertion of an airway.

TWO-PERSON RESCUE
- If another rescuer arrives, and the EMS team hasn't arrived, tell the second rescuer to repeat the call for help.
- If the second rescuer isn't a health care professional, ask him to stand by. Then, after about 2 minutes or five cycles of compressions and ventilations, you could switch. The switch should occur within 5 seconds.
- If the rescuer is another health care professional, you can perform two-person CPR. He should start assisting after you've finished five cycles of 30 compressions, two ventilations, and a pulse check.
- The second rescuer should be opposite you.
- While you're checking for a pulse, he should find the proper hand placement for delivering chest compressions (as shown below).

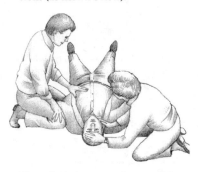

- If you don't detect a pulse, say, "No pulse, continue CPR."
- The second rescuer should begin giving compressions at a rate of 100 per minute.

- Compressions and ventilations should be given at a ratio of 30 to 2.
- The "compressor" should count out loud so that the "ventilator" can anticipate when to ventilate.
- To ensure ventilations are effective, they should cause a visible chest rise.
- As the "ventilator," you must check for breathing and a pulse.
- The compressor role should switch after five cycles of compressions and ventilations. The switch should take no more than 5 seconds.
- Both rescuers should continue giving CPR until an AED or defibrillator arrives, the ACLS providers take over, or the victim starts to move.

SPECIAL CONSIDERATIONS

◆ Acquired immunodeficiency syndrome (AIDS) isn't known to be transmitted in saliva, but some health care professionals may hesitate to give rescue breaths if the patient has AIDS. AHA recommends health care professionals learn how to use disposable airway equipment.

COMPLICATIONS

◆ Fractured ribs
◆ Lacerated liver
◆ Punctured lungs
◆ Gastric distention

PATIENT TEACHING

None

DOCUMENTATION

◆ Note why you initiated CPR.
◆ Report whether the patient suffered cardiac or respiratory arrest.
◆ Record when you found the patient and started CPR.
◆ Document how long the patient received CPR.
◆ Note the patient's response and complications.
◆ Note the interventions taken to correct complications.
◆ If the patient received ACLS, document interventions performed, who performed them, when they were performed, and what equipment was used.

SELECTED REFERENCES

American Heart Association. "2005 AHA Guidelines for Cardiopulmonary Care: Interventional Consensus on Science," *Circulation* 112(22 Suppl):IV-1-IV-221, November 2005.

Cooper, S., et al. "A Decade of In-hospital Resuscitation: Outcomes and Prediction of Survival?" *Resuscitation* 68(2):231-37, February 2006.

Hajbaghery, M.A., et al. "Factors Influencing Survival After In-hospital Cardiopulmonary Resuscitation," *Resuscitation* 66(3):317-21, September 2005.

Jevon, P. "An Overview of the New Resuscitation Guidelines," *Nursing Times* 102(3):25-27, January 2006.

Kellum, M.J., et al. "Cardiocerebral Resuscitation Improves Survival of Patients With Out-of-hospital Cardiac Arrest," *American Journal of Medicine* 119(4):335-40, April 2006.

Kim, S.H., and Kjervik, D. "Deferred Decision Making: Patients' Reliance on Family and Physicians for CPR Decisions in Critical Care," *Nursing Ethics* 12(5):493-506, September 2005.

Cardiopulmonary resuscitation, child (age 1 to puberty)

OVERVIEW

DESCRIPTION
- A child needing cardiopulmonary resuscitation (CPR) typically suffers from hypoxia caused by respiratory difficulty or respiratory arrest.
- Common causes of respiratory arrest include car accidents, drowning, burns, smoke inhalation, falls, poisoning, suffocation, and choking.
- Causes of cardiopulmonary arrest in children include laryngospasm and edema from upper respiratory infections and sudden infant death syndrome.
- CPR in the adult, child, and infant aims to restore cardiopulmonary function by ventilating the lungs and pumping the patient's heart until natural function resumes.
- CPR techniques differ depending on whether the patient is an adult, child, or infant. For CPR purposes, the American Heart Association defines a patient by age. An infant is younger than age 1; a child is age 1 to the onset of adolescence or puberty.
- Survival chances improve the sooner CPR begins and the faster advanced life support systems are implemented.

CONTRAINDICATIONS
None known

EQUIPMENT

Hard surface (to place the patient on) ◆ child-size bag-valve mask, if available

KEY STEPS

- Gently shake the child's shoulders and shout at her to get a response.
- If the child is conscious but has difficulty breathing, help her into the best position to ease her breathing. A responsive child with respiratory distress will often assume a position that maintains airway patency and optimizes ventilation. Allow the child to remain in a position that's most comfortable to her.
- Call for help to alert others and enlist emergency assistance.
- If you're alone and the child is unresponsive and isn't moving, shout for help and begin CPR. Continue CPR for five cycles (about 2 minutes or 30 compressions and two breaths).
- Position the child supine on a firm, flat surface.
- If you must turn the child from a prone position, support her head and neck and turn her as a unit to avoid injuring her spine (as shown below).

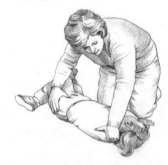

ESTABLISHING A PATENT AIRWAY
- Kneel beside the child's shoulder.
- Place one hand on the child's forehead; gently lift her chin with your other hand to open the airway (as shown below). In infants, this is called the sniffing position.

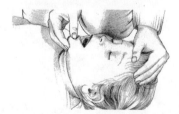

- Avoid fingering the soft neck tissue to avoid obstructing the airway.
- Never let the child's mouth close completely.
- If you suspect a neck injury, use the jaw-thrust maneuver to avoid moving the child's neck while you open her airway.
- To prepare for the maneuver, kneel beside the child's head.
- With your elbows on the ground, rest your thumbs at the corners of the child's mouth, and place two or three fingers of each hand under the lower jaw.
- Lift the jaw upward.
- While maintaining an open airway, place your ear near the child's mouth and nose to evaluate her breathing status (as shown below).

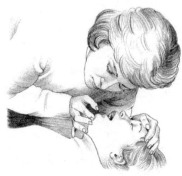

- Look for chest movement, listen for exhaled air, and feel for exhaled air on your cheek.
- If the child is breathing, maintain an open airway and monitor respirations.

⚡ **WARNING** *If you suspect that a mechanical airway obstruction blocks respiration (whether the child is conscious or not), attempt to clear the airway as you would in an adult, but with two exceptions: Don't use the blind finger-sweep maneuver (which could compound or relodge the obstruction) and adjust your technique to the child's size. Perform a finger sweep only when you can see the object in the child's mouth.*

RESTORING VENTILATION
- If the child isn't breathing, maintain

the open airway position and take a normal breath.
- Pinch the child's nostrils shut and cover her mouth with your mouth (as shown below).

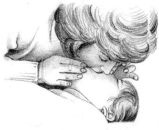

- Give two breaths that make the chest rise, pausing briefly after the first breath.
- While maintaining an open airway, take no more than 10 seconds to check breathing (rhythmic chest or abdominal movement, hearing exhaled breaths, or feeling exhaled air on your cheek).
- If your first attempt at ventilation fails to restore the child's breathing, reposition her head to open the airway and try again.

⚡ **WARNING** *If you're still unsuccessful, the airway may be obstructed by a foreign body.*

- Repeat the steps for establishing a patent airway.
- After you free the obstruction, check for breathing and a pulse.
- If breathing or a pulse is absent, proceed with chest compressions.
- If the child is breathing and there's no evidence of trauma, turn her on her side or place her in the recovery position.

RESTORING HEARTBEAT AND CIRCULATION
- Assess circulation by palpating the carotid artery for a pulse.
- Locate the carotid artery with two or three fingers of one hand. (You'll need the other hand to maintain the head-tilt position that keeps the airway open.)
- Place your fingers in the center of the child's neck on the side closest to you, and slide your fingers into the groove formed by the trachea and the

sternocleidomastoid muscles (as shown below).

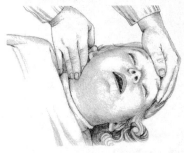

- Palpate the artery for no more than 10 seconds to confirm the child's pulse status. The pulse should be greater than or equal to 60 beats/minute.
- If you feel the child's pulse and it's greater than or equal to 60 beats/minute, continue rescue breathing, giving one breath every 3 seconds (20 breaths per minute), and recheck for a pulse every 2 minutes.
- If you can't feel a pulse or the pulse is less than 60 beats/minute, and there are signs of poor perfusion, begin cardiac compressions.
- Kneel next to the child's chest.
- Hold your middle and index fingers together and move them up the rib cage to the notch where the ribs and sternum join.
- Put your middle finger on the notch and your index finger next to it (as shown below).

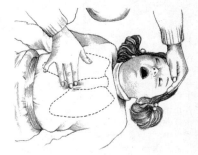

(continued)

- Lift your hand and place the heel just above the spot where your index finger was (as shown below).

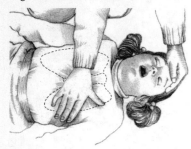

- The heel of your hand should be aligned with the long axis of the sternum.
- Using the heel of one hand or two hands, apply enough pressure to compress the child's chest downward approximately one-third to one-half the depth of the chest (as shown below).

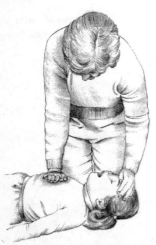

- Compressions should be hard and fast at a rate of 100 compressions/minute.
- If you can't detect a pulse, or if the pulse is less than 60 beats/minute and there are signs of poor perfusion, continue chest compressions and rescue breathing.
- If not already done, call 911 (call a code) and use an automated external defibrillator or defibrillator after five cycles of CPR.

- If the child begins breathing spontaneously, keep the airway open and place her in a side-lying position to prevent aspiration.

⚫ **WARNING** *If trauma is suspected, logroll the patient to avoid injury.*

- Monitor both the respirations and pulse.

SPECIAL CONSIDERATIONS

- A child's small airway can be easily blocked by her tongue. If this occurs, simply opening the airway may eliminate the obstruction.
- Take care to ensure smooth motions when performing cardiac compressions.
- Keep your fingers off, and the heel of your hand on, the child's chest at all times.
- Time your motions so that the compression and relaxation phases are equal to promote effective compressions.
- If the child has breathing difficulty and a parent is present, find out whether the child recently had a fever or an upper respiratory tract infection.

⚫ **WARNING** *If the child recently had a fever or an upper respiratory tract infection, suspect epiglottiditis. In this instance, don't attempt to manipulate the airway because laryngospasm may occur and completely obstruct the airway. Allow the child to assume a comfortable position, and monitor her breathing until additional assistance arrives.*

- Persist in attempts to remove an obstruction.
- As hypoxia develops, the child's muscles will relax, allowing you to remove the foreign object.
- Make sure that someone communicates support and information to the parents during resuscitation efforts.
- Place a bag-valve mask, if available, over the child's nose and mouth when performing ventilations.

COMPLICATIONS
- Fractured ribs
- Lacerated liver
- Punctured lungs
- Gastric distention

PATIENT TEACHING

None

DOCUMENTATION

◆ Record the events of resuscitation and the names of individuals present.
◆ Report whether the child had cardiac or respiratory arrest.
◆ Note where the arrest occurred, the time CPR began, and how long the procedure continued.
◆ Document the outcome.
◆ Report complications and actions taken to correct them.
◆ If the child received advanced cardiac life support, document interventions performed, who performed them, when they were performed, and what equipment was used.

SELECTED REFERENCES

American Heart Association. "2005 AHA Guidelines for Cardiopulmonary Care: Inerventional Consensus on Science," *Circulation* 112(22 Suppl):IV-156-IV-166, November 2005.

Jevon, P. "An Overview of the New Resuscitation Guidelines," *Nursing Times* 102(3):25-27, January 2006.

Olympia, P.R., et al. "The Preparedness of Schools to Respond to Emergencies in Children: A National Survey of School Nurses," *Pediatrics* 116(6):e738-45, December 2005.

Plunkett, J. "Resuscitation Injuries Complicating the Interpretation of Premortem Trauma and Natural Disease in Children," *Journal of Forensic Sciences* 51(1):127-30, January 2006.

Srikantan, S.K., et al. "Effect of One-Rescuer Compression/Ventilation Ratios on Cardiopulmonary Resuscitation in Infant, Pediatric, and Adult Manikins," *Pediatric Critical Care Medicine* 6(3):293-97, May 2005.

Stevenson, A.G., et al. "CPR for Children: One Hand or Two?" *Resuscitation* 64(2):205-208, February 2005.

Cardiopulmonary resuscitation, infant (0 to 1 year)

OVERVIEW

DESCRIPTION
♦ The objective of cardiopulmonary resuscitation (CPR) in an infant is the same as in a child or adult, but the techniques for an infant vary.

CONTRAINDICATIONS
None known

EQUIPMENT

Hard surface (to place the patient on) ♦ infant-sized bag-valve mask, if available

KEY STEPS

♦ Gently tap the foot of the apparently unconscious infant and call out his name.
♦ For a sudden, witnessed collapse, call for help or call emergency medical services. If you didn't witness the collapse, perform resuscitation measures for 2 minutes; then call for help.
♦ If you're alone, perform resuscitation measures for 2 minutes, then call for help.
♦ You may move an uninjured infant close to a telephone, if necessary.
♦ Place the infant supine on a hard surface.
♦ Open the airway using the head-tilt, chin-lift maneuver, unless contraindicated by trauma; don't hyperextend the infant's neck.
♦ Place your ear next to the infant's mouth and nose to evaluate his breathing status. Look for chest movement, listen for exhaled air, and feel for exhaled air on your cheek.
♦ If the infant is breathing, maintain an open airway and monitor respirations.

CLEARING THE AIRWAY
♦ If you're unable to ventilate the infant, reposition the head and try again.
♦ To remove an airway obstruction, place the infant facedown on your forearm, with his head lower than his trunk.
♦ Support your forearm on your thigh.
♦ Give five blows between the infant's shoulder blades using the heel of your free hand.

⚡ **WARNING** *Back blows are safer than abdominal thrusts in infants because of the size of the infant's liver, the close proximity of vital organs, and the poor abdominal muscle tone.*

♦ If the airway remains obstructed, sandwich the infant between your hands and forearms and flip him over onto his back.

⚡ **WARNING** *Don't do a blind finger-sweep to find or remove an obstruction. In an infant, the maneuver may push the object back into the airway and cause further obstruction. Only place your fingers in the infant's mouth if you see an object to remove.*

♦ Keeping the infant's head lower than his trunk, give five midsternal chest thrusts, using your middle and ring fingers only (as shown below), to raise intrathoracic pressure enough to force a cough that will expel the obstruction.

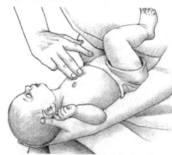

♦ Remember to hold the infant's head firmly to avoid injury.
♦ Repeat this sequence until the obstruction is dislodged or the infant loses consciousness.
♦ If the infant loses consciousness, start CPR. Every time you open the airway to deliver breaths, check the mouth and remove any object you see.

RESTORING VENTILATION
♦ If the infant isn't breathing, take a breath and tightly seal your mouth over the infant's nose and mouth (as shown below).

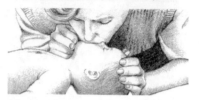

⚡ **WARNING** *Give a gentle puff of air because an infant's lungs hold less air than an adult's lungs.*

♦ If the infant's chest rises and falls, then the amount of air is probably adequate.
♦ Continue rescue breathing with one breath every 3 seconds (20 breaths per minute) if you can detect a pulse.
♦ Give each breath over 1 second.

RESTORING HEARTBEAT AND CIRCULATION
♦ Assess the infant's pulse by palpating the brachial artery, located inside his upper arm between the elbow and the shoulder (as shown below).

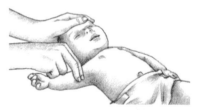

♦ If you find a pulse, continue rescue breathing but don't initiate chest compressions.
♦ Begin chest compressions if you find no pulse.
♦ To locate the correct position on the infant's sternum for chest compressions, draw an imaginary horizontal line between the infant's nipples.
♦ Place your middle and ring fingers on the sternum, directly below — and perpendicular to — the nipple line.
♦ Use these two fingers to depress the sternum here one-third to one-half the depth of the chest at least 100 compressions/minute (as shown top of next page).

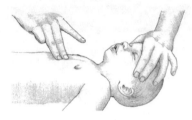

- When two rescuers are present, use a two-thumb encircling technique to provide chest compressions.
- In this technique, use both hands to encircle the infant's chest with both thumbs together over the lower half of the sternum.
- Forcefully compress the sternum with your thumbs as you squeeze the thorax with your fingers.
- Give two breaths for every 30 compressions if you're working alone, or two breaths for every 15 compressions if you're working with a partner.
- Maintain this ratio whether you're the helper or the lone rescuer.
- This ratio allows for 100 compressions and 20 breaths per minute for an infant.

⚡ WARNING *Be aware that, if available, you should use a bag-valve mask over the infant's nose and mouth when performing ventilations.*

SPECIAL CONSIDERATIONS

- An infant's small airway can be easily blocked by his tongue. If this occurs, simply opening the airway may eliminate the obstruction.
- Take care to ensure smooth motions when performing cardiac compressions.
- Time your motions so that the compression and relaxation phases are equal to promote effective compressions.
- If the infant has breathing difficulty and a parent is present, find out whether the infant recently had a fever or an upper respiratory tract infection.

⚡ WARNING *If the infant recently had a fever or an upper respiratory tract infection, suspect epiglottiditis. In this instance, don't attempt to manipulate the airway because laryngospasm may occur and completely obstruct the airway. Place the infant in a comfortable position, and monitor his breathing until additional assistance arrives.*

- Persist in attempts to remove an obstruction.
- As hypoxia develops, the infant's muscles will relax, allowing you to remove the foreign object.
- Make sure that someone communicates support and information to the parents during resuscitation efforts.
- Place a bag-valve mask, if available, over the infant's nose and mouth when performing ventilations.

COMPLICATIONS

- Lacerated liver
- Punctured lungs
- Gastric distention

PATIENT TEACHING

None

DOCUMENTATION

- Document events of resuscitation and names of individuals present.
- Record whether the infant had cardiac or respiratory arrest.
- Note where the arrest occurred, time CPR began, and how long the procedure continued.
- Note the outcome.
- If the infant received advanced cardiac life support, document advanced interventions performed, who performed them, when they were performed, and what equipment was used.

SELECTED REFERENCES

American Heart Association. "2005 AHA Guidelines for Cardiopulmonary Care: Interventional Consensus on Science," *Circulation* 112(22 Suppl):IV-1-IV-221, November 2005.

Cooper, S., et al. "A Decade of In-hospital Resuscitation: Outcomes and Prediction of Survival?" *Resuscitation* 68(2): 231-37, February 2006.

Hajbaghery, M.A., et al. "Factors Influencing Survival After In-hospital Cardiopulmonary Resuscitation," *Resuscitation* 66(3):317-21, September 2005.

Jevon, P. "An Overview of the New Resuscitation Guidelines," *Nursing Times* 102(3):25-27, January 2006.

Srikantan, S.K., et al. "Effect of One-Rescuer Compression/Ventilation Ratios on Cardiopulmonary Resuscitation in Infant, Pediatric, and Adult Manikins," *Pediatric Critical Care Medicine* 6(3): 293-97, May 2005.

Wyckoff, M.H., et al. "Use of Volume Expansion During Delivery Room Resuscitation in Near-Term and Term Infants," *Pediatrics* 115(4):950-55, April 2005.

Cardioversion, synchronized

DESCRIPTION

- Synchronized cardioversion delivers an electric charge to the myocardium at the peak of the R wave to treat tachyarrhythmias.
- This technique causes immediate depolarization, interrupting reentry circuits and allowing the sinoatrial node to resume control.
- Synchronizing the electric charge with the R wave ensures that the current won't be given on a vulnerable T wave and disrupt repolarization.
- Synchronized cardioversion is the treatment of choice for arrhythmias that don't respond to vagal massage or drug therapy, such as unstable supraventricular tachycardia, unstable atrial fibrillation, unstable atrial flutter, and monomorphic ventricular tachycardia.
- This may be an elective or urgent procedure, depending on how well the patient tolerates the arrhythmia.
- When preparing for cardioversion, the patient's condition can deteriorate quickly, necessitating immediate defibrillation.
- Indications include stable paroxysmal atrial tachycardia, unstable paroxysmal supraventricular tachycardia, atrial fibrillation, atrial flutter, and ventricular tachycardia.

CONTRAINDICATIONS

None known

Cardioverter-defibrillator ◆ conductive gel pads ◆ anterior, posterior, or transverse paddles ◆ electrocardiogram (ECG) monitor with recorder ◆ sedative ◆ oxygen therapy equipment ◆ airway ◆ handheld resuscitation bag ◆ emergency pacing equipment ◆ emergency cardiac drugs ◆ automatic blood pressure cuff (if available) ◆ pulse oximeter

- Confirm the patient's identity using two patient identifiers according to facility policy.
- Explain the procedure to the patient and make sure he has signed a consent form.
- Check his recent serum potassium and magnesium levels and arterial blood gas results.
- Check recent digoxin levels.
- Digitalized patients may undergo cardioversion, but tend to require lower energy levels to convert.

WARNING *If the patient takes digoxin, withhold the dose on the day of the procedure.*

- Withhold food and fluids for 6 to 12 hours before the procedure.
- Obtain a 12-lead ECG to serve as a baseline.
- Check to see if the physician has ordered cardiac drugs before the procedure.
- Verify that the patient has a patent I.V. site in case drugs become necessary.
- Connect the patient to a pulse oximeter and automatic blood pressure cuff, if available.
- Consider giving oxygen for 5 to 10 minutes before cardioversion to promote myocardial oxygenation.
- If the patient wears dentures, evaluate whether they support his airway or may cause airway obstruction. If they may cause an obstruction, remove them.
- Place the patient in the supine position and assess vital signs, level of consciousness (LOC), cardiac rhythm, and peripheral pulses.
- Remove the oxygen delivery device before cardioversion to prevent combustion.
- Have epinephrine (Adrenalin), lidocaine (Xylocaine), and atropine at the patient's bedside.
- Make sure the resuscitation bag is at the bedside.
- Give a sedative, as ordered. The sedation is considered moderate to deep with reflexes intact and with the patient still able to breathe adequately.

- Carefully monitor blood pressure and respiratory rate until he recovers.
- Press the POWER button to turn on the defibrillator.
- Push the SYNC button to synchronize the machine with the patient's QRS complexes. Make sure the SYNC button flashes with each of the patient's QRS complexes.
- You should see a bright green flag flash on the monitor.
- Turn the ENERGY SELECT dial to the ordered amount of energy.

⚡ **WARNING** *Advanced cardiac life support protocols call for a monophasic energy dose of 50 to 100 joules for a patient with unstable supraventricular tachycardia, 100 to 200 joules for a patient with atrial fibrillation, 50 to 100 joules for a patient with atrial flutter, and 100 joules for a patient who has monomorphic ventricular tachycardia with a pulse. If there's no response with the first shock, the health care provider should increase the joules in a step-wise manner.*

- Remove paddles from machine and prepare them as if you were defibrillating the patient.
- Place conductive gel pads or paddles in the same positions you would to defibrillate.
- Make sure everyone stands away from the bed; push the discharge buttons.
- Hold the paddles in place and wait for energy to be discharged — the machine has to synchronize the discharge with the QRS complex.
- Check the waveform on the monitor.
- If the arrhythmia fails to convert, repeat the procedure two or three more times at 3-minute intervals.
- Gradually increase the energy level with each additional countershock.
- After cardioversion, frequently assess the patient's LOC and respiratory status, including airway patency, respiratory rate and depth, and need for supplemental oxygen.

⚡ **WARNING** *The patient may require airway support because he's heavily sedated.*

- Record a postcardioversion 12-lead ECG, and monitor the patient's ECG rhythm for 2 hours or per facility sedation protocol.
- Check for electrical burns and treat as needed.

SPECIAL CONSIDERATIONS

- Improper synchronization may result if the patient's ECG tracing contains artifact-like spikes, such as peaked T waves or bundle-branch heart blocks when the R′ wave may be taller than the R wave.

COMPLICATIONS

- Transient, harmless arrhythmias (common), such as atrial, ventricular, and junctional premature beats
- Serious ventricular arrhythmias such as ventricular fibrillation resulting from high amounts of electrical energy, digoxin toxicity, severe heart disease, electrolyte imbalance, or improper synchronization with the R wave

PATIENT TEACHING

- Explain the procedure to the patient and answer any questions.

DOCUMENTATION

- Document the procedure.
- Record voltage given with each attempt.
- Provide rhythm strips before and after the procedure.
- Note how the patient tolerated the procedure.

SELECTED REFERENCES

American Heart Association. "2005 AHA Guidelines for Cardiopulmonary Care: Interventional Consensus on Science," *Circulation* 112(22 Suppl):IV-1-IV-221, November 2005.

Jacoby, J.L., et al. "Synchronized Emergency Department Cardioversion of Atrial Dysrhythmias Saves Time, Money and Resources," *Journal of Emergency Medicine* 28(1):27-30, January 2005.

Stellbrink, C., and Schimpf, T. "Anticoagulation During Cardioversion in Patients With Atrial Fibrillation: Current Clinical Practice," *American Journal of Cardiovascular Drugs* 5(3):155-62, 2005.

Wazni, O., et al. "C Reactive Protein Concentration and Recurrence of Atrial Fibrillation After Electrical Cardioversion," *Heart* 91(10):1303-05, October 2005.

Xavier, L.C., and Memon, A. "Synchronized Cardioversion of Unstable Supraventricular Tachycardia Resulting in Ventricular Fibrillation," *Annals of Emergency Medicine* 44(2):178-80, August 2004.

Casts

DESCRIPTION
- Casts are hard molds that encase a body part, usually an extremity, to provide immobilization of bones and surrounding tissue.
- They can be used to treat injuries (including fractures), correct orthopedic conditions (such as deformities), or promote healing after general or plastic surgery, amputation, or nerve and vascular repair.
- May be constructed of fiberglass or other synthetic materials.
- Fiberglass is lighter, stronger, and more resilient than plaster, but is more difficult to mold because it dries rapidly. It can bear body weight immediately, if necessary. (See *Types of cylindrical casts*.)
- A physician usually applies a cast; nurses prepare the patient and equipment and assist during the procedure.
- With proper preparation, a nurse may apply or change a standard cast after an orthopedist reduces and sets the fracture.

CONTRAINDICATIONS
- Skin diseases
- Peripheral vascular disease
- Diabetes mellitus
- Open or draining wounds
- Overwhelming edema
- Susceptibility to skin irritations

APPLYING A CAST
Casting material ◆ plaster rolls ◆ tubular stockinette ◆ plaster splints (if necessary) ◆ bucket of water ◆ sink equipped with plaster trap ◆ linen-saver pad ◆ sheet ◆ wadding ◆ sponge or felt padding (if necessary)

REMOVING A CAST
Cast scissors, cast saw, and cast spreader (if necessary) ◆ pillows or bath blankets ◆ rubber gloves ◆ cast stand ◆ moleskin or adhesive tape (optional) ◆ tubular stockinette, cast material, and plaster splints in appropriate sizes

PREPARATION
- Gently squeeze packaged casting material to make sure envelopes don't have air leaks.
- Room temperature or slightly warmer water is best because it allows the cast to set in about 7 minutes without excessive exothermia.
- Cold water slows the rate of setting and may be used to facilitate difficult molding.
- Warm water speeds the rate of setting and raises skin temperature under the cast.

- Explain the procedure to allay patient's fears.
- Begin explaining aspects of proper cast care.
- Cover the patient's bedding and gown with a linen-saver pad.
- If the cast is applied to the wrist or arm, remove the patient's rings to prevent circulation problems.
- Assess the condition of the patient's skin in the affected area, noting redness, contusions, or open wounds, to aid in evaluating complaints he may have after the cast is applied.
- If the patient has an open wound, prepare him for a local anesthetic, as ordered.
- Clean the wound.
- Assist the physician as he closes the wound and applies a dressing.
- To establish baseline measurements, assess the patient's neurovascular status.
- Palpate the distal pulses, assess color, temperature, and capillary refill of appropriate fingers or toes.
- Check neurologic function, including sensation and motion in extremities.
- Help the physician position the limb as ordered. Commonly, the limb is immobilized in a neutral position.
- Support the limb in the prescribed position while the physician applies the tubular stockinette and sheet wadding. The stockinette, if used, should extend past the cast's ends to pad the edges.

PREPARING A COTTON AND POLYESTER CAST
WARNING Open these casting materials one roll at a time because cotton and polyester casting must be applied within 3 minutes — before humidity in the air hardens the tape.
- Immerse the roll in cold water, and squeeze it four times to ensure uniform wetness.
- Remove the dripping wet material from the bucket.
- Warn the patient that the material will feel warm, giving off heat as it sets.

PREPARING A FIBERGLASS CAST

◆ If using water-activated fiberglass, immerse the tape rolls in tepid water for 10 to 15 minutes to initiate the chemical reaction that causes the cast to harden.

◆ Open one roll at a time.

⚡ **WARNING** *Avoid squeezing out excess water before application.*

◆ If you're using light-cured fiberglass, unroll the material more slowly. Light-cured fiberglass casting remains soft and malleable until it's exposed to ultraviolet light, which sets it.

COMPLETING THE CAST

◆ As necessary, "petal" the cast's edges to reduce roughness and cushion pressure points. (See *How to petal a cast,* page 88.)

◆ Use a cast stand or your palm to support the cast in the therapeutic position until it becomes firm (6 to 8 minutes) to prevent indentations.

◆ Place the cast on a firm, smooth surface to continue drying.

◆ Place pillows under joints to maintain flexion, if necessary.

◆ To check circulation in the casted limb, palpate the distal pulse and assess color, temperature, and capillary refill of the fingers or toes.

◆ Determine neurologic status by asking the patient if he's experiencing paresthesia in the extremity or decreased motion of the extremity's uncovered joints.

◆ Assess the unaffected extremity and compare findings.

◆ Elevate the limb above heart level with pillows or bath blankets, as ordered, to facilitate venous return and reduce edema.

◆ The physician will send the patient for X-rays to ensure proper positioning.

◆ Tell the patient to notify the physician of pain, foul odor, drainage, or burning sensation under the cast.

Types of cylindrical casts

Made of fiberglass or other synthetic material, casts may be applied almost anywhere on the body to support a single finger or the entire body. Common casts are shown here.

HANGING ARM CAST

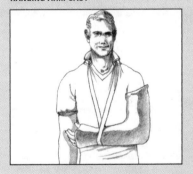

SHOULDER SPICA

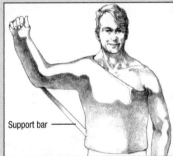

Support bar

SHORT ARM CAST

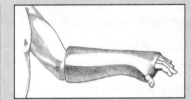

ONE- AND ONE-HALF HIP-SPICA

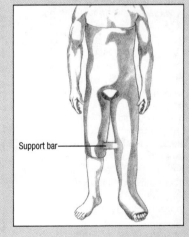

Support bar

LONG LEG CAST

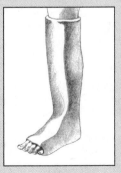

SHORT LEG CAST

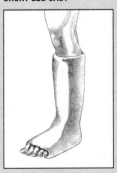

SINGLE HIP-SPICA

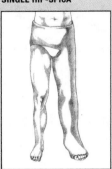

(continued)

- A fiberglass cast dries immediately after application.
- During the drying period, the cast must be properly positioned to prevent a surface depression that could cause pressure areas or dependent edema.
- Neurovascular status must be assessed, drainage monitored, and the condition of the cast checked periodically.
- After the cast dries completely, it looks white and shiny and no longer feels damp or soft.
- Care consists of monitoring for changes in drainage pattern, preventing skin breakdown near the cast, and dealing with immobility.
- Patient teaching must start right after the cast is applied and continue until the patient or a family member can care for the cast.
- Never use the bed or a table to support the cast as it sets because molding can result, causing pressure necrosis of the underlying tissue.
- Don't use rubber- or plastic-covered pillows before the cast hardens because they can trap heat under the cast.
- If a cast is applied after surgery or traumatic injury, remember the most accurate way to assess for bleeding is to monitor vital signs.
- ⚡ **WARNING** *A visible blood spot on the cast can be misleading: One drop of blood can produce a circle 3″ (7.6 cm) in diameter.*
- Casts may need to be opened to assess underlying skin or pulses or to relieve pressure in a specific area.
- In a windowed cast, an area is cut out to allow inspection of the skin.
- A bivalved cast is split medially and laterally, creating anterior and posterior sections, and one section may be removed to relieve pressure while the other maintains immobilization.
- The physician removes the cast at the appropriate time, with a nurse assisting.
- Tell the patient when the cast is removed, the limb will appear thinner than the uncasted limb and the skin will appear yellowish or gray.
- Reassure the patient that exercise and skin care will return it to normal.

COMPLICATIONS

- Compartment syndrome
- Palsy
- Paresthesia
- Ischemia
- Ischemic myositis
- Pressure necrosis
- Misalignment or nonunion of fractured bones

- Teach the patient how to care for his cast.
- Tell the patient to keep the limb above heart level to minimize swelling.
- Elevate the casted leg by having the patient lie down with his leg propped on pillows.
- Prop a casted arm so the hand and elbow are higher than the shoulder.
- ⚡ **WARNING** *Tell the patient to call the physician if he can't move his fingers or toes, if he has numbness or tingling in the affected limb, or has symptoms of infection, such as fever, unusual pain, or a foul odor from the cast.*
- Tell the patient to maintain muscle strength by doing recommended exercises.
- If the cast needs repair or if the patient has questions about cast care, tell him to notify his physician.
- Warn the patient not to get the cast wet, because moisture will weaken or ruin it.
- If the physician approves, have the patient cover the cast with a plastic

How to petal a cast

Rough cast edges can be cushioned by petaling them with adhesive tape or moleskin. To do this, cut several 4″ × 2″ (10 × 5 cm) strips. Round off one end of each strip to keep it from curling. Then, making sure the rounded end of the strip is on the outside of the cast, tuck the straight end just inside the cast edge (as shown below).

Smooth the moleskin with your finger until you're sure it's secured inside and out. Repeat the procedure, overlapping the moleskin pieces until you've covered the cast's edge (as shown below).

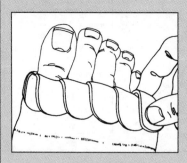

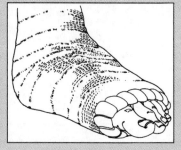

bag or cast cover for showering or bathing.

◆ Urge the patient not to insert anything into the cast to relieve itching because foreign matter can damage skin and cause infection. Instead, advise the patient to use alcohol on the skin at the cast edges.

● **WARNING** *Warn the patient not to chip, crush, cut, or otherwise break any area of the cast and not to bear weight on the cast unless told to do so by the physician.*

◆ If the patient must use crutches, tell him to remove throw rugs and rearrange furniture to reduce the risk of tripping.

◆ If he has a cast on his dominant arm, the patient may need help bathing, using the toilet, eating, and dressing.

DOCUMENTATION

◆ Document date and time of application and the patient's skin condition before the cast was applied.

◆ Note contusions, redness, or open wounds.

◆ Record the results of neurovascular checks, before and after application, for affected and unaffected limbs.

◆ Describe the location of special devices, such as felt pads or plaster splints.

◆ Note patient teaching.

SELECTED REFERENCES

Altizer, L. "Casting for Immobilization," *Orthopaedic Nursing* 23(2):136-41, March-April 2004.

Bhatia, M., and Housden, P.H. "Re-Displacement of Paediatric Forearm Fractures: Role of Plaster Moulding and Padding," *Injury* 37(3):259-68, March 2006.

Carmichael, K.D., and Goucher, N.R. "Cast Abscess: A Case Report," *Orthopaedic Nursing* 25(2):137-39, March-April 2006.

Cassinelli, E.H., et al. "Spica Cast Application in the Emergency Room for Select Pediatric Femur Fractures," *Journal of Orthopaedic Trauma* 19(10):709-16, November-December 2005.

Guyton, G.P. "An Analysis of Iatrogenic Complications From the Total Contact Cast," *Foot & Ankle International* 26(11):903-907, November 2005.

Catheter, urinary (indwelling), care and removal

DESCRIPTION

- Urinary catheter care is intended to prevent infection and other complications by keeping the catheter site clean.
- Care is performed daily after the morning bath and right after perineal care.
- Bedtime care may be performed before perineal care.
- Equipment and the patient's genitalia require inspection twice daily.
- The catheter is removed when bladder decompression is no longer needed, when the patient can resume voiding, or when the catheter is obstructed.
- The physician may order bladder retraining before catheter removal, depending on length of time of catheterization.
- Some facilities don't recommend daily care because of increased infection risk and other complications.

CONTRAINDICATIONS

None known

EQUIPMENT

URINARY CATHETER CARE

Soap and water ◆ sterile gloves ◆ sterile 4″×4″ gauze pads ◆ povidone-iodone or other antiseptic cleaning agent ◆ basin ◆ washcloth ◆ leg bag ◆ collection bag ◆ adhesive tape or leg band ◆ waste receptacle ◆ optional: safety pin, rubber band, gooseneck lamp or flashlight, adhesive remover, and specimen container

PERINEAL CLEANING

Washcloth ◆ additional basin ◆ soap and water

URINARY CATHETER REMOVAL

Gloves ◆ alcohol pad ◆ 10-ml syringe with a luer-lock ◆ bedpan ◆ linen-saver pad ◆ clamp for bladder retraining (optional)

PREPARATION

- Wash your hands and bring equipment to the bedside.
- Open gauze pads, place several in first basin, and pour povidone-iodine or other cleaning agent over them.

🔰 **WARNING** *Some facilities specify, after wiping the urinary meatus with cleaning solution, you should wipe it off with wet, sterile gauze pads to prevent irritation from cleaning solution. If your facility has this policy, pour water into second basin and moisten three more gauze pads.*

- Confirm the patient's identity using two patient identifiers according to facility policy.
- Explain the procedure and its purpose to the patient.
- Provide privacy.

URINARY CATHETER CARE

- Make sure lighting is adequate so you can see the perineum and catheter tubing clearly. Place a lamp or flashlight at bedside if needed.
- Inspect the catheter for problems and check urine drainage for mucus, blood clots, sediment, and turbidity.
- Pinch the catheter between two fingers to determine if the lumen contains any material.

🔰 **WARNING** *If you notice mucus, blood clots, sediment, or turbidity in the urine drainage or lumen (or facility policy requires it), obtain a urine specimen (collect at least 3 ml of urine, but don't fill the specimen cup more than halfway) and notify the physician.*

- Inspect the outside of the catheter where it enters the urinary meatus for encrusted material and suppurative drainage.
- Inspect tissue around the meatus for irritation or swelling.
- Remove the leg band or adhesive tape used to secure the catheter.
- Inspect the area for signs and symptoms of adhesive burns — redness, tenderness, or blisters.
- Put on the gloves.

- Clean the outside of the catheter and tissue around the meatus, using soap and water.

🔰 **WARNING** *To avoid contaminating the urinary tract, always clean by wiping away from — never toward — the urinary meatus.*

- Use a dry gauze pad to remove encrusted material.

🔰 **WARNING** *Don't pull on the catheter while cleaning it. This can injure the urethra and bladder wall. It can also expose a section of the catheter that was inside the urethra, so when you release the catheter, the newly contaminated section will reenter the urethra, introducing potentially infectious organisms.*

- Remove your gloves, reapply the leg band, and reattach the catheter to the leg band. If a leg band isn't available, use adhesive tape.
- To prevent skin hypersensitivity or irritation, retape the catheter on the opposite side.

🔰 **WARNING** *Provide enough slack before securing the catheter to prevent tension on the tubing, which could injure the urethral lumen or bladder wall.*

🔲 **TROUBLESHOOTER** *Most drainage bags have a plastic clamp on the tubing to attach them to the sheet. If a plastic clamp isn't provided, wrap a rubber band around the drainage tubing, insert the safety pin through a loop of the rubber band, and pin the tubing to the sheet below bladder level.*

- Attach the collection bag, below bladder level, to the bed frame.
- Clean residue from the previous tape site with adhesive remover, if necessary.
- Dispose of all used supplies in a waste receptacle.

URINARY CATHETER REMOVAL

- Wash your hands.
- Assemble equipment at the patient's bedside.
- Explain the procedure and tell the patient he may feel slight discomfort.
- Tell him that you'll check periodically during the first 6 to 24 hours after

catheter removal to make sure he resumes voiding.
◆ Put on gloves.
◆ Place a linen-saver pad under the patient's buttocks.
◆ Attach the syringe to the luer-lock mechanism on the catheter.
◆ Pull back on the plunger of the syringe to deflate the balloon by aspirating the injected fluid. The amount of fluid injected is usually indicated on the tip of the catheter's balloon lumen and recorded on the care plan or Kardex and the patient's chart.
◆ Offer him a bedpan because urine may leak as the catheter is removed.
◆ Grasp the catheter and pinch it firmly with your thumb and index finger to prevent urine from flowing back into the urethra.
◆ Gently pull the catheter from the urethra.
◆ If there's resistance, don't apply force; notify the physician.
◆ Remove the bedpan.
◆ Measure and record the amount of urine in the collection bag before discarding.
◆ Remove and discard gloves, and wash your hands.
◆ For the first 24 hours after catheter removal, note the time and amount of each voiding.

SPECIAL CONSIDERATIONS

◆ Your facility may require use of specific cleaning agents for urinary catheter care; check policy before beginning procedure.
◆ A physician's order will be needed to apply antibiotic ointments to the urinary meatus after cleaning.
◆ Avoid raising the drainage bag above bladder level to prevent reflux of urine, which may contain bacteria.
◆ To avoid damaging the urethral lumen or bladder wall, disconnect the drainage bag and tubing from the bed linen and bed frame before helping the patient out of bed.
◆ When possible, attach a leg bag to allow him greater mobility.
◆ If he will be discharged with an indwelling urinary catheter, teach him how to use a leg bag.
◆ Encourage patients with unrestricted fluid intake to increase intake to at least 3 qt (3 L)/day to help flush the urinary system and reduce sediment formation.
◆ To prevent urinary sediment and calculi from obstructing the drainage tube, some patients are placed on an acid-ash diet to acidify the urine.
◆ After catheter removal, report to the physician incidents of incontinence (or dribbling), urgency, persistent dysuria or bladder spasms, fever, chills, or palpable bladder distention.
◆ When changing the catheter after long-term use (usually 30 days), you may need a larger catheter because the meatus enlarges, causing urine to leak around the catheter.

COMPLICATIONS

◆ Dehydration

WARNING *Be alert for sharply reduced urine flow from the catheter. Acute renal failure may result from a catheter obstructed by sediment.*

◆ Bladder discomfort or distention
◆ Urinary tract infection
◆ Failure of the balloon to deflate, causing it to rupture during removal

PATIENT TEACHING

◆ Tell the patient discharged with an indwelling urinary catheter to wash the urinary meatus and perineal area with soap and water twice daily and the anal area after each bowel movement.

DOCUMENTATION

◆ Record care performed, modifications, patient complaints, and condition of the perineum and urinary meatus.
◆ Note the character of the urine in the drainage bag.
◆ Report sediment buildup.
◆ Note whether a specimen was sent for laboratory analysis.
◆ Record fluid intake and output.
◆ Provide an hourly record (usually necessary) for critically ill patients and those with renal insufficiency who are hemodynamically unstable.
◆ For bladder retraining, give the date and time the catheter was clamped, time it was released, and volume and appearance of urine.
◆ For urinary catheter removal, give the date and time and the patient's tolerance of the procedure.
◆ Report when and how much the patient voided after catheter removal and associated problems.

SELECTED REFERENCES

Gilbert, R., and Henderson, S. "Catheter Specimens of Urine: An Audit of Practice," *Nursing Times* 101(47):56, 58, 60-61, November 2005.
Rew, M. "Caring for Catheterized Patients: Urinary Catheter Maintenance," *British Journal of Nursing* 14(2):87-92, January-February 2005.
Tew, L., et al. "Infection Risks Associated With Urinary Catheters," *Nursing Standard* 20(7):55-61, October-November 2005.
Webster, J., et al. "Does Evening Removal of Urinary Catheters Shorten Hospital Stay Among General Hospital Patients? A Randomized Controlled Trial," *Journal of Wound, Ostomy, and Continence Nursing* 33(2):156-63, March-April 2006.

Catheter, urinary (indwelling), insertion

OVERVIEW

DESCRIPTION

◆ Also known as a *Foley* or *retention catheter,* an indwelling urinary catheter remains in the bladder to provide continuous urine drainage.

◆ A balloon inflated at the catheter's distal end prevents it from slipping out of the bladder after insertion.

◆ Urinary catheters are most commonly used to relieve bladder distention caused by urine retention and allow continuous urine drainage when the urinary meatus is swollen from childbirth, surgery, or local trauma.

◆ They're also used to treat urinary tract obstruction (by a tumor or enlarged prostate), urine retention or infection from neurogenic bladder paralysis caused by spinal cord injury or disease, and illness in which the patient's urine output must be monitored closely.

◆ They're used during bladder retraining for patients with neurologic disorders, such as stroke or spinal cord injury, to determine post-void residual urine volume and the need for intermittent catheterization.

◆ An indwelling urinary catheter is inserted only when absolutely necessary.

◆ Insertion should be performed with extreme care and sterile technique to prevent injury and infection.

CONTRAINDICATIONS

None known

EQUIPMENT

Sterile indwelling urinary catheter (latex or silicone #10 to #22 French [average adult sizes #16 to #18 French]) ◆ syringe filled with 5 to 8 ml of sterile water (normal saline solution is sometimes used) ◆ washcloth ◆ towel ◆ soap and water ◆ two linen-saver pads ◆ sterile gloves ◆ sterile drape ◆ sterile fenestrated drape ◆ sterile cotton-tipped applicators (or cotton balls and plastic forceps) ◆ povidone-iodine or other antiseptic cleaning agent ◆ urine receptacle ◆ sterile water-soluble lubricant ◆ sterile drainage collection bag ◆ intake and output sheet ◆ adhesive tape ◆ urine-specimen container and laboratory request form, leg band with Velcro closure, gooseneck lamp or flashlight, pillows or rolled blankets or towels (optional)

PREPARATION

◆ Check the order on the patient's chart to determine if the catheter size or type has been specified.

◆ Wash your hands, select appropriate equipment, and assemble at the bedside.

KEY STEPS

◆ Confirm the patient's identity using two patient identifiers according to facility policy.

◆ Explain the procedure to the patient and provide privacy.

◆ Check the patient's chart and ask when he voided last.

◆ Put on gloves.

◆ Percuss and palpate the bladder to establish baseline data.

◆ Ask if he feels the urge to void.

◆ In poor lighting, have a coworker hold a flashlight or place a lamp next to patient's bed so you can see the urinary meatus clearly.

◆ Place the female patient in the supine position, with her knees flexed and separated and her feet flat on the bed, about 2′ (61 cm) apart.

◆ If she finds this position uncomfortable, have her flex one knee and keep the other leg flat on the bed.

🌸 **AGE FACTOR** *Elderly patients may need pillows, rolled towels, or blankets to provide positioning support.*

◆ Get assistance as needed to help the patient stay in position or to direct light.

◆ Place the male patient in the supine position with the legs extended and flat on the bed.

◆ Ask him to hold the position to give a clear view of the urinary meatus and prevent contamination of the sterile field.

◆ Use the washcloth to clean the patient's genital area and perineum thoroughly with soap and water.

◆ Dry the area with the towel.

◆ Remove gloves and wash your hands.

◆ Place the linen-saver pads on the bed between the patient's legs and under the hips.

◆ To create a sterile field, open the prepackaged kit or equipment tray and place it between the female patient's legs or next to the male patient's hip.

◆ If sterile gloves are the first item on the tray, put them on.

◆ Place the sterile drape under the patient's hips.

- Drape the patient's lower abdomen with the sterile fenestrated drape so only the genital area remains exposed.
- Take care not to contaminate gloves.
- Open the rest of the kit or tray and put on sterile gloves if you haven't already.

⚡ **WARNING** *Make sure the patient isn't allergic to iodine solution; if he's allergic, use another antiseptic cleaning agent.*

- Tear open the packet of povidone-iodine or other antiseptic cleaning agent and saturate sterile cotton balls or applicators, being careful not to spill solution on the equipment.
- Open the packet of water-soluble lubricant and apply it to the catheter tip.
- Attach the drainage bag to the other end of the catheter.
- If using a commercial kit, the drainage bag may be attached.
- Make sure all tubing ends remain sterile; be sure the clamp at the emptying port of the drainage bag is closed to prevent urine leakage from the bag.
- Some drainage systems have an airlock chamber to prevent bacteria from traveling to the bladder from urine in the drainage bag.

⚡ **WARNING** *Some urologists and nurses use a syringe prefilled with a water-soluble lubricant and instill the lubricant directly into the male urethra, instead of on the catheter tip. This method helps prevent trauma to the urethral lining and possible urinary tract infection (UTI). Check facility policy.*

- Before inserting the catheter, inflate the balloon with sterile water or normal saline solution to inspect for leaks.
- Attach the prefilled syringe to the Luer-lock, then push the plunger and check for seepage as the balloon expands.
- Aspirate the solution to deflate the balloon.
- Inspect the catheter for resiliency. Rough, cracked catheters can injure the urethral mucosa during insertion, which can predispose the patient to infection.

FEMALE PATIENT

- Separate the labia majora and labia minora as widely as possible with the thumb, middle, and index fingers of your nondominant hand so you have a full view of the urinary meatus.
- Keep the labia separated throughout procedure, so they don't obscure the urinary meatus or contaminate the area after it's cleaned.
- Wipe one side of the urinary meatus with a sterile, cotton-tipped applicator (or pick up a sterile cotton ball with the plastic forceps) with a single downward motion.
- Wipe the other side with another sterile applicator or cotton ball in same way.
- Wipe directly over the meatus with a third sterile applicator or cotton ball.
- Take care not to contaminate your sterile glove.

MALE PATIENT

- Hold the penis with your nondominant hand.
- If the patient is uncircumcised, retract the foreskin.
- Lift and stretch the penis to a 60- to 90-degree angle.
- Hold the penis this way throughout procedure to straighten the urethra and maintain a sterile field.
- Use your dominant hand to clean the glans with a sterile cotton-tipped applicator or a sterile cotton ball held in forceps.
- Clean in a circular motion, starting at the urinary meatus and working outward.
- Repeat the procedure using another sterile applicator or cotton ball and taking care not to contaminate your sterile glove.
- Pick up the catheter with your dominant hand and prepare to insert the lubricated tip into the urinary meatus.
- To facilitate insertion by relaxing the sphincter, ask him to cough as you insert the catheter. Tell him to breathe deeply and slowly to further relax the sphincter.
- Hold the catheter close to its tip to ease insertion and control direction.

⚡ **WARNING** *Never force a catheter during insertion. Maneuver it gently as the patient bears down or coughs. If you meet resistance, stop and notify physician. Sphincter spasms, strictures, misplacement in the vagina (in females), or an enlarged prostate (in males) may cause resistance.*

URINARY CATHETER ADVANCEMENT

- For the female patient, advance the catheter 2″ to 3″ (5 to 7.5 cm) — while continuing to hold the labia apart — (as shown below) until urine begins to flow.

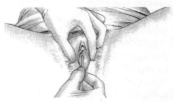

- If the catheter is inadvertently inserted into the vagina, leave it there as a landmark. Then begin the procedure over again using new supplies.
- For the male patient, advance the catheter to the bifurcation 5″ to 7½″ (12.5 to 19 cm) and check for urine flow (as shown below).

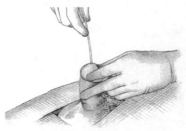

- If the foreskin was retracted, replace it to prevent compromised circulation and painful swelling.
- When urine stops flowing, attach the pre-filled syringe to the luer-lock.
- Push the plunger and inflate the balloon to keep the catheter in place in the bladder.

⚡ **WARNING** *Never inflate a balloon without establishing urine flow, which assures that the catheter is in the bladder.*

(continued)

- Hang the collection bag below bladder level to prevent urine reflux into the bladder, which can cause infection, and to facilitate gravity drainage of the bladder.

⚡ **WARNING** *Make sure the tubing doesn't get tangled in the bed rails.*

- Tape the catheter to the female patient's thigh to prevent possible tension on the urogenital trigone.
- Tape the catheter to the male patient's abdomen or anterior thigh to prevent pressure on the urethra at the penoscrotal junction, which can lead to formation of urethrocutaneous fistulas.
- Securing the catheter with tape prevents traction on the bladder and alteration in the normal direction of urine flow in males.
- As an alternative, secure the catheter to his thigh using a leg band with a Velcro closure.
- Using the patient's thigh to secure the catheter decreases skin irritation, especially in those with long-term indwelling catheters.
- Dispose of all used supplies properly.

SPECIAL CONSIDERATIONS

- Several catheters are available with balloons of various sizes; each type has its own method of inflation and closure.
- Methods of balloon inflation and closure include:
  – sterile solution or air may be injected through the inflation lumen; then, the end of the injection port is folded over itself and fastened with a clamp or rubber band
  – the catheter may be inflated when a seal in the end of the inflation lumen is penetrated with a needle or the tip of the solution-filled syringe
  – the catheter may be self-inflatable when a prepositioned clamp is loosened.
- Injecting a catheter with air makes identifying leaks difficult and doesn't guarantee deflation of the balloon for removal.
- Balloon size determines the amount of solution needed for inflation; the exact amount is usually printed on the distal extension of the catheter used for inflating the balloon.

✿ **AGE FACTOR** *Ask the elderly or disabled female patient, such as one with severe contractures, to lie on her side with her knees drawn up to her chest during the catheter procedure to help facilitate catheter insertion.*

- If the physician orders a urine specimen, obtain it from the urine receptacle with a specimen collection container at the time of catheterization, and send it to the laboratory with the appropriate laboratory request form.
- Connect the drainage bag when urine stops flowing.
- Inspect the catheter and tubing periodically to detect compression or kinking that could obstruct urine flow.
- Explain gravity drainage so the patient realizes the importance of keeping the drainage tubing and collection bag lower than the bladder at all times.

- If necessary, provide the patient with detailed instructions for performing clean intermittent self-catheterization.
- For monitoring purposes, empty the collection bag at least every 8 hours.
- Excessive fluid volume may require more frequent emptying to prevent injury to the urethra and bladder wall, and prevent traction on the catheter, which may cause discomfort.
- Some health care facilities encourage changing catheters at regular intervals, such as every 30 days, if the patient has long-term continuous drainage.

⚡ **WARNING** *Observe the patient carefully for adverse reactions caused by removing excessive volumes of residual urine, such as hypovolemic shock.*

⚡ **WARNING** *Check facility policy to determine the maximum amount of urine that may be drained at one time (some facilities limit the amount to 700 to 1,000 ml). Clamp the catheter at the first sign of an adverse reaction, and notify the physician.*

COMPLICATIONS

- UTI (due to introduction of bacteria into bladder)
- Improper insertion (causing traumatic injury to urethral and bladder mucosa)
- Bladder atony or spasms (resulting from rapid decompression of a severely distended bladder)

PATIENT TEACHING

◆ If the patient will be discharged with long-term indwelling catheter, teach him and his family the aspects of daily catheter maintenance, including:
- care of skin and urinary meatus
- signs and symptoms of UTI or obstruction
- how to irrigate the catheter (if appropriate)
- importance of adequate fluid intake to maintain patency
- need for a home care nurse to visit every 4 to 6 weeks, or as needed, to change catheter.

DOCUMENTATION

◆ Record the date, time, size, and type of indwelling catheter used.
◆ Describe the amount, color, and other characteristics of urine emptied from bladder. (Your facility may require only intake and output sheet for fluid-balance data.)
◆ If large volumes of urine have been emptied, describe patient's tolerance of procedure.
◆ Note whether a urine specimen was sent for laboratory analysis.

SELECTED REFERENCES

Abadi, S., et al. "Misleading Positioning of a Foley Catheter Balloon," *British Journal of Radiology* 79(938):175-76, February 2006.

Addison, R. "Choosing a Urinary Catheter for Short and Long-Term Use," *Professional Nurse* 19(12):41-44, August 2004.

Bardsley, A. "Use of Lubricant Gels in Urinary Catheterization," *Nursing Standard* 20(8):41-46, November 2005.

Morey, A.F. "Consensus Statement on Urethral Trauma," *Journal of Urology* 174(3):968-69, September 2005.

Ribby, K.J. "Decreasing Urinary Tract Infections Through Staff Development, Outcomes, and Nursing Process," *Journal of Nursing Care Quality* 21(2):194-98, April-June 2006.

Catheter, urinary, irrigation

OVERVIEW

DESCRIPTION

◆ To avoid introducing microorganisms into the bladder, urinary catheter irrigation is only done to remove an obstruction such as a blood clot that develops after bladder, kidney, or prostate surgery.

CONTRAINDICATIONS

None known

EQUIPMENT

Ordered irrigating solution (such as normal saline solution) ◆ sterile graduated receptacle or emesis basin ◆ sterile bulb syringe or 50-ml catheter tip syringe ◆ two alcohol pads ◆ sterile gloves ◆ linen-saver pad ◆ intake-output sheet ◆ basin of warm water (optional)

PREPARATION

◆ Check expiration date on irrigating solution and warm solution to room temperature to prevent vesical spasms during instillation.
◆ If necessary, place container in a basin of warm water.

⚡ **WARNING** *Never heat the solution on a burner or in a microwave oven. Hot irrigating solution can injure the patient's bladder.*

KEY STEPS

◆ Confirm the patient's identity using two patient identifiers according to facility policy.
◆ Wash your hands and assemble equipment at the bedside.
◆ Explain the procedure to the patient and provide privacy.
◆ Place the patient in the dorsal recumbent position.
◆ Place a linen-saver pad under the patient's buttocks to protect bed linens.
◆ Create a sterile field at the patient's bedside by opening the sterile equipment tray or commercial kit.
◆ Clean the lip of solution bottle by pouring a small amount into the sink or waste receptacle, using aseptic technique.
◆ Pour the prescribed amount of solution into the graduated receptacle or emesis basin.
◆ Place the tip of the syringe into the solution.
◆ Squeeze the bulb or pull back the plunger (depending on type of syringe), and fill the syringe with the appropriate amount of solution (usually 30 ml).
◆ Open the package of alcohol pads and put on sterile gloves.
◆ Clean the juncture of the catheter and drainage tube with an alcohol pad to remove as many bacterial contaminants as possible.
◆ Disconnect the catheter and drainage tube by twisting them in opposite directions and carefully pulling them apart without creating tension on the catheter.
◆ Don't let go of the catheter — hold it in your nondominant hand.
◆ Place the end of the drainage tube on the sterile field, making sure not to contaminate the tube.
◆ Keep the end of the drainage tube sterile by placing sterile gauze over it and securing the gauze with a piece of tape.
◆ Twist the bulb syringe or catheter-tip syringe onto the catheter's distal end.

- Squeeze the bulb or slowly push the plunger of the syringe to instill the irrigating solution through the catheter. Don't force the irrigant through the catheter.
- Refill the syringe and repeat this step until you've instilled the prescribed amount of irrigating solution, if necessary.
- Remove the syringe and direct the return flow from the catheter into a graduated receptacle or emesis basin.
- Don't let the catheter end touch the drainage in the receptacle or become contaminated in any way.
- Wipe the end of the drainage tube and catheter with the remaining alcohol pad.
- Wait a few seconds until the alcohol evaporates, then reattach the drainage tubing to the catheter.
- Dispose of all used supplies properly.

SPECIAL CONSIDERATIONS

- Catheter irrigation requires strict aseptic technique to prevent bacteria from entering the bladder.
- The ends of the catheter and drainage tube and tip of the syringe must be kept sterile throughout procedure.

WARNING If you encounter resistance during instillation of the irrigating solution, don't try to force the solution into the bladder. Instead, stop the procedure and notify the physician.

WARNING If an indwelling catheter becomes totally obstructed, obtain an order to remove it and replace it with a new one to prevent bladder distention, acute renal failure, urinary stasis, and subsequent infection.

- The physician may order a continuous irrigation system, which decreases the risk of infection by eliminating the need to disconnect the catheter and drainage tube repeatedly.
- Encourage the patient not on restricted fluid intake to increase intake to 3,000 ml per day to help flush the urinary system and reduce sediment formation.
- To keep the patient's urine acidic and help prevent calculus formation, tell him to eat foods containing ascorbic acid, including citrus fruits and juices, cranberry juice, and dark green and deep yellow vegetables.

COMPLICATIONS
None known

PATIENT TEACHING

- Explain the procedure to the patient and answer any questions.

DOCUMENTATION

- Note the amount, color, and consistency of return urine flow, and document the patient's tolerance of the procedure.
- Note resistance during instillation of the solution.
- If the return flow volume is less than the amount of solution instilled, note this on the intake and output balance sheets and in your notes.

SELECTED REFERENCES
Braasch, M., et al. "Irrigation and Drainage Properties of Three-Way Urethral Catheters," *Urology* 67(1):40-44, January 2006.
Castledine, G. "Nurse Whose Inexperience and Negligence in Bladder Washout Put Her Patient at Risk," *British Journal of Nursing* 15(3):141, February 2006.

Central venous catheter use

DESCRIPTION

- A central venous catheter (CVC) is a sterile catheter made of polyurethane, or silicone rubber (Silastic).
- It's inserted through a large vein such as the subclavian vein or the jugular vein; the tip of the catheter is placed in the superior vena cava. (See *Central venous catheter pathways*.)
- A CVC offers several benefits, including:
- monitoring of central venous pressure to determine blood volume or pump efficiency
- administering blood products or aspiration of blood samples for diagnostic tests
- long-term venous access
- giving I.V. fluids in emergencies
- I.V. access when decreased peripheral circulation makes peripheral vein access difficult
- prolonged I.V. therapy doesn't reduce number of accessible peripheral veins
- I.V. access for diluted solutions or large fluid volumes
- I.V. access for irritating or hypertonic fluids such as total parenteral nutrition solutions.
- The CVC line reduces patient anxiety and preserves peripheral veins because multiple blood samples can be drawn without repeated venipuncture.
- Central venous therapy increases the risk of pneumothorax, sepsis, thrombus formation, and vessel and adjacent organ perforation (all life-threatening conditions).
- The CVC reduces patient mobility, is difficult to insert, and costs more than a peripheral I.V. catheter.
- Removal of a CVC is usually done by a physician or nurse either at the end of therapy or at the onset of complications.
- If the patient may have an infection, removal procedure includes swabbing the catheter tip over an agar plate for culture.

CONTRAINDICATIONS

- Subclavian venous thrombosis or stenosis
- Surface infection at the insertion site
- Coagulopathies

EQUIPMENT

INSERTING THE CVC

Skin preparation kit, if necessary ◆ cap ◆ sterile gloves and gowns ◆ blanket ◆ linen-saver pad ◆ sterile towel ◆ large sterile drape ◆ masks ◆ chlorhexidine applicators or other antimicrobial solution ◆ alcohol pads ◆ normal saline solution ◆ 3-ml syringe with 25G 1″ needle ◆ 1% or 2% injectable lidocaine ◆ dextrose 5% in water ◆ syringes for blood sample collection ◆ suture material ◆ two 14G or 16G CVCs ◆ I.V. solution with administration set prepared for use ◆ infusion pump or controller as needed ◆ 1″ adhesive tape ◆ sterile scissors ◆ heparin or normal saline flushes as needed ◆ transparent semipermeable dressing ◆ sterile marker ◆ sterile labels

FLUSHING THE CATHETER

Normal saline solution or heparin flush solution ◆ alcohol pad ◆ 70% alcohol solution

CHANGING THE INJECTION CAP

Alcohol ◆ injection cap ◆ padded clamp

REMOVING THE CVC

Clean gloves ◆ sterile suture removal set ◆ alcohol pads ◆ sterile 2″×2″ gauze pads ◆ forceps ◆ tape ◆ sterile, transparent semipermeable dressing ◆ agar plate, if culture needed ◆ povidone-iodine ointment

Type of catheter selected depends on type of therapy used. Some facilities have prepared trays containing most equipment.

PREPARATION

- Confirm catheter type and size (usually 14G or 16G) with the physician.
- Set up I.V. solution and prime the administration set using strict aseptic technique.
- Recheck all connections to make sure they're tight.
- Notify the radiology department that a chest X-ray will be needed.

KEY STEPS

- Wash your hands.

INSERTING THE CVC

- Confirm the patient's identity using two patient identifiers according to facility policy.
- Reinforce physician's explanation of procedure and answer the patient's questions.
- Make sure that the patient has signed a consent form, and check his history for hypersensitivity to latex, or the local anesthetic.
- Place the patient in Trendelenburg's position to dilate veins and reduce the risk of air embolism.
- For subclavian access, place a rolled blanket lengthwise between the patient's shoulders to increase venous distention.
- For jugular access, place a rolled blanket under the opposite shoulder to extend the neck, making the anatomic landmarks more visible.
- Place a linen-saver pad under the patient.
- Turn his head away from the site to prevent possible contamination from airborne pathogens and make the site more accessible.
- Prepare the insertion site.
- Make sure the skin is free from hair because hair can harbor microorganisms.

WARNING It's recommended to clip hair close to the skin rather than shaving. Shaving may cause skin irritation and create multiple small open wounds, increasing risk of infection. If physician orders that area be shaved, shave the evening before catheter insertion to allow minor skin irritations to heal partially.

- Wash the skin with soap and water first, if necessary.
- Establish a sterile field on a table, using a sterile towel or wrapping from the instrument tray.
- Label all medications, medication containers, and other solutions on and off the sterile field.
- Put on a mask, sterile gloves, and gown (maximum barrier precautions).
- Clean the area around the insertion site with a chlorhexidine swab using a vigorous side-to-side motion.
- After the physician puts on a sterile cap, mask, gown, and gloves and drapes the area with a large sterile drape to create a sterile field, open packaging of the 3-ml syringe and 25G needle and give it to him using sterile technique.
- Wipe the top of the lidocaine vial with an alcohol pad and invert it.
- The physician fills the 3-ml syringe and injects the anesthetic into the site.
- Open the catheter package and give catheter to the physician using aseptic technique.
- The physician inserts the catheter.
- Prepare the I.V. administration set for immediate attachment to the catheter hub.
- Ask the patient to perform Valsalva's maneuver while the physician attaches the I.V. line to the catheter hub. Valsalva's maneuver increases intrathoracic pressure, reducing the possibility of an air embolus.
- After the physician attaches the I.V. line to the catheter hub, set the flow rate at a keep-vein-open rate to maintain venous access.
- Alternatively, the catheter may be capped and flushed with heparin.
- The physician sutures the catheter in place.
- After an X-ray confirms correct catheter placement in the superior vena cava, set the flow rate as ordered.
- Use normal saline solution to remove dried blood that could harbor microorganisms.
- Secure the catheter with 1″ adhesive tape, and use a transparent semipermeable dressing.

Central venous catheter pathways

The illustrations below show several common pathways for central venous catheter insertion. Typically, a central venous catheter is inserted in the subclavian vein or the internal jugular vein. The catheter typically terminates in the superior vena cava. The central venous catheter is tunneled when long-term placement is required.

Insertion: Subclavian vein
Termination: Superior vena cava

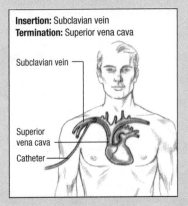

Insertion: Subclavian vein
Termination: Right atrium

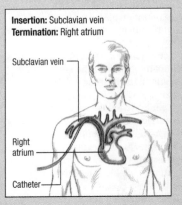

Insertion: Internal jugular vein
Termination: Superior vena cava

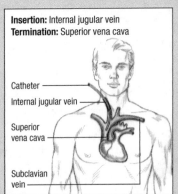

Insertion: Basilic vein (peripheral)
Termination: Superior vena cava

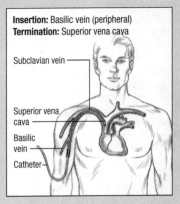

Insertion: Through a subcutaneous tunnel to the subclavian vein (Dacron cuff helps hold catheter in place)
Termination: Superior vena cava

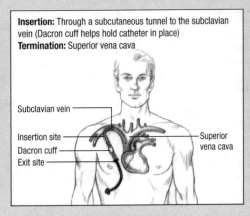

(continued)

- Expect some serosanguineous drainage during the first 24 hours.
- Place the patient in a comfortable position and reassess his status.
- Label the dressing with the time and date of catheter insertion.

FLUSHING THE CATHETER

- To maintain patency, flush the catheter routinely according to facility policy.
- If the system is being maintained as a heparin lock and infusions are intermittent, the flushing procedure will vary according to policy, drug administration schedule, and type of catheter.
- All lumens of a multilumen catheter must be flushed regularly.
- Most facilities use a heparin flush solution available in premixed 10-ml multidose vials.
- Recommended heparin concentrations vary from 10 to 100 units per milliliter.
- Use normal saline solution instead of heparin to maintain patency in two-way valved devices, such as the Groshong type, because research suggests that heparin isn't needed to keep the line open.
- Recommended frequency for flushing CVCs varies from once every 12 hours to once weekly. Recommended amount of flushing solution also varies.
- Some facilities recommend using twice the volume of the capacity of the cannula and the add-on devices if this volume is known.
- Most facilities recommend 3 ml of solution to flush the catheter.
- Different catheters require different amounts of solution.
- To perform flushing, start by cleaning the cap with an alcohol pad.
- Allow the cap to dry.
- If using the needleless system, follow manufacturer's guidelines.
- Access the cap and aspirate 3 to 5 ml blood to confirm proper catheter function and patency of the CVC.
- Inject the recommended type and amount of flush solution.

- After flushing the catheter, maintain positive pressure by keeping your thumb on the plunger of the syringe while withdrawing the syringe. This prevents blood backflow and clotting in the line.
- If flushing a valved catheter, close the clamp just before the last of the flush solution leaves the syringe.

CHANGING THE INJECTION CAP

- CVCs used for intermittent infusions have needle-free injection caps (short luer-lock devices similar to heparin lock adapters used for peripheral I.V. infusion therapy).
- Injection caps must be luer-lock types to prevent disconnection and air embolism.
- Luer-lock injection caps contain minimal empty space, so you don't have to preflush before connecting it.
- Frequency of cap changes varies according to facility policy and how often the cap is used, but once weekly is recommended.
- Use strict aseptic technique when changing the cap.
- Clean the connection site with an alcohol pad.
- Tell the patient to perform Valsalva's maneuver while you quickly disconnect the old cap and connect the new cap using aseptic technique.
- If he can't perform this maneuver, use a padded clamp to prevent air from entering the catheter.

REMOVING THE CVC

- Make sure assistance is available in case a complication, such as uncontrolled bleeding, occurs.
- Some vessels, such as the subclavian vein, can be difficult to compress.
- Explain the procedure to the patient before removing the catheter.
- Wash your hands and put on clean gloves and a mask.
- Turn off all infusions.
- Remove and discard the old dressing and change to sterile gloves.
- Inspect the site for signs of drainage or inflammation.

- Clip the sutures and, using forceps, remove the catheter in a slow, even motion.
- To prevent an air embolism, have the patient perform Valsalva's maneuver as the catheter is withdrawn.
- Apply pressure with a dry sterile gauze pad immediately after removing the catheter.
- Apply ointment to the catheter exit site to seal it and prevent an embolism.
- Cover the site with a gauze pad, and place a transparent semipermeable dressing over the gauze.
- Label the dressing with the date and time of removal and your initials.
- Keep the site covered until site epithelization has occurred.

WARNING *If you suspect the catheter hasn't been completely removed, notify the physician immediately and monitor the patient closely for signs of distress.*

WARNING *If you suspect an infection, swab the catheter on a fresh agar plate and send it to the laboratory for culture.*

- Dispose of I.V. tubing and equipment properly.

SPECIAL CONSIDERATIONS

◆ While awaiting chest X-ray confirmation of the proper catheter placement, infuse an I.V. solution such as dextrose 5% in water or normal saline solution at a keep-vein-open rate until correct placement is assured. Or, use heparin to flush the line.

⚡ **WARNING** *Watch for signs of air embolism: sudden onset of pallor, cyanosis, dyspnea, coughing, and tachycardia, progressing to syncope and shock. If any occur, place the patient on his left side in Trendelenburg's position and notify the physician.*

⚡ **WARNING** *After insertion, watch for signs and symptoms of pneumothorax: shortness of breath, uneven chest movement, tachycardia, and chest pain. Notify the physician immediately if signs and symptoms appear.*

◆ Change the dressing every 48 hours if a gauze dressing is used or every 3 to 7 days if a transparent semipermeable dressing is used, according to facility policy, or whenever it becomes moist or soiled.

◆ Change the tubing every 72 hours and solution every 24 hours, or according to facility policy, while the CVC is in place.

◆ Dressing, tubing, and solution changes for a CVC should be performed using aseptic technique.

◆ Assess the site for signs and symptoms of infection, such as discharge, inflammation, and tenderness.

◆ To prevent an air embolism, close the catheter clamp or have the patient perform Valsalva's maneuver each time the catheter hub is open to air.

◆ A Groshong catheter doesn't require clamping because it has an internal valve.

COMPLICATIONS

◆ Pneumothorax (typically occurring during insertion but may not be noticed until after procedure is done)
◆ Sepsis (typically occurring later during infusion therapy)
◆ Cardiac dysrhythmias that may necessitate catheter repositioning
◆ Phlebitis (especially in peripheral central venous therapy), thrombus formation, and air embolism

PATIENT TEACHING

◆ Care procedures in the home are the same as those in the facility, except the home therapy patient uses clean instead of aseptic technique. Teach the caregiver proper patient care techniques.

◆ Overall goal of home therapy is patient safety, so patient teaching must begin well before discharge.

◆ After discharge, a home therapy coordinator provides follow-up care until the patient or caregiver can provide catheter care and infusion therapy.

◆ Many home therapy patients learn to care for the catheter themselves and infuse their own drugs and solution.

DOCUMENTATION

◆ Document the time and date of insertion.
◆ Note the length and location of catheter.
◆ Report the solution infused.
◆ Record the physician's name.
◆ Describe the patient's response to the procedure.
◆ Document the time of X-ray, its results, and notification of the physician.
◆ Record the time and date of removal and type of antimicrobial ointment and dressing applied.
◆ Note the condition of catheter insertion site and collection of culture specimen.

SELECTED REFERENCES

Earsing, K.A., et al. "Best-Practice Protocols: Preventing Central Line Infection," *Nursing Management* 36(10): 18-24, October 2005.

Hadaway, L.C. "Caring for a Nontunneled CVC Site," *Nursing* 35(12):54-56, December 2005.

McInally, W. "Whose Line Is It Anyway? Management of Central Venous Catheters in Children," *Paediatric Nursing* 17(5):14-18, June 2005.

van der Hoogen, A., et al. "In-Line Filters in Central Venous Catheters in a Neonatal Intensive Care Unit," *Journal of Perinatal Medicine* 34(1):71-74, 2006.

Central venous pressure monitoring

DESCRIPTION

- Central venous pressure (CVP) is an index of right ventricular function.
- The physician inserts a catheter through a vein and advances it until its tip lies in or near the right atrium.
- Because no major valves lie at the junction of the vena cava and right atrium, pressure at end diastole reflects back to the catheter.
- When connected to a manometer, the catheter measures CVP.
- CVP monitoring helps assess cardiac function, evaluate venous return to the heart, and indirectly gauges how well the heart is pumping.
- The central venous line also provides access to a large vessel for rapid, high-volume fluid administration and allows easy blood withdrawal for laboratory samples.
- CVP monitoring can be done intermittently or continuously.
- The catheter is inserted percutaneously or using a cutdown method.
- To measure the patient's volume status, a disposable plastic water manometer may be attached between the I.V. line and the central catheter with a three- or four-way stopcock.
- CVP may also be monitored continuously through a central venous catheter attached to a pressure transducer.
- CVP is recorded in millimeters of mercury (mm Hg).
- Normal CVP ranges from 2 to 6 mm Hg.
- Any condition that alters venous return, circulating blood volume, or cardiac performance may affect CVP.
- If circulating volume increases (such as with enhanced venous return to the heart), CVP rises.
- If circulating volume decreases (such as with reduced venous return), CVP drops.

CONTRAINDICATIONS

None known

INTERMITTENT CVP MONITORING

Disposable CVP manometer set ◆ leveling device (such as a rod from a reusable CVP pole holder or a carpenter's level or rule) ◆ additional stopcock (to attach the CVP manometer to the catheter) ◆ extension tubing (if needed) ◆ I.V. pole ◆ I.V. solution ◆ I.V. drip chamber and tubing

CONTINUOUS CVP MONITORING

Pressure monitoring kit with disposable pressure transducer ◆ leveling device ◆ bedside pressure module ◆ continuous I.V. flush solution ◆ pressure bag

WITHDRAWING BLOOD SAMPLES THROUGH THE CV LINE

Appropriate number of syringes for ordered tests ◆ 5- or 10-ml syringe for discard sample (syringe size depends on tests ordered)

USING AN INTERMITTENT CV LINE

Syringe with normal saline solution ◆ syringe with heparin flush solution

REMOVING A CV CATHETER

Sterile gloves ◆ suture removal set ◆ sterile gauze pads ◆ povidone-iodine ointment ◆ dressing ◆ tape

- Gather the necessary equipment.
- Explain the procedure to the patient to reduce anxiety.
- Assist the physician as he inserts the central venous catheter.
- The procedure is similar to that used for pulmonary artery pressure monitoring, except the catheter is advanced only as far as the superior vena cava.

OBTAINING INTERMITTENT CVP READINGS WITH A WATER MANOMETER

- With the central venous line in place, position the patient flat.
- Align the base of the manometer with the previously determined zero reference point by using a leveling device.
- Because CVP reflects right atrial pressure, you must align the right atrium (the zero reference point) with the zero mark on the manometer.
- To find the right atrium, locate the fourth intercostal space at the midaxillary line.
- Mark the appropriate place on the patient's chest so all subsequent recordings will be made using the same location.
- If the patient can't tolerate a flat position, place him in semi-Fowler's position.
- When the head of the bed is elevated, the phlebostatic axis remains constant but the midaxillary line changes. Use the same degree of elevation for all subsequent measurements.
- Attach the water manometer to an I.V. pole or place it next to the patient's chest.
- Make sure the zero reference point is level with the right atrium.
- Verify that the water manometer is connected to the I.V. tubing.
- Typically, markings on the manometer range from −2 to 38 cm H_2O.
- Manufacturer's markings may differ; be sure to read directions before setting up the manometer and obtaining readings.

◆ Turn the stopcock off to the patient and slowly fill the manometer with I.V. solution until the fluid level is 10 to 20 cm H_2O higher than the patient's expected CVP value.

⚡ **WARNING** *Don't overfill the tube; fluid that spills over the top can cause contamination.*

◆ Turn the stopcock off to the I.V. solution and open to the patient.
◆ The fluid level in the manometer will drop.
◆ After the fluid level comes to rest, it will fluctuate slightly with respirations.
◆ Expect the fluid level to drop during inspiration and rise during expiration.
◆ Record CVP at the end of expiration, when intrathoracic pressure has a negligible effect.
◆ Depending on the type of water manometer used, note the value either at the bottom of the meniscus or at the midline of the small floating ball.
◆ After obtaining the CVP value, turn the stopcock to resume I.V. infusion.
◆ Adjust the I.V. drip rate as required.
◆ Place the patient in a comfortable position.

OBTAINING CONTINUOUS CVP READINGS WITH A WATER MANOMETER

◆ Make sure the stopcock is turned so the I.V. solution port, CVP column port, and patient port are all open.

⚡ **WARNING** *Be aware that with this stopcock position, infusion of the I.V. solution increases CVP. Therefore, expect higher readings than those taken with the stopcock turned off to the I.V. solution.*

◆ If the I.V. solution infuses at a constant rate, the CVP will change as the patient's condition changes, although the initial reading will be higher.
◆ Assess the patient closely for changes.

OBTAINING CONTINUOUS CVP READINGS WITH A PRESSURE MONITORING SYSTEM

◆ Make sure the central venous line or the proximal lumen of a pulmonary artery catheter is attached to the system.
◆ If the patient has a central venous line with multiple lumens, one lumen may be dedicated to continuous CVP monitoring and the others used for fluid administration.
◆ Set up a pressure transducer system.
◆ Connect the pressure tubing from the CVP catheter hub to the transducer.
◆ Connect the flush solution container to a flush device.
◆ To obtain values, position the patient flat. If the patient can't tolerate this position, use semi-Fowler's position.
◆ Locate the level of the right atrium by identifying the phlebostatic axis.
◆ Zero the transducer, leveling the transducer air-fluid interface stopcock with the right atrium.
◆ Read the CVP value from the digital display on the monitor and note the waveform.
◆ Make sure the patient is still when the reading is taken to prevent artifact; be sure to use the same position for all subsequent readings. (See *Identifying hemodynamic pressure monitoring problems,* pages 104 and 105.)

REMOVING A CENTRAL VENOUS LINE

◆ You may assist the physician in removing a central venous line.
◆ A nurse may be permitted to remove the catheter with a physician's order or when acting under advanced collaborative standards of practice.
◆ Elevate the head of the bed to minimize the risk of air embolism during catheter removal — for instance, place the patient in Trendelenburg's position if the line was inserted using a superior approach. If he can't tolerate this, position him flat.
◆ Turn the patient's head to the side opposite the catheter insertion site.
◆ The physician removes the dressing and exposes the insertion site.
◆ If sutures are in place, remove them.
◆ Turn the I.V. solution off.
◆ The physician pulls the catheter out in a slow, smooth motion, then applies pressure to the insertion site.
◆ Put on sterile gloves.
◆ Clean the insertion site, apply povidone-iodine ointment, and cover with a sterile gauze dressing.
◆ Remove gloves, and wash your hands.
◆ Assess for signs of respiratory distress, which may indicate an air embolism.

(continued)

Identifying hemodynamic pressure monitoring problems

PROBLEM	POSSIBLE CAUSES	NURSING INTERVENTIONS
No waveform	◆ Power supply turned off ◆ Monitor screen pressure range set too low ◆ Loose connection in line ◆ Transducer not connected to amplifier ◆ Stopcock off to patient ◆ Catheter occluded or out of blood vessel	◆ Check the power supply. ◆ Raise the monitor screen pressure range, if necessary. ◆ Rebalance and recalibrate the equipment. ◆ Tighten loose connections. ◆ Check and tighten the connection. ◆ Position the stopcock correctly. ◆ Use the fast-flush valve to flush the line, or try to aspirate blood from the catheter. If the line remains blocked, notify the physician and prepare to replace the line.
Drifting waveforms	◆ Improper warm-up ◆ Electrical cable kinked or compressed ◆ Temperature change in room air or I.V. flush solution	◆ Allow the monitor and transducer to warm up for 10 to 15 minutes. ◆ Place the monitor's cable where it can't be stepped on or compressed. ◆ Zero and calibrate the equipment 30 minutes after setting it up. This allows I.V. fluid to warm to room temperature.
Line fails to flush	◆ Stopcocks positioned incorrectly ◆ Inadequate pressure from pressure bag ◆ Kink in pressure tubing ◆ Blood clot in catheter	◆ Make sure the stopcocks are positioned correctly. ◆ Make sure the pressure bag gauge reads 300 mm Hg. ◆ Check the pressure tubing for kinks. ◆ Try to aspirate the clot with a syringe. If the line still won't flush, notify the physician and prepare to replace the line, if necessary. *Important:* Never use a syringe to flush a hemodynamic line.
Artifact (waveform interference)	◆ Patient movement ◆ Electrical interference ◆ Catheter fling (tip of pulmonary artery [PA] catheter moving rapidly in large blood vessel in heart chamber)	◆ Wait until the patient is relaxed before taking the reading. ◆ Make sure the electrical equipment is connected and grounded correctly. ◆ Notify physician; he may try to reposition the catheter.
False-high readings	◆ Transducer balancing port positioned below patient's right atrium ◆ Flush solution flow rate is too fast ◆ Air in system ◆ Catheter fling (tip of PA catheter moving rapidly in large blood vessel in heart chamber)	◆ Position the balancing port level with the patient's right atrium. ◆ Check the flush solution flow rate. Maintain it at 3 to 4 ml/hour. ◆ Remove air from the lines and the transducer. ◆ Notify physician; he may try to reposition the catheter.
False-low readings	◆ Transducer balancing port positioned above right atrium ◆ Transducer imbalance ◆ Loose connection	◆ Position the balancing port level with the patient's right atrium. ◆ Make sure transducer's flow system isn't kinked or occluded; rebalance and recalibrate the equipment. ◆ Tighten loose connections.
Damped waveform	◆ Air bubbles ◆ Blood clot in catheter ◆ Blood flashback in line ◆ Incorrect transducer position ◆ Arterial catheter out of blood vessel or pressed against vessel wall	◆ Secure all connections. ◆ Remove air from the lines and the transducer. ◆ Check for and replace cracked equipment. ◆ Refer to "Line fails to flush" (earlier in this chart). ◆ Make sure stopcock positions are correct; tighten loose connections and replace cracked equipment; flush the line with the fast-flush valve; replace the transducer dome if blood backs up into it. ◆ Make sure the transducer is kept at the level of the right atrium at all times. Improper levels give false-high or false-low pressure readings. ◆ Reposition the catheter if it's against the vessel wall. ◆ Try to aspirate blood to confirm proper placement in the vessel. If you can't aspirate blood, notify the physician and prepare to replace the line. *Note:* Bloody drainage at the insertion site may indicate catheter displacement. Notify the physician immediately.

(continued)

SPECIAL CONSIDERATIONS

- Arrange for daily chest X-rays to check catheter placement, as ordered.
- Care for the insertion site according to facility policy.
- Change the dressing every 24 to 48 hours.
- Be sure to wash your hands before dressing changes; use aseptic technique and sterile gloves when redressing the site.
- When removing the old dressing, observe for signs of infection, such as redness, and note patient complaints of tenderness.
- Apply ointment if directed by facility policy, then cover the site with a sterile gauze dressing or a clear occlusive dressing.
- After the initial CVP reading, reevaluate readings frequently to establish a baseline for the patient.
- Authorities recommend obtaining readings at 15-, 30-, and 60-minute intervals to establish a baseline.
- If the patient's CVP fluctuates by more than 2 cm H_2O, suspect a change in his clinical status and report this finding to the physician.
- Change the I.V. solution every 24 hours and the I.V. tubing every 96 hours, according to facility policy.
- Expect the physician to change the catheter every 96 hours.
- Label the I.V. solution, tubing, and dressing with the date, time, and your initials.

COMPLICATIONS

- Pneumothorax (typically occurs upon catheter insertion)
- Sepsis
- Thrombus
- Vessel or adjacent organ puncture
- Air embolism

PATIENT TEACHING

- Explain the procedure to the patient and answer any questions.

DOCUMENTATION

- Record all dressing, tubing, and solution changes.
- Document the date and time of catheter removal.
- Note the type of dressing applied.
- Report the condition of the catheter insertion site and whether a culture specimen was collected.
- Note complications and actions taken.
- Describe the patient's tolerance of the procedure.

SELECTED REFERENCES

Craig, J., and Mathieu, S. "Is Central Venous Pressure Monitoring Appropriate for Assessment of Perioperative Fluid Balance?" *British Journal of Hospital Medicine* 67(2):108, February 2006.

Higgins, D. "CVP Monitoring," *Nursing Times* 100(43):32-33, November 2004.

Ho, A.M., et al. "Accuracy of Central Venous Pressure Monitoring During Simultaneous Continuous Infusion Through the Same Catheter," *Anaesthesia* 60(10):1027-1030, October 2005.

Identifying hemodynamic pressure monitoring problems *(continued)*

PROBLEM	POSSIBLE CAUSES	NURSING INTERVENTIONS
Pulmonary artery wedge pressure tracing unobtainable	◆ Ruptured balloon	◆ If you feel no resistance when injecting air, or if you see blood leaking from the balloon inflation lumen, stop injecting air and notify the physician. If the catheter is left in, label the inflation lumen with a warning not to inflate.
	◆ Incorrect amount of air in balloon	◆ Deflate the balloon. Check the label on the catheter for correct volume. Reinflate slowly with the correct amount. To avoid rupturing the balloon, never use more than the stated volume.
	◆ Catheter malpositioned	◆ Notify the physician. Obtain a chest X-ray.

Cerebral blood flow monitoring

DESCRIPTION
◆ This procedure permits continuous regional blood flow monitoring at bedside.
◆ A sensor placed on the cerebral cortex calculates the cerebral blood flow in the capillary bed by thermal diffusion.
◆ Thermistors within the sensor detect the temperature differential between two metallic plates — one heated, one neutral.
◆ The differential relates inversely to cerebral blood flow.
◆ As the differential decreases, cerebral blood flow increases — as the differential increases, cerebral blood flow decreases.
◆ Monitoring yields important information about the effects of interventions on cerebral blood flow, and gives continuous real-time values for cerebral blood flow, essential in conditions where compromised blood flow may put the patient at risk for ischemia and infarction.
◆ Monitoring is indicated whenever cerebral blood flow alterations are anticipated.
◆ Monitoring is used commonly in patients with subarachnoid hemorrhage (in which a vasospasm may restrict blood flow), trauma associated with high intracranial pressure, or vascular tumors.

CONTRAINDICATIONS
None known

Special sensor that attaches to a computer data system

SITE CARE
Sterile 4″ × 4″ gauze pads ◆ clean gloves ◆ sterile gloves ◆ povidone-iodine solution or ointment ◆ adhesive tape

SENSOR REMOVAL
Sterile suture removal tray ◆ 1″ adhesive tape ◆ sterile 4″ × 4″ gauze pads ◆ clean gloves ◆ sterile gloves ◆ suture material

PREPARATION
◆ Make sure that the patient or a family member is fully informed about procedures involved; verify that a consent form has been signed.
◆ Explain the procedure to the patient.

Setting up the sensor monitor
◆ Assemble a monitor and a sensor cable with an attached sensor at the bedside.
◆ Attach the distal end of the sensor cable (from the patient's head) to the SENSOR CONNECT port on the monitor.
◆ When the sensor cable is securely in place, press the ON key to activate the monitor.
◆ Calibrate the system by pressing the CAL key.
◆ You should see the red light appear on the CAL button.
◆ Begin by calibrating the sensor to 00.0 by pressing the directional arrows.
◆ Sensor readouts of plus or minus 0.1 are acceptable.

◆ The surgeon typically inserts the sensor in the operating room during or after a craniotomy.
◆ Occasionally, the surgeon may insert the sensor through a burr hole.
◆ The surgeon implants the sensor far from major blood vessels and verifies that the metallic plates have good contact with the brain surface. (See *Inserting a cerebral blood flow sensor.*)
◆ Press the RUN key to display the cerebral blood flow reading.
◆ Observe the monitor's digital display, and document the baseline value.
◆ Record the cerebral blood flow hourly.
◆ Be sure to watch for trends and correlate sensor values with the patient's clinical status.

⚡ *WARNING Stimulation or activity may cause a 10% increase or decrease in cerebral blood flow. If you detect a 20% increase or decrease, suspect poor contact between the sensor and cerebral cortex.*

CARING FOR THE INSERTION SITE
◆ Confirm the patient's identity using two patient identifiers according to facility policy.
◆ Explain the procedure to the patient.
◆ Wash your hands.
◆ Put on clean gloves and remove the dressing from the sensor insertion site.
◆ Observe the site for cerebrospinal fluid (CSF) leakage, a potential complication.
◆ Remove and discard your gloves.
◆ Put on sterile gloves.
◆ Using aseptic technique, clean the insertion site with a gauze pad soaked in povidone-iodine solution.
◆ Clean the site, starting at the center and working outward in a circular pattern.
◆ Using a new gauze pad soaked with povidone-iodine solution, clean the exposed part of the sensor from the insertion site to the end of the sensor.
◆ Completely cover the insertion site with sterile 4″ × 4″ gauze pads.

- Tape all edges securely to create an occlusive dressing.

REMOVING THE SENSOR
- The cerebral blood flow sensor usually remains in place for about 3 days for postoperative monitoring.
- Explain the procedure to the patient and wash your hands.
- Put on clean gloves, remove the dressing, and dispose of gloves and dressing properly.
- Open the suture removal tray and package of suture material.
- The surgeon removes the anchoring sutures, then gently removes the sensor from insertion site.
- After the surgeon closes the wound, put on sterile gloves, apply a folded gauze pad to the site, and tape in place.
- Observe the condition of the site, including leakage.

SPECIAL CONSIDERATIONS

- Cerebral blood flow fluctuates with the brain's metabolic demands, ranging from 60 to 90 ml/100 g/minute. Normally, the patient's neurologic condition dictates the acceptable range. In the patient in a coma, cerebral blood flow may be one-half the normal value; in a patient in a barbiturate-induced coma with burst suppression on the electrocardiogram, cerebral blood flow may be as low as 10 ml/100 g/minute. Vasospasm secondary to subarachnoid hemorrhage may result in cerebral blood flow below 40 ml/100 g/minute. In an awake patient, cerebral blood flow above 90 ml/100 g/minute may indicate hyperemia.

TROUBLESHOOTER *If you suspect poor contact between the sensor and cerebral cortex, turn the patient toward the side of the sensor or gently wiggle the catheter back and forth (using a sterile-gloved hand). To determine whether contact between the sensor and cortex improves, observe the cerebral blood flow value on the monitor as you make the adjustment.*

- If your patient has low cerebral blood flow but no neurologic symptoms that indicate ischemia, suspect a fluid layer (a small hematoma) between the sensor and the cortex.
- Cerebral blood flow monitoring may lead to infection. Give prophylactic antibiotics as ordered, and maintain a sterile dressing around the insertion site.
- Change the dressing at the insertion site daily, using sterile technique, to reduce the risk of infection.

COMPLICATIONS
- CSF leakage (at the sensor insertion site)

PATIENT TEACHING

- If the patient will need cerebral blood flow monitoring after surgery, tell him that a sensor will be in place for about 3 days.
- Tell the patient that the insertion site will be covered with a dry, sterile dressing, and the sensor may be removed at the bedside.

DOCUMENTATION

- Document cleaning of the site.
- Describe appearance of the site.
- Record dressing changes.
- After sensor removal, report leakage from the site.

SELECTED REFERENCES
Albano, C., et al. "Innovations in the Management of Cerebral Injuries," *Critical Care Nursing Quarterly* 28(2):135-49, April-June 2005.
Kirkness, C.J. "Cerebral Blood Flow Monitoring in Clinical Practice," *AACN Clinical Issues* 16(4):476-87, October-December 2005.
Marcoux, K.K. "Management of Increased Intracranial Pressure in the Critically Ill Child With an Acute Neurological Injury," *AACN Clinical Issues* 16(2):212-31, April-June 2005.

Inserting a cerebral blood flow sensor

Typically, the surgeon inserts a cerebral blood flow sensor during a craniotomy. He tunnels the sensor toward the craniotomy site and then carefully inserts the metallic plates of the thermistor to make sure that they continuously contact the surface of the cerebral cortex. After closing the dura and replacing the bone flap, he closes the scalp.

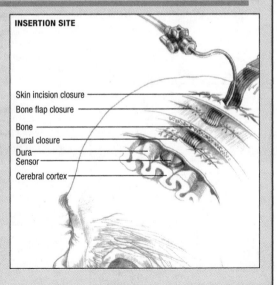

INSERTION SITE

Skin incision closure
Bone flap closure
Bone
Dural closure
Dura
Sensor
Cerebral cortex

Cerebrospinal fluid drains

OVERVIEW

DESCRIPTION

- Cerebrospinal fluid drains are used to reduce cerebrospinal fluid (CSF) pressure to the desired level, then maintain it.
- CSF can be withdrawn from the lateral ventricle (ventriculostomy) or lumbar subarachnoid space, depending on indication and desired outcome.
- Ventricular drainage is used to reduce increased intracranial pressure (ICP), whereas lumbar drainage is used to aid healing of the dura mater.
- External CSF drainage is commonly used to manage increased ICP and facilitate spinal or cerebral dural healing after traumatic injury or surgery.
- CSF is drained by a catheter or a ventriculostomy tube in a sterile, closed drainage collection system.
- CSF drainage is used for ICP monitoring via the ventriculostomy, for direct instillation of drugs, contrast media, or air for diagnostic radiology, and for aspiration of CSF for laboratory analysis.
- To place the ventricular drain, the physician inserts a ventricular catheter through a burr hole in the patient's skull.
- Insertion is usually done in the operating room under general anesthesia.
- To place the lumbar subarachnoid drain, the physician may give a local spinal anesthetic at bedside or in the operating room. (See *Using a cerebrospinal fluid drainage system*.)

CONTRAINDICATIONS

None known

EQUIPMENT

Overbed table ◆ sterile gloves ◆ sterile cotton-tipped applicators ◆ povidone-iodine solution ◆ alcohol pads ◆ sterile fenestrated drape ◆ 3-ml syringe for local anesthetic ◆ 25G ¾″ needle for injecting anesthetic ◆ local anesthetic (usually 1% lidocaine) ◆ 18G or 20G sterile spinal needle or Tuohy needle ◆ #5 French whistle-tip catheter or ventriculostomy tube external drainage set (includes drainage tubing and sterile collection bag) ◆ suture material ◆ 4″×4″ dressings ◆ paper tape ◆ lamp or other light source ◆ I.V. pole ◆ ventriculostomy tray and twist drill ◆ sterile marker ◆ sterile labels ◆ analgesic and anti-infective agent (optional)

PREPARATION

- Open all equipment using sterile technique.

Using a cerebrospinal fluid drainage system

Cerebrospinal fluid (CSF) drainage aims to control intracranial pressure (ICP) during treatment for traumatic injury or other conditions that cause a rise in ICP.

VENTRICULAR DRAIN

For a ventricular drain, the physician makes a burr hole in the patient's skull and inserts the catheter into the ventricle. The distal end of the catheter is connected to a closed drainage system.

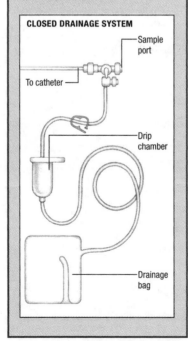

CLOSED DRAINAGE SYSTEM

Sample port

To catheter

Drip chamber

Drainage bag

- Check all packaging for breaks in seals and for expiration dates.
- After the physician places the catheter, connect it to the external drainage system tubing.
- Secure the connection points with tape or a connector.
- Place the collection system, including drip chamber and collection bag, on an I.V. pole.

KEY STEPS

- Explain the procedure to the patient and his family.
- Confirm the patient's identity using two patient identifiers according to facility policy.
- Documented consent should be obtained by the physician.
- Wash your hands.
- Perform a baseline neurologic assessment, including vital signs, to help detect alterations or signs of deterioration.

INSERTING A VENTRICULAR DRAIN

- Place the patient in the supine position.
- Place the equipment tray on the overbed table and unwrap it.
- Label all medications, medication containers, and other solutions on and off the sterile field.
- Adjust the height of the bed so the physician can perform the procedure comfortably.
- Illuminate the insertion site.
- The physician will shave around the insertion site, clean the insertion site, and give a local anesthetic.
- The physician will put on sterile gloves and drape the insertion site.
- To insert the drain, the physician will request a ventriculostomy tray with a twist drill.
- After completing the ventriculostomy, the physician will connect the drainage system and suture the ventriculostomy in place.
- The physician will cover the insertion site with a sterile dressing.

INSERTING A LUMBAR SUBARACHNOID DRAIN

◆ Position the patient in a side-lying position with his chin tucked to his chest and knees drawn up to his abdomen, as for a lumbar puncture.
◆ Urge the patient to remain as still as possible during the procedure.
◆ An alternate position for the patient is sitting up at the bedside, leaning forward over a bedside table.
◆ To insert the drain, the physician attaches a Tuohy needle (or spinal needle) to the whistle-tip catheter.
◆ After the physician removes the needle, he connects the drainage system, sutures or tapes the catheter securely in place, and covers it with a sterile dressing.

MONITORING CEREBROSPINAL FLUID DRAINAGE

◆ Maintain a continuous hourly output of CSF by raising or lowering the drainage system drip chamber.
◆ To maintain CSF outflow, the drip chamber should be slightly lower than or at the level of the lumbar drain insertion site.
◆ You may need to carefully raise or lower the drip chamber to increase or decrease CSF flow.
◆ For ventricular drains, ensure that the flow chamber of the ICP monitoring setup remains positioned as ordered.
◆ Correlate changes in ICP readings to the drainage.
◆ To drain CSF as ordered, put on gloves, and turn the main stopcock on to drainage to allow CSF to collect in the graduated flow chamber.
◆ Document the time and the amount of CSF obtained, and turn the stopcock off to drainage.
◆ To drain the CSF from this chamber into the drainage bag, release the clamp below the flow chamber.
◆ Check the dressing frequently for drainage, which could indicate CSF leakage.
◆ Check the tubing for patency by watching the CSF drops in the drip chamber.

◆ Observe CSF for color, clarity, amount, blood, and sediment.
◆ CSF specimens for laboratory analysis should be obtained from the collection port attached to the tubing, not from the collection bag.
◆ Change the collection bag when it's full or every 24 hours, according to facility policy.

⚡ WARNING *Never empty the drainage bag. Instead, replace it when full, using sterile technique.*

SPECIAL CONSIDERATIONS

◆ Maintenance of a continual hourly output of CSF is essential to prevent overdrainage or underdrainage.
◆ Underdrainage or lack of CSF may reflect kinked tubing, catheter displacement, or a drip chamber placed higher than the catheter insertion site.
◆ Overdrainage can occur if the drip chamber is placed too far below the catheter insertion site.
◆ Raising or lowering the head of the bed can affect the CSF flow rate.
◆ When changing the patient's position, reposition the drip chamber.
◆ Patients with lumbar drains are generally kept in a flat position, especially if the drain is placed for a spinal dural tear.
◆ Patients may experience chronic headache during continuous CSF drainage.
◆ Assess for signs of overdrainage, which may include headache.
◆ Reassure him that overdrainage isn't unusual; give analgesics as appropriate.
◆ To prevent infection, maintain a sterile closed system and a dry, sterile dressing over the site; give antibiotics as ordered.

COMPLICATIONS

◆ Headache, tachycardia, diaphoresis, and nausea (due to excessive CSF drainage)
◆ Collapsed ventricles, tonsillar herniation, and medullary compression (due to acute overdrainage)

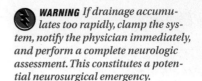 **WARNING** *If drainage accumulates too rapidly, clamp the system, notify the physician immediately, and perform a complete neurologic assessment. This constitutes a potential neurosurgical emergency.*
◆ Clot formation (due to cessation of drainage)

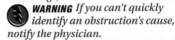 **WARNING** *If you can't quickly identify an obstruction's cause,* notify the physician.
◆ Signs of increased ICP (if drainage is blocked)
◆ Infection that may cause meningitis

PATIENT TEACHING

◆ Explain the procedure to the patient and answer any questions.

DOCUMENTATION

◆ Record the time and date of insertion, and the patient's response.
◆ Record vital signs and neurologic assessment findings at least every 4 hours.
◆ Document the color, clarity, and amount of CSF at least every 8 hours.
◆ Record hourly and 24-hour CSF output, and describe the condition of the dressing.

SELECTED REFERENCES

Anderson, R.C., et al. "Complications of Intracranial Pressure Monitoring in Children With Head Trauma," *Journal of Neurosurgery* 101(Suppl 1):53-58, August 2004.
Hughes, S.A., et al. "Prolonged Jackson-Pratt Drainage in the Management of Lumbar Cerebrospinal Fluid Leaks," *Surgical Neurology* 65(4):410-14, April 2006.
Macsween, K.F., et al. "Lumbar Drainage for Control of Raised Cerebrospinal Fluid Pressure in Cryptococcal Meningitis: Case Report and Review," *Journal of Infection* 51(4):e221-24, November 2005.

Cervical collar

DESCRIPTION

◆ A cervical collar may be used for an acute injury (such as strained cervical muscles) or a chronic condition (such as arthritis or cervical metastasis).
◆ A cervical collar may augment such splinting devices as a spine board to prevent potential cervical spine fracture or spinal cord damage.
◆ It may prevent further injury and promote healing.
◆ The collar immobilizes the cervical spine, decreases muscle spasms, and reduces pain by holding the neck straight with the chin slightly elevated and tucked in.
◆ As symptoms of an acute injury subside, the patient may gradually discontinue wearing the collar, alternating periods of wear with increasing periods of removal, until she no longer needs the collar.

CONTRAINDICATIONS
None known

Cervical collar in the appropriate size ◆ cotton for padding (optional) (see *Types of cervical collars*)

Types of cervical collars

Cervical collars are used to support an injured or weakened cervical spine and to maintain alignment during healing.
   Made of rigid plastic, the molded cervical collar holds the patient's neck firmly, keeping it straight, with the chin slightly elevated and tucked in.

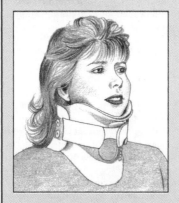

The soft cervical collar, made of spongy foam, provides gentler support and reminds the patient to avoid cervical spine motion.

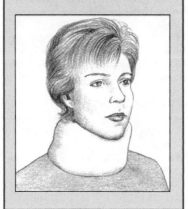

◆ Check the patient's neurovascular status before application.
◆ Tell her to position her head slowly to face directly forward.
◆ Place the cervical collar in front of her neck to ensure that the size is correct.
◆ Fit the collar snugly around the neck and attach the Velcro fasteners or buckles at the back of the neck.
◆ Check her airway and neurovascular status to ensure that the collar isn't too tight.

SPECIAL CONSIDERATIONS

◆ For a sprain or a potential cervical spine fracture, make sure the collar isn't too high in front because this may hyperextend the neck.
◆ Hard collar application usually requires log rolling the patient to prevent injury to the spinal cord.
◆ With a neck sprain, hyperextension may cause ligaments to heal in a shortened position.
◆ With a potential cervical spine fracture, hyperextension may cause serious neurologic damage.
◆ If the patient complains of pressure, the collar may be too tight and should be removed and reapplied.

TROUBLESHOOTER *If the patient complains of skin irritation or friction, the collar itself may be irritating her. Apply protective cotton padding between the irritated skin and the collar.*

COMPLICATIONS
None known

PATIENT TEACHING

◆ Teach the patient how to apply the collar and how to do a neurovascular check.
◆ Have the patient demonstrate how to apply the collar after you have instructed her.
◆ Some collars are complex and the patient (or caregiver) may need to practice if she'll be responsible for application.
◆ Advise sleeping without a pillow, if indicated.

DOCUMENTATION

◆ Record the type and size of the cervical collar and the time and date of application in your notes.
◆ Record the results of neurovascular checks.
◆ Document patient comfort, the collar's snugness, and all patient instructions.

SELECTED REFERENCES

Chi, C.H., et al. "Effect of Hair and Clothing on Neck Immobilization Using a Cervical Collar," *American Journal of Emergency Medicine* 23(3):386-90, May 2005.

Chin, K.R., et al. "Mastication Causing Segmental Spinal Motion in Common Cervical Orthoses," *Spine* 31(4):430-34, February 2006.

Iizuka, H., et al. "Clinical Results After Cervical Laminoplasty: Differences Due to the Duration of Wearing a Cervical Collar," *Journal of Spinal Disorders & Techniques* 18(6):489-91, December 2005.

Chemotherapeutic drug administration

DESCRIPTION

- Chemotherapeutic drug administration requires specific skills in addition to those used giving other drugs.
- Some drugs require specialized equipment or must be given through an unusual route, some become unstable, and others must be protected from light.
- The drug dosage must be exact to avoid potentially fatal complications.
- Only specially trained nurses and physicians should give these drugs.
- These drugs may be given through a number of routes.
- Although I.V. (using peripheral or central veins) is used most commonly, they may be given orally, subcutaneously, I.M., intra-arterially, into a body cavity, through a central venous catheter, or through an Ommaya reservoir into the spinal canal. They may also be given into an artery, the peritoneal cavity, or the pleural space.
- The administration route depends on drug pharmacodynamics and tumor characteristics.
- If a malignant tumor is confined to one area, the drug may be given through a localized or regional method, which allows delivery of a high dose directly to the tumor.
- Regional administration is advantageous because many solid tumors don't respond to drug levels that are safe for systemic administration.
- Adjuvant chemotherapy helps ensure no undetectable metastasis exists in patients who have had surgery or radiation therapy.
- Induction chemotherapy (or neoadjuvant or synchronous chemotherapy) occurs before surgery or radiation therapy. It improves survival rates by shrinking a tumor before surgical excision or radiation therapy.

CONTRAINDICATIONS

None known

EQUIPMENT

Prescribed drug ◆ aluminum foil or brown paper bag (if drug is photosensitive) ◆ normal saline solution ◆ syringes and needleless adapters ◆ infusion pump or controller ◆ gloves ◆ impervious containers labeled CAUTION: BIOHAZARD

PREPARATION

- Verify the drug, dosage, and administration route.
- Make sure you know the immediate and delayed adverse effects.
- Follow administration guidelines.

KEY STEPS

- Confirm the patient's identity using two patient identifiers according to facility policy.
- Explain the procedure to the patient.
- Assess the patient's physical condition and medical history.
- Make sure you understand what drug needs to be given and by what route.
- Determine the best site to give the drug.
- When selecting the site, consider drug compatibilities, frequency of administration, and the vesicant potential of the drug.
- Continuous infusion of a vesicant drug should be done through a central venous line or a vascular access device.
- Nonvesicant agents (including irritants) may be given by direct I.V. push, through the side port of an infusing I.V. line, or as a continuous infusion.
- Because vein integrity decreases with time, some facilities require that vesicants be given before other drugs. Also, because vesicants increase vein fragility, some facilities require vesicants be given after other drugs (check facility policy).
- Evaluate the patient, paying attention to recent laboratory studies, including complete blood count, blood urea nitrogen level, platelet count,

urine creatinine level, and liver function studies.
- Determine if he has received chemotherapy before, and note severity of adverse effects.
- Check his history for drugs that might interact with chemotherapy.

⚡ **WARNING** *Don't mix chemotherapeutic drugs with other drugs. If you have questions or concerns, talk with the physician or pharmacist before giving the drug.*

- Double-check the chart for the complete chemotherapy protocol order, including the patient's name, drug's name, dosage, route, rate, and frequency of administration.
- Check if the drug's dosage depends on certain laboratory values.
- Some facilities require two nurses to read the dosage order and check the drug and amount given.
- Check to see if an antiemetic, fluids, a diuretic, or electrolyte supplements are to be given before, during, or after chemotherapy.
- Evaluate the patient's understanding and make sure a consent form has been signed.
- Wear gloves through all stages of handling the drug.
- Before giving the drug, perform a new venipuncture proximal to the old site.

⚡ **WARNING** *Avoid using an existing peripheral I.V. line.*

- To identify an administration site, examine the patient's veins, starting with his hand then his forearm.
- After an appropriate line is in place, infuse 10 to 20 ml of normal saline solution to test vein patency.

⚡ **WARNING** *Never test vein patency with a chemotherapeutic drug.*

- Give the drug as appropriate: nonvesicants by I.V. push or admixed in a bag of I.V. fluid; vesicants by I.V. push through a piggyback set connected to a rapidly infusing I.V. line.
- During I.V. administration, closely monitor for signs of hypersensitivity or extravasation.
- Check for adequate blood return after 5 ml of drug has been infused or according to facility guidelines.
- Infuse 20 ml of normal saline solution after infusion of the drug, be-

tween administration of different chemotherapeutic drugs, and before discontinuing the I.V. line.
◆ Dispose of used needles and syringes carefully in a sharps container.
◆ To prevent aerosol dispersion of chemotherapeutic drugs, don't clip needles.
◆ Place the needles intact in an impervious container for incineration.
◆ Dispose of I.V. bags, bottles, gloves, and tubing in a properly labeled, covered trash container.
◆ Wash your hands thoroughly after giving chemotherapeutic drugs, even though you wore gloves.

SPECIAL CONSIDERATIONS

◆ Check frequently for signs of extravasation and allergic reaction (swelling, redness, and urticaria).
◆ **WARNING** *If you suspect extravasation, stop infusion immediately. Leave I.V. catheter in place and notify the physician. A conservative method for treating extravasation involves aspirating residual drug from the tubing and I.V. catheter, instilling an I.V. antidote, and then removing the I.V. catheter. Afterward, apply heat or cold to the site and elevate the limb.*
◆ To avoid breakdown, some drugs shouldn't be exposed to direct sunlight. To protect from sunlight, cover vial with a brown paper bag or aluminum foil.
◆ When giving vesicants, avoid sites where damage to underlying tendons or nerves may occur (veins in the antecubital fossa, near the wrist, or the dorsal surface of the hand).
◆ If you're unable to stay with the patient, use an infusion pump or controller to ensure drug delivery within the prescribed time and rate.
◆ Observe him regularly during and after treatment for adverse reactions.
◆ Monitor vital signs throughout infusion.
◆ Record the types and amounts of drugs the patient received.
◆ Maintaining a list is especially important if he has received drugs that have a cumulative effect and that can

be toxic to such organs as the heart or kidneys.

COMPLICATIONS

◆ Nausea and vomiting, ranging from mild to debilitating
◆ Bone marrow suppression, leading to neutropenia and thrombocytopenia
◆ Intestinal irritation
◆ Stomatitis
◆ Pulmonary fibrosis
◆ Cardiotoxicity
◆ Nephrotoxicity
◆ Neurotoxicity
◆ Hearing loss
◆ Anemia
◆ Alopecia
◆ Urticaria
◆ Radiation recall (if drugs are given with, or soon after, radiation therapy)
◆ Anorexia
◆ Esophagitis
◆ Diarrhea
◆ Constipation
◆ I.V. administration that may also cause extravasation, inflammation, ulceration, necrosis, loss of vein patency

PATIENT TEACHING

◆ Teach the patient about possible adverse reactions to chemotherapy.
◆ Let the patient know that drugs can be given to treat some of the adverse reactions.
◆ Explain to the patient the type and sequence of drugs he'll receive.

DOCUMENTATION

◆ Record location and description of the I.V. site before treatment and presence of blood return during bolus administration.
◆ Note drugs and dosages given.
◆ Document the sequence of drug administration.
◆ Indicate needle type and size.
◆ Report the amount and type of flushing solution.
◆ Describe the site's condition after treatment.
◆ Document adverse reactions.
◆ Note the patient's tolerance of the treatment.
◆ Record topics discussed with patient and his family.

SELECTED REFERENCES

Hendershot, E., et al. "Outpatient Chemotherapy Administration: Decreasing Wait Times for Patients and Families," *Journal of Pediatric Oncology Nursing* 22(1):31-37, January-February 2005.

Schulmeister, L. "Look-alike, Sound-alike Oncology Medications," *Clinical Journal of Oncology Nursing* 10(1):35-41, February 2006.

Treleaven, J., et al. "Obtaining Consent for Chemotherapy," *British Journal of Haematology* 132(5):552-59, March 2006.

Wyatt, A., et al. "Cutaneous Reactions to Chemotherapy and Their Management," *American Journal of Clinical Dermatology* 7(1):45-63, 2006.

Chemotherapeutic drug preparation

OVERVIEW

DESCRIPTION

- Chemotherapeutic drug preparation requires extra care, for the safety of you and the patient.
- The patient receiving drugs risks teratogenic, mutagenic, and carcinogenic effects; health care professionals who prepare and handle the drugs are also at risk.

CONTRAINDICATIONS

- Pregnancy
- Breast-feeding

WARNING *Although danger from handling these drugs hasn't been fully determined, chemotherapeutic drugs can increase the handler's risk of reproductive abnormalities. These drugs also pose environmental threats, and the best method for handling them hasn't been determined.*

EQUIPMENT

Prescribed drugs ◆ patient's medication record and chart ◆ long-sleeved gown ◆ powder-free latex surgical gloves ◆ face shield or goggles ◆ eyewash ◆ plastic absorbent pad ◆ alcohol pads ◆ sterile gauze pads ◆ shoe covers ◆ impervious container with CAUTION: BIOHAZARD label for disposal of unused drug and equipment ◆ I.V. solution ◆ diluent (if necessary) ◆ compatibility reference source ◆ medication labels ◆ class II biological safety cabinet ◆ disposable towel ◆ hydrophobic filter or dispensing pin ◆ 18G needle ◆ syringes and needles of various sizes ◆ I.V. tubing with Luer-lock fittings ◆ I.V. controller pump (if available)

Have a chemotherapeutic spill kit available that includes water-resistant, nonpermeable, long-sleeved gown with cuffs and back closure ◆ shoe covers ◆ two pairs of gloves for double gloving ◆ goggles ◆ mask ◆ disposable dustpan ◆ plastic scraper for collecting broken glass ◆ plastic-backed or absorbable towels ◆ desiccant powder or granules to absorb wet contents ◆ two disposable sponges ◆ puncture-proof, leak-proof container labeled BIOHAZARD WASTE ◆ container of 70% alcohol for cleaning the spill area

KEY STEPS

- Wash your hands before and after preparation and administration.
- Prepare drugs in a class II biological safety cabinet with an air-removal hood.
- Wear protective garments: long-sleeved gown, powder-free gloves, a face shield or goggles, and shoe covers, as indicated by facility policy.
- Don't wear the protective garments outside the preparation area.
- Don't eat, drink, smoke, or apply cosmetics in the drug preparation area.
- Before and after you prepare the drug, clean the internal surfaces of the cabinet with 70% alcohol and a disposable towel.
- Discard the towel in a leak-proof chemical waste container.
- Cover the work surface with a clean plastic absorbent pad to minimize contamination by droplets or spills.
- Change the pad at the end of the shift or when a spill occurs.
- Consider all of the equipment used in drug preparation, as well as unused drug, as hazardous waste and dispose according to facility policy.
- Place all chemotherapeutic waste products in labeled, leak-proof, sealable plastic bags or other appropriate impervious containers.

- Prepare drugs using current product instructions, paying attention to compatibility, stability, and reconstitution technique.
- Label the prepared drug with the patient's name, dosage, date, and time of preparation.

⚠️ **WARNING** *Reduce your exposure to chemotherapeutic drugs. Systemic absorption can occur through ingestion of contaminated materials, contact with skin, or inhalation. You can inhale a drug without realizing it, such as while opening a vial, clipping a needle, expelling air from a syringe, or discarding excess drug. You can also absorb a drug from handling contaminated stools or body fluids.*

- Prime all I.V. bags that contain chemotherapeutic drugs under the hood.
- The hood blower should run 24 hours per day.
- If a hood isn't available, prepare drugs in a well-ventilated workspace, away from heating or cooling vents and other personnel.
- Vent vials with a hydrophobic filter, or use negative-pressure techniques.
- Use a needle with a hydrophobic filter to remove the solution from the vial.
- To break an ampule, wrap a sterile pad around the neck of the ampule to decrease risk of contamination.
- Check that the cabinet is certified for safe use, if necessary.
- Use only syringes and I.V. sets that have Luer-lock fittings.
- Label all chemotherapeutic drugs with a chemotherapy hazard label.
- Don't clip needles, break syringes, or remove needles from syringes.
- Use a gauze pad when removing chemotherapy syringes and needles from I.V. bags of chemotherapeutic drugs.
- Place used syringes or needles in a punctureproof container, along with other sharp or breakable items.
- When mixing drugs, wear latex surgical gloves and a gown of low-permeability fabric with a closed front and cuffed long sleeves.

- Change gloves every 30 minutes.
- If you spill the drug or puncture or tear a glove, remove gloves immediately.
- Wash your hands before putting on new gloves and after removing gloves.
- If the drug comes in contact with your skin, wash the area thoroughly with soap (not a germicidal agent) and water.
- If eye contact occurs, flood the eye with water or an isotonic eyewash for at least 5 minutes while holding the eyelid open.
- Obtain a medical evaluation as soon as possible after exposure.
- If a major spill occurs, clean it with the chemotherapeutic spill kit.
- Discard disposable gowns and gloves in an appropriately marked, waterproof receptacle when contaminated or when you leave the work area.
- Don't place food or drinks in the same refrigerator as chemotherapeutic drugs.
- Become familiar with drug excretion patterns, and take precautions when handling a chemotherapy patient's body fluids.
- Provide the male patient with a urinal with a tight-fitting lid.
- Wear disposable latex surgical gloves when handling body fluids.
- Before flushing the toilet, place a waterproof pad over it to avoid splashing.
- Wear gloves and a gown when handling linens soiled with body fluids.
- Place soiled linens in isolation linen bags.

⚠️ **WARNING** *Women who are pregnant, trying to conceive, or breast-feeding should exercise caution when handling chemotherapeutic drugs.*

COMPLICATIONS

- Damage to the liver or chromosomes (due to chronic exposure)
- Burning or damage to skin (due to direct exposure)

- Discuss safety if the patient will be using the drugs at home.
- Teach the patient how to dispose of contaminated equipment.
- Tell the patient and his family to wear gloves when handling chemotherapy equipment or contaminated linens or gowns and pajamas.
- Tell the patient and his family to put soiled linens in a pillowcase and launder it twice, with soiled linens inside, separate from other linens.
- Tell the patient and his family to empty waste into the toilet, close to the water to minimize splashing, and close the lid and flush twice.
- Tell the patient and his family that all treatment materials need to be placed in a leak-proof container and taken to a disposal site. Arrangements can be made with a hospital or private company for pickup and disposal of contaminated waste.

- Document each incident of exposure according to facility policy.

SELECTED REFERENCES

Martin, S., and Larson, E. "Chemotherapy-Handling Practices of Outpatient and Office-Based Oncology Nurses," *Oncology Nursing Forum* 30(4):575-81, July-August 2003.

Saria, M.G., and Rome, S.I. "The ACE Project: Avoiding Chemotherapy Errors in a Blended Medical/Surgical/Oncology Unit," *Clinical Nurse Specialist* 19(2): 80, March-April 2005.

Schulmeister, L. "Look-alike, Sound-alike Oncology Medications," *Clinical Journal of Oncology Nursing* 10(1):35-41, February 2006.

Chest physiotherapy

DESCRIPTION

- Chest therapy techniques include postural drainage, chest percussion and vibration, and coughing and deep-breathing exercises.
- Techniques mobilize and eliminate secretions, reexpand lung tissue, and promote efficient use of respiratory muscles.
- Technique is important for the bedridden patient; helps prevent or treat atelectasis and may prevent pneumonia, which can seriously impede recovery.
- Postural drainage done with percussion and vibration causes peripheral pulmonary secretions to empty into the major bronchi or trachea. It's accomplished by sequential repositioning of the patient.
- Secretions drain best with the patient positioned so the bronchi are perpendicular to the floor.
- Lower and middle lobe bronchi empty best with the patient in the head-down position; upper lobe bronchi, in the head-up position.
- Percussing the chest with cupped hands mechanically dislodges thick, tenacious secretions from the bronchial walls.
- Vibration can be used with percussion or as an alternative to it in the patient who's frail, in pain, or recovering from thoracic surgery or trauma.
- Chest physiotherapy is used on the patient who expectorates large amounts of sputum, such as those with bronchiectasis and cystic fibrosis.
- It hasn't proven effective in the patient with status asthmaticus, lobar pneumonia, or acute exacerbations of chronic bronchitis when he has scant secretions and is being mechanically ventilated.
- It has little value for treating the patient with stable, chronic bronchitis.

CONTRAINDICATIONS

- Active pulmonary bleeding with hemoptysis (at immediate posthemorrhage stage)
- Fractured ribs
- Unstable chest wall
- Lung contusions
- Pulmonary tuberculosis
- Untreated pneumothorax
- Acute asthma
- Bronchospasm
- Lung abscess
- Tumor
- Bony metastasis
- Head injury
- Recent myocardial infarction

Stethoscope ♦ pillows ♦ tilt or postural drainage table (if available) or adjustable hospital bed ♦ emesis basin ♦ facial tissues ♦ suction equipment ♦ oral care equipment ♦ trash bag ♦ sterile specimen container ♦ mechanical ventilator ♦ supplemental oxygen (optional)

PREPARATION

- Gather equipment at the patient's bedside.
- Set up and test the suction equipment.

Performing percussion and vibration

Instruct the patient to breathe slowly and deeply, using the diaphragm, to promote relaxation. Percuss each segment with a cupped hand for 1 to 2 minutes. Listen for a hollow sound on percussion to verify correct performance of technique.

To perform vibration, ask him to inhale deeply, then exhale slowly. During exhalation, firmly press your hands against the chest wall. Tense the muscles of your arms and shoulders in an isometric contraction to send fine vibrations through the chest wall. Do this during five exhalations over each chest segment.

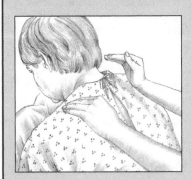

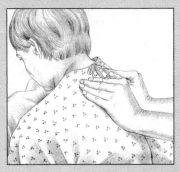

KEY STEPS

- Confirm the patient's identity using two patient identifiers according to facility policy.
- Explain the procedure to the patient, provide privacy, and wash your hands.
- Auscultate his lungs to determine baseline respiratory status.
- Position him as ordered.
- In generalized disease, drainage begins with lower lobes, continues with middle lobes, and ends with upper lobes.
- In localized disease, drainage begins with affected lobes and proceeds to other lobes to avoid spreading disease to uninvolved areas.
- Tell him to remain in each position for 10 to 15 minutes.
- Perform percussion and vibration as ordered. (See *Performing percussion and vibration.*)
- After postural drainage, percussion, or vibration, tell him to cough to remove loosened secretions.
- Tell him to inhale deeply through his nose, then exhale in three short huffs.
- Have him inhale deeply again and cough through a slightly open mouth.
- Three consecutive coughs are highly effective.
- An effective cough sounds deep, low, and hollow; an ineffective cough sounds high-pitched.
- Have him perform exercises for about 1 minute, then rest for 2 minutes.
- Gradually progress to a 10-minute exercise period four times daily.
- Provide oral hygiene because secretions may have a foul taste or stale odor.
- Auscultate his lungs to evaluate effectiveness of therapy.

SPECIAL CONSIDERATIONS

- For effectiveness and safety, modify chest physiotherapy as needed.
- Suction the patient who has an ineffective cough reflex.
- If he tires quickly during therapy, shorten the sessions because fatigue leads to shallow respirations and increased hypoxia.
- Maintain adequate hydration if he's receiving chest physiotherapy to prevent mucus dehydration and promote mobilization.
- Avoid postural drainage immediately before or within 1½ hours after meals to avoid nausea, vomiting, and aspiration of food or vomitus.
- To prevent bronchospasm, adjunct treatments (intermittent positive-pressure breathing, aerosol, or nebulizer therapy) should precede chest physiotherapy.
- To avoid injury, don't percuss over the spine, liver, kidneys, or spleen.
- Avoid percussion on bare skin or on the female patient's breasts.
- Percuss over soft clothing (but not over buttons, snaps, or zippers) or place a thin towel over the chest wall.

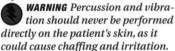 **WARNING** *Percussion and vibration should never be performed directly on the patient's skin, as it could cause chaffing and irritation.*

- Remove jewelry before percussing.

COMPLICATIONS

- Hypoxia or orthostatic hypotension (occurring during postural drainage in the head-down position, where pressure on the diaphragm can impair respiratory excursion)
- Increased intracranial pressure (caused by the head-down position, which precludes use in a patient with acute neurologic impairment)
- Vigorous percussion or vibration that causes rib fracture (especially in the patient with osteoporosis)
- Pneumothorax (caused by coughing in an emphysematous patient with blebs)

PATIENT TEACHING

- Explain coughing and deep-breathing exercises preoperatively so the patient can practice them when he's pain-free and better able to concentrate.
- Postoperatively, splint the patient's incision using your hands, or teach him to splint it himself to minimize pain during coughing.

DOCUMENTATION

- Record the date and time of chest physiotherapy.
- Note the positions for secretion drainage and length of time for each.
- Document the chest segments percussed or vibrated.
- Report the color, amount, odor, and viscosity of secretions produced and presence of blood.
- Record complications and nursing actions taken.
- Note the patient's tolerance of treatment.

SELECTED REFERENCES

Bagley, C.E., et al. "Routine Neonatal Postextubation Chest Physiotherapy: A Randomized Controlled Trial," *Journal of Paediatrics and Child Health* 41(11):592-97, November 2005.

McCool, F.D., and Rosen, M.J. "Nonpharmacologic Airway Clearance Therapies: ACCP Evidence-Based Clinical Practice Guidelines," *Chest* 129(1 Suppl):250S-59S, January 2006.

Soni, R., et al. "Acute Effects of Chest Physiotherapy on Gas Exchange and Wellbeing in Severe Cystic Fibrosis," *Respirology* 9(Suppl 2):A51, March 2004.

Varela, G., et al. "Cost-Effectiveness Analysis of Prophylactic Respiratory Physiotherapy in Pulmonary Lobectomy," *European Journal of Cardiothoracic Surgery* 29(2):216-20, February 2006.

Chest tube insertion and removal

DESCRIPTION

◆ Pleural space contains a thin layer of lubricating fluid that allows visceral and parietal pleura to move without friction during respiration.

◆ Excess fluid (hemothorax or pleural effusion), air (pneumothorax), or both, in the pleural space changes intrapleural pressure and causes partial or complete lung collapse.

◆ Chest tube insertion allows drainage of air or fluid from the pleural space.

◆ It's usually performed by the physician with nurse assistance, and requires sterile technique.

◆ Insertion sites vary, depending on the patient's condition and physician's judgment.

◆ For pneumothorax, the second to third intercostal space is the usual site because air rises to the top of the intrapleural space.

◆ For hemothorax or pleural effusion, the fourth to sixth intercostal spaces are common sites because fluid settles to the lower levels of the intrapleural space.

◆ For removal of air and fluid, chest tubes are inserted into high and low sites.

◆ After insertion, chest tubes are connected to a thoracic drainage system that removes air, fluid, or both from pleural space, prevents backflow, and promotes lung reexpansion.

CONTRAINDICATIONS

None known

EQUIPMENT

Two pairs of sterile gloves ◆ sterile drape ◆ povidone-iodine solution ◆ vial of 1% lidocaine ◆ 10-ml syringe ◆ alcohol pad ◆ 22G 1″ needle ◆ 25G ⅜″ needle ◆ sterile scalpel (usually with #11 blade) ◆ sterile forceps ◆ two rubber-tipped clamps ◆ sterile 4″ × 4″ gauze pads ◆ two sterile 4″ × 4″ drain dressings (gauze pads with slit) ◆ 3″ or 4″ sturdy, elastic tape ◆ 1″ adhesive tape for connections ◆ chest tube of appropriate size (#16 to #20 French catheter for air or serous fluid; #28 to #40 French catheter for blood, pus, or thick fluid), with or without a trocar ◆ sterile Kelly clamp ◆ suture material (usually 2-0 silk with cutting needle) ◆ thoracic drainage system: sterile drainage tubing, 6′ (1.8 m) long, and connector ◆ sterile Y connector (for two chest tubes on the same side) ◆ petroleum gauze ◆ sterile marker or sterile label

PREPARATION

◆ Check the expiration date on the sterile packages and inspect for tears.

◆ In the nonemergency situation, make sure the patient has signed consent form.

◆ Assemble equipment in the patient's room and set up the thoracic drainage system.

◆ Place it by the patient's bed below chest level to facilitate drainage.

KEY STEPS

◆ Confirm the patient's identity using two patient identifiers according to facility policy.

◆ Explain the procedure to the patient, provide privacy, and wash your hands.

◆ Record baseline vital signs and respiratory assessment.

◆ Position the patient.

◆ If he has pneumothorax, place him in high Fowler's, semi-Fowler's, or supine position.

◆ The physician will insert the tube in the anterior chest at the midclavicular line in the second to third intercostal space.

◆ If he has hemothorax, have him lean over the overbed table or straddle a chair with his arms dangling over the back.

◆ The physician will insert the tube in the fourth to sixth intercostal space at the midaxillary line.

◆ For either pneumothorax or hemothorax, the patient may lie on his unaffected side with arms extended over his head.

◆ When you've positioned him properly, place the chest tube tray on the overbed table.

◆ Open the equipment using sterile technique.

◆ Label all medications, medication containers, and other solutions on and off the sterile field.

◆ The physician will prepare the insertion site by cleaning the area with povidone-iodine solution.

◆ Wipe the rubber stopper of the lidocaine vial with an alcohol pad.

◆ Invert the bottle and hold it for the physician to withdraw the anesthetic.

◆ After anesthetizing the site, he'll make a small incision, insert the chest tube, and connect it to the thoracic drainage system.

◆ As the chest tube is inserted, reassure the patient and assist the physician as needed.

◆ The physician may secure the tube to the skin with a suture.

◆ Open the packages containing the petroleum gauze, 4″ × 4″ drain dressings, and gauze pads, and put on sterile gloves.

◆ Place the petroleum gauze and two 4″ × 4″ drain dressings around the insertion site, one from the top and one from the bottom.

◆ Place several 4″ × 4″ gauze pads on top of the drain dressings.

◆ Tape the dressings, covering them completely.

◆ Securely tape the chest tube to the patient's chest distal to the insertion site to prevent accidental dislodgment.

◆ Securely tape the junction of the chest tube and the drainage tube to prevent separation.

- Make sure the tubing remains level with the patient and there are no dependent loops.
- Immediately after the drainage system is connected, tell him to take a deep breath, hold it momentarily, and slowly exhale to assist drainage of the pleural space and lung reexpansion.
- A portable chest X-ray is done to check tube position.
- Check patient's vital signs every 15 minutes for 1 hour, then as indicated.
- Auscultate his lungs at least every 4 hours following the procedure to assess air exchange in the affected lung.

⚡ **WARNING** *Diminished or absent breath sounds indicate that the lung hasn't reexpanded.*

- Monitor and record the drainage in the drainage collection chamber.

SPECIAL CONSIDERATIONS

- Clamping the chest tube isn't recommended because of the risk of tension pneumothorax.
- During patient transport, keep the thoracic drainage system below chest level.

▣ **TROUBLESHOOTER** *If the chest tube comes out, cover the site immediately with 4″ × 4″ gauze pads and tape in place. Stay with the patient, and monitor vital signs every 10 minutes. Look for signs and symptoms of tension pneumothorax (hypotension, distended jugular veins, absent breath sounds, tracheal shift, hypoxemia, weak and rapid pulse, dyspnea, tachypnea, diaphoresis, chest pain). Have another staff member notify the physician and gather equipment needed to reinsert tube.*

- Place the rubber-tipped clamps at bedside.

▣ **TROUBLESHOOTER** *If the drainage system cracks, or a tube disconnects, clamp the chest tube as close to the insertion site as possible.*

⚡ **WARNING** *No air or liquid can escape from the pleural space while the tube is clamped, observe the patient closely for signs and symptoms*

of tension pneumothorax while clamp is in place.

- The tube may be clamped with the large, smooth, rubber-tipped clamps for several hours before removal.
- As an alternative to clamping the tube, submerge the distal end in a container of normal saline solution to create a temporary water seal while you replace the drainage system. Follow facility policy.
- Look for signs and symptoms of respiratory distress, an indication that air or fluid remains trapped in the pleural space.
- Chest tubes are usually removed within 7 days to prevent infection. (See *Removing a chest tube.*)

COMPLICATIONS
None known

PATIENT TEACHING

- Explain the procedure to the patient and answer any questions.
- Instruct him to report increased pain or increased or sudden dyspnea.

DOCUMENTATION

- Document the date and time of chest tube insertion.
- Note the insertion site.
- Indicate the drainage system used.
- Report the presence of drainage and bubbling.
- Record vital signs.
- Note auscultation findings.

SELECTED REFERENCES
Allibone, L. "Nursing Management of Chest Drains," *Nursing Standard* 17(22):45-54, February 2003.
Coughlin, A.M., and Parchinsky, C. "Go With the Flow of Chest Tube Therapy," *Nursing* 36(3):36-41, March 2006.
Giacomini, M., et al. "How to Avoid and Manage a Pneumothorax," *Journal of Vascular Access* 7(1):7-14, January-March 2006.
Roman, M., and Mercado, D. "Review of Chest Tube Use," *Medsurg Nursing* 15(1):41-43, February 2006.

Removing a chest tube

After the patient's lung has reexpanded, you may assist the physician in removing a chest tube. First, check vital signs and perform a respiratory assessment. After explaining the procedure, give an analgesic, as ordered, 30 minutes before tube removal. Then follow these steps:

- Place him in semi-Fowler's position or on unaffected side.
- Place a linen-saver pad under the affected side.
- Put on clean gloves, remove chest tube dressings — being careful not to dislodge the chest tube, and discard soiled dressings.
- The physician holds the chest tube in place with sterile forceps, and cuts the suture anchoring the tube.
- Make sure the chest tube is securely clamped, then instruct the patient to perform Valsalva's maneuver by exhaling fully and bearing down. Valsalva's maneuver effectively increases intrathoracic pressure.

- The physician holds an airtight dressing, usually petroleum gauze, so he can cover the insertion site immediately after removing the tube.
- After the tube is removed and the site is covered, secure the dressing with tape. Cover the dressing completely to make it as airtight as possible.
- Dispose of the chest tube, soiled gloves, and equipment according to facility policy.
- Check vital signs as ordered, and assess depth and quality of respirations. Assess carefully for signs and symptoms of pneumothorax, subcutaneous emphysema, or infection.

Clavicle strap

OVERVIEW

DESCRIPTION

- A clavicle strap, or figure-eight strap, reduces and immobilizes fractures of the clavicle by elevating, extending, and supporting the shoulders in position for healing, known as the position of attention.
- A commercially available figure-eight strap or a 4″ elastic bandage may serve as a clavicle strap. (See *Types of clavicle straps*.)

CONTRAINDICATIONS

- Uncooperative patient

EQUIPMENT

Powder or cornstarch ◆ figure-eight clavicle strap or 4″ elastic bandage ◆ safety pins (optional) ◆ tape ◆ cotton batting or padding ◆ marking pen ◆ analgesics, as ordered ◆ scissors (optional)

KEY STEPS

- Confirm the patient's identity using two patient identifiers according to facility policy.
- Explain the procedure to the patient and provide privacy.
- Help the patient take off his shirt or cut the shirt off if movement is too painful.
- Assess neurovascular integrity by:
  - palpating skin temperature
  - noting the color of the hand and fingers
  - palpating the radial, ulnar, and brachial pulses bilaterally
  - comparing the affected side with the unaffected side.
- Ask the patient about numbness or tingling distal to the injury, and assess his motor function.
- Ask the patient if he's comfortable and give analgesics, as ordered.
- Show the patient how to assume the position of attention.
- Tell the patient to sit upright gradually to minimize pain.
- Apply powder, as needed, to the axillae and shoulder area to reduce friction.
- Use cornstarch if the patient is allergic to powder.

APPLYING A FIGURE-EIGHT STRAP

- Place the apex of the triangle between the scapulae and drape the straps over his shoulders.
- Bring the strap with the Velcro or buckle end under one axilla and through the loop and pull the other strap under the other axilla and through the loop.
- Gently adjust straps so they support the shoulders in the position of attention.
- Bring the straps back under the axillae toward the anterior chest, making sure they maintain the position of attention.

APPLYING A 4″ ELASTIC BANDAGE

- Roll both ends of the elastic bandage toward the middle, leaving between 12″ and 18″ (30.5 to 45.5 cm) unrolled.
- Place the unrolled portion diagonally across the patient's back, from the right shoulder to the left axilla.
- Bring the lower end of the bandage under the left axilla and back over the left shoulder, and loop the upper end over the right shoulder and under the axilla.
- Pull the two ends together snugly at the center of the back so the bandage supports the position of attention.

COMPLETING A FIGURE-EIGHT STRAP OR ELASTIC BANDAGE

- Secure the ends using safety pins, Velcro pads, or a buckle, depending on the equipment.
- Make sure a buckle or any sharp edges face away from the skin.
- Tape the secured ends to the underlying strap or bandage.
- Place cotton batting or padding under the straps as well as under the buckle or pins, to avoid skin irritation.
- Use a pen to mark the strap at the site of the loop of the figure-eight strap or the site where the elastic bandage crosses on the patient's back.
- If the strap loosens, marking the strap helps you tighten it to the original position.
- Assess neurovascular integrity, which may be impaired by a strap that's too tight.

WARNING *If neurovascular integrity is compromised when the strap is correctly applied, notify the physician. He may want to change the treatment.*

SPECIAL CONSIDERATIONS

◆ If possible, perform the procedure with the patient standing.
◆ Standing may not be feasible because the pain from the fracture can cause syncope.
◆ If the patient can't stand, have him sit upright.
◆ The adult with a clavicle strap made from an elastic bandage may require a triangular sling to help support the weight of the arm, enhance immobilization, and reduce pain.

⚘ **AGE FACTOR** *For the small child or confused adult, a well-molded plaster jacket is needed to ensure immobilization. Inadequate immobilization can cause improper healing.*

◆ For the hospitalized patient, monitor the position of the strap by checking the pen markings every 8 hours.
◆ Assess neurovascular integrity.
◆ Clavicle straps are typically worn for 4 to 8 weeks.

COMPLICATIONS
None known

PATIENT TEACHING

◆ Tell the patient not to remove the clavicle strap.
◆ Explain that, with help, the patient can maintain proper hygiene by lifting segments of the strap to remove the cotton and by washing and powdering the skin daily.
◆ Explain to the patient that fresh cotton should be applied after cleaning.
◆ Teach the patient how to assess his own neurovascular integrity and to recognize symptoms and report them promptly to the physician.

DOCUMENTATION

◆ Record information in the appropriate section of the emergency department sheet or in your notes.
◆ Record the date and time of strap application.
◆ Note the type of clavicle strap used.
◆ Document the use of powder and padding.
◆ Describe the bilateral neurovascular integrity before and after the procedure.
◆ Note instructions to the patient.

SELECTED REFERENCES
Beals, R.K., and Sauser, D.D. "Nontraumatic Disorders of the Clavicle," *Journal of the American Academy of Orthopaedic Surgeons* 14(4):205-14, April 2006.
Lazarides, S., and Zafiropoulos, G. "Conservative Treatment of Fractures at the Middle Third of the Clavicle: The Relevance of Shortening and Clinical Outcome," *Journal of Shoulder and Elbow Surgery* 15(2):191-94, March-April 2006.
Meyer, D.C., and Hertel, R. "Prevention of Pressure-Induced Skin Ischemia and Impending Skin Penetration in a Displaced Clavicle Fracture," *Orthopedics* 28(10):1151-152, October 2005.

Types of clavicle straps

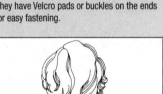

Clavicle straps provide support to the shoulder to help heal a fractured clavicle. These straps are available ready-made. They can also be created from a bandage.

Commercially made clavicle straps have a short back panel and long straps that extend around the patient's shoulders and axillae. They have Velcro pads or buckles on the ends for easy fastening.

When making a clavicle strap with a wide elastic bandage, start in the middle of the patient's back. After wrapping the bandage around the shoulders, fasten the ends with safety pins.

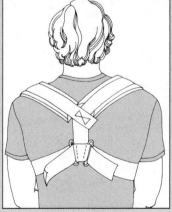
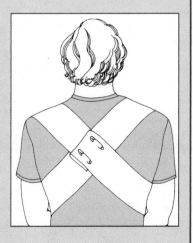

Clinitron therapy bed

OVERVIEW

DESCRIPTION

◆ The Clinitron bed was originally designed for managing burns; now it's used for the patient with various debilities.

◆ It promotes comfort and healing by allowing harmless contact between the bed's surface and grafted sites.

◆ It's actually a large tub that supports the patient on a thick layer of silicone-coated microspheres of lime glass. (See *A look at the Clinitron therapy bed.*)

◆ A monofilament polyester filter sheet covers the microsphere-filled tub.

◆ Warmed air, propelled by a blower beneath the bed, passes through the sheet.

◆ The bed reduces pressure on the skin to avoid obstructing capillary blood flow, prevent pressure ulcers, and promote wound healing.

◆ The bed's air temperature can be adjusted to help control hypothermia and hyperthermia.

CONTRAINDICATIONS

◆ The patient with an unstable spine

◆ The patient unable to mobilize and expel pulmonary secretions (because lack of back support impairs productive coughing)

EQUIPMENT

Clinitron therapy bed with microspheres (about 1,650 lb [748 kg]) ◆ filter sheet ◆ six aluminum rails (for restraining and sealing filter sheet) ◆ flat sheet ◆ elastic cord

PREPARATION

◆ A manufacturer's representative or trained staff member should prepare the bed.

◆ During preparation, make sure the microspheres reach to within ½″ (1.3 cm) of the top of the tank.

◆ Position the filter sheet on the bed with printed side up.

◆ Match the holes in the sheet to the holes in the edge of the bed's frame.

◆ Place the aluminum rails on the frame, with the studs in the proper holes.

◆ Depress the rails firmly and secure them by tightening the knurled knobs to seal the filter sheet.

◆ Place a flat sheet over the filter sheet and secure it with the elastic cord.

◆ Turn on the air current to activate microspheres and ensure the bed is working properly, and then turn it off.

KEY STEPS

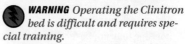 **WARNING** *Operating the Clinitron bed is difficult and requires special training.*

◆ With the help of several coworkers, transfer the patient to the bed using a lift sheet.

◆ Turn on the air pressure to activate the bed and adjust temperature as necessary.

◆ Set the room temperature to 75° F (23.9° C); the bed operates within 10° to 12° F (5.5° to 6.6° C) of ambient air temperature.

◆ If the microsphere temperature reaches 105° F (40.6° C), the bed automatically shuts off, and restarts after 30 minutes.

A look at the Clinitron therapy bed

This tub-shaped bed filled with microspheres suspended by air pressure gives the patient fluidlike support. The bed provides advantages of flotation without disadvantages of instability, patient positioning difficulties, and immobility.

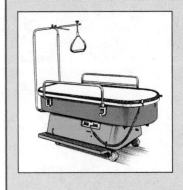

- Monitor fluid and electrolytes; the bed increases evaporative water loss.
- If the patient has excessive upper respiratory tract dryness, use a humidifier and mask, as ordered.
- Encourage coughing and deep breathing.
- After prolonged use of the bed, watch for hypocalcemia and hypophosphoremia.
- To position a bedpan, roll him away from you, place the bedpan on the flat sheet, push it into the microspheres, and reposition the patient.
- To remove the bedpan, hold it steady and roll him away from you, turn off the air pressure and remove the bedpan, then turn the air pressure on and reposition the patient.
- Don't wear a watch when handling microspheres; it can damage the mechanism.
- Don't secure the filter sheet with pins or clamps; they may puncture the sheet and release microspheres.
- Take care to avoid puncturing the bed when giving injections.
- Holes or tears may be repaired with iron-on patching tape.
- Sieve the microspheres monthly or between patients to remove clumped microspheres.
- Handle microspheres carefully to avoid spills, which may cause falls.
- Treat a soiled filter sheet and clumped microspheres as contaminated items, and handle according to policy.
- Assess the patient's skin and reposition him every 2 hours. If the patient is at risk for skin breakdown, consider using an air therapy bed as an alternative. (See *Air therapy bed*.)
- Specialty beds don't eliminate the need for frequent assessment and position changes.

COMPLICATIONS
None known

- Explain to the patient, and demonstrate if possible, how the bed works.
- Tell the patient why it's used and that he'll feel as though he's floating.

- Record the duration of therapy and the patient's response to it.
- Document the condition of the patient's skin, pressure ulcers, and other wounds.

SELECTED REFERENCES
Barillo, D.J., et al. "Tracking the Daily Availability of Burn Beds for National Emergencies," *Journal of Burn Care and Rehabilitation* 26(2):174-82, March-April 2005.

Hickerson, W.L., et al. "Comparison of Total Body Tissue Interface Pressure of Specialized Pressure-Relieving Mattresses," *Journal of Long-Term Effects of Medical Implants* 14(2):81-94, 2004.

Air therapy bed

Patients at risk for skin breakdown may benefit from an air therapy bed without the microspheres as an alternative to the Clinitron bed. This type of bed has air-filled compartments that can be inflated to varying degrees, providing different levels of support to different body parts.

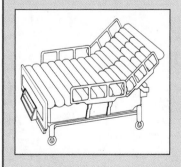

Closed-wound drain management

DESCRIPTION

- Promotes healing and prevents swelling by suctioning serosanguineous fluid that accumulates at the wound site.
- It's typically inserted during surgery in anticipation of substantial postoperative drainage.
- It reduces the risk of infection and skin breakdown and frequency of dressing changes by removing postoperative fluid.
- Hemovac and Jackson-Pratt closed drainage systems are most commonly used.
- The system consists of perforated tubing connected to a portable vacuum unit.
- The distal end of the tubing lies inside the wound and usually exits the body from a site other than the primary suture line, to preserve integrity of the surgical wound.
- The drain is usually sutured to the skin and the tubing exit site is treated as an additional surgical wound.
- If the wound produces heavy drainage, the closed-wound drain may be left in place for longer than 1 week.

- Drainage must be emptied and measured frequently to maintain maximum suction and prevent strain on the suture line.

CONTRAINDICATIONS
None known

EQUIPMENT

Graduated biohazard cylinder ◆ sterile laboratory container, if needed ◆ alcohol pads ◆ gloves ◆ gown ◆ face shield ◆ trash bag ◆ sterile gauze pads ◆ antiseptic cleaning agent ◆ prepackaged povidone-iodine swabs ◆ label (optional)

KEY STEPS

- Check the physician's order and assess the patient's condition.
- Confirm the patient's identity using two patient identifiers according to facility policy.
- Explain the procedure, provide privacy, and wash your hands.
- Unclip the vacuum unit from the patient's bed or gown.
- Using aseptic technique, release the vacuum by removing the spout plug on the collection chamber.
- The container expands completely as it draws in air.
- Empty the unit's contents into a graduated biohazard cylinder, and note the amount and appearance of drainage.
- If diagnostic tests will be performed on the specimen, pour the drainage directly into a sterile laboratory container, note amount and appearance, label the specimen pad, and send it to the laboratory.
- Clean the unit's spout and plug with an alcohol pad using aseptic technique.
- To reestablish the vacuum that creates the drain's suction power, fully compress the vacuum unit.

Using a closed-wound drainage system

This system draws drainage from a wound site, such as the chest wall postmastectomy shown at left, by means of a Y-tube. To empty the drainage, remove plug and empty into a graduated cylinder. To reestablish suction, compress the drainage unit against a firm surface to expel air and, while holding it down, replace the plug, as shown. The same principle is used for the Jackson-Pratt bulb drain, shown here (far right).

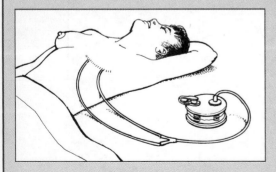
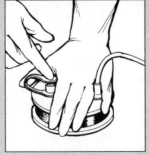
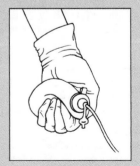

- Compress the unit with one hand to maintain the vacuum and replace the spout plug. (See *Using a closed-wound drainage system.*)
- Check the patency of equipment.
- Make sure the tubing is free from twists, kinks, and leaks; the drainage system must be airtight to work properly.
- The vacuum unit should remain compressed when you release the manual pressure.

  TROUBLESHOOTER *If rapid reinflation occurs, indicating an air leak, recompress the unit and resecure the spout plug.*
- Fasten the vacuum unit to the patient's gown below wound level to promote drainage.
- To prevent dislodgment, don't apply tension on drainage tubing when fastening the unit.
- Remove and discard gloves and wash your hands.
- Check the sutures that secure the drain to the patient's skin.
- Look for signs of pulling or tearing and swelling or infection.
- Gently clean the sutures with sterile gauze pads soaked in an antiseptic cleaning agent or with a povidone-iodine swab.
- Properly dispose of drainage, solutions, and trash bag, and clean or dispose of soiled equipment and supplies according to facility policy.

SPECIAL CONSIDERATIONS

- Empty drain and measure contents once during each shift, more often if drainage is excessive.
- Removing excess drainage maintains maximum suction and avoids straining the drain's suture line.
- Empty and measure before the patient ambulates to prevent the weight of the drainage from pulling on the drain.

  WARNING *Be careful not to mistake chest tubes for closed-wound drains because the vacuum of a chest tube should never be released.*

COMPLICATIONS
- Reduction or obstruction of drainage (due to occlusion of tubing by fibrin, clots, or other particles)

PATIENT TEACHING

- Explain the procedure to the patient and answer any questions.
- If the patient will be discharged with the drain in place, teach her and her caregivers how to drain the pump.

DOCUMENTATION

- Record the date and time when you empty the drain.
- Describe the appearance of the drain site.
- Note the presence of swelling or signs of infection.
- Document equipment malfunction and nursing action.
- Note the patient's tolerance of the treatment.
- Record drainage color, consistency, type, and amount on the input and output sheet.
- If there's more than one closed-wound drain, number the drains and record the information above separately for each drainage site.

SELECTED REFERENCES
Langer, S., et al. "Does Fibrin Sealant Reduce Drain Output and Allow Earlier Removal of Drainage Catheters in Women Undergoing Operation for Breast Cancer?" *American Surgeon* 69(1):77-81, January 2003.

Parker, M.J., et al. "Closed Suction Drainage for Hip and Knee Arthroplasty. A Meta-analysis," *Journal of Bone and Joint Surgery* 86-A(6):1146-152, June 2004.

Reid, R.R., and Dumanian, G.A. "A Minimalist Approach to the Care of the Indwelling Closed Suction Drain: A Prospective Analysis of Local Wound Complications," *Annals of Plastic Surgery* 51(6):575-78, December 2003.

Code management

DESCRIPTION

- Goals of a code are to restore the patient's spontaneous heartbeat and respirations and prevent hypoxic damage to the brain and other vital organs.
- A team approach is required; it should include health care workers trained in advanced cardiac life support (ACLS) or, at least, basic life support (BLS).
- The ACLS course, sponsored by the American Heart Association, incorporates BLS skills with advanced resuscitation techniques.
- ACLS-trained nurses usually provide first resuscitative efforts to cardiac arrest patients, giving cardiac drugs and defibrillating before the physician's arrival.
- Ventricular fibrillation commonly precedes sudden cardiac arrest; initial resuscitative efforts involve rapid recognition of arrhythmias and defibrillation, as needed.
- If monitoring equipment isn't available, only perform BLS measures.

WARNING The scope of your responsibilities depends on facility policies and procedures and your state's nurse practice act.

- A code may be called for the patients with an absent pulse, apnea, ventricular fibrillation, ventricular tachycardia, and asystole.

CONTRAINDICATIONS

- Do-not-resuscitate (DNR) order

EQUIPMENT

Oral, nasal, and endotracheal (ET) airways ◆ one-way valve masks ◆ oxygen source ◆ oxygen flowmeter ◆ intubation supplies ◆ handheld resuscitation bag ◆ suction supplies ◆ nasogastric (NG) tube ◆ goggles, masks, and gloves ◆ cardiac arrest board ◆ peripheral I.V. supplies: 16G, 18G, and 20G peripheral I.V. catheters ◆ central I.V. supplies, including an 18G thin-wall catheter, a 6-cm needle catheter, and a 16G 15- to

20-cm catheter ◆ I.V. administration sets (including microdrip and minidrip) ◆ I.V. fluids, including dextrose 5% in water (D_5W), normal saline solution, and lactated Ringer's solution ◆ electrocardiogram (ECG) monitor and leads ◆ cardioverter-defibrillator ◆ conductive medium ◆ cardiac drugs: adenosine, amiodarone, atropine, calcium chloride, dobutamine, dopamine, epinephrine, isoproterenol, lidocaine, procainamide, and vasopressin ◆ transthoracic pacemaker, percutaneous transvenous pacer, cricothyrotomy kit, and end-tidal carbon dioxide detector (optional)

PREPARATION

- Personnel and equipment must be ready for a code at any time.
- Familiarize yourself with the cardiac drugs you may have to give.

AGE FACTOR Pediatric equipment use is based on weight and size of the patient. Some facilities have equipment for infants and children in color-coded bags or similar arrangements using color-coded resuscitation tape (Broselow tape). This simplifies the selection of appropriate equipment for an infant or child.

- Be aware of your patient's code status as defined by physician's orders, patient's advance directives, and family wishes.
- If physician has ordered a DNR, make sure he has written and signed the order; if possible, have the patient or a family member co-sign the order.

KEY STEPS

- If you're first to arrive at the site of a code, assess the patient's level of consciousness (LOC).
- Call for help, assess airway, breathing, and circulation; begin cardiopulmonary resuscitation (CPR) as needed.
- Use a pocket mask to ventilate the patient.
- When a second BLS provider arrives, have them call a code and retrieve emergency equipment.

- When emergency equipment arrives, have the second BLS provider place the cardiac arrest board under the patient and assist with two-person CPR.
- If possible, get the patient's medical history and description of events leading to cardiac arrest from his nurse.
- A third person, either a BLS certified nurse or respiratory therapist, will attach the handheld resuscitation bag to the oxygen source and begin to ventilate the patient with 100% oxygen.
- When an ACLS-trained nurse arrives, she'll expose the patient's chest and apply defibrillator pads.
- The ACLS-trained nurse will apply the paddles to his chest to obtain a "quick look" at his cardiac rhythm.
- If he's in ventricular fibrillation, ACLS protocol calls for defibrillation as soon as possible.
- The ACLS-trained nurse acts as code leader until the physician arrives.
- If not already in place, apply ECG electrodes and attach them to the defibrillator's cardiac monitor.
- Avoid placing electrodes on bony prominences or hairy areas.
- Avoid areas where defibrillator pads will be placed and where chest compressions will be given.
- As CPR continues, you or an ACLS-trained nurse will start two peripheral I.V. lines with large-bore I.V. catheters.

WARNING Use only a large vein, such as the antecubital vein, to allow for rapid fluid administration and prevent drug extravasation.

- As soon as the I.V. catheter is in place, begin an infusion of normal saline solution to help prevent circulatory collapse.

WARNING D_5W is acceptable, but the latest ACLS guidelines encourage using normal saline solution because D_5W can produce hyperglycemic effects during cardiac arrest.

- While one nurse starts the I.V. lines, the other sets up portable or wall suction equipment and suctions the oral secretions to maintain an open airway.

- The ACLS-trained nurse prepares and gives emergency cardiac drugs, as needed.
- Drugs given through a central line reach the myocardium quicker than drugs given through a peripheral line.
- If the patient doesn't have an accessible I.V. line, give drugs such as epinephrine, lidocaine, and atropine through an ET tube. To do so, dilute the drugs in 10 ml of normal saline solution or sterile water, and then instill them into the patient's ET tube.
- Ventilate the patient manually to improve absorption by distributing the drug throughout the bronchial tree.
- The ACLS-trained nurse also prepares, and assists with, ET intubation.

WARNING *During intubation, don't interrupt CPR longer than 30 seconds.*

- Suction the patient as needed.
- After he has been intubated, assess his breath sounds to ensure proper tube placement.
- If he has diminished or absent breath sounds over the left lung field, the physician will pull back the ET tube slightly and reassess.
- When the tube is correctly positioned, tape it securely.
- As a reference, mark the point on the tube that's level with the patient's lips.
- Throughout the code, check the carotid or femoral pulses before and after each defibrillation.
- Check pulses frequently during the code to evaluate the effectiveness of cardiac compressions.
- Other members of the code team should keep a written record of events.
- If the family is at the facility during the code, have someone, such as a clergy member or social worker, remain with them.
- Keep the family informed of patient's status; if they aren't at the facility, contact them as soon as possible.

SPECIAL CONSIDERATIONS

- When the patient's condition has stabilized, assess his LOC, breath sounds, heart sounds, peripheral perfusion, bowel sounds, and urine output.
- Take the patient's vital signs every 15 minutes, and monitor cardiac rhythm continuously.
- Make sure the patient receives adequate oxygen through a mask or ventilator.
- Check the infusion rates of all I.V. fluids; use infusion pumps to give vasoactive drugs.
- To check fluid therapy effectiveness, insert an indwelling catheter if the patient doesn't already have one.
- Insert an NG tube to relieve or prevent gastric distention.
- Reassure the patient and explain what's happening, if appropriate.
- Allow his family to visit as soon as possible.
- If the patient dies, notify the family and let them see him as soon as possible.
- To make sure your code team performs optimally, schedule a time to review the code.

COMPLICATIONS
- Fractured ribs, liver laceration, lung puncture, and gastric distention
- Electric shock caused by defibrillation
- Esophageal or tracheal laceration, subcutaneous emphysema, or accidental right mainstem bronchus intubation (due to emergency intubation)

PATIENT TEACHING

None

DOCUMENTATION

- Document events in as much detail as possible.
- Note whether the arrest was witnessed or unwitnessed, time of the arrest, time CPR was begun, time the ACLS-trained nurse arrived, and total resuscitation time.
- Document the number of defibrillations, times performed, joule level, patient's cardiac rhythm before and after defibrillation, and if the patient had a pulse.
- Document drug therapy, including dosages, routes of administration, and patient response.
- Record procedures, such as peripheral and central line insertion, pacemaker insertion, and ET tube insertion with the time performed and the patient's tolerance.
- Keep track of all arterial blood gas results.
- Record if the patient was transferred to another unit or facility along with his condition at the time of transfer and whether his family was notified.
- Document complications and corrective measures.
- When documentation is complete, have the physician and ACLS nurse review and sign.

SELECTED REFERENCES

Heath, J., et al. "Critical Care Providers' Perception of the Use of Vasopressin in Cardiac Arrest," *American Journal of Critical Care* 14(6):481-92, November 2005.

Marett, B.E. "American Heart Association Releases New Guidelines," *Journal of Emergency Nursing* 32(1):63-64, February 2006.

Scholle, C.C., and Mininni, N.C. "Best-Practice Interventions: How a Rapid Response Team Saves Lives," *Nursing* 36(1):36-40, January 2006.

Strzyzewski, N. "Common Errors Made in Resuscitation of Respiratory and Cardiac Arrest," *Plastic Surgical Nursing* 26(1):10-14, January-March 2006.

Weil, M.H., and Fries, M. "In-hospital Cardiac Arrest," *Critical Care Medicine* 33(12):2825-830, December 2005.

Cold application

DESCRIPTION

- Cold constricts blood vessels; inhibits local circulation, suppuration, and tissue metabolism; relieves vascular congestion; slows bacterial activity in infections; reduces body temperature; and acts as temporary anesthetic during brief, painful procedures. (See *Reducing pain with ice massage.*)
- Cold relieves inflammation, reduces edema, and slows bleeding; may provide effective initial treatment after eye injuries, strains, sprains, bruises, muscle spasms, and burns.
- Cold doesn't reduce existing edema because it inhibits the reabsorption of excess fluid.
- Cold may be applied in dry or moist forms, but ice shouldn't be placed directly on the skin because it may damage tissue.
- Moist application is more penetrating than dry because moisture facilitates conduction.
- Devices for applying cold include an ice bag or collar, K pad (which can produce cold or heat), and chemical cold packs.
- Devices for applying moist cold include cold compresses for small body areas and cold packs for large areas.
- **AGE FACTOR** *Apply cautiously on patients with impaired circulation, on children, and on elderly or arthritic patients because of ischemic tissue damage risk.*

CONTRAINDICATIONS

None known

EQUIPMENT

Patient thermometer ◆ towel ◆ adhesive tape or roller gauze ◆ gloves (optional)

ICE BAG OR COLLAR

Ice bag or collar ◆ tap water ◆ ice chips ◆ absorbent, protective cloth covering

K PAD

Device ◆ distilled water ◆ temperature-adjustment key ◆ absorbent, protective cloth covering

CHEMICAL COLD PACK

Single-use pack or reusable pack

COLD COMPRESS OR PACK

Basin of ice chips ◆ tap water ◆ bath thermometer ◆ compress material (4" × 4" gauze pads or washcloths) or pack material (towels or flannel) ◆ linen-saver pad ◆ waterproof covering

PREPARATION

Ice bag or collar

- Select a correct-sized device, fill it with tap water, and check for leaks.
- Empty the device, and then fill it halfway with crushed ice.
- Small pieces of ice help the device mold to the patient's body.
- Squeeze the device to expel air that might reduce conduction.
- Fasten the cap and wipe moisture from outside of the device.
- Wrap the bag or collar in a cloth covering and secure it with tape or roller gauze.
- The cover prevents tissue trauma and absorbs condensation.

K pad

- Check the cord for damage.

- Fill the control unit two-thirds with distilled water or to the level recommended by the manufacturer.
- **WARNING** *Don't use tap water; it leaves mineral deposits.*
- Check for leaks, then tilt the unit several times to clear the pad's tubing of air.
- Tighten the cap.
- After ensuring that hoses between the control unit and pad aren't tangled, place the unit on a bedside table, slightly above the patient so gravity can assist water flow.
- If the central supply department hasn't preset the temperature, use the temperature-adjustment key to adjust the control unit to the lowest temperature.
- Cover the pad with an absorbent, protective cloth and secure the cover with tape or roller gauze.
- Plug the unit in and turn it on.
- Allow the pad to cool for 2 minutes before placing it on the patient.

Chemical cold pack

- Select an appropriate size pack (single-use packs are lightweight, plastic packs used to apply dry cold; reusable packs are filled with an alcohol-based solution and may be stored frozen until used); follow manufacturer's directions to activate the cold-producing chemicals (some

---

Reducing pain with ice massage

Ice shouldn't be applied directly to skin because it can damage the surface and underlying tissues. However, carefully performed, this technique may help patients tolerate brief, painful procedures such as bone marrow aspiration, catheterization, chest tube removal, injection into joints, lumbar puncture, and suture removal.

Prepare by gathering the ice, a porous covering to hold it in (if desired), and a cloth for wiping water as ice melts. Water may be frozen in a paper cup ahead of time. Remove one-half the cup, exposing the ice.

Before starting the procedure, rub the ice over the appropriate area to numb it. Assess

the site frequently; stop immediately if you detect signs of tissue intolerance.

As the procedure begins, rub the ice on a point near the site. This distracts the patient from the procedure and gives another stimulus to concentrate on.

If the procedure is longer than 10 minutes, or you think tissue damage may occur, move the ice to a different site and continue.

If you know in advance that the procedure will last longer than 10 minutes, massage the site intermittently (2 minutes of massage alternating with a rest period) until skin regains normal color. You can also divide the area into several sites and apply ice to each one for several minutes.

are activated by striking, squeezing, or kneading).
- Make certain the container hasn't been broken during activation.
- Wrap the pack in a cloth cover; secure the cover with tape or roller gauze.

Cold compress or pack
- Cool a container of tap water by adding ice or putting it in a basin of ice.
- Using a bath thermometer for guidance, adjust the water temperature to 59° F (15° C) or as ordered.
- Immerse the compress material or pack material in the water.

KEY STEPS

- Check the physician's order and assess the patient.
- Confirm the patient's identity using two patient identifiers according to facility policy.
- Explain the procedure, provide privacy, and make sure the room is warm and free of drafts.
- Wash your hands.
- Record the patient's temperature, pulse, and respirations to serve as baseline.
- Expose only the treatment site to avoid chilling the patient.

APPLYING AN ICE BAG OR COLLAR, A K PAD, OR A CHEMICAL COLD PACK
- Place the covered device on the treatment site and time the application.
- **WARNING** *Watch for signs of tissue intolerance, such as blanching, mottling, cyanosis, maceration, or blisters. Be alert for shivering and complaints of burning or numbness. If these signs or symptoms develop, discontinue and notify the physician.*
- Refill or replace the cold device as necessary to maintain correct temperature.
- Change the protective cover if it becomes wet.
- Remove the device after the prescribed treatment period (usually 30 minutes).

APPLYING A COLD COMPRESS OR PACK
- Place a linen-saver pad under the site.
- Remove the compress or pack from the water, and wring it out to stop dripping.
- Apply to the treatment site and time the application.
- Cover the compress or pack with a waterproof covering to provide insulation and keep the surrounding area dry.
- Secure the covering with tape or roller gauze to prevent slippage.
- Change the compress or pack as needed to maintain correct temperature.
- Remove after the prescribed treatment period (usually 20 minutes).

CONCLUDING ALL COLD APPLICATIONS
- Dry the patient's skin and redress treatment site according to the physician's orders.
- Position him comfortably and take his temperature, pulse, and respirations for comparison with baseline.
- Dispose of liquids and soiled materials.
- If treatment will be repeated, clean and store equipment in the patient's room; if not, return it to storage.

SPECIAL CONSIDERATIONS

- Apply cold immediately after an injury to minimize edema.
- To avoid vasodilation don't apply cold longer than one hour.
- Application of temperatures below 59° F (15° C) may cause local reflex vasodilation.
- Use sterile technique when applying cold to an open wound or lesion that may open.
- Maintain sterile technique during eye treatment, with separate sterile equipment for each eye to prevent cross-contamination.
- Avoid securing cooling devices with pins because accidental puncture could allow extremely cold fluids to leak and burn skin.

- If the patient is unconscious, anesthetized, neurologically impaired, irrational, or otherwise insensitive to cold, stay with him throughout treatment and check the application site frequently for complications.

COMPLICATIONS
- Thrombi due to hemoconcentration
- Pain, burning, or numbness due to intense cold

PATIENT TEACHING

- Warn the patient against putting ice directly on the skin; extreme cold can cause burns.

DOCUMENTATION

- Record the time, date, and duration of cold application.
- Note the type of device used.
- Note the application site.
- Record the temperature or temperature setting.
- Provide the patient's temperature, pulse, and respirations before and after application.
- Describe the patient's skin appearance before, during, and after application.
- Note the complications and patient's tolerance of treatment.

SELECTED REFERENCES
Cheing, G.L., et al. "Ice and Pulsed Electromagnetic Field to Reduce Pain and Swelling After Distal Radius Fractures," *Journal of Rehabilitation Medicine* 37(6):372-77, November 2005.

Dover, G., et al. "Cold Urticaria Following an Ice Application: A Case Study," *Clinical Journal of Sport Medicine* 14(6): 362-64, November 2004.

Howatson, G., et al. "The Efficacy of Ice Massage in the Treatment of Exercise-Induced Muscle Damage," *Scandinavian Journal of Medicine & Science in Sports* 15(6):416-22, December 2005.

Colostomy and ileostomy care

DESCRIPTION

◆ A patient with an ascending or transverse colostomy or ileostomy must wear an external pouch to collect emerging fecal matter.

◆ The external pouch also helps control odor and protect the stoma and peristomal skin.

◆ Most disposable pouching systems can be used for 2 to 7 days; some models last longer.

◆ Pouches need to be emptied when one-third to one-half full.

◆ Pouching systems need to be changed immediately if a leak develops.

◆ A patient with an ileostomy may need to empty his pouch four or five times daily.

◆ It's best to change the pouching system when the bowel is least active, usually between 2 and 4 hours after meals.

◆ After a few months, most patients can predict the best changing time.

◆ Consider which system provides the best adhesive seal and skin protection, when selecting a pouching system.

◆ Type of pouch also depends on stoma location and structure, availability of supplies, wear time, consistency of effluent, personal preference, and finances.

◆ Pouching systems may be drainable or closed-bottomed, disposable or reusable, adhesive-backed, and one- or two-piece.

CONTRAINDICATIONS

None known

Pouching system ◆ stoma measuring guide ◆ stoma paste (if drainage is watery to pasty or stoma secretes excess mucus) ◆ plastic bag ◆ washcloth and towel ◆ closure clamp ◆ toilet or bedpan ◆ water or pouch cleaning solution ◆ gloves ◆ facial tissues ◆ ostomy belt, paper tape, mild nonmoisturizing soap, skin shaving equipment, liquid skin sealant, and pouch deodorant (optional)

◆ Provide privacy and emotional support.

◆ Confirm the patient's identity using two patient identifiers according to facility policy.

FITTING THE POUCH AND SKIN BARRIER

◆ Explain the procedure to the patient.

◆ To fit a pouch with an attached skin barrier, use the stoma-measuring guide.

◆ Select the opening size that matches the stoma.

◆ To fit an adhesive-backed pouch with a separate skin barrier, measure the stoma and select the opening that matches.

◆ Trace the selected size opening onto the paper back of the skin barrier's adhesive side and cut out the opening, as needed.

◆ If the pouch has precut openings, which are handy for a round stoma, select an opening that's ⅛″ larger than the stoma.

◆ If the pouch comes without an opening, cut the hole ⅛″ wider than the measured tracing.

◆ The cut-to-fit system works best for an irregularly shaped stoma.

◆ Avoid fitting the pouch too tightly. A constrictive opening could injure the stoma or skin tissue without discomfort.

◆ Avoid cutting the opening too big; it may expose the skin to fecal matter and moisture.

◆ A patient with a descending or sigmoid colostomy who has formed stools and whose ostomy doesn't secrete much mucus may wear only a pouch. In this case, make sure the pouch opening closely matches the stoma size.

◆ Between 6 weeks and 1 year after surgery, the stoma will shrink to its permanent size. Pattern-making preparations will then be unnecessary unless the patient gains weight, has additional surgery, or injures the stoma.

APPLYING OR CHANGING THE POUCH

◆ Collect all equipment.

◆ Wash your hands and provide privacy.

◆ Explain the procedure to the patient.

◆ As you perform each step, explain what you're doing and why so the patient learns to perform the procedure.

◆ Put on gloves.

◆ Remove and discard the old pouch.

◆ Wipe the stoma and peristomal skin gently with a facial tissue.

◆ Carefully wash with mild soap and water and dry the peristomal skin by patting gently and allow the skin to dry.

◆ Inspect the peristomal skin and stoma.

◆ If necessary, shave surrounding hair away from the stoma to promote a better seal and avoid skin irritation from hair pulling against the adhesive.

◆ If applying a separate skin barrier, peel the paper backing off the prepared skin barrier, center the barrier over the stoma, and press to ensure adhesion.

◆ You may outline the stoma on the back of the skin barrier (depending on product) with a thin ring of stoma paste for extra skin protection (skip this step if he has a sigmoid or descending colostomy, formed stools, and little mucus).

◆ Remove the paper backing from the adhesive side of the pouching system, center the pouch opening over the stoma, and press gently to secure.

- For a pouching system with flanges, align the lip of the pouch flange with the bottom edge of the skin barrier flange.
- Gently press around the circumference of the pouch flange, beginning at the bottom, until the pouch adheres to the barrier flange (the pouch will click into secured position).
- Holding the barrier against the skin, pull on the pouch to confirm the seal.
- Have him stay still for about 5 minutes to improve adherence.
- Body warmth also helps improve adherence and soften a rigid skin barrier.
- Attach an ostomy belt to further secure the pouch, if desired. Some pouches have belt loops; others have plastic adapters for belts.
- Leave some air in the pouch to allow drainage to fall to the bottom.
- Apply the closure clamp, if necessary.
- If desired, apply paper tape to the pouch edges for additional security.

EMPTYING THE POUCH

- Put on gloves.
- Tilt the bottom of the pouch upward and remove the closure clamp.
- Turn up a cuff on the lower end of the pouch and allow it to drain into the toilet or bedpan.
- Wipe the bottom of the pouch and reapply the closure clamp.
- The bottom part of the pouch may be rinsed with water.
  - **WARNING** *Don't aim water near the top of the pouch because this may loosen the seal on the skin.*
- A two-piece flanged system can also be emptied by unsnapping the pouch.
- Let drainage flow into the toilet.
- Release flatus through the gas release valve if the pouch has one, or release flatus by tilting the pouch bottom upward, releasing the clamp, and expelling the flatus.
- To release flatus from a flanged system, loosen the seal between the flanges.
  - **WARNING** *Never make a pinhole in a pouch to release gas. This destroys the odor-proof seal.*
- Remove gloves.

SPECIAL CONSIDERATIONS

- Use adhesive solvents and removers only after patch-testing his skin; some products may irritate the skin or cause hypersensitivity.
- Consider using a liquid skin sealant, if available, to give skin tissue additional protection from drainage and adhesive irritants.
- Remove the pouching system if the patient reports burning or itching or purulent drainage around the stoma.
  - **WARNING** *Notify the physician or therapist of skin irritation, breakdown, rash, or unusual appearance of the stoma or peristomal area.*
- Most pouches are odor-free; odor should only be evident when you empty the pouch or if it leaks.
- Use commercial pouch deodorants, if desired.
- If he wears a reusable pouching system, suggest that he get two or more systems so he can wear one while the other dries after cleaning.

COMPLICATIONS

- Injury to the stoma (due to failure to fit the pouch properly or improper use of a belt)
- Allergic reaction to adhesives and other ostomy products

PATIENT TEACHING

- After performing and explaining the procedure, teach the patient self-care.
- Before discharge, suggest that the patient avoid odor-causing foods, such as fish, eggs, onions, and garlic.

DOCUMENTATION

- Record the date and time of the pouching system change.
- Note the character of the drainage, including color, amount, type, and consistency.
- Describe the appearance of the stoma and peristomal skin.
- Document patient teaching.
- Describe the teaching content.
- Record the patient's response to self-care, and evaluate his learning progress.

SELECTED REFERENCES

Berg, K., and Seidler, H. "Randomized Crossover Comparison of Adhesively Coupled Colostomy Pouching Systems," *Ostomy/Wound Management* 51(3):30-32, 34, 36, March 2005.

Cronin, E. "Best Practice in Discharging Patients With a Stoma," *Nursing Times* 101(47):67-68, November 2005.

Notter, J., and Burnard, P. "Preparing for Loop Ileostomy Surgery: Women's Accounts From a Qualitative Study," *International Journal of Nursing Studies* 43(2):147-59, February 2006.

Palmieri, B., et al. "The Anal Bag: A Modern Approach to Fecal Incontinence Management," *Ostomy/Wound Management* 51(12):44-52, December 2005.

Ratliff, C.R., et al. "Descriptive Study of Peristomal Complications," *Journal of Wound, Ostomy, and Continence Nursing* 32(1):33-37, January-February 2005.

Colostomy irrigation

DESCRIPTION

◆ Irrigation allows the patient with a descending or sigmoid colostomy to regulate bowel function and cleans the large bowel before and after tests, surgery, or other procedures.

◆ Irrigation may begin as soon as bowel function resumes after surgery.

◆ It may be advisable to wait until bowel movements are more predictable before beginning colostomy irrigation.

◆ The nurse or patient initially irrigates the colostomy at the same time every day, recording amount of output and any spillage between irrigations.

◆ After 4 to 6 weeks a predictable elimination pattern is established.

CONTRAINDICATIONS
None known

Colostomy irrigation set (contains irrigation drain or sleeve, ostomy belt [if needed] to secure drain or sleeve, water-soluble lubricant, drainage pouch clamp, irrigation bag with clamp, tubing, and cone tip) ◆ 1,000 ml of tap water irrigant warmed to about 100° F (37.8° C) ◆ normal saline solution (for cleansing enemas) ◆ I.V. pole or wall hook ◆ washcloth and towel ◆ water ◆ ostomy pouching system ◆ linen-saver pad ◆ gloves ◆ bedpan or chair, mild nonmoisturizing soap, rubber band or clip, small dressing or bandage, and stoma cap (optional)

PREPARATION

◆ Depending on patient's condition, colostomy irrigation may be performed in bed using a bedpan or in the bathroom using a chair and the toilet.

◆ Set up irrigation bag with tubing and cone tip.

◆ If irrigation is done with him in bed, place a bedpan beside the bed and elevate the head of the bed past 45 degrees, if allowed.

◆ If irrigation is done in the bathroom, have the patient sit on the toilet or on a chair facing the toilet, whichever is more comfortable.

◆ Fill the irrigation bag with warm tap water (or normal saline solution, if the irrigation is for bowel cleaning).

◆ Hang the bag on the I.V. pole or wall hook.

◆ The bottom of the bag should be at his shoulder level to prevent fluid from entering the bowel too quickly.

◆ Most irrigation sets also have a clamp that regulates flow rate.

◆ Prime the tubing with irrigant to prevent air from entering the colon and possibly causing cramps and gas pains.

◆ Provide privacy and wash your hands.

◆ Confirm the patient's identity using two patient identifiers according to facility policy.

◆ Explain the procedure to the patient.

◆ If the patient is in bed, place a linen-saver pad under him to protect the sheets.

◆ Put on gloves.

◆ Remove the ostomy pouch if he uses one.

◆ Place the irrigation sleeve over the stoma.

◆ If the sleeve doesn't have an adhesive backing, secure the sleeve with an ostomy belt.

◆ If he has a two-piece pouching system with flanges, snap off the pouch and save it.

◆ Snap on the irrigation sleeve.

◆ Place the open-ended bottom of the irrigation sleeve in the bedpan or toilet to promote drainage by gravity.

◆ If necessary, cut the sleeve so it meets the water level inside the bedpan or toilet.

◆ Effluent may splash from a short sleeve or may not drain from a long sleeve.

◆ Lubricate your gloved small finger with water-soluble lubricant and insert it into the stoma. If you're teaching the patient, have him do this to determine the bowel angle at which to insert the cone safely.

◆ Expect the stoma to tighten when the finger enters the bowel; it relaxes after a few seconds.

◆ Lubricate the cone with water-soluble lubricant to prevent it from irritating the mucosa.

◆ Gently insert the cone into the top opening of the irrigation sleeve, then into the stoma. Never force it in place.

◆ Angle the cone to match the bowel angle.

◆ Unclamp the irrigation tubing and allow the water to flow slowly.

◆ If you don't have a clamp to control the irrigant's flow rate, pinch the tubing to control the flow. The water should enter the colon over 10 to 15 minutes.

● **WARNING** *If he gets cramps, slow or stop the flow, keep the cone in place, and have him take a few deep breaths until the cramping stops. Cramping during irrigation may result from a bowel that's ready to empty, water that's too cold, a rapid flow rate, or air in the tubing.*

◆ Have him remain still for 15 to 20 minutes so the initial effluent can drain.

◆ If he's ambulatory, he can stay in the bathroom until all effluent empties, or he can clamp the bottom of the drainage sleeve with a rubber band or clip and return to bed.

◆ Explain that ambulation and activity stimulate elimination.

◆ Suggest that the nonambulatory patient lean forward or massage his abdomen to stimulate elimination.

◆ Wait about 45 minutes for the bowel to finish eliminating the irrigant and effluent, and remove the irrigation sleeve.

◆ If the irrigation was intended to clean the bowel, repeat the procedure with warmed normal saline solution until the return solution appears clear, or per facility policy.

◆ Gently clean the area around the stoma using a washcloth, mild soap, and water.

◆ Rinse and dry the area thoroughly with a clean towel.

◆ Inspect the skin and stoma for changes in appearance.

◆ Stoma color is usually dark pink to red but may change with patient's status.

◆ Notify the physician of stoma color changes because a pale hue may indicate anemia, and darkening may indicate a change in blood flow to the stoma.

◆ Apply a clean pouch.

◆ If he has a regular bowel elimination pattern, he may prefer a small dressing, bandage, or commercial stoma cap.

◆ Discard a disposable irrigation sleeve.

◆ Rinse a reusable irrigation sleeve and hang it to dry with the irrigation bag, tubing, and cone.

SPECIAL CONSIDERATIONS

◆ Irrigating a colostomy to establish a regular bowel elimination pattern doesn't work for all patients.

◆ If the bowel continues to move between irrigations, try decreasing the volume of irrigant.

● **WARNING** *Increasing the irrigant won't help; it will only stimulate peristalsis.*

◆ Keep a record of results.

◆ Also consider irrigating every other day.

◆ Irrigation may help regulate bowel function in patients with a descending or sigmoid colostomy because this is the bowel's stool storage area.

◆ A patient with an ascending or transverse colostomy won't benefit from irrigation.

◆ A patient with a descending or sigmoid colostomy who's missing part of the ascending or transverse colon may not be able to irrigate successfully because his ostomy may function like an ascending or transverse colostomy.

◆ If diarrhea develops, discontinue irrigations until stools form again.

◆ Keep in mind that irrigation alone won't achieve regularity for the patient. He must observe a complementary diet and exercise regimen.

◆ If he has a strictured stoma that prohibits cone insertion, remove the cone from the irrigation tubing and replace it with a soft silicone catheter.

◆ Angle the catheter gently 2″ to 4″ (5 to 10 cm) into the bowel to instill the irrigant.

● **WARNING** *Don't force the catheter into the stoma and don't insert it further than the recommended length because you may perforate the bowel.*

COMPLICATIONS

◆ Fluid and electrolyte imbalances may result from using too much irrigant.

PATIENT TEACHING

◆ Explain every step of the procedure to the patient so that he can perform colostomy irrigation himself.

DOCUMENTATION

◆ Record the date and time of irrigation and type and amount of irrigant.

◆ Note the stoma's color and character of drainage, including color, consistency, and amount.

◆ Report patient teaching.

◆ Describe teaching and patient response to self-care instruction.

◆ Evaluate the patient's learning progress.

SELECTED REFERENCES

Karadag, A., et al. "Colostomy Irrigation: Results of 25 Cases With Particular Reference to Quality of Life," *Journal of Clinical Nursing* 14(4):479-85, April 2005.

O'Bichere, A., et al. "Randomized Cross-Over Trial of Polyethylene Glycol Electrolyte Solution and Water for Colostomy Irrigation," *Diseases of the Colon and Rectum* 47(9):1506-509, September 2004.

Turnbull, G.B. "Managing Oversight of Colostomy Irrigation in Long Term-Care," *Ostomy/Wound Management* 49(10):13-14, October 2003.

Woodhouse, F. "Colostomy Irrigation: Are We Offering It Enough?" *British Journal of Nursing* 14(16):S14-15, September 2005.

Contact lens care

DESCRIPTION

- Illness or emergency treatment may require that you insert or remove and store a patient's contact lenses.
- Proper handling and lens care techniques help prevent eye injury and infection as well as lens loss or damage.
- Lens-handling techniques depend on what type of lenses the patient wears.
- All contact lenses float on the corneal tear layer.
- Rigid lenses typically have a smaller diameter than the cornea, and soft lens diameters typically exceed that of the cornea.
- Because soft lenses are larger and more pliable, they tend to mold themselves more closely to the eye for a more stable fit than rigid lenses.
- Most patients remove and clean lenses daily, but some wear lenses overnight or for several days without removing them for cleaning.
- Some patients wear disposable lenses that they replace at regular intervals (a few days to a few months), possibly without removing them for cleaning between replacements.
- Improper handling of lenses can result in eye contamination or infection.

CONTRAINDICATIONS
None known

Lens storage case or two small medicine cups and adhesive tape ◆ gloves ◆ patient's lens care equipment, if available ◆ sterile normal saline solution or soaking solution ◆ flashlight, if needed ◆ suction cup (optional)

PREPARATION

- If a lens storage case isn't available, put normal sterile saline solution into two medicine cups and submerge a lens in each one.
- To avoid confusing the right and left lenses, which may have different prescriptions, mark one cup "L" and the other "R" before placing lenses.

- Confirm the patient's identity using two patient identifiers according to facility policy.
- Tell the patient what you're about to do, wash your hands, and put on gloves to help prevent ocular infection.

INSERTING RIGID LENSES

- Wet one lens with solution and gently rub it between your thumb and index finger, or place it on your palm and rub it with your opposite index finger.
- Rinse well with the solution, leaving a small amount on the lens.
- Place the lens, convex side down, on the tip of the index finger of your dominant hand.
- Tell him to gaze upward slightly.
- Separate the eyelids with your other thumb and index finger, and gently place the lens on the cornea.
- You don't need to press the lens to the eye; the tear film will attract it naturally at first touch.
- Insert the opposite lens using the same procedure.

INSERTING SOFT LENSES

- To see if the lens is inside out, bend it between your thumb and index fin-

ger or fill it with saline or soaking solution.

- If the lens rolls inward or the edge points slightly inward, it's oriented correctly.
- If the edge points out or the lens collapses over your fingertip, it's probably inside out and needs to be reversed.
- Wet the lens with fresh normal saline solution and rub it gently between your thumb and index finger, or place it on your palm and rub it with your opposite index finger.
- Rinse well.
- Place the lens, convex side down, on the tip of the index finger of your dominant hand.
- Tell the patient to gaze upward slightly.
- Separate the eyelids with your other thumb and index finger, and place the lens on the sclera, just below the cornea.
- Slide the lens gently upward with your finger until it centers on the cornea.
- Insert the opposite lens using the same procedure.

REMOVING RIGID LENSES

- Before removing a lens, place the patient in a supine position to prevent the lens from popping out onto the floor, risking loss or damage.
- Place one thumb against his upper eyelid and the other thumb against his lower eyelid.
- Move the lids toward each other while gently pressing inward against the eye to trap the lens edge and break the suction.
- Extract the lens from his eyelashes.
- Depending on lens type and thickness, it may pop out when the suction breaks. You may want to try to break the suction with one hand while cupping the other hand below the patient's eye to catch the lens as it falls.
- Sometimes the lens will pop out on its own if you ask the patient to blink after stretching the corner of the eyelids toward the temporal bone, thus tightening the lid edges against the globe of the eye.

- Place the lens in the proper well of a storage case with enough solution to cover it, or place the lens in a labeled medicine cup with solution and secure adhesive tape over the top to prevent loss of the lens.
- Remove and care for the opposite lens using the same technique.

REMOVING SOFT LENSES

- Place the patient in the supine position.
- Using your nondominant hand, raise his upper eyelid and hold it against the orbital rim.
- Lightly place the forefinger of your other hand on the lens and move it down onto the sclera below the cornea.
- Pinch the lens between your forefinger and thumb and expect it to pop off.
- Place the lens in the proper well of a storage case with enough solution to cover it, or place the lens in a labeled medicine cup with solution and secure adhesive tape over the top to prevent loss of the lens.
- Remove and care for the other lens using the same technique.

CLEANING LENSES

- Because lens-cleaning steps vary with lens type and each manufacturer's and physician's instructions, ask the patient to guide you step-by-step through his normal cleaning routine.
- If he's unable to tell you how to clean his lenses properly, remember that most lens types require two steps: cleaning and disinfection.
- Cleaning involves rubbing the lens with a surfactant solution designed to remove surface deposits.
- For some patients, especially those who wear soft lenses, the cleaning step may also include use of an enzyme agent to remove protein deposits against which surfactant cleaners typically are ineffective.
- Enzyme cleaning involves soaking the lenses overnight in a solution in which you've dissolved special enzyme tablets.
- For patients who use a storage solution that contains a disinfectant, cleaning with an enzyme agent isn't necessary.
- Disinfection, which doesn't require rubbing, may be accomplished through chemical means or by heat. This step aims to rid the lens of infectious organisms.
- If you must clean a patient's lenses, use his regular solutions. This minimizes the risk of allergic reactions to substances included in other solutions.

⚡ **WARNING** *To avoid solution contamination, never touch the nozzle opening of a solution bottle to the lens, your fingers, or other objects.*

SPECIAL CONSIDERATIONS

⬛ **TROUBLESHOOTER** *If the patient's eyes appear dry or you have difficulty moving the lens on the eye, instill several drops of sterile normal saline solution and wait a few minutes before trying again; this helps prevent corneal damage.*

- If you can't remove the lens easily, notify the physician.
- Avoid instilling eye drugs while the patient is wearing lenses. The lenses can trap a drug, possibly causing eye irritation or lens damage.
- Don't allow soft lenses, which are 40% to 60% water, to dry out.
- If soft lenses dry out, soak them in sterile normal saline solution and they may return to their natural shape.

⚡ **WARNING** *If an unconscious patient is admitted to the emergency department, check for contact lenses by opening each eyelid and searching with a small flashlight. If you detect lenses, remove them immediately because tears can't circulate freely beneath the lenses with eyelids closed, possibly leading to corneal oxygen depletion or infection.*

- If a patient can't provide adequate care for his lenses during hospitalization, encourage him to send them home with a family member.

COMPLICATIONS
None known

PATIENT TEACHING

- Tell contact lens wearers to carry appropriate identification to speed lens removal and ensure proper care in an emergency.

DOCUMENTATION

- Record eye condition before and after removal of lenses.
- Record the time of lens insertion, removal, and cleaning.
- Note the location of stored lenses.
- If applicable, record removal of lenses from the facility by a family member.

SELECTED REFERENCES

Foulks, G.N. "Prolonging Contact Lens Wear and Making Contact Lens Wear Safer," *American Journal of Ophthalmology* 141(2):369-73, February 2006.

Roberts, A., et al. "Informed Consent and Medical Devices: The Case of the Contact Lens," *British Journal of Ophthalmology* 89(6):782-83, June 2005.

Szczotka-Flynn, L.B. "Medical Contact Lens Practice," *Optometry & Vision Science* 82(10):873, October 2005.

Yildirim, N., et al. "Prosthetic Contact Lenses: Adventure or Miracle," *Eye & Contact Lens* 32(2):102-103, March 2006.

Contact precautions

DESCRIPTION

- Contact precautions prevent the spread of infectious diseases transmitted by contact with body substances or contaminated items containing infectious agents.
- Contact precautions apply to patients infected or colonized (presence of microorganism without clinical signs or symptoms of infection) with epidemiologically important organisms that can be transmitted by direct or indirect contact. (See *Diseases requiring contact precautions.*)
- Effective contact precautions require a single room and the use of gloves and gowns by anyone having contact with the patient, the patient's support equipment, or items soiled with body substances containing the infectious agent.
- Thorough hand washing and proper handling and disposal of articles contaminated by the body substance containing the infectious agent are also essential.

CONTRAINDICATIONS
None known

Gloves ◆ gowns or aprons ◆ masks, if necessary ◆ isolation door card ◆ plastic bags ◆ thermometer ◆ stethoscope ◆ blood pressure cuff

PREPARATION

- Keep all contact precaution supplies outside the patient's room in a cart or anteroom.

- Confirm the patient's identity using two patient identifiers according to facility policy.
- Situate the patient in a single room with private toilet facilities and an anteroom, if possible.
- Two patients with the same infection may share a room, if necessary.
- Explain isolation procedures to the patient and his family.
- Place a contact precautions card on the door to notify anyone entering the room.
- Wash your hands before entering and after leaving the patient's room and after removing gloves.
- Place laboratory specimens in impervious, labeled containers, and send them to the laboratory at once.
- Attach requisition slips to the outside of the container.
- Tell visitors to wear gloves and a gown while visiting the patient and to wash their hands after removing the gown and gloves.
- Place all items that have come in contact with the patient in a single impervious bag, and arrange for their disposal or disinfection and sterilization.
- Limit the patient's movement from the room.
- If he must be moved, cover draining wounds with clean dressings.
- Notify the receiving department of the patient's isolation precautions so they can be maintained and the patient can be returned to the room promptly.

- Cleaning and disinfecting equipment between patients is essential.
- Try to dedicate certain reusable equipment (thermometer, stethoscope, blood pressure cuff) for the patient in contact precautions to reduce the risk of transmitting infection to other patients.
- Remember to change gloves during patient care as indicated by the procedure or task.
- Wash your hands after removing gloves and before putting on new gloves.
- Prior planning is advised before entering a patient's room to ensure complete and efficient care.

COMPLICATIONS
None known

- Inform the patient of the need for contact precautions.
- Make sure the patient understands that all visitors must wear gloves and a gown while visiting, and that they should wash their hands when leaving after removing the gown and gloves.
- Instruct the patient that he isn't to leave his room.

DOCUMENTATION

- ◆ Record the need for contact precautions on the nursing care plan and as indicated by your facility.
- ◆ Document the initiation and maintenance of precautions.
- ◆ Note the patient's tolerance of the procedure.
- ◆ Describe the patient or family teaching.
- ◆ Record the date contact precautions were discontinued.

SELECTED REFERENCES

Cromer, A.L., et al. "Impact of Implementing a Method of Feedback and Accountability Related to Contact Precautions Compliance," *American Journal of Infection Control* 32(8):451-55, December 2004.

Stirling, B., et al. "Nurses and the Control of Infectious Disease. Understanding Epidemiology and Disease Transmission Is Vital to Nursing Care," *Canadian Nurse* 100(9):16-20, November 2004.

Trick, W.E., et al. "Comparison of Routine Glove Use and Contact-Isolation Precautions to Prevent Transmission of Multidrug-Resistant Bacteria in a Long-Term Care Facility," *Journal of the American Geriatrics Society* 52(12):2003-2009, December 2004.

Diseases requiring contact precautions

DISEASE	PRECAUTIONARY PERIOD
Acute viral (acute hemorrhagic) conjunctivitis	Duration of illness
Clostridium difficile enteric infection	Duration of illness
Diphtheria (cutaneous)	Duration of illness
Enteroviral infection, in diapered or incontinent patient	Duration of illness
Escherichia coli disease, in diapered or incontinent patient	Duration of illness
Hepatitis A, in diapered or incontinent patient	Duration of illness
Herpes simplex virus infection (neonatal or mucocutaneous)	Duration of illness
Impetigo	Until 24 hours after initiation of effective therapy
Infection or colonization with multidrug-resistant bacteria	Until off antibiotics and culture negative
Major abscesses, cellulitis, or decubitus	Until 24 hours after initiation of effective therapy
Parainfluenza virus infection, in diapered or incontinent patient	Duration of illness
Pediculosis (lice)	Until 24 hours after initiation of effective therapy
Respiratory syncytial virus infection, in infants and young children	Duration of illness
Rotavirus infection, in diapered or incontinent patient	Duration of illness
Rubella, congenital syndrome	Place infant on precautions during any admission until 1 year old, unless nasopharyngeal and urine culture are negative for virus after age 3 months
Scabies	Until 24 hours after initiation of effective therapy
Shigellosis, in diapered or incontinent patient	Duration of illness
Smallpox	Duration of illness; requires airborne precautions
Staphylococcal furunculosis in infants and young children	Duration of illness
Viral hemorrhagic infections (Ebola, Lassa, Marburg)	Duration of illness
Zoster (chickenpox, disseminated zoster, or localized zoster in immunodeficient patient)	Until all lesions are crusted; requires airborne precautions

Continent ileostomy care

DESCRIPTION

- The continent, or pouch, ileostomy (also called a *Koch ileostomy* or an *ileal pouch*) has an internal reservoir fashioned from the terminal ileum.
- Continent ileostomy is an alternative to conventional ileostomy.
- Continent ileostomy may be used for a patient who requires proctocolectomy for chronic ulcerative colitis or multiple polyposis.
- Others may have a traditional ileostomy converted to a continent ileostomy.

CONTRAINDICATIONS

- Crohn's disease
- Gross obesity
- Patients needing emergency surgery
- Patients who can't care for the pouch

EQUIPMENT

Leg drainage bag ◆ bedside drainage bag ◆ normal saline solution ◆ 50-ml catheter-tip syringe ◆ extra continent ileostomy catheter ◆ 20-ml syringe with adapter ◆ 4″ × 4″ × 1″ foam dressing and Montgomery straps ◆ precut drain dressing ◆ gloves ◆ water-soluble lubricant ◆ graduated container ◆ skin sealant ◆ commercial catheter securing device (optional)

KEY STEPS

- Length of preoperative hospitalization varies with the patient's condition.
- Nursing responsibilities include providing bowel preparation, antibiotic therapy, and emotional support.
- After surgery, nursing includes ensuring patency of drainage catheter, assessing GI function, stoma and peristomal skin care, managing pain, and perineal skin care.
- Daily teaching on pouch intubation and drainage begins soon after surgery.
- Continuous drainage is maintained for 2 to 6 weeks to allow suture lines to heal.
- During healing, a drainage catheter is attached to low intermittent suction.
- After the suture line heals, the patient learns to drain the pouch himself.
- Nursing interventions for a patient having a continent ileostomy range from standard preoperative and postoperative care to pouch care and patient teaching.

PREOPERATIVE CARE

- Reinforce and supplement the physician's explanation of the procedure and implications for the patient.
- Assess the patient and family attitudes related to the operation and forthcoming changes in the patient's body image.
- Provide encouragement and support.

POSTOPERATIVE CARE

- When he returns to his room, attach the drainage catheter emerging from the ileostomy to continuous gravity drainage.
- A leg drainage bag may be attached to his thigh during ambulation.
- Irrigate the catheter with 30 ml of normal saline solution, as ordered, to prevent obstruction and allow fluid return by gravity.
- Immediately after surgery, keep the pouch empty because drainage will be serosanguineous.
- Monitor fluid intake and output.

- Check the catheter frequently when the patient begins eating solid food to ensure neither mucus nor undigested food block it.

> **TROUBLESHOOTER** *If the patient complains of abdominal cramps, distention, and nausea — symptoms of bowel obstruction — the catheter may be clogged. Gently irrigate with 20 to 30 ml of water or normal saline solution until the catheter drains freely. Move the catheter slightly or rotate gently to help clear obstruction. Try milking the catheter to clear the obstruction and notify the physician, if this fails. Check the stoma frequently for color, edema, and bleeding.*

> **WARNING** *Normally pink to red, a stoma that turns dark red or blue-red may have a compromised blood supply.*

- To care for the stoma and peristomal skin, put on gloves.
- Remove dressing, gently clean peristomal area with water, and pat dry.
- Use skin sealant around the stoma to prevent skin irritation.
- A stoma dressing can be applied by slipping a precut drain dressing around the catheter.
- Cut a hole slightly larger than the lumen of the catheter in the center of a 4″ × 4″ × 1″ piece of foam.
- Disconnect the catheter from the drainage bag and insert the distal end of the catheter through the hole in the foam and slide it onto the dressing.
- Secure it with Montgomery straps.
- Secure the catheter by wrapping the strap ties around it or use a commercial catheter-securing device.
- Reconnect the catheter to the drainage bag.
- The drainage catheter will be removed by the surgeon when he determines that the suture line has healed.
- Assess the peristomal skin for irritation from moisture.
- To reduce gas discomfort, encourage ambulation.
- To minimize gas pains, recommend he avoid swallowing air by chewing food well, limiting talking while eating, and not drinking from a straw.

DRAINING THE POUCH

- Provide privacy, explain procedure, and wash your hands.
- Put on gloves.
- Have the patient sit on the toilet to put him more at ease during the procedure.
- Remove the stoma dressing.
- Encourage him to relax his abdominal muscles to allow the catheter to slide easily into the pouch.
- Lubricate the tip of the drainage catheter with the water-soluble lubricant and insert it in the stoma.
- Gently push the catheter downward.
- Direction of insertion may vary by patient.
- When the catheter reaches the nipple valve of the internal pouch or reservoir (after 2" or 2½" [5 or 6.5 cm]), you'll feel resistance.
- Tell him to take a deep breath as you exert gentle pressure on the catheter to insert it through the valve.
- If this fails, have him lie supine and rest a few minutes, then try again.
- Advance the catheter to the suture marking made by the surgeon.
- Let the pouch drain completely. It usually takes 5 to 10 minutes, but with thick drainage or a clogged catheter, it may take 30 minutes.

TROUBLESHOOTER *If the tube clogs, irrigate with 30 ml of water or normal saline solution using the 50-ml catheter-tip syringe. Rotate and milk the tube. If these steps fail, remove, rinse, and reinsert the catheter.*

- Remove the catheter after completing drainage.
- Measure output, subtracting the amount of irrigant used.
- Rinse the catheter thoroughly with warm water.
- Clean the peristomal area and apply a fresh stoma dressing.

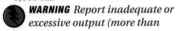

SPECIAL CONSIDERATIONS

- Never aspirate fluid from the catheter because resulting negative pressure may damage inflamed tissue.
- The first few times you intubate, the patient may be tense, making insertion difficult.
- Encourage him to relax.
- To shorten drainage time, have him cough, press gently on his abdomen over the pouch, or suddenly tighten and relax his abdominal muscles.
- Keep a record of intake and output to ensure fluid and electrolyte balance.
- Average daily output should be 1,000 ml.

WARNING *Report inadequate or excessive output (more than 1,400 ml daily).*

COMPLICATIONS

- Obstruction
- Fistula
- Pouch perforation
- Nipple valve dysfunction
- Abscesses
- Diarrhea
- Skin irritation
- Stenosis of the stoma
- Bacterial overgrowth in the pouch

PATIENT TEACHING

- Make sure the patient can properly intubate and drain the pouch himself.
- Provide the patient with appropriate equipment.
- If the postoperative drainage catheter is still in place, teach the patient proper care.
- Make sure the patient has a pouch-draining schedule, and give him appropriate pamphlets or video instructions.
- Make sure the patient feels comfortable calling the physician, nurse, or other caregiver to ask questions or discuss problems.
- Tell the patient where to obtain supplies.
- Refer the patient to a local ostomy group.
- Provide dietary counseling.

DOCUMENTATION

- Describe preoperative and postoperative care.
- Note the condition of stoma and peristomal skin.
- Record diet, drugs, and intubations.
- Note patient teaching.
- Document discharge planning.

SELECTED REFERENCES

Berndtsson, I., et al. "Thirty Years of Experience Living With a Continent Ileostomy," *Journal of Wound, Ostomy & Continence Nursing* 32(5):321-26, September-October 2005.

Nessar, G., et al. "Long-Term Outcome and Quality of Life After Continent Ileostomy," *Diseases of the Colon and Rectum* 49(3):336-44, March 2006.

Remzi, F.H., et al. "Long-Term Outcome and Quality of Life After Continent Ileostomy," *Colorectal Disease Supplement* 7(Suppl 1):112, July 2005.

Coronary angioplasty

OVERVIEW

DESCRIPTION

- Percutaneous transluminal coronary angioplasty (PTCA) is a nonsurgical approach to opening coronary vessels narrowed by arteriosclerosis. It involves inserting a balloon-tipped catheter into a narrowed coronary artery.
- PTCA is done in the cardiac catheterization laboratory under local anesthesia and moderate sedation.
- Cardiac catheterization is also done to assess stenosis and the efficacy of angioplasty.
- Catheterization is used as a visual tool to direct the balloon-tipped catheter through the vessel's area of stenosis.
- As the balloon is inflated, plaque is compressed against the vessel wall, allowing coronary blood to flow more freely.
- PTCA provides an alternative for patients who are poor surgical risks.
- It's also useful for those who have total coronary occlusion, unstable angina, plaque buildup in several areas, and those with poor left ventricular function.
- The ideal candidate for PTCA has single- or double-vessel disease excluding the left main coronary artery with at least 50% proximal stenosis.
- The lesion should be discrete, uncalcified, concentric, and not located near a bifurcation.
- Laser-enhanced angioplasty, shows promise in vaporizing occlusions in atherosclerosis.
- Your responsibilities include teaching the patient and family about the procedure and assessing for complications.

CONTRAINDICATIONS

- Left main coronary artery disease (especially when patient is a poor surgical risk)
- Variant angina or critical valvular disease
- Vessels occluded at the aortic wall orifice

EQUIPMENT

Povidone-iodine solution ◆ local anesthetic ◆ I.V. solution and tubing ◆ electrocardiogram (ECG) monitor and electrodes ◆ oxygen ◆ nasal cannula ◆ hair clippers ◆ sedative ◆ pulmonary artery (PA) catheter ◆ contrast medium ◆ emergency medications ◆ heparin for injection ◆ 5-lb (2.3-kg) sandbag ◆ introducer kit for PTCA catheter ◆ sterile gown, gloves, and drapes ◆ nitroglycerin, soft restraints (optional)

KEY STEPS

- Confirm the patient's identity using two patient identifiers according to facility policy.
- Explain the procedure to reduce the patient's fear and promote cooperation.
- Inform him that the procedure lasts from 1 to 4 hours and he may feel some discomfort from lying on a hard table that long.
- Tell him that a catheter will be inserted into an artery or vein in his groin and he may feel pressure as it moves along the vessel.
- Reassure him that although he'll be awake during the procedure, he'll be given a sedative.
- Explain that the physician or nurse may ask him how he's feeling and that he should tell them if he experiences angina.
- Explain that a contrast medium will be used to outline the lesion's location.
- Warn him that he'll feel a hot, flushing sensation or transient nausea during the injection.

BEFORE ANGIOPLASTY

- Check his history for allergies.
- If he's allergic to shellfish, iodine, or contrast media, notify the physician.
- Give 650 mg of aspirin the evening before the procedure, as ordered, to prevent platelet aggregation.
- Make sure a consent form has been signed.
- Restrict food and fluids for at least 6 hours before the procedure or as ordered.
- Ensure that results of coagulation studies, complete blood count, serum electrolyte studies, and blood typing and screening are available.
- Insert an I.V. line for emergency drugs.
- Clip hair from the insertion site as needed.
- Clean the area with povidone-iodine solution.
- Give him a sedative, as ordered.
- Take baseline peripheral pulses in all extremities.

DURING ANGIOPLASTY

- When the patient arrives at the cardiac catheterization laboratory, apply ECG electrodes and ensure I.V. line patency.
- Give oxygen through a nasal cannula.
- The physician will put on a sterile gown and gloves.
- Open the sterile supplies.
- The physician will prepare and drape the site and inject a local anesthetic.
- If the patient doesn't already have a PA catheter, the physician may insert one if the patient meets specified criteria (check facility policy).
- The physician will insert a large guide catheter into the artery and thread an angioplasty catheter through the guide catheter.
- Using a thin, flexible guide wire, the physician threads the catheter retrograde through the aorta, into the coronary artery to the area of stenosis.
- He will inject a contrast medium through the angioplasty catheter, into the obstructed coronary artery to outline the lesion's location and assess blockage.
- He will also inject heparin to prevent clotting, and intracoronary nitroglycerin to dilate coronary vessels and prevent spasm, if needed.
- The physician will inflate the catheter's balloon; gradually increasing the amount of time and pressure.
- The expanding balloon compresses the atherosclerotic plaque against the arterial wall, expanding the arterial lumen.

WARNING *Because balloon inflation deprives the myocardium distal to the inflation area of blood, the patient may experience angina.*

- If balloon inflation fails to decrease stenosis, a larger balloon may be used.
- Serial angiograms are done to determine the effectiveness of treatment.
- The physician removes the angioplasty catheter, leaving the guide catheter in place, in case the procedure needs repeating because of vessel occlusion.

AFTER ANGIOPLASTY

- When he returns to the unit, he may receive I.V. heparin or nitroglycerin.
- If he's bleeding at the catheter insertion site, a sandbag may be placed on it to prevent a hematoma.
- Assess vital signs every 15 minutes for the first hour, and every 30 minutes for 4 hours, unless more frequent checks are warranted.
- Assess peripheral pulses distal to the catheter insertion site and color, sensation, temperature, and capillary refill of the affected extremity.
- Monitor ECG rhythm and arterial pressures.

WARNING *Because coronary spasm may occur during or after PTCA, monitor the ECG for ST- and T-wave changes, and take vital signs frequently. Coronary artery dissection may occur with no early symptoms, but can cause restenosis of the vessel. Watch for symptoms of ischemia, which requires emergency coronary revascularization.*

- Tell the patient to stay in bed and keep the affected extremity straight per physician's orders.
- If he's restless and moving the extremity, apply soft restraints if necessary.
- Elevate the head of the bed 15 to 30 degrees.
- Assess the catheter site for hematoma, ecchymosis, and hemorrhage.

WARNING *If an area of expanding hematoma appears, mark the site and alert the physician. If bleeding occurs, locate the artery and apply manual pressure; then notify the physician.*

- Give I.V. fluids as ordered, usually 100 ml/hour, to help contrast medium excretion.

WARNING *Assess for fluid overload (distended jugular veins, atrial and ventricular gallops, dyspnea, pulmonary congestion, tachycardia, hypertension, and hypoxemia).*

- After the physician removes the catheter, apply direct pressure for at least 10 minutes and monitor the site frequently.

SPECIAL CONSIDERATIONS

- Monitor the patient carefully before, during, and after procedure.
- Vascular stents may be inserted to prevent vessel closure.
- Coronary spasm may occur during or after PTCA; monitor the ECG for ST- and T-wave changes, and take vital signs frequently.
- Coronary artery dissection may occur with no early symptoms, but can cause restenosis of the vessel.
- Watch for symptoms of ischemia, which requires emergency coronary revascularization.

COMPLICATIONS

- Prolonged angina (most common)
- Coronary artery perforation
- Balloon rupture
- Reocclusion (necessitating coronary artery bypass graft)
- Myocardial infarction
- Pericardial tamponade
- Hematoma
- Hemorrhage
- Reperfusion arrhythmias
- Closure of the vessel

PATIENT TEACHING

- Provide information about coronary anatomy, coronary artery disease, and any new medications prescribed to the patient.

DOCUMENTATION

- Note the patient's tolerance of the procedure and condition afterwards.
- Record vital signs and the condition of the extremity distal to the insertion site.
- Document complications and interventions.

SELECTED REFERENCES

Berger, J.S., et al. "Comparison of Outcomes in Acute Myocardial Infarction Treated With Coronary Angioplasty Alone Versus Coronary Stent Implantation," *American Journal of Cardiology* 97(7):977-80, April 2006.

Chlan, L.L., et al. "Effects of Three Groin Compression Methods on Patient Discomfort, Distress, and Vascular Complications Following a Percutaneous Coronary Intervention Procedure," *Nursing Research* 54(6):391-98, November-December 2005.

Tagney, J., and Lackie, D. "Bed-rest Post-femoral Arterial Sheath Removal — What Is Safe Practice? A Clinical Audit," *Nursing in Critical Care* 10(4):167-73, July-August 2005.

Vlasic, W. "Nursing Care of the Client Requiring Percutaneous Coronary Intervention," *Nursing Clinics of North America* 39(4):829-44, December 2004.

Credé's maneuver

DESCRIPTION

- When lower motor neuron damage impairs the voiding reflex, the bladder may become flaccid or areflexic.
- Because the bladder fails to contract properly, urine collects inside it, causing distention.
- Credé's maneuver (application of manual pressure over the lower abdomen) helps empty the bladder completely.
- After instruction, the patient can perform the maneuver herself, unless she can't reach her lower abdomen or lacks sufficient strength and dexterity.
- The maneuver isn't always successful and doesn't always eliminate the need for catheterization.
- Don't use after abdominal surgery if the incision isn't completely healed.
- When using Credé's maneuver, closely monitor urine output to help detect possible infection from the accumulation of residual urine.

CONTRAINDICATIONS

- Normal bladder tone
- Bladder spasms
- After abdominal surgery if incision isn't completely healed

Bedpan, urinal, or bedside commode

- Confirm the patient's identity using two patient identifiers according to facility policy.
- Explain the procedure to the patient and wash your hands.
- If allowed, place the patient in Fowler's position and position the bedpan or urinal.
- If her condition permits, assist her onto the bedside commode.
- Place your hands flat on her abdomen just below the umbilicus.
- Firmly stroke downward toward the bladder about 6 times to stimulate the voiding reflex.
- Place one hand on top of the other above the pubic arch.
- Press firmly inward and downward to compress the bladder and expel residual urine. (See *Credé's maneuver*.)

Credé's maneuver

Place one hand on top of the other above the patient's pubic arch. Press firmly inward and downward to compress the bladder and expel residual urine.

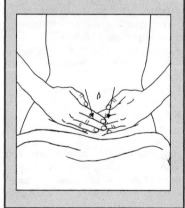

SPECIAL CONSIDERATIONS

◆ Some facilities require a physician's order for performance of Credé's maneuver.
◆ An ultrasound bladder scanner, if available, may be used to document residual urine volume after the procedure.
◆ After the patient has learned the procedure and can use it successfully, measuring the expelled urine may not be necessary.
◆ The patient may use the maneuver to void directly into the toilet.

COMPLICATIONS

◆ Infection caused by accumulation of residual urine

PATIENT TEACHING

◆ Explain to the patient that Credé's maneuver is a simple exercise that can be done at home.
◆ Tell the patient that she can start a stream of urine from her bladder by performing this easy-to-do maneuver.
◆ Tell the male patient to void directly into the toilet from a standing position if possible.
◆ The female patient should sit on the toilet as she normally would.
◆ Show the female patient how to lean forward and bend at the hips to increase pressure on the bladder.
◆ Have the patient place one hand on top of the other in a return demonstration.
◆ Explain that the stroking movement compresses the bladder and expels urine.

DOCUMENTATION

◆ Record the date and time of the procedure.
◆ Record the amount of urine expelled.
◆ Note the patient's tolerance of the procedure.

SELECTED REFERENCES

Almeida, F.G., et al. "Correlation Between Urethral Sphincter Activity and Valsalva Leak Point Pressure at Different Bladder Distentions: Revisiting the Urethral Pressure Profile," *Journal of Urology* 174(4 Pt 1):1312-315, October 2005.

Fitzpatrick, J.M., and Kirby, R.S. "Management of Acute Urinary Retention," *BJU International* 97(Suppl 2):16-20, April 2006.

Cricothyrotomy

DESCRIPTION

◆ When endotracheal (ET) intubation or a tracheotomy can't be performed quickly to establish an airway, an emergency cricothyrotomy may be necessary.

◆ Performed rarely, this procedure involves puncturing the trachea through the cricothyroid membrane.

◆ Your role will be to assist the physician, but if you have received special training, you may have to perform the procedure in an emergency.

◆ Cricothyrotomy should be performed using sterile technique, but in an emergency this may not be possible.

CONTRAINDICATIONS

None known

EQUIPMENT

WARNING *Have one person stay with the patient while another collects the necessary equipment.*

SCALPEL CRICOTHYROTOMY

Sterile gloves ◆ goggles ◆ povidone-iodine solution ◆ sterile 4″ × 4″ gauze pads ◆ dilator ◆ tape ◆ oxygen source ◆ scalpel ◆ #6 or smaller tracheostomy tube (if available) ◆ handheld resuscitation bag or T tube and wide-bore oxygen tubing

NEEDLE CRICOTHYROTOMY

Sterile gloves ◆ goggles ◆ povidone-iodine solution ◆ sterile 4″ × 4″ gauze pads ◆ dilator ◆ tape ◆ oxygen source ◆ 14G (or larger) through-the-needle or over-the-needle catheter ◆ 10-ml syringe ◆ tape ◆ I.V. extension tubing ◆ hand-operated release valve or pressure-regulating adjustment valve

KEY STEPS

◆ Put on sterile gloves and personal protective equipment.

◆ Hyperextend the patient's neck to expose the area of the incision site.

◆ Hold the patient's head in the correct position while the physician performs the procedure. (See *Performing an emergency cricothyrotomy.*)

SPECIAL CONSIDERATIONS

◆ Immediately after the procedure, check for bleeding at the insertion site, subcutaneous emphysema or inadequate ventilation, and tracheal or vocal cord damage.

AGE FACTOR *Scalpel cricothyrotomy isn't recommended for children younger than age 12 because it could damage the cricoid cartilage — the only circumferential support to the upper trachea.*

COMPLICATIONS

◆ Hemorrhage

◆ Perforation of the thyroid or esophagus

◆ Subcutaneous or mediastinal emphysema

◆ Infection may occur several days after procedure

None

DOCUMENTATION

- Document the date, time, and circumstances requiring the procedure.
- Record the patient's vital signs.
- Note whether the patient initiated spontaneous respirations after the procedure.
- Record how much oxygen was given and what method was used.
- Note procedures, such as ET intubation, performed after the airway was established.

SELECTED REFERENCES

Borg, P. "Emergency Cricothyrotomy," *Anaesthesia* 60(4):412-13, April 2005.

Fikkers, B.G., et al. "Emergency Cricothyrotomy: A Randomized Crossover Trial Comparing the Wire-guided and Catheter-over-needle Techniques," *Anaesthesia* 59(10):1008-1011, October 2004.

Keane, M.F., et al. "A Laboratory Comparison of Emergency Percutaneous and Surgical Cricothyrotomy by Prehospital Personnel," *Prehospital Emergency Care* 8(4):424-26, October-December 2004.

Melker, J.S., and Gabrielli, A. "Melker Cricothyrotomy Kit: An Alternative to the Surgical Technique," *Annals of Otology, Rhinology, and Laryngology* 114(7):525-28, July 2005.

Performing an emergency cricothyrotomy

- The physician puts on sterile gloves and cleans the patient's neck with a gauze pad soaked in povidone-iodine solution using a circular motion, working outward from the incision site.
- The physician locates the precise insertion site by sliding his thumb and fingers down to the thyroid gland. The outer borders are located when the space between the physician's fingers and thumb widens.
- The physician will move his fingers across the center of the gland, over the anterior edge of the cricoid ring.

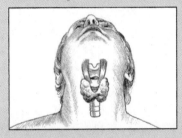

USING A SCALPEL

- A horizontal incision, less than ½" (1.3 cm) long, is made in the cricothyroid membrane just above the cricoid ring.
- A dilator is inserted to prevent tissue from closing around the incision.
- If a dilator isn't available, the handle of the scalpel is inserted and rotated 90 degrees (as shown).

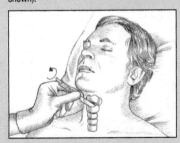

- If a small tracheostomy tube (#6 or smaller) is available, it's inserted into the opening and secured to help maintain a patent airway.
- If a tracheostomy tube isn't available, the dilator or scalpel handle is taped in place until a tracheostomy tube is available.
- If the patient can breathe spontaneously, a humidified oxygen source is taped to the tracheostomy tube with a T tube; if he can't, a handheld resuscitation bag is used.

- The cuff of the tracheostomy tube is inflated with a syringe to provide positive-pressure ventilation.
- Auscultate bilaterally for breath sounds, and take the patient's vital signs.
- Dispose of gloves properly and wash your hands.

USING A NEEDLE

- A 10-ml syringe is attached to a 14G (or larger) through-the-needle or over-the-needle catheter, then the catheter is inserted into the cricothyroid membrane just above the cricoid ring.
- The catheter is directed downward at a 45-degree angle to the trachea (as shown) to avoid damaging the vocal cords.

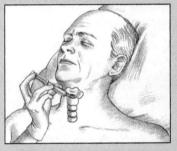

- Negative pressure is maintained by pulling back the syringe plunger as the catheter is advanced. Air entering the syringe indicates that the catheter has entered the trachea.
- When the catheter reaches the trachea, it's advanced and the needle and syringe are removed.
- The catheter is taped in place.
- The catheter hub is attached to one end of the I.V. extension tubing.
- At the other end, attach a hand-operated release valve or a pressure-regulating adjustment valve.
- Connect the entire assembly to an oxygen source.
- Press the release valve to introduce oxygen into the trachea and inflate the lungs.
- When you can see that they're inflated, release the valve to allow passive exhalation.
- Adjust the pressure-regulating valve to the minimum pressure needed for adequate lung inflation.
- Auscultate bilaterally for breath sounds, and take the patient's vital signs.
- Dispose of gloves properly and wash your hands.

Crutches

DESCRIPTION

- Crutches remove weight from one or both legs, enabling the patient to support himself with his hands and arms.
- They're typically prescribed for the patient with lower-extremity injury or weakness.
- Use of crutches requires balance, stamina, and upper-body strength.
- Crutch selection and walking gait depend on the patient's condition.
- The patient who can't use crutches may be able to use a walker.
- Three types of crutches are commonly used:
- Standard aluminum or wooden crutches are used by the patient with a sprain, strain, or cast. They require stamina and upper-body strength.
- Aluminum forearm crutches are used by the paraplegic or other patient using the swing-through gait. They have a collar that fits around the forearm and a horizontal handgrip that provides support.
- Platform crutches are used by the arthritic patient who has an upper-extremity deficit that prevents weight bearing through the wrist. They provide padded surfaces for the upper extremities.

CONTRAINDICATIONS
None known

EQUIPMENT

Crutches with axillary pads, handgrips, and rubber suction tips ◆ walking belt (optional)

PREPARATION

- After choosing the appropriate crutches, adjust their height with the patient standing or, if necessary, recumbent. (See *Fitting a patient for a crutch*.)

Fitting a patient for a crutch

Position the crutch so it extends from a point 4″ to 6″ (10 to 15 cm) to the side and 4″ to 6″ in front of the patient's feet, to 1½″ to 2″ (4 to 5 cm) below the axillae (about the width of two fingers). Adjust the handgrips so that the patient's elbows are flexed at a 15-degree angle when he's standing with the crutches in the resting position

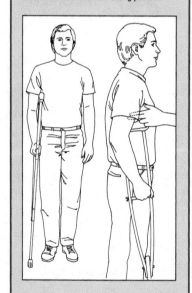

KEY STEPS

- Consult with the physician and physical therapist to coordinate rehabilitation orders and teaching.
- Confirm the patient's identity using two patient identifiers according to facility policy.
- Describe the gait you'll teach and the reason for your choice.
- Demonstrate the gait, as necessary.
- Have the patient give a return demonstration.
- Place a walking belt around his waist, if necessary, to help prevent falls.
- Tell him to position the crutches and shift his weight from side to side.
- Use a full-length mirror to facilitate learning and coordination.

FOUR-POINT GAIT

- Teach the four-point gait to the patient who can bear weight on both legs.
- The four-point is the safest gait because three points are always in contact with the floor.
- The four-point gait requires greater coordination than others because of its constant shifting of weight.
- Use this sequence: right crutch, left foot, left crutch, right foot.
- Suggest counting to help develop rhythm, and make sure each short step is of equal length.
- If he gains proficiency at this gait, teach him the faster two-point gait.

TWO-POINT GAIT

- Teach the two-point gait to the patient with weak legs but good coordination and arm strength.
- The two-point gait is the most natural crutch-walking gait because it mimics walking, with alternating swings of the arms and legs.
- Tell him to advance the right crutch and left foot simultaneously, followed by the left crutch and right foot.

THREE-POINT GAIT

- Teach the three-point gait to the patient who can bear only partial or no weight on one leg.

- Tell him to advance both crutches 6″ to 8″ (15 to 20 cm) along with the involved leg.
- Tell him to bring the uninvolved leg forward and bear the bulk of his weight on the crutches and some of it on the involved leg, if possible.
- Stress the importance of taking steps equal in length and duration with no pauses.

SWING-TO AND SWING-THROUGH GAITS
- Teach the swing-to or swing-through gaits — the fastest ones — to the patient with complete paralysis of the hips and legs.
- Tell him to advance both crutches simultaneously and swing the legs parallel to (swing-to) or beyond the crutches (swing-through).

USING A CHAIR
- To sit down, have him support himself with the crutches in one hand and lower himself with the other.
- To stand up, tell him to hold both crutches in one hand, with the tips resting firmly on the floor.
- Have him push up from the chair with his free hand, supporting himself with the crutches.

USING STAIRS
- To go up stairs using the three-point gait, tell him to lead with the uninvolved leg and follow with both the crutches and the involved leg.
- To go down stairs, he should lead with the crutches and the involved leg and follow with the good leg.
- He may find it helpful to remember, "The good goes up, the bad goes down."

SPECIAL CONSIDERATIONS
- Encourage arm- and shoulder-strengthening exercises to prepare the patient for crutch walking.
- If possible, consult physical therapy to teach two techniques — one fast and one slow — so the patient can alternate between them to prevent excessive muscle fatigue and can adjust more easily to various walking conditions.

COMPLICATIONS
- Atrophy of the hips and legs (from the swing-to and swing-through gaits with chronic conditions)
- Damage to brachial nerves causing brachial nerve palsy (due to prolonged pressure on the axillae from leaning on crutches)

PATIENT TEACHING
- Provide appropriate instruction based on patient's needs and condition.

DOCUMENTATION
- Record the type of gait the patient is taught.
- Report the amount of assistance required.
- Note the distance walked.
- Describe the patient's tolerance of crutches.

SELECTED REFERENCES
Dula, D.J., et al. "Use of Modified Wooden Crutches as an Adjunct in the Radiographic Evaluation of the Cervical Spine," *Journal of Trauma Injury Infection & Critical Care* 54(6):1250-252, June 2003.

Haubert, L.L., et al. "A Comparison of Shoulder Joint Forces During Ambulation With Crutches Versus a Walker in Persons With Incomplete Spinal Cord Injury," *Archives of Physical Medicine and Rehabilitation* 87(1):63-70, January 2006.

Youdas, J.W., et al. "Partial Weight-Bearing Gait Using Conventional Assistive Devices," *Archives of Physical Medicine and Rehabilitation* 86(3):394-98, March 2005.

Defibrillation

DESCRIPTION

- Standard treatment involves using electrode paddles to direct an electric current through the patient's heart.
- Current causes the myocardium to depolarize, encouraging the sinoatrial node to resume control of the heart's electrical activity.
- Current may be delivered by a monophasic or biphasic defibrillator.
- Electrode paddles delivering current may be placed on the patient's chest or, during cardiac surgery, directly on the myocardium.
- Because ventricular fibrillation leads to death if not corrected, success depends on early recognition and quick treatment of arrhythmias.
- Besides treating ventricular fibrillation, it may also be used to treat ventricular tachycardia that doesn't produce a pulse.
- Patients with history of ventricular fibrillation may need an implantable cardioverter-defibrillator (ICD), a sophisticated device that automatically discharges an electric current when it senses a ventricular tachyarrhythmia.

CONTRAINDICATIONS

- None known

Defibrillator (monophasic or biphasic) ◆ external paddles or internal paddles (sterilized for cardiac surgery) ◆ conductive medium pads ◆ electrocardiogram (ECG) monitor with recorder ◆ oxygen therapy equipment ◆ handheld resuscitation bag ◆ airway equipment ◆ emergency pacing equipment ◆ emergency cardiac drugs

Biphasic defibrillators

Most hospital defibrillators are monophasic. They deliver a single current of electricity that travels in one direction between the two pads or paddles on the patient's chest. For monophasic defibrillation to be effective, a high amount of electrical current is required.

Biphasic defibrillators are now used at some hospitals. Pad or paddle placement is the same as with the monophasic defibrillator. However, during biphasic defibrillation, the electrical current discharged from the pads or paddles travels in a positive direction for a specified duration, then reverses and flows in a negative direction during the rest of the electrical discharge. It delivers two currents of electricity and lowers the defibrillation threshold of the heart muscle, making it possible to successfully defibrillate ventricular fibrillation with less energy. Instead of 200 joules, an initial shock of 120 joules is commonly effective.

Biphasic defibrillators can adjust for differences in impedance or resistance of current through the chest. This helps lessen the number of shocks needed to terminate ventricular fibrillation. By using less energy and fewer shocks, damage to the myocardial muscle is reduced. Biphasic defibrillators, when used at the clinically appropriate energy level, may be used for defibrillation and, when placed in the synchronized mode, may be used for synchronized cardioversion.

- Assess the patient to determine lack of a pulse.
- Call for help and perform cardiopulmonary resuscitation (CPR) until defibrillator and emergency equipment arrive.
- Work with other healthcare professionals to make sure the time between stopping chest compressions and shock delivery is minimized.
- If the defibrillator has "quick-look" capability, place paddles on the patient's chest to quickly view the cardiac rhythm.
- Connect the monitoring leads of the defibrillator to the patient and assess his cardiac rhythm.
- Expose the patient's chest and apply conductive pads at the paddle placement positions.
- For anterolateral placement, position one paddle to the right of the upper sternum, just below the right clavicle, and the other over the fifth or sixth intercostal space at the left anterior axillary line.
- For anteroposterior placement, position the anterior paddle directly over the heart at the precordium, to the left of the lower sternal border.
- Place the flat posterior paddle under the patient's body beneath the heart and immediately below the scapulae (not under the vertebral column).
- Turn on the defibrillator and, if performing external defibrillation, set the energy level for 360 joules for an adult patient when using a monophasic defibrillator.
- Use clinically appropriate energy levels for a biphasic defibrillator. (See *Biphasic defibrillators*.)
- Charge the paddles by pressing the charge buttons, located either on the machine or on the paddles themselves.
- Place the paddles over the conductive pads and press firmly against the patient's chest, using 25 lb of pressure.
- Reassess the patient's cardiac rhythm.

- If the patient remains in ventricular fibrillation or pulseless ventricular tachycardia, tell all personnel to stand clear of the patient and the bed.
- Discharge the current by pressing both paddle charge buttons simultaneously.
- Perform five cycles (2 minutes) of CPR, and then check the patient's rhythm.
- Tell someone to reset the energy level on the defibrillator (or on the paddles) to 360 joules, or the biphasic energy equivalent, if necessary.
- Announce that you're preparing to defibrillate, and repeat the procedure.
- Perform five cycles (2 minutes) of CPR, and then check the patient's rhythm.
- If defibrillation is again necessary, tell someone to reset the energy level to 360 joules, or the biphasic energy equivalent.
- Follow the same procedure.
- When possible, secure an airway and confirm placement. Always minimize the amount of time chest compressions must be stopped.
- When availabe, give epinephrine or vasopressin.
- Consider possible causes for failure of the patient's rhythm to convert, such as acidosis or hypoxia.
- If defibrillation restores a normal rhythm, check the patient's central and peripheral pulses and obtain a blood pressure reading, heart rate, and respiratory rate.
- Assess the patient's level of consciousness, cardiac rhythm, breath sounds, skin color, and urine output.
- Obtain baseline arterial blood gas levels and a 12-lead ECG.
- Provide supplemental oxygen, ventilation, and drugs as needed.
- Check the patient's chest for electrical burns and treat them, as ordered, with corticosteroid or lanolin-based creams.
- Prepare the defibrillator for immediate reuse.

SPECIAL CONSIDERATIONS

- Defibrillators vary by manufacturer; familiarize yourself with your facility's equipment.
- Defibrillator operation should be checked at least every 8 hours and after each use.
- Defibrillation can be affected by several factors, including paddle size and placement, condition of the patient's myocardium, duration of the arrhythmia, chest resistance, and number of countershocks.

COMPLICATIONS
- Accidental electric shock to those providing care
- Skin burns from using an insufficient amount of conductive medium

PATIENT TEACHING

- During defibrillation, have someone with the patient's family, explaining the events.

DOCUMENTATION

- Document the procedure, including the patient's ECG rhythm both before and after defibrillation.
- Report the number of times defibrillation was performed.
- Document the voltage used with each attempt.
- Note whether a pulse returned.
- Record the dosage, route, and time of drug administration.
- Report whether CPR was used and how the airway was maintained.
- Document the patient's outcome.

SELECTED REFERENCES
Bubien, R.S., et al. "Cardiac Defibrillation and Resynchronization Therapies: Principles, Therapies, and Management Implications," *AACN Clinical Issues* 15(3):340-61, July-September 2004.

Germano, J.J., et al. "Frequency and Causes of Implantable Cardioverter-Defibrillator Therapies: Is Device Therapy Proarrhythmic?" *American Journal of Cardiology* 97(8):1255-61, April 2006.

Gullick, J. "A Study into Safe and Efficient Use of Defibrillators by Nurses," *Nursing Times* 100(44):42-44, November 2004.

Gura, M.T. "Implantable Cardioverter Defibrillator Therapy," *Journal of Cardiovascular Nursing* 20(4):276-87, July-August 2005.

Marett, B.E. "American Heart Association Releases New Guidelines," *Journal of Emergency Nursing* 32(1):63-64, February 2006.

Doppler blood flow detector use

OVERVIEW

DESCRIPTION
- The Doppler ultrasound blood flow detector is more sensitive than palpation for determining pulse rate.
- It's especially useful when a pulse is faint or weak.
- Doppler ultrasound detects the motion of red blood cells (RBCs), unlike palpation, which detects arterial wall expansion and retraction.

CONTRAINDICATIONS
- None known

EQUIPMENT

Doppler ultrasound blood flow detector ◆ coupling or transmission gel ◆ soft cloth ◆ antiseptic solution or soapy water

KEY STEPS

- Confirm the patient's identity using two patient identifiers according to facility policy.
- Apply a small amount of coupling gel or transmission gel (not water-soluble lubricant) to the ultrasound probe.
- Position the probe on the skin directly over the selected artery. (See *Pulse points*.)
- When using a Doppler model with a speaker, turn the instrument on and, moving counter-clockwise, set the volume control to the lowest setting.
- If your model doesn't have a speaker, plug in the earphones and slowly raise the volume.
- The Doppler ultrasound stethoscope is basically a stethoscope fitted with an audio unit, volume control, and transducer, which amplifies the movement of RBCs. (See *Doppler ultrasound blood flow detector.*)
- To obtain the best signals with either device, tilt the probe 45 degrees from the artery, making sure you put gel between the skin and the probe.
- Slowly move the probe in a circular motion to locate the center of the artery and the Doppler signal, which will produce a swishing sound at the heartbeat.
- Count the signals for 60 seconds to determine the pulse rate.
- After you've measured the pulse rate, clean the probe with a soft cloth soaked in antiseptic solution or soapy water.

Pulse points

This illustration shows the locations where an artery crosses bone or firm tissue and can be palpated for a pulse or assessed by using a Doppler ultrasound device.

Temporal

Carotid

Apical

Brachial

Ulnar

Radial

Femoral

Popliteal

Posterior tibial

Pedal

SPECIAL CONSIDERATIONS

◆ Don't immerse the probe in water or solution or bump it against a hard surface.
◆ Avoid rapid movements of the probe because this distorts the signal.

COMPLICATIONS
◆ None known

PATIENT TEACHING

◆ Explain the procedure to the patient as you are performing it.

DOCUMENTATION

◆ Record the location and quality of the pulse as well as the pulse rate and time of measurement.

SELECTED REFERENCES

Blaivas, M. "Ultrasound-Guided Peripheral I.V. Insertion in the ED," *American Journal of Nursing* 105(10):54-57, October 2005.

French, L. "Community Nurse Use of Doppler Ultrasound in Leg Ulcer Assessment," *British Journal of Community Nursing* 10(9):S6-S10, passim, September 2005.

Ozbudak, O., et al. "Doppler Ultrasonography Versus Venography in the Detection of Deep Vein Thrombosis in Patients with Pulmonary Embolism," *Journal of Thrombosis and Thrombolysis* 21(2):159-62, April 2006.

Patel, U. "The Potential Value of Power Doppler Ultrasound Imaging Compared With Grey-Scale Ultrasound Findings in the Diagnosis of Local Recurrence After Prostatectomy," *Clinical Radiology* 61(4):323-24, April 2006.

Doppler ultrasound blood flow detector

The Doppler ultrasound blood flow detector detects the motion of red blood cells within the vessel.

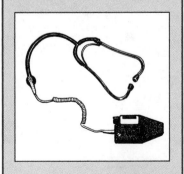

Droplet precautions

DESCRIPTION

- Droplet precautions prevent the spread of infectious diseases (including some formerly included in respiratory isolation) transmitted when nasal or oral secretions from an infected patient come in contact with mucous membranes of another person.
- Droplets of moisture, which arise from coughing or sneezing, are heavy and generally fall to the ground within 3' (0.9 m)
- Organisms contained in droplets don't become airborne or suspended in air. (See *Diseases requiring droplet precautions*.)
- Requires a single room (not necessarily a negative-pressure room), and the door doesn't need to be closed.
- Persons with direct contact or within 3' of the patient should wear a surgical mask to cover the nose and mouth.

   AGE FACTOR *When handling infants or young children who require droplet precautions, you may also need to wear gloves and a gown to prevent soiling of clothing with nasal and oral secretions.*

CONTRAINDICATIONS

- None known

Masks ◆ gowns (if necessary) ◆ gloves ◆ plastic bags ◆ DROPLET PRECAUTIONS door card ◆ thermometer ◆ stethoscope ◆ blood pressure cuff

PREPARATION

- Keep supplies outside the patient's room in a cart or anteroom.

- Put the patient in a single room with private toilet facilities and an anteroom, if possible.
- Explain isolation procedures to the patient and his family.
- Put a DROPLET PRECAUTIONS card on the door to notify anyone entering the room.
- Wash your hands before entering the room, during patient care as indicated, and after leaving the room.
- Pick up your mask by the top strings, adjust it around your nose and mouth, and tie the strings for a comfortable fit.
- If the mask has a flexible metal nose strip, adjust it to fit firmly but comfortably.
- Tape a plastic bag to the patient's bedside so he can properly dispose of facial tissues.
- Make sure all visitors wear masks when near the patient (within 3') and, if necessary, gowns, and gloves.
- Make sure the patient wears a surgical mask over his nose and mouth when he leaves the room.
- Notify receiving department of isolation precautions so they can be maintained and the patient can be returned to his room promptly.
- Two patients with the same infection, and no other, may share a room, if necessary.

SPECIAL CONSIDERATIONS

◆ Before removing your mask, remove gloves (if worn), and wash your hands.
◆ Untie the strings and dispose of the mask, handling it by the strings only.

COMPLICATIONS
◆ None known

PATIENT TEACHING

◆ Instruct the patient to cover his nose and mouth with a facial tissue while coughing or sneezing.

DOCUMENTATION

◆ Record the need for droplet precautions on the care plan and as indicated by your facility.
◆ Document initiation and maintenance of precautions.
◆ Describe the patient's tolerance of procedure.
◆ Report patient or family teaching.
◆ Document the date droplet precautions were discontinued.

SELECTED REFERENCES
Gamage, B., et al. "Protecting Health Care Workers from SARS and Other Respiratory Pathogens: A Review of the Infection Control Literature," *American Journal of Infection Control* 33(2):114-21, March 2005.
Muller, M.P., and McGeer, A. "Febrile Respiratory Illness in the Intensive Care Unit Setting: An Infection Control Perspective," *Current Opinion in Critical Care* 12(1):37-42, February 2006.
Sweeney, A.M., et al. "Nursing and Infection-Control Issues During High-Frequency Oscillatory Ventilation," *Critical Care Medicine* 33(3 Suppl):S204-208, March 2005.

Diseases requiring droplet precautions

DISEASE	PRECAUTIONARY PERIOD
Invasive *Haemophilus influenzae* type b disease, including meningitis, pneumonia, and sepsis	Until 24 hours after initiation of effective therapy
Invasive *Neisseria meningitidis* disease, including meningitis, pneumonia, epiglottis, and sepsis	Until 24 hours after initiation of effective therapy
Diphtheria (pharyngeal)	Until off antibiotics and two cultures taken at least 24 hours apart are negative
Mycoplasma pneumoniae infection	Duration of illness
Pertussis	Until 5 days after initiation of effective therapy
Pneumonic plague	Until 72 hours after initiation of effective therapy
Streptococcal pharyngitis, pneumonia, or scarlet fever in infants and young children	Until 24 hours after initiation of effective therapy
Adenovirus infection in infants and young children	Duration of illness
Influenza	Duration of illness
Mumps	For 9 days after onset of swelling
Parvovirus B19	Maintain precautions for duration of hospitalization when chronic disease occurs in an immunodeficient patient (For patients with transient aplastic crisis or red-cell crisis, maintain precautions for 7 days.)
Rubella (German measles)	Until 7 days after onset of rash

Drug administration, pediatric

DESCRIPTION
◆ Because a child responds more rapidly — and unpredictably — to drugs than an adult does, pediatric drug administration requires special care.
◆ Such factors as age, weight, body surface area, and drug form and route may dramatically affect a child's response to a drug.

AGE FACTOR *Because of his thin epithelium, a neonate absorbs topical medications much faster than an older child does.*

◆ Certain disorders also affect a child's response to medication. For example, gastroenteritis increases gastric motility, which in turn impairs absorption of certain oral medications; liver or kidney disorders may hinder the metabolism of some medications.
◆ Usual drug administration techniques may need adjustment to account for the child's age, size, and developmental level. A tablet for a young child, for example, may be crushed and mixed with a liquid for oral administration. In addition, the injection site and needle size will vary depending on the child's age and physical development.

CONTRAINDICATIONS
◆ Vary based on administration route, medication, and child's condition

ORAL MEDICATIONS
Prescribed medication ◆ plastic disposable syringe ◆ plastic medicine dropper or spoon ◆ medication cup ◆ water, syrup, or jelly (for tablets) ◆ optional: fruit juice

INJECTABLE MEDICATIONS
Prescribed medication ◆ appropriately sized syringe and needle ◆ alcohol pads or povidone-iodine solution ◆ gloves ◆ gauze pads ◆ adhesive bandage ◆ optional: cold compress, EMLA cream, transparent occlusive dressing

PREPARATION
◆ Check the prescriber's order for the prescribed drug, dosage, and route.
◆ Compare the order with the drug label, check the drug expiration date, and review the patient's chart for drug allergies. Also check any relevant laboratory values.
◆ Carefully calculate the dosage, if necessary, and have another nurse verify it. Typically, you'll double-check dosages for potentially hazardous or lethal drugs, such as insulin, heparin, digoxin, epinephrine, and opioids. Check facility policy to learn which drugs must be calculated and checked by two nurses.
◆ For giving an injection, select the appropriate needle. Typically, for I.M. injections in infants, you'll use a 25G ¾" needle, and in older children, a 23G 1" needle. For subcutaneous injections, select a ¾" or ½" needle and, for intradermal medications, a 27G ½" needle. To administer viscous medications, select a larger-gauge needle.

◆ Assess the child's condition to determine the need for medication.
◆ Carefully observe the child for a rash, pruritus, cough, or other signs of an adverse reaction to a previously administered drug.
◆ Confirm the child's identity using two patient identifiers according to facility policy.
◆ If your facility uses a bar code scanning system, be sure to scan your ID badge, the patient's ID bracelet, and the medication's bar code.
◆ Explain the procedure to the child and his parents. Use terms the child can understand. Give the child choices, if possible. For example, ask the child if he wants the medication mixed with chocolate or strawberry syrup.
◆ Provide privacy — especially for an older child.

GIVING ORAL MEDICATION TO AN INFANT
◆ Use either a plastic syringe without a needle or a drug-specific medicine dropper to measure the dose.
◆ If the medication comes in tablet form, first crush the tablet (if appropriate) and mix it with water or syrup. Then draw the mixture into the syringe or dropper.
◆ Pick up the infant, raising his head and shoulders or turning his head to one side to prevent aspiration. Hold the infant close to your body to help restrain him.
◆ Using your thumb, press down on the infant's chin to open his mouth.
◆ Slide the syringe or medicine dropper into the infant's mouth alongside his tongue. Release the medication slowly to let the infant swallow and to prevent choking. If appropriate, allow him to suck on the syringe as you expel the medication.
◆ If not contraindicated, give fruit juice after giving medication.
◆ If the infant is particularly small or seemingly inactive, place him on his side or back to decrease the risk of sudden infant death syndrome, as

recommended by the American Academy of Pediatrics. Allow an active infant to assume a position that's comfortable for him; avoid forcing him into a side-lying position to prevent agitation.

GIVING ORAL MEDICATION TO A TODDLER

- Use a plastic, disposable syringe or dropper to measure liquid medication. Then transfer the fluid to a medication cup.
- Elevate the toddler's head and shoulders to prevent aspiration.
- If possible, ask him to help hold the cup to enlist his cooperation. Otherwise, hold the cup to the toddler's lips, or use a syringe or a spoon to administer the liquid. Make sure that the toddler ingests all of the medication.
- If the medication is in tablet form, first crush the tablet, if appropriate, and mix it with water, syrup, or jelly.

GIVING ORAL MEDICATION TO AN OLDER CHILD

- If possible, let the child choose both the liquid medication mixer and a beverage to drink after taking the medication.
- If appropriate, allow him to choose where he'll take the medication; for example, sitting in bed or sitting on a parent's lap.
- If the medication comes in tablet or capsule form, and if the child is old enough (between ages 4 and 6), teach him how to swallow it. (If he already knows how to swallow solid medication, review the procedure with him for safety's sake.) Tell him to place the pill on the back of his tongue and to swallow it immediately by drinking water or juice. Focus most of your explanation on the water or juice to draw the child's attention away from the pill. Make sure the child drinks enough water or juice to keep the pill from lodging in his esophagus.
- Afterward, look inside the child's mouth to confirm that he swallowed the pill.

- If the child can't swallow the pill whole, crush it (if appropriate) and mix it with water, syrup, or jelly. Or, after checking with the child's practitioner, order the medication in liquid form.

⚡ **WARNING** *When administering medication to infants and children, remember that not all pills can be crushed for easier administration. Consult a pharmacist (or an appropriate drug reference book) to make sure that crushing the tablet won't interfere with its effectiveness.*

GIVING AN I.M. INJECTION

- Choose an injection site that's appropriate for the child's age and muscle mass. (See *I.M. injection sites in children,* page 157.)
- If time allows, place EMLA cream on the intended skin site at least 1 hour before the procedure, but don't spread the cream or rub it in. Cover with a transparent occlusive dressing.

❀ **AGE FACTOR** *EMLA cream isn't approved for use in infants younger than age 1 month.*

- Immediately before the procedure, remove the dressing and wipe the skin with a gauze pad to remove the cream.
- Position the patient appropriately for the site chosen, and locate key landmarks, for example, the posterior superior iliac spine and the greater trochanter.
- Have someone help you restrain an infant; seek an older child's cooperation before enlisting assistance.
- Put on gloves.
- Clean the injection site with an alcohol or povidone-iodine pad. Wipe outward from the center with a spiral motion to avoid contaminating the clean area.
- Grasp the tissue surrounding the site between your index finger and thumb to immobilize the site and to create a muscle mass for the injection.
- Insert the needle quickly, using a darting motion. If you're using the ventrogluteal site, insert the needle at a 45-degree angle toward the knee.

- Aspirate the plunger to ensure that the needle isn't in a blood vessel. If no blood appears, inject the medication slowly so the muscle can distend to accommodate the volume.
- Withdraw the needle and gently massage the area with a gauze pad to stimulate circulation and enhance absorption.
- Provide comfort and praise.

GIVING A SUBCUTANEOUS INJECTION

- Select from these possible sites: the middle third of the upper outer arm; the middle third of the upper outer thigh, or the abdomen.
- You may apply a cold compress or EMLA cream, as described above, to the injection site to minimize pain.
- Put on gloves, and prepare the injection site with alcohol or povidone-iodine solution according to the patient's needs and facility policy.
- Pinch the tissue surrounding the site between your index finger and thumb to ensure injection into the subcutaneous tissue.
- Holding the needle at a 45- to 90-degree angle, quickly insert it into the tissue.
- Release your grasp on the tissue, and slowly inject the medication.
- Remove the needle quickly to decrease discomfort.
- Unless contraindicated, gently massage the area to facilitate absorption.

GIVING AN INTRADERMAL INJECTION

- Put on gloves and pull the patient's skin taut (the site of choice is the inner aspect of the forearm).
- Insert the needle, bevel up, at a 10- to 15-degree angle just beneath the outer skin layer.
- Slowly inject the medication, and watch for a bleb to appear.
- Quickly remove the needle, being careful to maintain the injection angle.
- If appropriate — for example, if the injection is related to allergy testing — draw a circle around the bleb, and avoid massaging the area so as not to interfere with test results.

(continued)

◆ Don't hesitate to consult the parents for tips on successfully administering medication to their child.

◆ If possible, have the parent administer prescribed oral medications while you supervise. However, avoid asking a parent to help with injections because the child may perceive the parent as a cause of pain.

◆ Aim for a trusting relationship with the child and his parents so you can offer support and promote cooperation even when a medication causes discomfort.

◆ If the child will receive one injection, allow him to choose from the appropriate sites. However, if the child will receive numerous injections, remember that site rotation must follow a set pattern.

◆ Allow the child to play with a medication cup or syringe and to pretend to give medication to a doll.

◆ When giving medication to an older child, be honest. Reassure him that distaste or discomfort will be brief.

◆ Emphasize that he must remain still to promote safety and minimize discomfort.

◆ Explain to the child and his parents that an assistant will help the child remain still, if necessary. Keep your explanations brief and simple.

◆ To divert the child's attention, have him start counting just before the injection, and challenge him to try to reach 10 before you finish the injection. If the child cries, don't scold him or allow the parents to scold him. Have one of the parents hold a younger child and praise him for allowing you to give him the injection. Apply an adhesive bandage to the injection site as a form of reward or badge.

◆ Avoid adding medication to a large amount of liquid, such as the child's milk or formula, because the child may not drink the entire amount, resulting in an inaccurate dose of medication.

◆ Compile a list of appropriate emergency drugs, calculating the dosages to the patient's weight. Post the list near the patient's bed for reference.

◆ If you have any doubt about proper medication dosage, always consult the prescriber who ordered the drug. Double-check information in a reliable drug reference.

COMPLICATIONS

◆ Adverse reactions to medication

◆ Teach the parents about the proper dosage and administration of all prescribed medications.

◆ If the parents will administer a liquid medication, advise them to use a commercially available, disposable oral syringe to measure the dose.

◆ To ensure an accurate dose, advise them to avoid using a teaspoon. Teach them how to use the oral syringe. Use written materials — a medication instruction sheet, for example — to reinforce your teaching.

- Note instructional activities related to the medications.

SELECTED REFERENCES

Rubin, B.K., and Fink, J.B. "The Delivery of Inhaled Medication to the Young Child," *Pediatric Clinics of North America* 50(3):717-31, June 2003.

Sullivan, J.E., and Buchino, J.J. "Medication Errors in Pediatrics —

The Octopus Evading Defeat," *Journal of Surgical Oncology* 88(3):182-88, December 2004.

Voirol, P., et al. "Impact of Pharmacists' Interventions on the Pediatric Discharge Medication Process," *Annals of Pharmacotherapy* 38(10):1597-602, October 2004.

I.M. injection sites in children

When selecting the best site for a child's I.M. injection, consider:
- the child's age, weight, and muscular development
- the type of drug you're administering
- the amount of subcutaneous fat over the injection site
- the drug's absorption rate.

VASTUS LATERALIS AND RECTUS FEMORIS

For a child younger than age 3, you'll typically use the vastus lateralis or rectus femoris muscle for an I.M. injection. Constituting the largest muscle mass in this age-group, the vastus lateralis and rectus femoris have fewer major blood vessels and nerves.

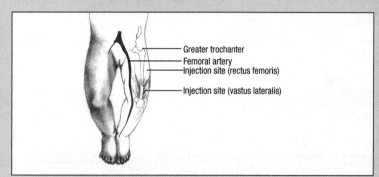

VENTROGLUTEAL AND DORSOGLUTEAL

For a child who can walk and is older than age 3, use the ventrogluteal and dorsogluteal muscles. Like the vastus lateralis, the ventrogluteal site is relatively free from major blood vessels and nerves. Before you select either site, make sure that the child has been walking for at least 1 year to ensure sufficient muscle development.

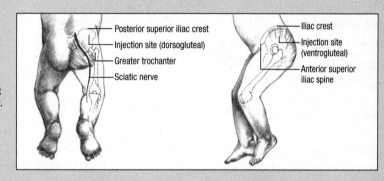

DELTOID

For a child older than 18 months who needs rapid medication results, consider using the deltoid muscle for the injection. Because blood flows faster in the deltoid muscle than in other muscles, drug absorption should be faster. However, be careful when using this site because the deltoid doesn't develop fully until adolescence. In a younger child, it's small and close to the radial nerve, which may be injured during needle insertion.

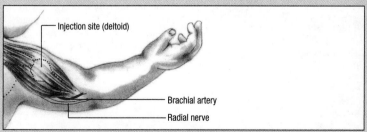

Drug implants

DESCRIPTION

◆ A method of advance drug delivery involves implanting drugs beneath the skin subcutaneously as well as targeting specific tissues with radiation implants.

◆ With subcutaneous implants, drug pellets are injected into the skin's subcutaneous layer. The drug is then stored in one area of the body, called a *depot.*

◆ A newer treatment for prostate cancer involves implants of goserelin acetate (Zoladex), a synthetic form of luteinizing hormone.

◆ Radiation drug implants with a short half-life may be placed inside a body cavity, within a tumor or on its surface, or in the area from which a tumor has been removed. These implants are usually inserted by a physician with a nurse assisting. However, some specially trained nurses may insert or inject intradermal implants. Radiation implants are usually put in place in an operating room or a radiation oncology suite.

CONTRAINDICATIONS

◆ Vary based on drug being implanted

EQUIPMENT

SUBCUTANEOUS IMPLANTS

Alcohol pad ◆ drug implant in a preloaded syringe ◆ local anesthetic (for some patients)

RADIATION IMPLANTS

RADIATION PRECAUTION sign for the patient's door ◆ warning labels for the patient's wristband and personal belongings ◆ film badge or pocket dosimeter ◆ lead-lined container ◆ long-handled forceps ◆ masking tape ◆ portable lead shield

KEY STEPS

◆ Confirm the patient's identity using two patient identifiers according to facility policy.

◆ Explain the procedure and its benefits and risks to the patient.

◆ Verify that an informed consent form has been signed.

INSERTING SUBCUTANEOUS IMPLANTS

◆ Help the patient into the supine position, and drape him so that his abdomen is accessible.

◆ Remove the syringe from the package, and make sure you can see the drug in the chamber.

◆ Put on gloves.

◆ Clean a small area on the patient's upper abdominal wall with the alcohol pad.

◆ As you stretch the skin at the injection site with one hand, grip the needle with the fingers of your other hand around the barrel of the syringe.

◆ Insert the needle into subcutaneous fat at a 45-degree angle.

◆ **WARNING** *Don't attempt to aspirate. If blood appears in the syringe, withdraw the needle and inject a new, preloaded syringe and needle at another site.*

◆ Change the direction of the needle so it's parallel to the abdominal wall.

◆ With the barrel hub touching the patient's skin, push the needle in, then withdraw it about ½" (1.3 cm) to create a space for the drug.

◆ Depress the plunger.

◆ Withdraw the needle and bandage the site with a sterile dressing and tape.

◆ Inspect the tip of the needle. If you can see the metal tip of the plunger, the drug has been discharged.

◆ Remove and discard gloves.

INSERTING RADIATION IMPLANTS

◆ To prepare for a radiation implant, place the lead-lined container and long-handled forceps in a corner of the patient's room. Also, place the lead shield in the back of the room so it can be worn when providing care.

◆ With masking tape, mark a safe line on the floor 6′ (1.8 m) from the bed to warn visitors of the danger of radiation exposure.

◆ Place a RADIATION PRECAUTION sign on the patient's door and warning labels on the patient's wristband and personal belongings.

◆ Place an emergency tracheotomy tray in the room if an implant will be inserted in the patient's mouth or neck.

◆ To insert the implant, the physician puts on gloves, makes a small incision in the skin, and creates a pocket in the tissue.

◆ He inserts the implant and closes the incision.

◆ The physician takes off the gloves and discards them.

◆ Your role in the implant procedure is to explain the treatment and its goals to the patient. Review radiation safety procedures and visitation policies. Talk with the patient about long-term physical and emotional aspects of the therapy and discuss home care.

- Special care may be necessary, depending on the type of implant used.

SUBCUTANEOUS IMPLANTS

- Be aware that if an implant must be removed, the physician will order an X-ray to locate it.
- Tell the patient to check the administration site for signs of infection or bleeding.
- Goserelin implants must be changed every 28 days. Female patients should be advised to use a nonhormonal form of contraception.

RADIATION IMPLANTS

- Know that if laboratory work is required during treatment, a technician wearing a film badge will obtain the specimen, affix a RADIATION PRECAUTION label to the specimen container, and alert laboratory personnel. If urine tests are needed, ask the radiation oncology department or laboratory technician how to transport the specimens safely.
- Minimize your own exposure to radiation. Wear a personal, nontransferable film badge or dosimeter at waist level during your entire shift. Turn in the film badge regularly. Pocket dosimeters measure immediate exposure.
- Use the principles of time, distance, and shielding.
- *Time:* Plan to give care in the shortest time possible. Less time equals less exposure.
- *Distance:* Work as far away from the radiation source as possible. Give care from the side opposite the implant or from a position that allows the greatest working distance possible. Prepare the patient's meal trays outside her room.
- *Shielding:* Wear a portable shield, if necessary.
- Make sure that the patient's room is monitored daily by the radiation oncology department and that disposable items are monitored and removed according to facility policy.

- Keep away staff members and visitors who are pregnant or trying to conceive or father a child. The gonads and a developing embryo or fetus are highly susceptible to the damaging effects of ionizing radiation.
- Collect a dislodged implant with long-handled forceps, and place it in a lead-lined container.
- If you must take the patient out of her room, notify the appropriate department of the patient's status to allow time for the necessary preparations.
- A patient with a permanent implant may not be released until her radioactivity level is less than 5 millirems/hour at a distance of about 3' (1 m).
- If a patient with an implant dies while on the unit, notify the radiation oncology staff so that a temporary implant can be properly removed and stored. If the implant was permanent, the staff will also determine which precautions should be followed after postmortem care measures.

COMPLICATIONS
Subcutaneous implants

- Goserelin implants: anemia, lethargy, pain, dizziness, insomnia, anxiety, depression, headache, chills, fever, edema, heart failure, arrhythmias, stroke, hypertension, peripheral vascular disease, nausea, vomiting, diarrhea, impotence, renal insufficiency, urinary obstruction, rash, sweating, hot flashes, gout, hyperglycemia, weight increase, or breast swelling and tenderness

Radiation implants

- Depending on implant site and dosage: implant dislodgment, tissue fibrosis, xerostomia, radiation pneumonitis, airway obstruction, muscle atrophy, sterility, vaginal dryness or stenosis, fistulas, altered bowel habits, diarrhea, hypothyroidism, infection, cystitis, myelosuppression, neurotoxicity, and secondary cancers

- Review radiation safety precautions, including time and distance restrictions, with the patient and his family, if the patient has a radiation drug implant.
- If the patient will be discharged with a radiation implant in place, instruct the patient and his family about the safe handling of waste materials.

- For subdermal and subcutaneous implants, document the name of the drug, the insertion or administration site, the date and time of insertion, and the patient's response to the procedure. Note the date that implants should be removed and a new set inserted or the date of the next administration, as appropriate.
- For radiation implants, document radiation precautions taken during treatment, adverse reactions, patient and family teaching and their responses, the patient's tolerance of isolation procedures and the family's compliance with procedures, and referrals to local cancer services.

SELECTED REFERENCES

Hirsch, H.J., et al. "The Histrelin Implant: A Novel Treatment for Central Precocious Puberty," *Pediatrics* 116(6):e798-802, December 2005.

Maloney, J.M., et al. "Electrothermally Activated Microchips for Implantable Drug Delivery and Biosensing," *Journal of Controlled Release* 109(1-3):244-55, December 2005.

Peterson, H.B., and Curtis, K.M. "Clinical Practice. Long-Acting Methods of Contraception," *New England Journal of Medicine* 353(20):2169-75, November 2005.

Yasukawa, T., et al. "Drug Delivery from Ocular Implants," *Expert Opinion on Drug Delivery* 3(2):261-73, March 2006.

Drug infusion through a secondary I.V. line

OVERVIEW

DESCRIPTION

- A secondary I.V. line is a complete I.V. set — container, tubing, and microdrip or macrodrip system — connected to the lower Y-port (secondary port) of a primary line instead of an I.V. catheter or needle.
- The secondary line permits constant or intermittent drug infusion and titration while the primary line maintains a constant total infusion rate.
- Most drugs can be piggybacked with a needle-free system through a "piggyback port." (See *Assembling a piggyback set*.)
- I.V. pumps may be used to maintain constant infusion rates, allow accurate titration of dosages, and maintain venous access.

CONTRAINDICATIONS

- None known

EQUIPMENT

Patient's medication record and chart ◆ I.V. medication ◆ I.V. solution ◆ administration set with secondary injection port ◆ needleless adapter ◆ alcohol pads ◆ 1″ adhesive tape ◆ time tape ◆ labels ◆ infusion pump ◆ extension hook and appropriate solution for intermittent piggyback infusion ◆ normal saline solution for infusion with incompatible solutions (optional)

INTERMITTENT INFUSION

- The primary line has a piggyback port with a backcheck valve that stops primary line flow during drug infusion and returns to primary line flow after infusion.

- A volume-control set can also be used with an intermittent infusion line.

PREPARATION

- Verify the order on the patient's drug record by checking against the prescriber's order.
- Wash your hands.
- Inspect the I.V. container for cracks, leaks, and contamination.
- Check drug compatibility with primary solution.
- Verify expiration date.
- Use an I.V. set with a secondary injection port if the drug is to be given regularly.
- Add the drug to the secondary I.V. solution as needed; remove any seals from the secondary container and

---

Assembling a piggyback set

A piggyback set is useful for intermittent drug infusion. To work properly, the secondary set's container must be positioned higher than the primary set's container.

- Extension hook
- Piggyback set
- Slide clamp
- Primary set
- Piggyback Y-port (with backcheck valve)
- Flow control clamp
- Secondary Y-port (to serve secondary set)

wipe the main port with an alcohol pad.
- ◆ Inject the drug into the port and gently agitate to mix the drug thoroughly.
- ◆ Properly label the I.V. mixture.
- ◆ Insert the administration set spike and attach the needle or use a needleless system.
- ◆ Open the flow clamp, prime the line, and then close the flow clamp.
- ◆ If the drug is in a vial ready for I.V. pole hanging, inject diluent directly into the drug vial, spike the vial, prime the tubing, and hang the set.

KEY STEPS

- ◆ Confirm the patient's identity using two patient identifiers according to facility policy.
- ◆ If your facility uses a bar code scanner, scan your ID badge, the patient's ID bracelet, and the drug's bar code.
- ◆ Assess the patient's I.V. site for pain, redness, or swelling and ensure patency.
- ⚡ **WARNING** *If the drug is incompatible with primary I.V. solution, replace the primary solution with normal saline solution and flush the line before starting the drug infusion.*
- ◆ If required, remove the primary I.V. solution and put in a sterile plug until it's rehung. This maintains the sterility and prevents use of the incompatible solution before the line is flushed with normal saline solution.
- ◆ Hang the secondary set's container and wipe the injection port of the primary line with an alcohol pad.
- ◆ Insert the needleless adapter from the secondary line into the injection port, and secure it to the primary line.
- ◆ To run the secondary set's container by itself, lower the primary set's container with an extension hook.
- ◆ To run both containers simultaneously, place them at the same height.
- ◆ Open the clamp and adjust the drip rate.

- ◆ For continuous infusion, set the secondary solution to the desired drip rate; adjust the primary solution to the desired total infusion rate.
- ◆ For intermittent infusion, adjust the primary drip rate, as required, on completion of the secondary solution.
- ◆ If secondary solution tubing is being reused, close the clamp on the tubing and follow facility policy.
- ◆ Remove the needleless adapter and replace it with a new one, or leave the system secured in the injection port and label it with the time of first use.
- ◆ Leave the empty container in place until you replace it with a new dose of drug at the prescribed time.
- ◆ If the tubing won't be reused, discard appropriately.

SPECIAL CONSIDERATIONS

- ◆ If facility policy allows, use a pump for drug infusion.
- ◆ Put a time tape on the secondary container.
- ◆ When reusing secondary tubing, change it according to facility policy (usually every 48 to 72 hours).
- ◆ Inspect the injection port for leakage with each use and change if needed.
- ◆ Unless you're piggybacking lipids, don't piggyback a secondary I.V. line to a total parenteral nutrition line because of risk of contamination. Check facility policy for any exceptions.

COMPLICATIONS
- ◆ Adverse reaction to infused drug
- ◆ Repeated punctures of secondary injection port damaging seal, possibly allowing leakage or contamination

PATIENT TEACHING

- ◆ Tell the patient to inform you of adverse reactions or problems, such as pain, redness, or swelling at the I.V. site.

DOCUMENTATION

- ◆ Record the amount and type of drug and I.V. solution on intake and output and drug records.
- ◆ Note the date, duration, and rate of infusion.
- ◆ Note patient response.

SELECTED REFERENCES
Briggs, B. "Pumped Up About I.V. System," *Health Data Management* 12(2):106-108, 110, February 2004.
Dulak, S.B. "Smart I.V. Pumps," *RN* 68(12):38-43, December 2005.
Fields, M., and Peterman, J. "Intravenous Medication Safety System Averts High-Risk Medication Errors and Provides Actionable Data," *Nursing Administration Quarterly* 29(1):78-87, January-March 2005.

Drug therapy, geriatric

OVERVIEW

DESCRIPTION

◆ Aging alters body composition that affects drug metabolism, absorption, distribution, and excretion, and may require altered drug dosage and administration.
◆ Adverse drug reactions that interfere with therapeutic compliance may commonly occur in the elderly patient. (See *How age affects drug action* and *Modifying I.M. injections.*)
◆ The elderly patient may have difficulty complying with his drug regimen.

How age affects drug action

With age, body structures and systems change, affecting how the body responds to drugs.

BODY COMPOSITION

As a person grows older, his total body mass and lean body mass tend to decrease while body fat tends to increase. These factors affect the relationship between a drug's concentration and solubility in the body.

DIGESTIVE SYSTEM

Decreases in gastric acid secretion and GI motility lead to a decreased ability to absorb many drugs. This can cause problems with certain drugs, such as digoxin, which has a narrow therapeutic range tied closely to absorption.

HEPATIC SYSTEM

Advancing age reduces blood supply, and certain liver enzymes become less active, resulting in the liver losing some of its ability to metabolize drugs. This results in intensified drug effects, as more of the drug remains in circulation, and increases occurrences of drug toxicity.

RENAL SYSTEM

Kidney function also diminishes with age. This alone may affect drug elimination by 50% or more. In many cases, decreased kidney function leads to increased blood levels of certain drugs.

CONTRAINDICATIONS

◆ None known

EQUIPMENT

Patient's drug record ◆ appropriate drugs ◆ written dosage instructions ◆

Modifying I.M. injections

Before you give an intramuscular (I.M.) injection to an elderly patient, remember the physical changes that accompany aging and choose your equipment, site, and technique accordingly.

CHOOSING A NEEDLE

An elderly patient usually has less subcutaneous tissue and less muscle mass than a younger patient — especially in the buttocks and deltoids. You may need to use a shorter needle than you would for a younger adult.

SELECTING A SITE

An elderly patient typically has more fat around the hips, abdomen, and thighs. This makes the vastus lateralis muscle and ventrogluteal area (gluteus medius and minimus, but not gluteus maximus) the primary injection sites.

You should be able to palpate the muscle in these areas easily. If the patient is extremely thin, gently pinch the muscle to elevate it and avoid putting the needle completely through it (which will alter absorption and distribution of the drug).

Never give an I.M. injection in an immobile limb because of poor drug absorption and the risk that a sterile abscess will form at the injection site.

CHECKING TECHNIQUE

To make sure the needle isn't in a blood vessel, pull back on the plunger, and look for blood before injecting the drug. Because of age-related vascular changes, elderly patients are also at greater risk for hematomas.

To stop bleeding after an I.M. injection, apply direct pressure for a longer time than usual. Gently massage the injection site to aid drug absorption and distribution. Avoid site massage with certain drugs given by the Z-track injection technique such as iron dextran.

---

compliance aids — pill containers, calendar, large-print teaching aids, premeasured injections (optional)

KEY STEPS

◆ Review the patient's complaint and obtain his health and drug histories.
◆ Ask him about the use of herbs or other therapies.
◆ Assess his physical ability to take drugs, such as reading labels, identifying drugs, and opening bottles.

AGE FACTOR *If the patient has dexterity problems, advise him to request snap or screw caps (rather than childproof closures) for his drug containers.*

◆ Evaluate his ability to take drugs on time and store them properly. Refer him to appropriate community resources for supervision if necessary.
◆ Assess his lifestyle and include family or friends in teaching sessions. Make referrals and contact appropriate social agencies if necessary.
◆ Assess his attitude toward drug use and willingness to take prescribed drugs.
◆ Ask whether his prescribed drug regimen interferes with his daily routine.
◆ Discuss his drug therapy with him. As he receives drugs, explain their intended effect, drug interactions, and possible adverse reactions to watch for and report. (See *Recognizing common adverse drug reactions in elderly patients.*)
◆ Ask him about the prescription and nonprescription drugs he takes, and has taken in the past. Also ask if he takes drugs prescribed for another person.
◆ Use an appropriate reference to assess possible drug interactions.

SPECIAL CONSIDERATIONS

◆ Monitor serum drug levels to avoid toxicity.
◆ When discontinuing a drug, instruct the patient to discard it in the toilet.
◆ Suggest that he store drugs as guided, or in a dry place out of sunlight.

WARNING *If the patient keeps drugs at the bedside, he may accidentally overdose by taking them before he's fully awake and alert. Suggest that he keep them in a medicine cabinet or kitchen.*

- If he's discharged with a new drug regimen, schedule visiting nurse follow-up care to make sure he's following the regimen and to monitor his response.
- If he can't afford drugs, suggest using generic equivalents, having his family help, or refer him to social service or community agencies.

COMPLICATIONS
- None known

- Advise the patient to contact you or his practitioner before taking nonprescription drugs.
- Advise the patient to use one pharmacy that maintains patient drug profiles and help him find a pharmacy that delivers or mails prescriptions.
- Inform the patient about food-drug interactions; provide a list of foods to avoid.
- Give dosage instructions in large print if necessary.
- Tell the patient which drugs to take with food and which to take without food.
- Check whether the patient eats regularly or skips meals; if he skips meals, he may skip doses, too. Help him schedule taking drugs with his eating habits.
- Help the patient find easier ways to take medicine, such as asking for liquid or powdered forms, or taking with soft food such as applesauce.
- Advise the patient which drugs shouldn't be crushed.
- Suggest the use of compliance aids, such as pill containers and premeasured injections.

DOCUMENTATION
- Document assessment findings and laboratory test results.
- Record instructions and teaching aids given to the patient or his caregivers.
- Record all drugs, dosages, adverse reactions, and interventions.
- Note the patient's understanding of his drug regimen.
- Note health and social service referrals.

SELECTED REFERENCES

Banning, M. "Medication Management: Older People and Nursing," *Nursing Older People* 17(7):20-23, October 2005.

Lynch, T. "Medication Costs as a Primary Cause of Nonadherence in the Elderly," *The Consultant Pharmacist* 21(2):143-46, February 2006.

Schmidt, K.S., and Lieto, J.M. "Validity of the Medication Administration Test Among Older Adults With and Without Dementia," *American Journal of Geriatric Pharmacotherapy* 3(4):255-61, December 2005.

Stuart, B., et al. "Coverage and Use of Prescription Drugs in Nursing Homes: Implications for the Medicare Modernization Act," *Medical Care* 44(3):243-49, March 2006.

Wang, P.S., et al. "Risk of Death in Elderly Users of Conventional vs. Atypical Antipsychotic Medications," *New England Journal of Medicine* 353(22):2335-41, December 2005.

Recognizing common adverse drug reactions in elderly patients

Signs and symptoms of adverse reactions to drugs include hives, impotence, incontinence, stomach upset, and rashes. Elderly patients are more likely to have serious adverse reactions, such as orthostatic hypotension, dehydration, altered mental status, anorexia, blood disorders, and tardive dyskinesia.

Some adverse reactions, such as anxiety, confusion, and forgetfulness, may be mistakenly dismissed as effects of aging.

ORTHOSTATIC HYPOTENSION
Marked by dizziness and poor balance, orthostatic hypotension is a common adverse effect of antidepressant, antihypertensive, antipsychotic, and sedative medications.

To prevent accidents, warn the patient not to sit up or get out of bed too quickly. Have him ask for assistance in walking if he feels dizzy or faint.

DEHYDRATION
If the patient is taking diuretics, be alert for dehydration and electrolyte imbalances. Monitor blood levels and provide potassium supplements, as ordered.

Many drugs cause dry mouth. If this occurs, suggest lozenges or sugarless hard candy.

ALTERED MENTAL STATUS
Agitation or confusion may follow ingestion of alcohol or anticholinergic, antidiuretic, antihypertensive, antipsychotic, antianxiety, and antidepressant drugs. Paradoxically, depression is a common adverse effect of antidepressant drugs.

ANOREXIA
Anorexia is a warning sign of toxicity — especially from cardiac glycosides, bronchodilators, and antihistamines. Low initial doses are prescribed and effects assessed.

BLOOD DISORDERS
If the patient takes an anticoagulant, watch for signs of easy bruising or bleeding. Drugs that may cause these reactions include antineoplastics, antibiotics, and anticonvulsants. These symptoms may indicate other problems, such as blood dyscrasias or thrombocytopenia. A patient with these symptoms should check with his physician immediately.

TARDIVE DYSKINESIA
Characterized by abnormal tongue movements, lip pursing, grimacing, blinking, and gyrating motions of the face and extremities, tardive dyskinesia may be triggered by psychotropic drugs.

Dying patient care

DESCRIPTION

- Emotional support for the dying patient and his family typically means the nurse's reassurance and presence to help ease fear and loneliness.
- Emotional support is important for patients with long-term progressive illnesses, to help them work through the stages of dying. (See *Five stages of dying*.)
- Signs of impending death include reduced respiratory rate and depth, decreased blood pressure, weak or erratic pulse, cooler skin, decreased consciousness, diminished sensory and neuromuscular control, diaphoresis, pallor, cyanosis, and mottling.
- Know that the patient may have signed a living will requesting no artificial support including defibrillators, respirators, life-sustaining drugs, and auxiliary hearts.

- Respect the patient's wishes, communicating the practitioner's "no code" order to all staff members.

CONTRAINDICATIONS

- None known

EQUIPMENT

Clean bed linens ◆ clean gowns ◆ gloves ◆ water-filled basin ◆ soap ◆ washcloth ◆ towels ◆ lotion ◆ linen-saver pads ◆ petroleum jelly ◆ suction equipment, as necessary ◆ optional: indwelling urinary catheter

KEY STEPS

- Take vital signs as needed, and observe for pallor, diaphoresis, and decreased consciousness.
- Reposition the patient in bed at least every 2 hours because sensation, reflexes, and mobility diminish first in the legs and gradually in the arms.
- Make sure bedding covers him loosely to reduce discomfort.
- When vision and hearing start to fail, turn his head toward the light and speak to him closely.
- Because hearing may be acute despite loss of consciousness, avoid whispering or speaking inappropriately in his presence.
- Change bed linens and gowns as needed.
- Provide skin care during gown changes; adjust the room temperature for patient comfort if necessary.
- Observe for incontinence or anuria. If necessary, obtain an order to catheterize the patient, or place linen-saver pads under him.
- Provide perineal care to prevent irritation.
- Suction his mouth and upper airway to remove secretions as needed.
- Elevate the head of his bed to decrease respiratory resistance.
- As his condition worsens, he may breathe mostly through his mouth.
- Offer fluids frequently, and lubricate his lips and mouth with petroleum jelly to counteract dryness.
- If a comatose patient's eyes are open, provide eye care to prevent corneal ulceration, which can cause blindness and prevent use of these tissues for potential transplantation.
- Provide analgesics as needed.
- As circulation diminishes, drugs given I.M. will be poorly absorbed. Give drugs I.V. for best results.
- Some drugs can be given sublingually or rectally if the patient can't swallow or has no I.V. access.
- Notify family members when the patient wishes to see them.
- Let the patient and his family discuss death at their own pace.

Five stages of dying

The dying patient may progress through five psychological stages in preparation for death. Patients experience these stages differently; understanding them will help you meet your patient's needs.

DENIAL

When the patient first learns of his terminal illness, he may not accept the diagnosis. He may experience physical symptoms similar to a stress reaction — shock, fainting, pallor, sweating, tachycardia, nausea, and GI disorders. Be honest with him, but not blunt or callous. Maintain communication so he can discuss his feelings when he accepts the reality of death. Don't force him to confront this reality.

ANGER

When he stops denying his impending death, he may resent those who will live on after he dies, including his family and caregivers around him. You may resent this behavior and want to avoid him; remember that he's dying and has a right to be angry. After you accept his anger, you can help him find different ways to express and understand it.

BARGAINING

Although he acknowledges his impending death, he may try to bargain for more time with God or fate. He may do this secretly. If he confides in you, don't urge him to keep any promises he makes.

DEPRESSION

He may experience regrets about his past or current condition. He may withdraw from friends, family, practitioner, and you. He may suffer from anorexia, increased fatigue, or self-neglect. You may find him alone and in tears. Accept his sorrow, and if he talks to you, listen. Provide comfort by touch, as appropriate. Avoid making optimistic remarks or cheerful small talk.

ACCEPTANCE

He accepts the inevitability and imminence of his death without emotion. He may desire the quiet company of family or friends. If they can't be present, stay with him to satisfy his final need. Remember, many patients die before reaching this stage.

- Offer to contact a member of the clergy or social services department, if appropriate.
- As the patient's death approaches, give his family emotional support.

SPECIAL CONSIDERATIONS

- If the patient signed a living will, the physician will write a "no code" order on his progress notes and order sheets. Transfer the "no code" order to the patient's chart or Kardex and inform other staff. (As needed, check your state's laws on living wills.)
- At an appropriate time, ask the patient's family if they have considered organ and tissue donation.
- Check the patient's records to determine whether he completed an organ donor card. (See *Understanding organ and tissue donation*.)

COMPLICATIONS
- None known

PATIENT TEACHING

- Explain care and treatment to the patient, even if he's unconscious. Answer any questions as candidly as possible, without sounding callous.
- Allow the patient to express his feelings, which may range from anger to loneliness. Take time to talk with him. Avoid looking rushed or unconcerned.
- If family members stay with the patient, show them the location of bathrooms, cafeterias, and other services.
- Explain the patient's needs, treatments, and care plan to family members.
- If appropriate, offer to teach family members specific skills so they can take part in nursing care.
- Emphasize that their efforts are important and effective.

Understanding organ and tissue donation

Federal regulations require facilities to report all deaths to the regional organ procurement organization. The law was enacted so that no potential donor is missed and ensures that families of potential donors understand the option to donate. About 25 different organs and tissues can be transplanted. Organ donors typically must be between infancy and age 60 and free of transmissible disease. Tissue donations are less restrictive; some tissue banks accept skin from donors up to age 75.

Collection of most organs (heart, liver, kidney, pancreas) requires that the patient be pronounced brain dead and kept physically alive until organs are harvested. Tissue such as eyes, skin, bone, and heart valves can be taken after death. Contact your regional organ procurement organization for specific organ donation criteria or to identify a potential donor. If you don't know the organization in your area, contact the United Network for Organ Sharing at (888) 894-6361 or at *www.unos.org*.

DOCUMENTATION

- Record changes in the patient's vital signs, intake and output, and level of consciousness.
- Note the times of cardiac arrest and the end of respiration, and notify the practitioner when these occur.

SELECTED REFERENCES
Copnell, B. "Death in the pediatric ICU: Caring for Children and Families at the End of Life," *Critical Care Nursing Clinics of North America* 17(4):349-60, December 2005.

Duffy, S.A., et al. "Racial/Ethnic Preferences, Sex Preferences, and Perceived Discrimination Related to End-of-Life Care," *Journal of the American Geriatrics Society* 54(1):150-57, January 2006.

Fairbrother, C.A., and Paice, J.A. "Life's Final Journey: The Oncology Nurse's Role," *Clinical Journal of Oncology Nursing* 9(5):575-79, October 2005.

Graham, I.W., et al. "Mutual Suffering: A Nurse's Story of Caring for the Living As They Are Dying," *International Journal of Nursing Practice* 11(6):277-85, December 2005.

Pier, J. "Care of Dying Patients," *Nursing Standard* 20(19):67-68, January 2006.

Touhy, T.A., et al. "Spiritual Caring: End of Life in a Nursing Home," *Journal of Gerontological Nursing* 31(9):27-35, September 2005.

Eardrop instillation

OVERVIEW

DESCRIPTION

◆ Eardrops may be instilled to treat infection and inflammation, soften cerumen for later removal, produce local anesthesia, or to facilitate removal of an insect trapped in the ear by immobilizing and smothering it.

CONTRAINDICATIONS

◆ Perforated eardrum, but might be allowed with certain drugs and sterile technique
◆ Eardrops containing hydrocortisone, if the patient has herpes, another viral infection, or a fungal infection

EQUIPMENT

Prescribed eardrops ◆ patient's drug record and chart ◆ light source ◆ facial tissue or cotton-tipped applicator ◆ cotton ball, bowl of warm water (optional)

PREPARATION

◆ Check the patient's drug record against the prescriber's order.
◆ To avoid adverse effects (such as vertigo, nausea, or pain) caused by eardrops that are too cold, put the eardrop container in a basin of warm water.
◆ Test the temperature of the drug by placing a drop on your wrist.

⚡ **WARNING** *If the drug is too hot, it may burn the patient's eardrum.*

KEY STEPS

◆ Wash your hands.
◆ Confirm the patient's identity using two patient identifiers according to facility policy.
◆ Provide privacy.
◆ Explain the procedure.
◆ Have the patient lie on the side opposite the affected ear.
◆ Straighten the patient's ear canal. For an adult, pull the auricle of the ear up and back. (See *Positioning the patient for eardrop instillation*.)

🔬 *AGE FACTOR For an infant or child younger than age 3, gently pull the auricle down and back because the ear canal is straighter at this age.*

◆ Using a light source, examine the ear canal for drainage.
◆ Clean the canal with the tissue or cotton-tipped applicator because drainage can reduce the drug's effectiveness.
◆ Compare the label on the eardrops with the order on the patient's drug record.
◆ Check the label again while drawing the drug into the dropper.
◆ To avoid damaging the ear canal with the dropper, support the hand holding the dropper against the patient's head.
◆ Straighten the patient's ear canal and instill the ordered number of drops.
◆ To prevent patient discomfort, instill the drops against the sides of the ear canal, not on the eardrum.
◆ Hold the ear canal in position until you see the drug disappear down the canal.
◆ Instruct the patient to remain on his side for 5 to 10 minutes to allow the drug to run further into the ear canal.
◆ If ordered, tuck the cotton ball loosely into the canal opening to prevent the drug from leaking out.

WARNING *Don't insert the cotton too deeply because this would prevent drainage of secretions and increase pressure on the eardrum.*
- Clean and dry the outer ear.
- Assist the patient into a comfortable position.
- Wash your hands.
- If ordered, repeat the procedure in the other ear after 5 to 10 minutes.

SPECIAL CONSIDERATIONS

- Some conditions, such as infection, make the normally tender ear canal even more sensitive; perform the procedure carefully.

    WARNING *To prevent eardrum injuries, never insert a cotton-tipped applicator into the ear canal past the point where you can see the tip.*
- After instilling eardrops to soften cerumen, irrigate the ear as ordered.
- If the patient has vertigo, keep the side rails of his bed up and assist him during the procedure.
- Move slowly and unhurriedly to avoid worsening vertigo.

COMPLICATIONS
- None known

PATIENT TEACHING

- Teach the patient to instill the eardrops correctly so that treatment can continue at home, if necessary.
- Review the procedure and let the patient try it himself while you observe.

DOCUMENTATION

- Note the name of the drug.
- Record which ear was treated.
- Record the date, time, and number of drops instilled.
- Note adverse reactions such as drainage, redness, vertigo, nausea, or pain.

SELECTED REFERENCES
Coates, H. "Ototoxic Eardrops and Tympanic Membrane Perforations: Time for a Change?" *Journal of Paediatric and Child Health* 41(8):401-404, August 2005.

Orr, C.F., and Rowe, D.B. "Eardrop Attacks: Seizures Triggered by Ciprofloxacin Eardrops," *Medical Journal of Australia* 178(7):343, April 2003.

Torum, B., et al. "Efficacy of Ofloxacin Otic Solution Once Daily for 7 Days in the Treatment of Otitis Externa: A Multicenter, Open-Label, Phase III Trial," *Clinical Therapeutics* 26(7): 1046-54, July 2004.

Wai, T.K., and Michael, C.F. "A Benefit-Risk Assessment of Ofloxacin Otic Solution in Ear Infection," *Drug Safety* 26(6):405-20, 2003.

Positioning the patient for eardrop instillation

Have the patient lie on his side. Straighten his ear canal to ensure medication reaches the eardrum. For an adult, gently pull the auricle up and back; for an infant or young child, gently pull down and back (as shown).

ADULT

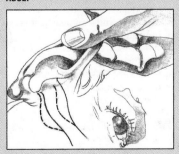

CHILD

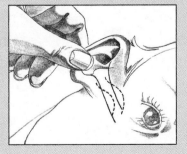

Ear irrigation

DESCRIPTION

- The external auditory canal is washed with a stream of solution to clean discharge from the ear canal, soften and remove impacted cerumen, or dislodge a foreign body.
- Irrigation is also used to relieve localized inflammation and discomfort.
- The procedure must be performed carefully to avoid causing discomfort or vertigo and avoid increasing the risk of otitis media.

⚡ **WARNING** *Irrigation can contaminate the middle ear if the tympanic membrane is ruptured; an otoscopic examination should be done before ear irrigation.*

CONTRAINDICATIONS

- Suspected tympanic membrane perforation
- Infectious process present

⚡ **WARNING** *Ear irrigation is contraindicated when a vegetable (such as a pea) obstructs the auditory canal because it can swell in contact with an irrigant, causing pain and complicating removal. Don't irrigate if a battery (or battery part) is lodged in the ear; if battery acid leaks, irrigation would spread caustic material throughout the canal.*

Ear irrigation syringe (rubber bulb) ◆ otoscope with aural speculum ◆ prescribed irrigant ◆ large basin ◆ linen-saver pad and bath towel ◆ cotton balls or cotton-tipped applicators ◆ 4″ × 4″ gauze pad ◆ adjustable light, container for irrigant, tubing, clamp, syringe with ear tip, normal saline solution, gloves, cotton (optional)

PREPARATION

- Wash your hands; wear gloves if you expect contact with infected matter.
- Select a syringe, and obtain prescribed irrigant.
- Put the container of irrigant in a large basin filled with hot water to warm the solution to body temperature (98.6° F [37° C]).
- Test the temperature of the irrigant by sprinkling some on your inner wrist.

⚡ **WARNING** *Avoid extreme temperature changes of the irrigant, which can affect inner ear fluids, causing nausea and dizziness.*

- Inspect equipment (syringe or catheter tips) for breaks or cracks; inspect metal tips for roughness.

- Confirm the patient's identity using two patient identifiers according to facility policy.
- Explain the procedure to the patient.
- Provide privacy.
- Inspect the auditory canal of the ear that will be irrigated using an otoscope.
- Help the patient to a sitting position with his head tilted slightly forward and toward the affected side.
- If the patient can't sit, lie him on his back and tilt his head slightly forward and toward the affected ear.
- Make sure you have adequate lighting.
- If the patient is sitting, place the linen-saver pad (covered with the bath towel) on his shoulder and upper arm, under the affected ear. If he's lying down, cover his pillow and the area under the affected ear.
- To avoid getting foreign matter into the ear canal, clean the auricle and the meatus of the auditory canal with a cotton-tipped applicator moistened with normal saline solution or the prescribed irrigating solution.
- Draw the irrigant into the syringe and expel any air.
- Straighten the auditory canal; then insert the syringe tip and start the flow. (See *How to irrigate the ear canal.*)

🌸 **AGE FACTOR** *To examine the ear canal of a child younger than age 3, pull the pinna down and back.*

- During irrigation, observe the patient for signs of pain or dizziness. If dizziness occurs, stop the procedure, recheck the temperature of the irrigant, inspect the patient's ear with the otoscope, and resume irrigation, as indicated.
- When the syringe is empty, remove it and inspect the return flow.
- Refill the syringe, and continue the irrigation until the return flow is clear.

⚡ **WARNING** *Never use more than 500 ml of irrigant during the procedure.*

- Remove the syringe, and inspect the ear canal for cleanliness with the otoscope.
- Dry the patient's auricle and neck.
- Remove the bath towel and linen-saver pad.
- Help the seated patient lie on his affected side with the 4″ × 4″ gauze pad under his ear to promote drainage of residual debris and solution.

How to irrigate the ear canal

- Gently pull the auricle up and back to straighten the ear canal. For a child, pull the ear down and back.
- Have the patient hold an emesis basin beneath the ear.
- Position the tip of the irrigating syringe at the meatus of the auditory canal (as shown).

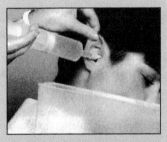

- Don't block the meatus; you'll impede backflow and raise pressure in the canal.
- Tilt the patient's head toward you, and point the syringe tip upward and toward the posterior ear canal (as shown). This angle prevents damage to the tympanic membrane and guards against pushing debris farther into the canal.

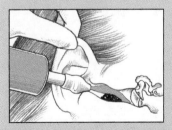

- Direct a steady stream of irrigant against the upper wall of the ear canal; inspect return fluid for cloudiness, cerumen, blood, or foreign matter.

SPECIAL CONSIDERATIONS

- Avoid dropping or squirting irrigant on the tympanic membrane, because this can startle the patient and cause discomfort.
- If you're using an irrigating catheter instead of a syringe, adjust the flow of solution to a steady, comfortable rate with a flow clamp.

⚡ **WARNING** *Don't raise the container more than 6″ (15.2 cm) above the ear because resulting pressure can damage the tympanic membrane.*

- If the practitioner directs you to place cotton in the ear canal to retain some of the solution, pack it loosely and tell the patient not to remove it.
- If impacted cerumen isn't dislodged, the practitioner may order several drops of glycerin or carbamide peroxide to be instilled two or three times daily for a few days, then irrigate the ear again.

COMPLICATIONS
- Trauma to the mucous membrane
- Pain
- Vertigo
- Infection
- Nausea
- Vomiting
- Tinnitus
- Ruptured tympanic membrane
- Otitis media

PATIENT TEACHING

- Inform the patient of signs and symptoms to report, such as abnormal discharge, pain, vertigo, or hearing problems.
- Explain proper ear care at home, such as preventing cerumen impaction and preventing insertion of foreign bodies.

DOCUMENTATION

- Note date and time, and which ear was irrigated.
- Record the volume and type of solution used.
- Note the appearance of the canal before and after irrigation.
- Note the appearance of the return flow.
- Note the patient's tolerance and comments about his condition, especially those related to his hearing acuity.

SELECTED REFERENCES
Baer, S. "Knowing When to Treat Ear Wax," *Practitioner* 249(1670):328, 330, 332, May 2005.
Dimmitt, P. "Cerumen Removal Products," *Journal of Pediatric Health Care* 19(5):332-36, September-October 2005.
Shefelbine, S.E., et al. "Mitigation of Hearing Loss from Semi-Circular Canal Transection in Pseudomonas Otitis Media with Ciprofloxacin-Dexamethasone Irrigation," *Otology & Neurotology* 27(2):265-69, February 2006.
Williams, D. "Does Irrigation of the Ear to Remove Impacted Wax Improve Hearing?" *British Journal of Community Nursing* 10(5):228-32, May 2005.

Elastic bandage application

DESCRIPTION

- An elastic bandage exerts gentle, even pressure on a body part.
- By supporting blood vessels, it promotes venous return and prevents pooling of blood in the legs.
- It can be used in place of antiembolism stockings to prevent thrombophlebitis and pulmonary embolism in postoperative or bedridden patients who can't stimulate venous return by muscle activity.
- It can be used to minimize joint swelling after trauma to the musculoskeletal system.
- Used with a splint, it immobilizes a fracture during healing.
- It can provide hemostatic pressure and anchor dressings over a fresh wound or after surgical procedures such as vein stripping.

CONTRAINDICATIONS

- None known

EQUIPMENT

Elastic bandage of appropriate width, typically 2″ to 6″ widths and 4″ and 6″ lengths (3″ width is adaptable to most applications) ◆ tape ◆ pins or self-closures ◆ gauze pads or absorbent cotton

PREPARATION

- Select a bandage that wraps the affected body part completely but isn't too long. Use a narrower bandage for wrapping the foot, lower leg, hand, or arm, and a wider bandage for the thigh or trunk.
- The bandage should be clean and rolled before application.

KEY STEPS

- **WARNING** *If the area to be wrapped has lesions or broken skin, consult the practitioner before applying an elastic bandage.*
- Confirm the patient's identity using two patient identifiers according to facility policy.
- Explain the procedure, provide privacy, and wash your hands.
- Put the body part to be bandaged in a normal position to promote circulation and prevent deformity and discomfort.
- **WARNING** *Avoid applying a bandage to a dependent extremity. If you're wrapping an extremity, elevate it for 15 to 30 minutes before application to facilitate venous return.*
- Apply the bandage so skin surfaces don't remain in contact when wrapped. Place gauze pads or cotton as needed between skin surfaces, such as between toes and fingers and under breasts and arms, to prevent skin irritation.
- Hold the bandage with the roll facing upward in one hand and the free end of the bandage in the other hand.
- Hold the bandage roll close to the part being bandaged to ensure even tension and pressure.
- Unroll the bandage as you wrap the body part in a spiral or spiral-reverse method.
- **WARNING** *Don't unroll the entire bandage before wrapping; this can cause uneven pressure, which interferes with blood circulation and cell nourishment.*
- Overlap each layer of bandage by one-half to two-thirds the width of the strip. (See *Bandaging techniques*.)
- Wrap firmly but not too tightly. Have the patient tell you if the bandage feels comfortable. If he complains of tingling, itching, numbness, or pain, loosen the bandage.
- When wrapping an extremity, first anchor the bandage by circling the body part twice.

- To prevent the bandage from slipping out of place on the foot, wrap it in a figure eight around the foot, the ankle and then the foot again before continuing. The same technique works on knees, wrists, and elbows.
- **WARNING** *Include the heel when wrapping the foot, but don't wrap toes or fingers, unless necessary; the distal extremities are used to detect impaired circulation.*
- When you're finished wrapping, secure the end of the bandage with tape, pins, or self-closures.
- **WARNING** *Avoid using metal clips; they can loosen when the patient moves, getting lost in bed linens and causing injury.*
- Check distal circulation after the bandage is in place because the elastic may tighten as you wrap.
- Check distal circulation periodically; an elastic bandage that's too tight may cause neurovascular damage.
- Lift the distal end of the bandage and assess the skin underneath for color, temperature, and integrity.
- Remove the bandage every 8 hours or whenever it's loose and wrinkled. Roll it up as you unwrap to prepare it for reuse.
- Observe the area and provide skin care before rewrapping the bandage.
- Change the bandage at least once daily.
- Bathe the skin, dry it thoroughly, and observe for irritation and breakdown before applying a fresh bandage.

- Wrap an elastic bandage from the distal area to the proximal area to promote venous return.
- Avoid leaving gaps in layers, which may cause uneven pressure.
- Observe for allergic reaction; some patients can't tolerate the sizing in a new bandage. Laundering reduces this risk.
- Wash the bandage daily or when it loses elasticity; laundering restores elasticity. Have two bandages on hand so one can be applied while the other is washed.

- When using an elastic bandage after a surgical procedure on an extremity (such as vein stripping) or with a splint to immobilize a fracture, remove it only as ordered rather than every 8 hours.

COMPLICATIONS

- Arterial obstruction, characterized by a decreased or absent distal pulse, blanching or bluish discoloration of skin, dusky nail beds, numbness and tingling or pain and cramping, and cold skin
- Edema from obstruction of venous return
- Allergic reaction
- Skin irritation

PATIENT TEACHING

- If the patient will be using an elastic bandage at home, teach him or a family member how to apply it correctly and assess for restricted circulation.
- Tell the patient to keep two bandages available so he'll have one on while the other is being laundered.

DOCUMENTATION

- Record the date and time of bandage application and removal.
- Note the application site.
- Record bandage size.
- Note skin condition before application.
- Note skin care after removal.
- Record complications.
- Document the patient's tolerance of the treatment.
- Note patient teaching.

SELECTED REFERENCES

Anderson, I. "Should Health Care Assistants Apply Compression Bandages?" *Nursing Times* 102(4):36-37, January 2006.

Fletcher, J. "The Importance of Correctly Choosing a Bandage and Bandaging Technique," *Nursing Times* 100(32):52-53, August 2004.

Pollard, A., and Cronin, G. "Compression Bandaging for Soft Tissue Injury of the Ankle: A Literature Review," *Emergency Nurse* 13(6):20-25, October 2005.

Bandaging techniques

You may have to apply an elastic bandage to an extremity or the patient's head to provide pressure or hold bandaging in place. Below are some common wrapping techniques.

CIRCULAR

Each turn encircles the previous one, covering it completely. Use this technique to anchor a bandage.

SPIRAL

Each turn partially overlaps the previous one. Use this technique to wrap a long, straight body part or one of increasing circumference.

SPIRAL-REVERSE

Anchor the bandage, and then reverse direction halfway through each spiral turn. Use this technique where there's increasing circumference of a body part.

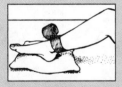 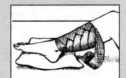

FIGURE EIGHT

Anchor below the joint, then use alternating ascending and descending turns to form a figure eight. Use this technique around joints.

RECURRENT

This technique includes a combination of recurrent and circular turns. Hold the bandage as you make each recurrent turn, then use the circular turns as a final anchor. Use this technique for a stump, a hand, or the scalp.

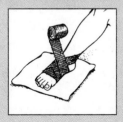 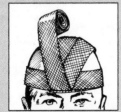 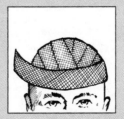

Electrocardiography, posterior chest lead placement

OVERVIEW

DESCRIPTION
- Because of the location of the heart's posterior surface, changes associated with myocardial damage aren't apparent on a standard 12-lead electrocardiography.
- The posterior chest lead electrocardiogram (ECG) can identify changes associated with the heart's posterior surface, which helps identify posterior wall infarction so that appropriate treatment can begin.
- It's typically performed with a standard ECG and involves recording only the additional posterior leads: V_7, V_8, and V_9.

CONTRAINDICATIONS
- None known

EQUIPMENT

Multichannel ECG machine with recording paper ◆ disposable pregelled electrodes ◆ 4″ × 4″ gauze pads ◆ clippers, marking pen, moist cloth (optional)

PREPARATION
- Place the ECG machine close to the patient and plug it in or confirm that the battery is charged.
- Keep the patient away from electrical fixtures and power cords to minimize electrical interference.
- Make sure paper speed is set at 25 mm/second and amplitude at 1 mV/10 mm.

KEY STEPS

- Confirm the patient's identity using two patient identifiers according to facility policy.
- Explain the procedure to the patient and his family.
- Wash your hands.
- Place the patient on his right side.
- Provide privacy and expose his arms, chest, and legs.
- Prepare the electrode sites according to the manufacturer's instructions.
- To ensure good skin contact, clip the sites if the patient has a lot of back hair.
- When using a multichannel ECG machine, begin by attaching a disposable electrode to the V_7 position on the left posterior axillary line, fifth intercostal space.
- Attach the V_4 leadwire to the V_7 electrode.
- Attach a disposable electrode at the V_8 position on the left midscapular line, fifth intercostal space.
- Attach the V_5 leadwire to this electrode.
- Attach a disposable electrode at the V_9 position, just left of the spinal column at the fifth intercostal space, and attach the V_6 leadwire to the V_9 electrode.

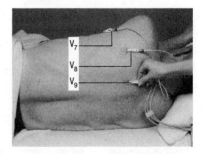

- If you're using a single-channel ECG machine, use electrodes and gel at locations for electrodes V_7, V_8, and V_9.
- Connect the brown leadwire to the V_7 electrode.
- Turn the machine on and make sure paper speed is set for 25 mm/second.
- Press AUTO.

- If you're using a multichannel ECG machine, all leads will print out as a straight line except the leads labeled V_4, V_5, and V_6, which should be relabeled V_7, V_8, and V_9, respectively.
- If you're using a single-channel ECG machine, turn the selector knob to "V" to record the V_7 lead.
- Stop the machine and reposition the electrode to the V_8 position and record that lead, repeating the procedure for the V_9 position.
- When the ECG is complete, remove the electrodes and clean the patient's skin with a gauze pad or moist cloth.
- If more than one posterior lead ECG may be needed, indicate the electrode sites on his skin with a marking pen to enable accurate comparison.

SPECIAL CONSIDERATIONS

- The number of leads may vary according to the practitioner's preference.
- If right posterior leads are requested, put the patient on his left side and use the corresponding landmarks on the right side for leads V_{7R}, V_{8R}, and V_{9R}.

TROUBLESHOOTER *If the ECG machine won't operate unless all leadwires are connected, you may need to connect the limb leadwires and the leadwires for V_1, V_2, and V_3.*

COMPLICATIONS
- Skin sensitivity reactions

PATIENT TEACHING

- Tell the patient why the procedure is needed and how it's performed.
- Advise the patient that the test doesn't hurt and won't cause an electrical shock.
- Explain to the patient that the test takes up to 10 minutes to perform.
- Tell the patient that electrodes will be attached to his arms, legs, chest, and back and the gel, if used, may feel cold.
- Tell the patient to lie still, relax, not talk, and breathe normally.

DOCUMENTATION

- Note the indications for posterior ECG.
- Record the date and time the procedure was performed.
- Include a copy of the relabeled ECG, if available.
- Note patient's tolerance of the procedure.
- Document on the ECG recording the date and time and patient's name, age, and gender.

SELECTED REFERENCES

Brown, D.F., and Nadel, E.S. "Posterior Wall Myocardial Infarction," *Journal of Emergency Medicine* 27(1):75-78, July 2004.

Docherty, B. "12-Lead Interpretation 2: Right Ventricular and Posterior Infarcts," *British Journal of Nursing* 12(22):1304-11, December 2003-January 2004.

Hoshino, Y., et al. "Electrocardiographic Abnormality of Pure Posterior Myocardial Infarction," *Internal Medicine* 43(9):883-85, September 2004.

Somers, M.P., et al. "Additional Electrocardiographic Leads in the ED Chest Pain Patient: Right Ventricular and Posterior Leads," *American Journal of Emergency Medicine* 21(7):563-73, November 2003.

Electrocardiography, right chest lead placement

OVERVIEW

DESCRIPTION
◆ Right chest lead placement electro-cardiography obtains information from the right side of the heart to as-sess interior and right ventricular is-chemia or infarction.
◆ It's also used to determine inferior wall myocardial infarction (MI) and suspected right ventricular involve-ment; 25% to 50% of MI patients have right ventricular involvement. Many also have high creatinine ki-nase levels.
◆ Early identification of a right ventric-ular MI is essential because it re-quires different treatment.

CONTRAINDICATIONS
◆ None known

EQUIPMENT

Multichannel electrocardiography ma-chine ◆ paper ◆ disposable pregelled electrodes ◆ several 4″ × 4″ gauze pads ◆ clippers

PREPARATION
◆ Place the electrocardiography ma-chine close to the patient and plug it in or confirm the battery is charged.
◆ Keep the patient away from electrical fixtures and power cords to minimize electrical interference.
◆ Make sure the paper speed is set at 25 mm/second and amplitude at 1 mV/10 mm.

KEY STEPS

◆ Confirm the patient's identity using two patient identifiers according to facility policy.
◆ Explain the procedure to the patient and his family.
◆ Reassure him that the test is painless and takes only a few minutes during which he'll need to lie quietly on his back.
◆ Wash your hands.
◆ Place him in a supine position or, if he has difficulty lying flat, in semi-Fowler's position.
◆ Provide privacy and expose his arms, chest, and legs.
◆ For a female patient, drape her chest until you apply the chest leads.
◆ Choose flat, fleshy (not bony or mus-cular), hairless areas such as the in-ner aspects of the wrist and ankles for placement of the extremity elec-trodes.
◆ Clean the sites with gauze pads to promote good skin contact.
◆ Connect the leadwires to the elec-trodes. The leadwires are color-coded and lettered.
◆ Attach the electrodes to the appro-priate extremities: white (RA) to the right arm, black (LA) to the left arm, green (RL) to the right leg, and red (LL) to the left leg.
◆ Locate the correct sites for chest lead placement (as shown below).

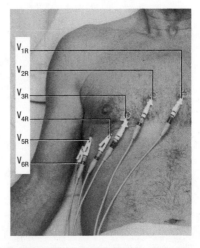

- If there's excessive hair in the area, clip it.
- For a female patient, place the electrodes under the breast tissue.
- Feel between the patient's ribs for the second intercostal space on the left (the notch at the top of the sternum, where the manubrium joins the body of the sternum), count down two spaces to the fourth intercostal space and apply an electrode to the site and attach leadwire V_{1R}.
- Move your fingers across the sternum to the fourth intercostal space on the right side of the sternum and apply an electrode to that site and attach lead V_{2R}.
- Move your fingers down to the fifth intercostal space and over to the midclavicular line and place an electrode here and attach lead V_{4R}.
- Visualize a line between V_{2R} and V_{4R}. Apply an electrode midway on the line and attach lead V_{3R}.
- Move your finger horizontally from V_{4R} to the right midaxillary line and apply an electrode to this site and attach lead V_{6R}.
- Move your fingers along the same horizontal line to the midpoint between V_{4R} and V_{6R} (the right anterior midaxillary line) and apply an electrode to this site and attach lead V_{5R}.
- Turn on the electrocardiography machine.
- Ask the patient to breathe normally but not talk during the recording so muscle movement won't distort the tracing.
- Enter appropriate patient information required by the machine you're using.
- If necessary, standardize the machine, causing a square tracing of 10 mm (two large squares) to appear on the electrocardiography paper when the machine is set for 1 mV (1 mV = 10 mm).
- Press the AUTO key to record all 12 leads automatically.
- Check facility policy for the number of readings to obtain. Some facilities require at least two ECGs so one can be sent for interpretation while the other stays in the patient's chart. If the ECG is to be put in the chart, it may need to be labeled "preliminary."
- After recording the ECG, turn off the machine.
- Clearly label the ECG with the patient's name, the date, and time.
- Label the tracing as "right chest ECG" to distinguish it from a standard 12-lead ECG.
- Remove the electrodes.

SPECIAL CONSIDERATIONS

- For best results, place the electrodes symmetrically on the limbs.
- If the patient's wrist or ankle is covered by a dressing, or if he's an amputee, choose an area that's available on both sides.

COMPLICATIONS
- Skin sensitivity reactions

PATIENT TEACHING

- Tell the patient why the procedure is needed and how it's performed.
- Inform the patient that the test doesn't hurt and won't cause an electrical shock.
- Tell the patient the test takes up to 10 minutes.
- Make the patient aware that electrodes will be attached to his arms, legs, and chest and that the gel may feel cold.
- Tell the patient to lie still, relax, not talk, and breathe normally.

DOCUMENTATION

- Document the indication for right chest lead ECG.
- Note the date and time the ECG was performed.
- Include a copy of the ECG, if available.
- Note the patient's tolerance.
- On the ECG tracing, note the date and time and patient's name, age, and gender.

SELECTED REFERENCES
Chockalingam, A., et al. "Right Ventricular Myocardial Infarction: Presentation and Acute Outcomes," *Angiology* 56(4): 371-76, July-August 2005.

Khan, S., et al. "Prevalence of Right Ventricular Myocardial Infarction in Patient with Acute Inferior Wall Myocardial Infarction," *International Journal of Clinical Practice* 58(4):354-57, April 2004.

Moye, S., et al. "The Electrocardiogram in Right Ventricular Myocardial Infarction," *American Journal of Emergency Medicine* 23(6):793-99, October 2005.

Rotondo, N., et al. "Electrocardiographic Manifestations: Acute Inferior Wall Myocardial Infarction," *Journal of Emergency Medicine* 26(4):433-40, May 2004.

Somers, M.P., et al. "Additional Electrocardiographic Leads in the ED Chest Pain Patient: Right Ventricular and Posterior Leads," *American Journal of Emergency Medicine* 21(7):563-73, November 2003.

Electrocardiography, signal-averaged

OVERVIEW

DESCRIPTION

◆ Signal-averaged electrocardiography identifies risk for sustained ventricular tachycardia in patients with malignant ventricular tachycardia, a history of myocardial infarction (MI), unexplained syncope, nonischemic congestive cardiomyopathy, or nonsustained ventricular tachycardia.

◆ Sustained ventricular tachycardia can be a precursor of sudden death after an MI. This procedure helps in establishing preventive measures.

◆ On a standard 12-lead ECG, noise from muscle tissue, electronic artifacts, and electrodes masks late potentials that have low amplitude.

◆ Signal-averaging detects low-amplitude signals or late electrical potentials that reflect slow conduction or disorganized ventricular activity through abnormal or infarcted regions of the ventricles.

◆ Signal-averaged ECG is performed by recording the noise-free surface ECG in three specialized leads for several hundred beats.

CONTRAINDICATIONS

◆ None known

EQUIPMENT

Signal-averaged electrocardiography machine ◆ signal-averaged computer ◆ record of patient's surface ECG for 200 to 300 QRS complexes ◆ three bipolar electrodes or leads ◆ alcohol pads ◆ clippers (optional)

Placing electrodes for signal-averaged electrocardiography

To prepare for signal-averaged electrocardiography, place the electrodes in the X, Y, and Z orthogonal positions shown here. These positions bisect one another to provide a three-dimensional, composite view of ventricular activation.

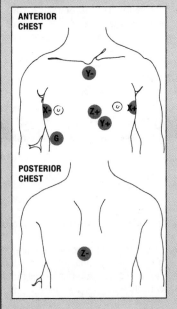

ANTERIOR CHEST

POSTERIOR CHEST

KEY
X+ Fourth intercostal space, midaxillary line, left side
X- Fourth intercostal space, midaxillary line, right side
Y+ Standard V_3 position (or proximal left leg)
Y- Superior aspect of manubrium
Z+ Standard V_2 position
Z- V_2 position, posterior
G Ground; eighth rib on right side

KEY STEPS

◆ Confirm the patient's identity using two patient identifiers according to facility policy.

◆ Place the patient in a supine position; have him lie as still as possible.

◆ Tell the patient to breathe normally, but not to speak during the procedure.

◆ If the patient has hair on his chest, clip the area, rub it with alcohol, and dry it before placing electrodes.

◆ Place the leads in the X, Y, and Z positions. (See *Placing electrodes for signal-averaged electrocardiography*.)

◆ The ECG machine gathers input from the leads and amplifies, filters, and samples the signals; the computer collects and stores data for analysis.

◆ Crucial values are those showing QRS complex duration, duration of the portion of the QRS complex with an amplitude under 40 microvolts, and the root mean square voltage of the last 40 msec.

SPECIAL CONSIDERATIONS

◆ Muscle movement may cause a false-positive result. Patients who are restless or in respiratory distress are poor candidates for signal-averaged electrocardiography.
◆ Proper electrode placement and skin preparation are essential.

⚡ **WARNING** *Low-amplitude signals are indicated by a QRS complex duration greater than 110 msec; a duration of more than 40 msec for the amplitude portion under 40 μV; and a root mean square voltage of less than 25 μV during the last 40 msec of the QRS complex. All three factors aren't needed to consider the result positive or negative. Final interpretation depends on individual patient factors.*

◆ Signal-averaged electrocardiography helps the physician determine if the patient needs an invasive procedure, such as electrophysiologic testing or angiography.
◆ Validity of signal-averaged electrocardiography in patients with bundle-branch heart block is unknown because myocardial activation doesn't follow the usual sequence in these patients.

COMPLICATIONS
◆ Skin sensitivity reactions

PATIENT TEACHING

◆ Tell the patient the procedure will take 10 to 30 minutes and will help the physician determine the risk for a certain type of arrhythmia.
◆ Inform the patient that it may be done along with other tests, such as echocardiography, Holter monitoring, electrophysiology studies, and stress testing.

DOCUMENTATION

◆ Document the time of the procedure.
◆ Note why the procedure was done.
◆ Note the patient's tolerance of the procedure.

SELECTED REFERENCES

Bennhagen, R.G., et al. "Serial Signal-Averaged Electrocardiography in Children After Cardiac Transplantation," *Pediatric Transplantation* 9(6):773-79, December 2005.

Budeus, M., et al. "Prediction of Atrial Fibrillation After Coronary Artery Bypass Grafting: The Role of Chemoreflex-Sensitivity and P Wave Signal Averaged ECG," *International Journal of Cardiology* 106(1):67-74, January 2006.

Haghjoo, M., et al. "Does the Abnormal Signal-Averaged Electrocardiogram Predict Future Appropriate Therapy in Patients with Implantable Cardioverter-Defibrillators?" *Journal of Electrocardiology* 39(2):150-55, April 2006.

Lee, K.L., and Lau, C.P. "The Use of Signal-Averaged Electrocardiogram in Risk Stratification after Acute Myocardial Infarction in the Modern Era," *European Heart Journal* 26(8):747-48, April 2005.

Electrocardiography, standard 12-lead

OVERVIEW

DESCRIPTION
◆ Electrocardiography identifies myocardial ischemia and infarction, rhythm and conduction disturbances, chamber enlargement, electrolyte imbalances, and drug toxicity.
◆ Electrocardiography is used during stress tests to monitor heart rate, blood pressure, and electrocardiogram (ECG) waveforms.
◆ Electrocardiography may be used at home to record heart activity 24 hours per day.
◆ An electrocardiography uses 10 electrodes to measure electrical potential from 12 different leads.
◆ The device measures and averages the difference between the electrical potential of electrode sites for each lead and graphs them over time. This creates the standard electrocardiography complex, called PQRST. (See *Reviewing electrocardiograph waveforms and components.*)

CONTRAINDICATIONS
◆ None known

EQUIPMENT

ECG machine ◆ recording paper ◆ disposable pregelled electrodes ◆ 4″×4″ gauze pads ◆ clippers, marking pen (optional)

PREPARATION
◆ Put the machine close to the bed and plug it in.
◆ If the patient is already connected to a cardiac monitor, notify the telemetry station, then remove the electrodes to accommodate the precordial leads and minimize electrical interference on the ECG tracing.
⚡ **WARNING** *Keep the patient away from electrical fixtures and power cords.*

KEY STEPS

◆ Confirm the patient's identity using two patient identifiers according to facility policy.
◆ Explain the procedure, provide privacy, and wash your hands.
◆ Put the patient in the supine position with his arms at his sides.
◆ Raise the head of the bed to make him comfortable.
◆ Expose his arms and legs.
◆ Have him relax his arms and legs to minimize muscle trembling, which can cause electrical interference and interfere with ECG tracing.
◆ Make sure his feet aren't touching the bed board.

◆ Select flat, fleshy areas for the electrodes; avoid muscular and bony areas.
⚡ **WARNING** *If the patient has an amputated limb, choose a site on the stump.*
◆ If an area is excessively hairy, clip it.
◆ Clean the skin to enhance electrode contact; allow it to dry.
◆ Peel off contact paper from the disposable electrodes and apply directly to the prepared site as recommended by the manufacturer.
◆ To get the best leadwire connection, position disposable electrodes on the legs with the lead connection pointing superiorly.
◆ Connect the limb leadwires to the electrodes.

Reviewing electrocardiograph waveforms and components

An electrocardiograph waveform has three basic components: the P wave, QRS complex, and T wave. These elements can be further divided into the PR interval, J point, ST segment, U wave, and QT interval.

P WAVE AND PR INTERVAL
The P wave represents atrial depolarization. The PR interval represents the time it takes an impulse to travel from the atria through the atrioventricular nodes and bundle of His; it measures from the beginning of the P wave to the beginning of the QRS complex.

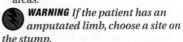

QRS COMPLEX
The QRS complex represents ventricular depolarization — the time it takes for the impulse to travel through the bundle branches to the Purkinje fibers.
The Q wave appears as the first negative deflection in the QRS complex; the R wave, as the first positive deflection. The S wave appears as the second negative deflection, or the first negative deflection after the R wave.

J POINT AND ST SEGMENT
The J point marks the end of the QRS complex and indicates the beginning of the ST segment. The ST segment represents part of ventricular repolarization.

T WAVE AND U WAVE
Usually following the same deflection pattern as the P wave, the T wave represents ventricular repolarization. The U wave follows the T wave, but isn't always seen.

QT INTERVAL
The QT interval represents ventricular depolarization and repolarization. It extends from the beginning of the QRS complex to the end of the T wave.

- Each leadwire is lettered and color-coded for easy identification: white (RA) goes to the right arm, green (RL) to the right leg, red (LL) to the left leg, black (LA) to the left arm, and brown (V_1 to V_6) to the chest.
- Expose the patient's chest and put an electrode at each position. (See *Positioning chest electrodes*.)
- For a woman, place chest electrodes below the breast tissue; laterally displace breast tissue of a large-breasted woman.
- Set the paper speed selector to the standard 25 mm/second and the machine to full voltage. The machine will record a normal standardization mark.
- Enter appropriate patient identification data as needed.

TROUBLESHOOTER If part of the waveform extends beyond the paper when recording, adjust the normal standardization to half-standardization and note the adjustment on the ECG strip.

- Ask the patient to relax, lie still, breathe normally, and not talk.
- Press the AUTO button and observe tracing quality. The machine records all 12 leads automatically, recording three consecutive leads simultaneously. (Some machines have a display screen so you can preview waveforms before the machine records them on paper.)
- When the machine finishes recording the 12-lead ECG, remove the electrodes and clean the patient's skin.
- After disconnecting the leadwires from the electrodes, dispose of the electrodes, as indicated.
- If serial ECGs are expected, consider marking the electrode placement on the patient's skin.

SPECIAL CONSIDERATIONS

- If the patient's respirations distort the recording, ask him to hold his breath briefly while you record the ECG.
- If the patient has a pacemaker, you can perform an ECG with or without a magnet (to temporarily change the pacemaker's mode), according to the physician's orders. Note the presence of a pacemaker and use of a magnet on the strip.

COMPLICATIONS
- Skin sensitivity reactions

Positioning chest electrodes

To ensure accurate test results, position chest electrodes as follows:

V_1: Fourth intercostal space at right sternal border
V_2: Fourth intercostal space at left sternal border
V_3: Halfway between V_2 and V_4
V_4: Fifth intercostal space at midclavicular line
V_5: Fifth intercostal space at anterior axillary line (halfway between V_4 and V_6)
V_6: Fifth intercostal space at midaxillary line, level with V_4

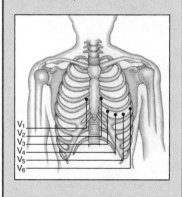

PATIENT TEACHING

- Explain to the patient that the test records the heart's electrical activity at certain intervals.
- Tell the patient why the procedure is being done.
- Explain to the patient that the test doesn't hurt and won't cause electrical shock.
- Advise the patient that the test takes up to 10 minutes to perform.
- Tell the patient where electrodes will be attached and explain that the gel may feel cold.
- Tell the patient to lie still, relax, not talk, and breathe normally.

DOCUMENTATION

- Label the ECG recording with patient's name and room number, date and time, facility identification number, and appropriate clinical information.
- Record in your notes the date and time of the ECG.
- Document significant patient responses.
- Note the patient's tolerance of the procedure.

SELECTED REFERENCES
Alinier, G., et al. "12-Lead ECG Training: The Way Forward," *Nurse Education Today* 26(1):87-92, January 2006.
Colyar, M. "Interpreting a 12-Lead ECG," *Advance for Nurse Practitioners* 12(4): 18, 21-23, April 2004.
Gregory, J. "Using the 12-Lead ECG to Assess Acute Coronary Patients," *British Journal of Nursing* 14(21):1135-40, November-December 2005.
Jahrsdoerfer, M., et al. "Clinical Usefulness of the EASI 12-Lead Continuous Electrocardiographic Monitoring System," *Critical Care Nurse* 25(5):28-30, 32-7, October 2005.
Pyne, C.C. "Classification of Acute Coronary Syndromes Using the 12-Lead Electrocardiogram as a Guide," *AACN Clinical Issues* 15(4):558-67, October-December 2004.

Endotracheal administration

DESCRIPTION

- If an I.V. line isn't available, drugs can be given via the respiratory system through an endotracheal (ET) tube.
- ET delivery allows uninterrupted resuscitation efforts and aids in avoiding coronary artery laceration, cardiac tamponade, and pneumothorax.
- ET drugs may be given using the syringe method or the adapter method.
- A swivel adapter can be placed on the end of the tube; while ventilation continues through a bag-valve device, the drug can be delivered with a needle through the closed stopcock.
- Drugs given endotracheally have a longer duration of action; repeat doses and continuous infusions must be adjusted to prevent adverse effects.
- The procedure is usually done in an emergency situation by a physician, an emergency medical technician, or a critical care nurse. (See *Administering endotracheal drugs*.)

CONTRAINDICATIONS

- None known

ET tube or swivel adapter ◆ gloves ◆ end-tidal carbon dioxide (CO_2) device or an esophageal detection device ◆ handheld resuscitation bag ◆ prescribed drug ◆ syringe or adapter ◆ sterile water or normal saline solution

PREPARATION

- Check the patient's drug record against the physician's order.

  WARNING *In an emergency, verify the physician's verbal order.*
- Wash your hands.
- Check ET tube placement by using an end-tidal CO_2 detector or an esophageal detection device.
- Calculate the drug dose.

  WARNING *Adult advanced cardiac life support guidelines recommend that drugs be administered at 2 to 2½ times the recommended I.V. dose.*
- Draw the drug into a syringe and dilute it in 10 ml of sterile water or normal saline solution. Dilution increases drug volume and contact with lung tissue.

- Put on gloves.
- Move the patient into a supine position, and make sure her head is level with or slightly higher than his body.
- Ventilate the patient three to five times with the resuscitation bag.
- Remove the bag.
- Remove the needle from the syringe, and insert the tip of the syringe into the ET tube or swivel adapter.
- Inject the drug deep into the tube.
- After injecting the drug, reattach the resuscitation bag and briskly ventilate the patient to propel the drug into the lungs, oxygenate the patient, and clear the tube.
- Discard the syringe in a sharps container.
- Remove and discard your gloves.

◆ The drug's onset of action is usually quicker than with I.V. administration.
◆ If the patient doesn't respond quickly, the physician may order a repeat dose.

COMPLICATIONS
◆ From the prescribed drug, not the administration route

◆ If appropriate, explain the procedure to the patient or his family.

◆ Note the date and time of drug administration.
◆ Record the drug administered.
◆ Document patient's response.

SELECTED REFERENCES

Aranda, J.V., et al. "Analgesia and Sedation during Mechanical Ventilation in Neonates," *Clinical Therapeutics* 27(6):877-99, June 2005.

Celik, S.A., and Kanan, N. "A Current Conflict: Use of Isotonic Sodium Chloride Solution on Endotracheal Suctioning in Critically Ill Patients," *Dimensions of Critical Care Nursing* 25(1):11-14, January-February 2006.

Dubus, J.C., et al. "Aerosol Deposition in Neonatal Ventilation," *Pediatric Research* 58(1):10-14, July 2005.

Klockare, M., et al. "Comparison Between Direct Humidification and Nebulization of the Respiratory Tract at Mechanical Ventilation: Distribution of Saline Solution Studies by Gamma Camera," *Journal of Clinical Nursing* 15(3):301-307, March 2006.

Administering endotracheal drugs

In an emergency, some drugs can be given through an endotracheal (ET) tube if I.V. access isn't available. They may be given using the syringe method or the adapter method. Before injecting any drug, check for proper placement of the ET tube using an end-tidal carbon dioxide detector or an esophageal detection device. Make sure the patient is in a supine position and her head is level with or slightly higher than her body.

SYRINGE METHOD

Remove the needle before injecting medication into the ET tube. Insert the tip of the syringe into the ET tube, and inject the drug deep into the tube (as shown).

ADAPTER METHOD

An adapter device for ET drug administration provides a more closed system of drug delivery than the syringe method. A special adapter placed on the end of the ET tube (as shown) allows drug delivery through the closed stopcock.

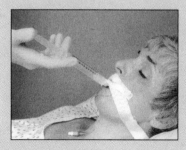

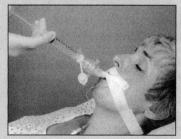

Endotracheal intubation

DESCRIPTION

- Procedure involves oral or nasal insertion of a flexible tube through the larynx into the trachea.
- Endotracheal (ET) intubation establishes and maintains a patent airway, protects against aspiration by sealing the trachea off from the digestive tract, permits removal of tracheobronchial secretions in patients who can't cough effectively, and provides a route for mechanical ventilation.
- Done by a physician, anesthetist, respiratory therapist, or trained nurse, it's usually performed in emergencies such as cardiopulmonary arrest or in diseases such as epiglottiditis, but may be done under more controlled circumstances such as just before surgery.

CONTRAINDICATIONS

Oral intubation

- Acute cervical spinal injury
- Degenerative spinal disorders

Nasal intubation

- Apnea
- Bleeding disorders
- Chronic sinusitis
- Nasal obstructions

Two ET tubes (one spare) ◆ 10-ml syringe ◆ stethoscope ◆ gloves ◆ lighted laryngoscope with a handle and various sized, curved and straight blades ◆ sedative ◆ local anesthetic spray ◆ mucosal vasoconstricting agent (for nasal intubation) ◆ overbed table ◆ water-soluble lubricant ◆ adhesive or other strong tape or Velcro tube holder ◆ compound benzoin tincture ◆ goggles ◆ oral airway or bite block (for oral intubation) ◆ suction equipment ◆ handheld resuscitation bag with sterile swivel adapter ◆ humidified oxygen source ◆ sterile gauze pad ◆ stylet ◆ Magill forceps ◆ sterile water ◆ sterile basin ◆ prepackaged intubation tray (optional) ◆ end-tidal carbon dioxide (CO_2) detector or an esophageal detection device.

PREPARATION

- Gather supplies or use a prepackaged intubation tray.
- Select an appropriate sized ET tube:
- Children ages 8 and younger: 2.5 to 5.5 mm, uncuffed
- Adolescents age 9 to 17: 7 to 8 mm
- Adults: 6 to 10 mm, cuffed (typically 7.5 mm for women or 9 mm for men)
- Select a slightly smaller tube for nasal intubation.
- Make sure the light in the laryngoscope works.
- Using sterile technique, open the ET tube package and other supplies on an overbed table.
- Pour the sterile water into the basin.
- To ease insertion, lubricate the first 1″ (2.5 cm) of the distal end of the ET tube with water-soluble lubricant using aseptic technique; squeeze the lubricant directly onto the tube.

  WARNING *Use only water-soluble lubricant because it can be absorbed by mucous membranes.*

- Attach the syringe to the port on the tube's exterior pilot cuff.
- Slowly inflate the cuff; watch for uniform inflation.
- Submerge the tube in the sterile water, watch for air bubbles, and then use the syringe to deflate the cuff.

- A stylet may be used on oral intubations to stiffen the tube. Lubricate the stylet and insert it into the tube until its distal tip is about ½″ (1.3 cm) from the distal end of the tube. Make sure the stylet doesn't protrude from the tube.
- Prepare the humidified oxygen source and the suction equipment for immediate use.
- Remove the headboard to provide easier access, if necessary.

- Administer a sedative as ordered to induce amnesia or analgesia; help calm and relax a conscious patient.
- Remove the patient's dentures or bridgework.
- To prevent hypoxia, hyperventilate the patient with 100% oxygen using a handheld resuscitation bag until the tube is inserted.
- Place the patient supine in the sniffing position so his mouth, pharynx, and trachea are extended. For blind intubation, place his head and neck in a neutral position.
- Put on gloves and personal protective equipment.
- For oral intubation, spray a local anesthetic, such as lidocaine, deep into the posterior pharynx to diminish the gag reflex and reduce patient discomfort.
- For nasal intubation, spray a local anesthetic and a mucosal vasoconstrictor into the nasal passages to anesthetize the nasal turbinates and lessen bleeding.
- If necessary, suction the patient's pharynx before tube insertion to improve visualization.

⚠ **WARNING** *To prevent hypoxia, limit intubation attempts to less than 30 seconds. Hyperventilate the patient between attempts, if necessary.*

INTUBATION WITH DIRECT VISUALIZATION

- With your right hand, hold the patient's mouth open by crossing your index finger over your thumb and putting your thumb on his upper teeth and index finger on his lower teeth.
- Slide the blade of the laryngoscope into the right side of his mouth.
- Center the blade and push his tongue to the left.
- Hold his lips away from his teeth to avoid trauma.

- Advance the blade to expose the epiglottis. With a straight blade, insert the tip under the epiglottis; with a curved blade, insert the tip between the base of the tongue and the epiglottis.
- Lift the laryngoscope handle upward and away from your body to reveal the vocal cords. Avoid hitting the patient's teeth.
- Have an assistant apply pressure to the cricoid ring to occlude the esophagus and minimize regurgitation.
- For oral intubation, insert the ET tube into the right side of his mouth. When performing nasotracheal intubation, insert the tube through the nostril and into the pharynx; use Magill forceps to guide the tube through the vocal cords.
- Guide the tube into the vertical openings of the larynx between the vocal cords; don't mistake the horizontal opening of the esophagus for the larynx.

⚠ **WARNING** *If the vocal cords are closed because of a spasm, wait for them to relax and then guide the tube past them.*

- Advance the tube until the cuff disappears beyond the vocal cords. Don't advance it further; you may occlude a major bronchus or cause lung collapse.
- Holding the ET tube in place, remove the stylet, if present.

BLIND NASOTRACHEAL INTUBATION

- Pass the ET tube along the floor of the nasal cavity. Use gentle force to pass the tube through the nasopharynx and into the pharynx.
- Listen and feel for air through the tube as it's advanced to ensure that it's properly placed in the airway.
- Slip the tube between the vocal cords when they separate as the patient inhales.
- When the tube is past the vocal cords, breath sounds become louder. If breath sounds stop during advancement, withdraw the tube until they reappear.

AFTER INTUBATION

- Inflate the tube's cuff with 5 to 10 cc of air until you feel resistance. For a mechanically ventilated patient, use the minimal-leak technique or minimal occlusive volume technique to establish correct inflation.
- For minimal-leak:
- Attach a 10-ml syringe to the port on the tube's exterior pilot cuff; place a stethoscope on the patient's neck.
- Inject small amounts of air with each breath until you don't hear a leak.
- Aspirate 0.1 cc of air from the cuff to create a minimal air leak.
- Record amount of air needed to inflate cuff.
- For minimal occlusive volume:
- Follow first two steps of the minimal-leak technique, but place the stethoscope over the trachea.
- Aspirate until you hear a small leak on inspiration; add just enough air to stop the leak.
- Record the amount of air needed to inflate the cuff for subsequent monitoring of tracheal dilation or erosion.
- Remove the laryngoscope.
- If the patient was intubated orally, insert an oral airway or bite block to prevent him from obstructing airflow or puncturing the tube with his teeth.
- To ensure correct tube placement, watch for chest expansion and auscultate for bilateral breath sounds. Also check placement using an end-tidal CO_2 detector or esophageal detection device.

⚠ **WARNING** *If you don't hear breath sounds, auscultate over the stomach while ventilating. Stomach distention, belching, or gurgling indicates esophageal intubation. Immediately deflate the cuff and remove the tube. After reoxygenating, repeat insertion using a sterile tube.*

- Auscultate bilaterally to exclude the possibility of endobronchial intubation.

(continued)

WARNING *If you don't hear breath sounds on both sides of the chest, you may have inserted the tube into one of the mainstem bronchi or the tube may be resting on the carina. This occludes the other bronchus and lungs, resulting in atelectasis on the obstructed side. To correct, deflate the cuff, withdraw the tube 1 to 2 mm, auscultate for bilateral breath sounds, and reinflate the cuff.*

◆ A chest X-ray is typically performed to confirm proper placement; check facility policy.
◆ When you've confirmed correct tube placement, give oxygen or start mechanical ventilation; suction if indicated.
◆ To secure tube position, apply compound benzoin tincture to each cheek and let it dry. Tape the tube firmly with adhesive or other strong tape or use a Velcro tube holder. (See *Securing an ET tube.*)

◆ Note the centimeter mark on the tube where it exits the patient's mouth or nose.
◆ Place a swivel adapter between the tube and the humidified oxygen source to allow for intermittent suctioning and reduce tube tension.
◆ Provide frequent care to prevent pressure ulcers and drying of oral mucous membranes.
◆ Suction secretions through the ET tube as indicated to prevent mucus plugs.

Securing an ET tube

Before securing an endotracheal (ET) tube, make sure the patient's face is clean, dry, and free from beard stubble. If possible, suction his mouth and dry the tube just before taping. Check the reference mark on the tube to ensure correct placement. After securing, always check for bilateral breath sounds to ensure that the tube hasn't been displaced by manipulation. To secure the tube, use one of the methods described below.

METHOD 1
◆ Cut one piece of 1″ cloth adhesive tape long enough to wrap around the patient's head and overlap in front, and then cut an 8″ (20.3-cm) piece of tape and center it on the longer piece, sticky sides together.
◆ Cut a 5″ (12.7-cm) slit in each end of the longer tape (as shown at right).
◆ Apply benzoin tincture to the patient's cheeks, under his nose, and under the lower lip. (Don't spray benzoin directly on the patient's face; the vapors can be irritating if inhaled and can harm the eyes.)
◆ Place the top half of one end of the tape under the patient's nose and wrap the lower half around the ET tube. Place the lower half of the other end of the tape along his lower lip and wrap the top half around the tube (as shown at right).

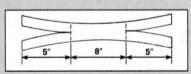

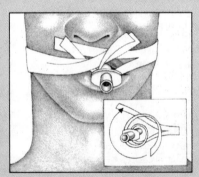

METHOD 2
◆ ET tube holders are available that can help secure a tracheal tube.
◆ Made of hard plastic or of softer materials, the tube holder secures the ET tube in place. The tube holder is available in adult and pediatric sizes. Some models come with bite blocks attached.
◆ Place the strap around the patient's neck and secure it around the tube with Velcro fasteners (as shown at right).
◆ Because each model is different, check the manufacturer's guidelines for correct placement and care.

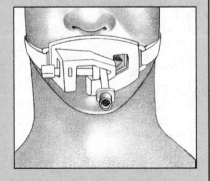

SPECIAL CONSIDERATIONS

◆ Nasotracheal intubation is preferred for elective insertion when the patient is capable of spontaneous ventilation for a short period.
◆ Nasotracheal intubation allows better tube placement, and less risk of dislodgment.
◆ Blind intubation is typically used in conscious patients who risk imminent respiratory arrest or have cervical spinal injury.
◆ Measure inflated cuff pressure at least every 8 hours to avoid overinflation. Normal cuff pressure is about 18 mm Hg.
◆ When neither method is possible, consider retrograde intubation — a technique in which a wire is inserted through the trachea and out the mouth; it's then used to guide the insertion of an ET tube.

COMPLICATIONS

◆ Apnea caused by reflex breath-holding
◆ Interruption of oxygen delivery
◆ Bronchospasm
◆ Aspiration of blood, secretions, or gastric contents
◆ Tooth damage or loss
◆ Injury to lips, mouth, pharynx, or vocal cords
◆ Laryngeal edema and erosion
◆ Tracheal stenosis, erosion, and necrosis
◆ Nasal bleeding
◆ Laceration
◆ Sinusitis
◆ Otitis media

PATIENT TEACHING

◆ Tell the patient that the tube will help him breathe easier.
◆ Tell the patient that he'll be given an anesthetic to numb his throat.
◆ Reassure the patient and provide a message board so he can communicate.

DOCUMENTATION

◆ Note the date and time of procedure.
◆ Record the indication and success or failure.
◆ Document the tube type and size.
◆ Note the cuff size. Record the depth of the ET tube by noting the measurement on the tube that corresponds with the patient's front teeth.
◆ Record the amount of inflation and technique used.
◆ Document administration of any drugs.
◆ Note initiation of supplemental oxygen or ventilation therapy.
◆ Record the results of chest auscultation.
◆ Document the results of chest X-rays.
◆ Note the complications and interventions.
◆ Record the patient's reaction to procedure.

SELECTED REFERENCES

Bair, A.E., et al. "An Assessment of a Tracheal Tube Introducer as an Endotracheal Tube Placement Confirmation Device," *American Journal of Emergency Medicine* 23(6):754-58, October 2005.

DeBoer, S., and Seaver, M. "End-Tidal CO_2 Verification of Endotracheal Tube Placement in Neonates," *Neonatal Network* 23(3):29-38, May-June 2004.

Pate, M.F. "Placement of Endotracheal and Tracheostomy Tubes," *Critical Care Nurse* 24(3):13, June 2004.

St. John, R.E. "Airway Management," *Critical Care Nurse* 24(2):93-96, April 2004.

Endotracheal tube care

DESCRIPTION

- Proper endotracheal tube (ET) care is important to ensure airway patency and prevent complications until the patient is off ventilation.
- Care includes assessing airway status, maintaining proper cuff pressure, and repositioning the tube as needed for patient comfort or if a chest X-ray shows improper placement.
- The tube should be moved frequently from one side of the mouth to the other to prevent pressure ulcers.
- For most intubated patients, the head of the bed should be kept at 35 to 40 degrees to prevent regurgitation and subsequent aspiration.

CONTRAINDICATIONS

- None known

EQUIPMENT

MAINTAINING THE AIRWAY

Stethoscope ◆ suction equipment ◆ gloves

REPOSITIONING THE ET TUBE

10-ml syringe ◆ compound benzoin tincture ◆ stethoscope ◆ adhesive, hypoallergenic tape, or Velcro tube holder ◆ suction equipment ◆ sedative or 2% lidocaine ◆ gloves ◆ handheld resuscitation bag with mask in case of accidental extubation

REMOVING THE ET TUBE

10-ml syringe ◆ suction equipment ◆ supplemental oxygen source with mask ◆ cool-mist, large-volume nebulizer ◆ handheld resuscitation bag with mask ◆ gloves ◆ equipment for reintubation

PREPARATION

- Wash your hands before all procedures.
- Assemble the equipment at the bedside.

- For repositioning the ET tube, set up the suction equipment using sterile technique.
- When removing the ET tube, set up the suction and supplemental oxygen equipment and have equipment for emergency reintubation ready.

KEY STEPS

- Confirm the patient's identity using two patient identifiers according to facility policy.
- Explain the procedure even if the patient doesn't seem alert.
- Provide privacy.
- Wear personal protective equipment, when necessary.
- Wear clean gloves.

MAINTAINING AIRWAY PATENCY

- Auscultate the patient's lungs regularly and at any sign of respiratory distress.
- If you detect an obstructed airway, determine the cause and treat it accordingly.
- If secretions obstruct the lumen of the tube, suction them.
- If the ET tube appears to have slipped from the trachea into the right or left mainstem bronchus, indicated by absent breath sounds over one lung, obtain a chest X-ray to verify tube placement and reposition if needed.

REPOSITIONING THE ET TUBE

- Get help from another nurse to prevent accidental extubation during the procedure if the patient coughs.

  ⚡ **WARNING** *To prevent traumatic manipulation of the tube, instruct the assisting nurse to hold it as you carefully untape the tube or unfasten the Velcro tube holder.*
- Hyperoxygenate the patient and then suction the trachea through the ET tube to remove secretions, which can cause the patient to cough during the procedure.
- To prevent aspiration during cuff deflation, suction the patient's pharynx to remove secretions that may have accumulated above the tube cuff.

- When freeing the tube, locate a landmark or measure from the patient's mouth to the top of the tube to get a reference point before moving the tube.
- Deflate the cuff by attaching a 10-ml syringe to the pilot balloon port and aspirating air until you meet resistance and the pilot balloon deflates.

  ⚡ **WARNING** *Deflate the cuff before moving the ET tube because the cuff forms a seal within the trachea; moving an inflated cuff can damage the tracheal wall and vocal cords.*
- Reposition the tube as needed, noting new landmarks or measuring the length.
- To reinflate the cuff, have the patient inhale, and slowly inflate the cuff using a 10-ml syringe attached to the pilot balloon port.
- As you do this, use your stethoscope to auscultate the patient's neck to determine presence of an air leak.
- When air leakage ceases, stop cuff inflation; while still auscultating the neck, aspirate a small amount of air until you detect a minimal air leak, indicating the cuff is inflated at the lowest possible pressure for an adequate seal.
- If the patient is mechanically ventilated, aspirate to create a minimal air leak during the inspiratory phase because the positive pressure of the ventilator during inspiration will create a larger leak around the cuff.
- Note the amount of air required to achieve a minimal air leak.
- Measure cuff pressure; compare the reading with previous ones to prevent overinflation.
- Verify placement of the ET by auscultating both lung fields to verify breath sounds; listen over the epigastric area to confirm that the ET wasn't positioned in the stomach. Carbon dioxide levels may also be monitored to verify placement, and a chest X-ray may be required.
- Use benzoin and tape to secure the tube, or refasten the Velcro tube holder.
- Make sure the patient is comfortable and the airway patent.
- Measure cuff pressure at least every 8 hours to avoid overinflation.

REMOVING THE ET TUBE

- Check the practitioner's order before removing the ET tube.
- To prevent traumatic manipulation of the tube, have another nurse help.
- Raise the head of the patient's bed to approximately 90 degrees.
- Suction the patient's oropharynx and nasopharynx to remove accumulated secretions and help prevent aspiration when the cuff is deflated.
- Using a handheld resuscitation bag or the mechanical ventilator, give the patient several deep breaths through the ET tube to hyperinflate his lungs and increase his oxygen reserve.
- Attach a 10-ml syringe to the pilot balloon port, and aspirate air until you meet resistance and the pilot balloon deflates.
- **WARNING** *If you don't detect an air leak around the deflated cuff, notify the practitioner immediately; don't proceed with extubation. Absence of an air leak can indicate marked tracheal edema, which can cause total airway obstruction if the ET tube is removed.*
- If you detect the proper air leak, untape or unfasten the ET tube while the assisting nurse stabilizes it.
- Insert a sterile suction catheter through the ET tube.
- Apply suction. To reduce risk of laryngeal trauma, ask the patient to take a deep breath, open his mouth fully, and pretend to cry out.
- Simultaneously remove the ET tube and suction catheter in one smooth, outward and downward motion, following the natural curve of the patient's mouth.
- **WARNING** *Suctioning during extubation removes secretions retained at the end of the tube and prevents aspiration.*
- Give the patient supplemental oxygen. For humidity, use a cool-mist, large-volume nebulizer to decrease airway irritation and laryngeal edema.
- Encourage him to cough and deep-breathe.
- Make sure he's comfortable and his airway is patent.
- After extubation, auscultate his lungs frequently and be alert for stridor or other evidence of upper airway obstruction.
- If ordered, draw an arterial sample for blood gas analysis.

SPECIAL CONSIDERATIONS

- Use sedation or instillation of 2% lidocaine (if ordered) to numb the airway when repositioning an ET tube in the patient with a sensitive airway.
- After extubation following a lengthy intubation, keep reintubation supplies available for at least 12 hours until you're sure he can tolerate extubation.
- Never extubate a patient unless someone skilled at intubation is available.
- If you inadvertently cut the pilot balloon on the cuff, leave the tube in place and immediately call the practitioner to remove and replace the damaged tube.

COMPLICATIONS

- Traumatic injury to the larynx or trachea
- Ventilatory failure
- Airway obstruction
- Laryngospasm
- Tracheal edema

PATIENT TEACHING

- Tell the patient why the ET tube is being repositioned and how it will be done.
- Tell the patient to keep his head still during repositioning.
- Explain to the patient how the ET tube will be removed and what he can do to help.
- Tell the patient that he'll be monitored closely after intubation.
- Tell the patient to expect a sore throat and temporary hoarseness.
- Explain the need for coughing and deep breathing.
- Inform the patient of the possible need for supplemental oxygen therapy.

DOCUMENTATION

- Note the date and time of tube repositioning.
- Record the reason for repositioning.
- Document the new tube position.
- Note the total amount of air in the cuff after procedure.
- Record complications and interventions.
- Record the date and time of extubation.
- Note the presence or absence of stridor or other signs of upper airway edema.
- Document the type of supplemental oxygen administered.
- Note any complications and required subsequent therapy.
- Record the patient's tolerance of the procedure.
- Document patient teaching.

SELECTED REFERENCES

Birkett, K.M., et al. "Reporting Unplanned Extubation," *Intensive & Critical Care Nursing* 21(2):65-75, April 2005.

O'Donnell, J.M. "A Comparison of Endotracheal Tube Cuff Pressures Using Estimation Techniques and Direct Intracuff Measurement," *AANA Journal* 72(4):250-51, August 2004.

Yeh, S.H., et al. "Implications of Nursing Care in the Occurrence and Consequences of Unplanned Extubation in Adult Intensive Care Units," *International Journal of Nursing Studies* 41(3): 255-62, March 2004.

End-tidal carbon dioxide monitoring

OVERVIEW

DESCRIPTION

◆ End-tidal carbon dioxide ($ETCO_2$) provides pulmonary, cardiac, and metabolic status information that helps in managing patients and preventing clinical compromise.

◆ $ETCO_2$ shows carbon dioxide (CO_2) concentration in exhaled gas by measuring amounts of infrared light absorbed by airway gas during inspiration and expiration. (See *How end-tidal carbon dioxide monitoring works.*)

◆ $ETCO_2$ is commonly used to wean a patient with a stable acid-base balance from mechanical ventilation.

◆ $ETCO_2$ monitoring allows less frequent arterial blood gas (ABG) measurements, especially when combined with pulse oximetry.

◆ It's used to confirm correct endotracheal (ET) tube placement.

◆ It's a standard procedure during anesthesia administration and mechanical ventilation.

CONTRAINDICATIONS

◆ None known

EQUIPMENT

Gloves ◆ mainstream or sidestream CO_2 monitor ◆ CO_2 sensor ◆ airway adapter ◆ $ETCO_2$ sensor

AGE FACTOR *Neonatal adapters may have a much smaller dead space, making it appropriate for a smaller patient.*

PREPARATION

◆ Calibrate the monitor as indicated by the manufacturer (unless self-calibrating).

◆ If you're using a sidestream CO_2 monitor (airway adapter is positioned at the airway), replace the water trap between patients, if directed. The trap allows humidity from exhaled gases to be condensed in an attached container.

◆ Newer sidestream models don't require water traps.

KEY STEPS

◆ Confirm the patient's identity using two patient identifiers according to facility policy.

◆ Wash your hands.

◆ Explain the procedure and expected duration to the patient and his family.

WARNING *The effects of manual resuscitation or ingestion of alcohol or carbonated beverages can alter the detector's findings.*

◆ Position the airway adaptor and sensor as indicated.

◆ Apply the $ETCO_2$ detector or monitor immediately after ET intubation; position the airway adapter directly on the ET tube.

◆ For a nonintubated patient, place the adapter at or near his airway.

◆ An oxygen-delivery cannula may have a sample port through which gas can be aspirated for monitoring.

◆ Turn on all alarms to appropriate settings; adjust volume so it can be heard.

SPECIAL CONSIDERATIONS

◆ Change the airway adapter with every breathing circuit and ET tube change.

◆ Place the adapter on the ET tube to avoid contaminating exhaled gases with fresh gas flow from the ventilator.

◆ If using a heat and moisture exchanger, you may position the airway adapter between the exchanger and breathing circuit.

◆ If your patient's $ETCO_2$ values differ from his partial pressure of arterial carbon dioxide, assess for factors that influence $ETCO_2$ — especially when the differential is above normal.

◆ $ETCO_2$ monitoring doesn't replace ABG measurements, because it doesn't assess oxygenation. Supplement with pulse oximetry.

How end-tidal carbon dioxide monitoring works

The optical part of an end-tidal carbon dioxide monitor contains an infrared light source, a sample chamber, a special carbon dioxide (CO_2) filter, and a photodetector. The infrared light passes through the sample chamber and is absorbed in varying amounts depending on the amount of CO_2 the patient exhales. The photodetector measures CO_2 content and relays information to the microprocessor in the monitor, which displays the CO_2 value and waveform.

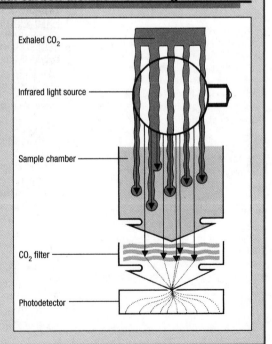

Exhaled CO_2

Infrared light source

Sample chamber

CO_2 filter

Photodetector

- If the CO_2 waveform is available, use it to help evaluate gas exchange.
- Make sure you know how to determine normal and abnormal waveforms. Print and document an abnormal waveform. (See *Carbon dioxide waveform*.)

⚡ **WARNING** *In a nonintubated patient, $ETCO_2$ values may be used to establish trends; exhaled gas is likely to mix with ambient air, and exhaled CO_2 may be diluted by fresh gas flow from the nasal cannula.*

- $ETCO_2$ monitoring is stopped after the patient is weaned from mechanical ventilation or is no longer at risk for respiratory compromise.

⚡ **WARNING** *Carefully assess tolerance for weaning. After extubation, continuous $ETCO_2$ monitoring may indicate a need for reintubation.*

- When using a disposable $ETCO_2$ detector, watch for changes indicating that the detector's life span is decreasing; for example, sluggish color changes from breath to breath.

COMPLICATIONS
- Inaccurate measurements (such as from poor sampling, calibration drift, moisture contamination, or equipment malfunction) leading to misdiagnosis and improper treatment
- Altered findings from the detector due to the effects of manual resuscitation or the ingestion of alcohol or carbonated beverages

SELECTED REFERENCES
Hillier, S.C., and Schamberger, M.S. "Transcutaneous and End-Tidal Carbon Dioxide Analysis: Complimentary Monitoring Strategies," *Journal of Intensive Care Medicine* 20(5):307-309, September-October 2005.

St. John, R.E. "End-Tidal Carbon Dioxide Monitoring," *Critical Care Nurse* 23(4): 83-88, August 2003.

Sullivan, K.J., et al. "End-Tidal Carbon Dioxide Monitoring in Pediatric Emergencies," *Pediatric Emergency Care* 21(5):327-32, May 2005.

Yosefy, C., et al. "End Tidal Carbon Dioxide as a Predictor of the Arterial PCO_2 in the Emergency Department Setting," *Emergency Medicine Journal* 21(5):557-59, September 2004.

Carbon dioxide waveform

The carbon dioxide (CO_2) waveform, or *capnogram*, produced in end-tidal carbon dioxide ($ETCO_2$) monitoring indicates CO_2 elimination during exhalation. A normal capnogram (shown below) consists of several segments that reflect various stages of exhalation and inhalation.

Normally, any gas eliminated from the airway during early exhalation is dead-space gas that hasn't undergone exchange at the alveolocapillary membrane. Measurements taken during this period contain no CO_2. As exhalation continues, CO_2 concentration rises sharply and

rapidly. The sensor now detects gas that has undergone exchange, producing measurable quantities of CO_2.

Final alveolar emptying occurs during late exhalation. During this plateau phase, CO_2 concentration rises more gradually because alveolar emptying is more constant.

The $ETCO_2$ value is derived at the end of exhalation, when CO_2 concentration peaks. Unless an alveolar plateau is present, the value doesn't accurately estimate alveolar CO_2. During inhalation, the CO_2 concentration declines sharply to zero.

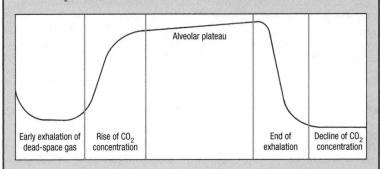

Alveolar plateau

| Early exhalation of dead-space gas | Rise of CO_2 concentration | | End of exhalation | Decline of CO_2 concentration |

Enema administration

DESCRIPTION

◆ An enema is given by instilling a solution into the rectum and colon to clean the lower bowel to:
– prepare for diagnostic or surgical procedures
– relieve distention and promote expulsion of flatus
– lubricate the rectum and colon
– soften hardened stool for removal.
◆ Enemas stimulate peristalsis by mechanically distending the colon and stimulating rectal wall nerves.

CONTRAINDICATIONS

◆ Recent colon or rectal surgery
◆ Myocardial infarction
◆ Acute abdominal conditions of unknown origin

EQUIPMENT

Prescribed solution ◆ bath thermometer ◆ enema administration bag with attached rectal tube and clamp ◆ I.V. pole ◆ gloves ◆ linen-saver pads ◆ bath blanket ◆ two bedpans with covers, or bedside commode ◆ water-soluble lubricant ◆ toilet tissue ◆ bulb syringe or funnel ◆ plastic bag for equipment ◆ water ◆ gown ◆ washcloth ◆ soap and water ◆ if observing enteric precautions: plastic trash bags, labels ◆ plastic rectal tube guard, indwelling urinary catheter or rectal catheter with 30-ml balloon and syringe (optional, for patients who can't retain solution)

PREPARATION

◆ Prepare the prescribed type and amount of solution, as indicated.
◆ Standard irrigating enema volume is 750 to 1,000 ml for an adult.

AGE FACTOR *Standard irrigating enema volumes for pediatric patients are 100 to 200 ml for infants weighing 11 to 23 lb (5 to 10 kg), 200 to 300 ml for children weighing 24 to 67 lb (11 to 30 kg), 300 to 500 ml for a child weighing 68 to 110 lb (31 to 50 kg), and 500 to 700 ml for an adolescent weighing over 110 lb.*

◆ Some ingredients may be mucosal irritants; make sure proportions are correct and agents thoroughly mixed to avoid localized irritation.
◆ Warm the solution to reduce patient discomfort. Administer an adult's enema at 100° to 105° F (37.8° to 40.6° C).

AGE FACTOR *Administer a child's enema at 100° F (37.8° C) to avoid burning rectal tissues.*

◆ Check the temperature of the solution with a bath thermometer.
◆ Clamp the tubing and fill the solution bag with prescribed solution.
◆ Unclamp tubing, flush solution, and then reclamp. Flushing detects leaks and removes air that could cause discomfort.
◆ Hang the container on an I.V. pole and take supplies to patient's room.
◆ If using an indwelling urinary catheter or rectal catheter, fill the syringe with 30 ml of water.

KEY STEPS

◆ Check the practitioner's order and assess the patient's condition.
◆ Confirm the patient's identity using two patient identifiers according to facility policy.
◆ Provide privacy and explain the procedure.

AGE FACTOR *If administering an enema to a child, familiarize him with the equipment and allow a parent to remain with him during the procedure.*

◆ Have the patient breathe through his mouth to relax the anal sphincter, which will facilitate catheter insertion.
◆ Ask if he has had previous difficulty retaining an enema to determine whether you need to use a rectal tube guard or a catheter.
◆ Wash your hands and put on gloves.
◆ Have the patient put on a hospital gown.
◆ Position the patient in the left-lateral Sims' position.

WARNING *If contraindicated, or if patient reports discomfort, reposition him on his back or right side.*

◆ Place linen-saver pads under his buttocks to prevent soiling linens.
◆ Replace the top bed linens with a bath blanket to provide privacy.
◆ Have a bedpan or commode nearby. If he can use the bathroom, make sure it's available when needed.
◆ Lubricate the distal tip of the rectal tube with water-soluble lubricant to facilitate rectal insertion and reduce irritation.
◆ Separate his buttocks and touch the anal sphincter with the rectal tube to stimulate contraction. As the sphincter relaxes, tell him to breathe deeply through the mouth as you advance the tube.

WARNING *If the patient feels pain or there's resistance, notify the physician. There may be an unknown stricture or abscess.*

◆ If he has poor sphincter control, use a plastic rectal tube guard.
◆ You can use an indwelling urinary or rectal catheter as a rectal tube if facility policy permits.
◆ Hold the solution container slightly above bed level and release the tubing clamp.
◆ Raise the container gradually to start flow; usually 75 to 100 ml/minute for an irrigating enema or slowest possible rate for a retention enema to avoid stimulating peristalsis and promote retention.
◆ Adjust the flow rate of an irrigating enema by raising or lowering the solution container according to the patient's retention ability and comfort.

AGE FACTOR *Don't raise container higher than 18" (45.7 cm) for an adult or 5" (12.7 cm) for a child. Excessive pressure can force colon bacteria into the small intestine or rupture the colon.*

WARNING *If the patient has discomfort or needs to defecate, clamp the tube and hold his buttocks together. Help him relax abdominal muscles and promote retention. Resume administration at a slower rate.*

◆ If flow slows or stops, the catheter tip may be clogged or pressed against the rectal wall. Turn it slightly to free it. If it remains clogged, withdraw it, flush with solution, and reinsert.

- After administering most of the prescribed solution, clamp the tubing. Stop before the container empties to avoid introducing air into the bowel.
- If the patient is apprehensive, position him on a bedpan and have him hold toilet tissue or a washcloth against his anus. Place the call signal within reach.
- Provide privacy while he expels the solution. Tell him not to flush the toilet.
- Remove and discard soiled linen and linen-saver pads. Place a clean linen-saver pad under him to absorb rectal drainage.
- Check the contents of the toilet or bedpan. Note fecal color, consistency, amount, and foreign matter such as blood, rectal tissue, worms, pus, or mucus.
- Send specimens to the laboratory if ordered.
- Properly dispose of the enema equipment. If additional enemas are scheduled, store clean, reusable equipment in a closed plastic bag.

SPECIAL CONSIDERATIONS

- For a flush enema, stop the flow by lowering the container below bed level and allowing gravity to siphon the enema from the colon. Continue to raise and lower until gas bubbles cease or abdominal distention subsides.
- For an irrigating enema, instruct the patient to retain the solution for 15 minutes, if possible.
- For a retention enema, instruct the patient not to defecate for the prescribed time or 30 minutes for oil retention; 15 to 30 minutes for anthelmintic and emollient enemas. If an indwelling catheter is in place, leave it to promote retention.
- Sodium may be absorbed from the saline enema solution; administer cautiously and monitor electrolyte status of patients with sodium restrictions.

- In patients with fluid and electrolyte disturbances, measure the amount of expelled solution to assess for retention of enema fluid.
- Give a retention enema before meals.
- Follow an oil-retention enema with a soap and water enema 1 hour later.
- Administer less solution when giving a hypertonic enema.
- If the patient has hemorrhoids, instruct him to bear down gently during tube insertion. This causes the anus to open and facilitates insertion.
- If he fails to expel the solution within 1 hour you may need to remove the enema solution.

⚡ **WARNING** *Inform the practitioner when a patient can't expel an enema spontaneously because of possible bowel perforation or electrolyte imbalance.*

- When siphoning the solution have the patient lie on his side. Place a bedpan on a chair. Disconnect tubing, place the distal end in the bedpan, and reinsert the rectal end. If gravity fails to drain the solution, instill 30 to 50 ml of warm water through the tube; quickly direct the distal end of the tube into the bedpan. Measure the return to make sure solution has drained.
- Double-bag and label enema equipment "isolation" if the patient is on enteric precautions.
- If the practitioner orders enemas until returns are clear, give no more than three to avoid excessive irritation of the rectal mucosa.

COMPLICATIONS

- Dizziness or faintness
- Excessive irritation of colonic mucosa
- Hyponatremia or hypokalemia from repeated use of hypotonic solutions
- Cardiac arrhythmias from vasovagal reflex stimulation
- Colonic water absorption or hypervolemia from prolonged retention

- Describe the procedure to the patient.
- Discuss relaxation techniques.
- Review measures for preventing constipation — regular exercise, dietary modifications, and adequate fluid intake.

DOCUMENTATION

- Record the date and time of enema.
- Record the type and amount of solution.
- Note the retention time.
- Record the approximate amount returned.
- Note the color, consistency, and abnormalities.
- Record the patient's tolerance of the procedure.

SELECTED REFERENCES

Jarman, L., and Coxsey, D. "Using the Benchmarking Process to Improve Care After Barium Enema," *Professional Nurse* 19(8):462-65, April 2004.

Mauk, K.L. "Preventing Constipation in Older Adults," *Nursing* 35(6):22-23, June 2005.

Ozkan, Z., et al. "Administration of a Single Dose of Sodium Phosphate Enema in Patients With Ingested Foreign Bodies: A Prospective Randomized Study," *European Journal of Emergency Medicine* 13(1):50, February 2006.

Schmelzer, M., et al. "Safety and Effectiveness of Large-Volume Enema Solutions," *Applied Nursing Research* 17(4): 265-74, November 2004.

Epidural analgesic administration

OVERVIEW

DESCRIPTION

- Helps manage acute or chronic pain, including postoperative pain; especially useful in patients with cancer or degenerative joint disease.
- Practitioner injects or infuses drug into epidural space outside subarachnoid space where cerebrospinal fluid (CSF) flows.
- Drug diffuses slowly into subarachnoid space of the spinal canal, then into the CSF and directly into the spinal area, bypassing the blood-brain barrier.
- In some cases, the physician injects the drug directly into the subarachnoid space. (See *Understanding intrathecal injections*.)
- Epidural catheter insertion is performed by an anesthesiologist using sterile technique.
- Nurses are responsible for monitoring the infusion and assessing the patient.

CONTRAINDICATIONS

- Local or systemic infection
- Neurologic disease
- Coagulopathy
- Spinal arthritis or deformity
- Hypotension
- Marked hypertension
- Allergy to prescribed drug
- Patients undergoing anticoagulant therapy

EQUIPMENT

Volume infusion device and epidural infusion tubing (depends on facility policy) ◆ patient's drug record and chart ◆ prescribed epidural solutions ◆ transparent dressing ◆ epidural tray ◆ labels for epidural infusion line ◆ silk tape ◆ emergency equipment: 0.4 mg I.V. naloxone (Narcan); 50 mg I.V. ephedrine; oxygen; intubation set; handheld resuscitation bag ◆ monitoring equipment for blood pressure and pulse, apnea monitor, pulse oximeter (optional)

PREPARATION

- Prepare device according to manufacturer's instructions and facility policy.
- Notify the pharmacy in advance; epidural solutions need special preparation.
- Check the drug concentration and infusion rate against the practitioner's order.

Understanding intrathecal injections

An intrathecal injection allows the physician to inject drugs into the subarachnoid space of the spinal canal. Certain drugs are administered by this route because they don't readily penetrate the blood-brain barrier through the bloodstream. This method is also used for regional anesthesia and pain management with drugs such as preservative-free morphine.

It's an invasive procedure that requires informed consent. The injection site is usually between the third and fourth (or fourth and fifth) lumbar vertebrae, well below the spinal cord to avoid risk of paralysis. The procedure may be preceded by aspiration of spinal fluid for laboratory analysis.

KEY STEPS

- Confirm the patient's identity using two patient identifiers according to facility policy.
- Make sure a consent form has been signed and witnessed.
- Position the patient on his side in the knee-chest position, or have him sit on the edge of the bed and lean over a bedside table.
- After catheter is in place, prime the infusion device, confirm appropriate drug and infusion rate and adjust accordingly.
- Help the anesthesiologist connect infusion tubing to the epidural catheter.
- Connect the tubing to the infusion pump.
- Bridge-tape all connection sites, and apply an "epidural infusion" label to the catheter, infusion tubing, and infusion pump to prevent infusion of other drugs.
- Start the infusion; tell the patient to report pain immediately.
- Have the patient use a 0 (least) to 10 (most) pain rating scale; 3 or less indicates tolerable pain. If he reports higher, the infusion rate may need to be increased. Call the practitioner or change rate within prescribed limits.
- If ordered, place the patient on an apnea monitor for the first 24 hours.
- Change the dressing over the exit site every 24 to 48 hours or as needed. Use transparent dressing to allow inspection of drainage.

⚡ **WARNING** *The epidural catheter is generally not sutured in place; don't manipulate the catheter during dressing changes.*

- Change infusion tubing every 48 hours and epidural solution every 24 hours or as specified by facility policy.

REMOVING AN EPIDURAL CATHETER

- The anesthesiologist orders analgesics and removes the catheter. Some facilities allow a specially trained nurse to remove the catheter.

WARNING *If you feel resistance, stop and call the physician for further orders.*

◆ Save the catheter. The physician will examine the tip to rule out damage during removal.

SPECIAL CONSIDERATIONS

◆ After starting infusion, assess respiratory rate, blood pressure, and oxygen saturation every 2 hours for 8 hours, then every 4 hours for the next 16 hours.
◆ Thereafter, assess the patient once per shift, depending on condition or facility policy.

WARNING *Notify the practitioner if the patient's respiratory rate is less than 10 breaths/minute or his systolic blood pressure is less than 90 mm Hg.*

◆ Assess his sedation level, mental status, and pain-relief status every hour initially, then every 2 to 4 hours until adequate pain control is achieved.

WARNING *Notify the practitioner if the patient appears drowsy, experiences nausea and vomiting, refractory itching, inability to void, or has pain. Drowsiness is an early indicator of respiratory depressant effects of opioids. Respiratory depression usually occurs during first 24 hours; treat it with I.V. naloxone (Narcan). For nausea, vomiting, and pruritus treat with low-dose I.V. naloxone.*

◆ Assess lower-extremity motor strength every 2 to 4 hours. If sensorimotor loss occurs, dosage may need to be decreased. Notify the practitioner; he may need to titrate the dosage to provide adequate pain control without excessive numbness and weakness.

WARNING *Drugs given epidurally diffuse slowly and may cause adverse effects, including excessive sedation up to 12 hours after infusion.*

◆ The patient should always have a peripheral I.V. line open to allow immediate administration of emergency drugs.

◆ Postural puncture headache may result from accidental puncture of the dura. The anesthesiologist may attempt again at a different lumbar interspace.
◆ If CSF leaks into the dura mater at the initial puncture site, the patient usually experiences a headache. This is treated with a "blood patch," blood (about 10 ml) withdrawn from a peripheral vein, then injected into the epidural space.

COMPLICATIONS
◆ Adverse reactions from opioids or local anesthetics
◆ Infection
◆ Epidural hematoma
◆ Catheter migration

WARNING *If catheter migration occurs notify the practitioner because the infusion needs to be stopped and the catheter removed.*

PATIENT TEACHING

◆ Explain the procedure and possible complications. Tell the patient that he'll feel some pain as the catheter is inserted.
◆ For home use, teach the patient or a family member the required care. The patient shouldn't use alcohol or other drugs that add to opioid action.

DOCUMENTATION

◆ Note the patient's response to treatment.
◆ Document the catheter's patency.
◆ Record the condition of the dressing and insertion site.
◆ Note vital signs.
◆ Record assessment results.
◆ Note the labeling of the epidural catheter.
◆ Document changing of the infusion bags.
◆ Note ordered analgesics and the patient's response.

SELECTED REFERENCES
Coyne, P.J., et al. "Effectively Starting and Titrating Intrathecal Analgesic Therapy in Patients with Refractory Cancer Pain," *Clinical Journal of Oncology Nursing* 9(5):581-83, October 2005.
De Pietri, L., et al. "The Use of Intrathecal Morphine for Postoperative Pain Relief after Liver Resection: A Comparison with Epidural Analgesia," *Anesthesia and Analgesia* 102(4):1157-63, April 2006.
Lieberman, E., et al. "Changes in Fetal Position During Labor and Their Association with Epidural Analgesia," *Obstetrics and Gynecology* 105(5 Pt 1):974-82, May 2005.
Mordecai, M.M., and Brull, S.J. "Spinal Anesthesia," *Current Opinion in Anaesthesiology* 18(5):527-33, October 2005.
Rathmell, J.P., et al. "The Role of Intrathecal Drugs in the Treatment of Acute Pain," *Anesthesia and Analgesia* 101(Suppl 5):S30-43, November 2005.
Viscusi, E.R. "Emerging Techniques in the Management of Acute Pain: Epidural Analgesia," *Anesthesia and Analgesia* 101(Suppl 5):S23-29, November 2005.

Esophageal airway insertion and removal

OVERVIEW

DESCRIPTION
◆ Esophageal airways, such as the esophageal gastric tube airway (EGTA), the esophageal obturator airway (EOA), and the Combitube are used to temporarily maintain ventilation in comatose patients during cardiac or respiratory arrest.
◆ These devices prevent tongue obstruction, keep air from entering the stomach, and keep stomach contents from entering the trachea.
◆ Health care providers must have special training to insert an EGTA or EOA; insertion is simpler than endotracheal intubation because visualization of the trachea or hyperextension of the neck isn't required.

CONTRAINDICATIONS
◆ Conscious or semiconscious patients
◆ Facial trauma preventing mask fit
◆ Absent or weak gag reflex
◆ Recent ingestion of toxic chemicals
◆ Esophageal disease
◆ Overdose of opioids that can be reversed by naloxone (Narcan)

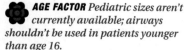 **AGE FACTOR** *Pediatric sizes aren't currently available; airways shouldn't be used in patients younger than age 16.*

EQUIPMENT

Esophageal tube ◆ face mask ◆ #16 or #18 French nasogastric (NG) tube (for EGTA) ◆ 35-ml syringe ◆ intermittent gastric suction equipment ◆ oral suction equipment ◆ gloves ◆ goggles ◆ handheld resuscitation bag, water-soluble lubricant (optional)

PREPARATION
◆ Fill the face mask with air and inflate the esophageal tube's cuff with 35 cc of air to check for leaks, then deflate.
◆ Connect the esophageal tube to the face mask (the lower opening on an EGTA); listen for a click that indicates proper placement.

KEY STEPS

◆ Determine if patient is a safe candidate for an esophageal airway.
◆ Put on gloves and personal protective equipment.
◆ Lubricate the first 1″ (2.5 cm) of the tube's distal tip. With an EGTA, also lubricate the first 1″ of the NG tube's distal tip.

INSERTING AN ESOPHAGEAL AIRWAY
◆ If his condition permits, place him in the supine position with his neck neutral or semiflexed.

⚡ **WARNING** *Hyperextension of the neck may cause the tube to enter the trachea instead of the esophagus.*
◆ Remove dentures, if applicable.
◆ Insert your thumb deep into the patient's mouth behind the base of his tongue.
◆ Put your index and middle fingers under his chin and lift his jaw straight up.
◆ With your other hand, grasp the esophageal tube (as you would hold a pencil) just below the mask. This enables gentle maneuvering of the tube and reduces risk of pharyngeal trauma.
◆ Insert the tip of the esophageal tube into the patient's mouth.
◆ Guide the airway over the tongue into the pharynx, then into the esophagus, following the natural pharyngeal curve.
◆ No force should be needed for proper insertion.
◆ If there's resistance, withdraw the tube slightly and readvance it. When fully advanced, the mask should fit snugly over the mouth and nose. The cuff must lie below the level of the carina.
◆ Deliver positive-pressure ventilation before inflating the cuff in case the tube entered the trachea. If his chest rises, the tube is in the esophagus.
◆ When the tube is properly in place, draw 35 cc of air into the syringe, connect the syringe to the tube's cuff-inflation valve, and inflate the cuff.

WARNING *Avoid overinflation; it can cause esophageal trauma.*

◆ If using an EGTA, insert the NG tube through the lower port on the face mask and into the esophageal tube; advance it to the second marking so it reaches 6″ (15.2 cm) beyond the distal end of the esophageal tube.

◆ Suction stomach contents using intermittent gastric suction to decompress the stomach.

◆ Attach a handheld resuscitation bag or a mechanical ventilator to the face mask port (upper port on EGTA). Up to 100% of inspired oxygen can be delivered this way.

WARNING *Monitor for adequate ventilation. Watch for chest movement and suction the patient if mucus blocks the EOA tube perforations or interrupts respiration.*

REMOVING AN ESOPHAGEAL AIRWAY

◆ Assess the patient's condition to determine if airway removal is appropriate. Respirations should be spontaneous and number 16 to 20 breaths/minute.

WARNING *After 2 hours, if respirations aren't spontaneous and at normal rate, switch to an endotracheal (ET) tube for long-term ventilation.*

◆ Detach the mask from the esophageal tube.

◆ If the patient is conscious, place him on his left side to avoid aspiration during tube removal. If he's unconscious and requires an ET tube, assist with its insertion. Inflate the ET tube's cuff before removing the esophageal tube.

◆ With the ET tube in place, stomach contents are less likely to be aspirated when the esophageal tube is removed.

◆ Deflate the cuff on the esophageal tube by removing air from the inflation valve with a syringe.

WARNING *Don't try to remove the tube with the cuff inflated; it may perforate the esophagus.*

◆ Turn the patient's head to the side to avoid aspiration.

◆ Remove the EGTA or EOA in one swift, smooth motion, following the natural pharyngeal curve to avoid esophageal trauma.

◆ Perform oropharyngeal suctioning to remove residual secretions.

◆ Assist the practitioner in monitoring and maintaining adequate ventilation.

SPECIAL CONSIDERATIONS

◆ Store EGTAs and EOAs in their packages to preserve the natural curve.

◆ Direct the airway along the right side of the patient's mouth because the esophagus is located to the right of and behind the trachea. Alternatively, advance the tube tip toward the hard palate, then invert it and glide it along the tongue into the pharynx. This helps avoid snagging on the sides of the throat and eases insertion in a patient with clenched jaws.

WARNING *If retching occurs, remove airway immediately; accumulation of vomitus blocked by the airway cuff may perforate the esophagus.*

◆ EOAs may be inferior to ET intubation in providing adequate oxygenation and ventilation.

COMPLICATIONS

◆ Esophageal injuries, including rupture

◆ Laryngospasm, vomiting, and aspiration in semiconscious patients

◆ Aspiration of foreign material from the mouth and pharynx into the trachea and bronchi

PATIENT TEACHING

◆ As the patient regains consciousness, restrain his hands if he tries to remove the airway. Explain the procedure to him to reduce anxiety.

DOCUMENTATION

◆ Note the date and time of the procedure.

◆ Record the type of airway inserted.

◆ Note the patient's vital signs and level of consciousness.

◆ Document the airway removal.

◆ Record the alternative airway inserted after extubation.

◆ Document the complications and nursing actions taken.

SELECTED REFERENCES

Bair, A.E., et al. "An Assessment of a Tracheal Tube Introducer as an Endotracheal Tube Placement Confirmation Device," *American Journal of Emergency Medicine* 23(6):754-58, October 2005.

Cady, C.E., and Pirrallo, R.G. "The Effect of Combitube Use of Paramedic Experience in Endotracheal Intubation," *American Journal of Emergency Medicine* 23(7):868-71, November 2005.

Genzwuerker, H.V., et al. "Comparison of Different Airway Devices in a Simulated Entrapped Car Accident Victim Scenario," *European Journal of Emergency Medicine* 13(1):60, February 2006.

Portereiko, J.V., et al. "Acute Upper Airway Obstruction by an Over-Inflated Combitube Esophageal Obturator Balloon," *Journal of Trauma* 60(2):426-27, February 2006.

Esophageal tube care

DESCRIPTION

◆ A physician inserts an esophageal tube; nurses care for the patient during and after intubation.

◆ The patient is held in the intensive care unit for close observation and constant care, which may help increase his tolerance for the procedure and help control bleeding.

◆ Traumatic injury from intubation or esophageal balloon inflation increases the chance of rupture.

◆ The patient with an esophageal tube to control variceal bleeding (typically from portal hypertension) must be observed closely for possible esophageal rupture, because varices weaken the esophagus.

◆ Emergency surgery is usually performed after a rupture, but has a low success rate.

CONTRAINDICATIONS

◆ None known

Manometer ◆ two 2-L bottles of normal saline solution ◆ irrigation set ◆ water-soluble lubricant ◆ several cotton-tipped applicators ◆ mouth-care equipment ◆ nasopharyngeal suction apparatus ◆ several #12 French suction catheters ◆ intake and output record sheets ◆ gloves ◆ goggles ◆ sedatives ◆ traction weights or football helmet scissors

◆ Provide privacy.
◆ Wash your hands and put on gloves and goggles.
◆ Monitor vital signs every 5 minutes to 1 hour as ordered.

⚡ **WARNING** *A change in vital signs may signal complications or recurrent bleeding.*

◆ If the patient has a Sengstaken-Blakemore or a Minnesota tube, check the pressure gauge on the manometer every 30 to 60 minutes to detect leaks in the esophageal balloon and verify set pressure.

⚡ **WARNING** *Fluid accumulating in the stomach may cause the patient to regurgitate the tube; fluid accumulating in the esophagus may lead to vomiting and aspiration. Maintain drainage and suction on gastric and esophageal aspiration ports.*

⚡ **WARNING** *Obstruction in the tube can lead to regurgitation of the tube and vomiting.*

◆ Irrigate the gastric aspiration port, as ordered, using the irrigation set and normal saline solution. Frequent irrigation keeps the tube from clogging.

◆ To prevent pressure ulcers, use warm water to loosen crusted nasal secretions, then apply lubricant with cotton-tipped applicators.

◆ Provide mouth care to remove foul-tasting matter and relieve dryness from mouth breathing.

◆ Use #12 French catheters to provide gentle oral suctioning, if necessary, to remove secretions.

◆ Offer emotional support. Keep the patient as quiet as possible; administer sedatives if ordered.

◆ A football helmet or traction weights may be used to secure the tube. Traction weights must hang from the foot of the bed at all times.

⚡ **WARNING** *Never rest weights on the bed. Instruct coworkers not to move weights; reduced traction may change the position of the tube.*

◆ Elevate the head of the bed about 25 degrees to ensure countertraction for the weights.

- Keep the patient on complete bed rest; exertion, coughing, or straining increases intra-abdominal pressure, which may trigger further bleeding.
- Keep the patient in semi-Fowler's position to reduce blood flow into the portal system and prevent reflux into the esophagus.
- Monitor intake and output as ordered.

SPECIAL CONSIDERATIONS

⚡ *WARNING Watch for signs and symptoms of esophageal rupture, including shock, increased respiratory difficulties, and increased bleeding.*
- Tape scissors to the head of the bed so the tube can be cut quickly to deflate the balloons if asphyxia develops. If this emergency intervention is needed, hold the tube firmly close to the nostril before cutting.
- If using traction, release the tension before deflating the balloons. If weights and pulleys supply traction, remove weights. If a football helmet supplies traction, untape the esophageal tube from the face guard before deflating balloons.

⚡ *WARNING Deflating the balloon under tension triggers a rapid release of the entire tube from the nose, which may injure mucous membranes, initiate recurrent bleeding, and obstruct the airway.*
- If an X-ray is ordered to check the tube's position or view the chest, lift the patient in the direction of the pulley, then place the X-ray film at his back.

⚡ *WARNING Never roll the patient from side to side; pressure exerted on the tube may shift its position. Lift the patient to make the bed or help with the bedpan.*

COMPLICATIONS

- Esophageal rupture, a serious, life-threatening complication occurring most commonly during intubation or inflation of the esophageal balloon
- Asphyxia, if the balloon moves up the esophagus and blocks the airway
- Aspiration of pooled esophageal secretions

PATIENT TEACHING

- Explain procedure to the patient and answer any questions.

DOCUMENTATION

- Read the manometer hourly; record esophageal pressures.
- Note when balloons are deflated and by whom.
- Record vital signs.
- Note the condition of the patient's nostrils.
- Document routine care.
- Record the drugs administered.
- Note the color, consistency, and amount of gastric returns.
- Record signs and symptoms of complications and nursing actions taken.
- Document gastric port and nasogastric tube irrigations.
- Maintain accurate intake and output records.

SELECTED REFERENCES

Chong, C.F. "Esophageal Rupture Due to Sengstaken-Blakemore Tube Misplacement," *World Journal of Gastroenterology* 11(41):6563-65, November 2005.

Greenwald, B. "Two Devices that Facilitate the Use of the Minnesota Tube," *Gastroenterology Nursing* 27(6):268-70, November-December 2004.

Ho, K.M. "Use of Sengstaken-Blakemore Tube to Stop Massive Upper Gastrointestinal Bleeding from Dieulafoy's Lesion in the Lower Oesophagus," *Anaesthesia and Intensive Care* 32(5): 711-14, October 2004.

Nakajima, M. "Intermittent Oro-Esophageal Tube Feeding in Acute Stroke Patients — A Pilot Study," *Acta Neurologica Scandinavica* 113(1):36-39, January 2006.

Noble, K.A. "Name That Tube," *Nursing* 33(3):56-63, March 2003.

Esophageal tube insertion and removal

DESCRIPTION

- An esophageal tube is inserted nasally or orally and advanced into the esophagus or stomach to control hemorrhage from esophageal or gastric varices.
- A physician inserts and removes the tube; in an emergency a nurse may remove it.
- When the tube is in place, a gastric balloon at the end can be inflated and drawn tightly against the cardia of the stomach. The balloon secures the tube and exerts pressure on the cardia, which controls the bleeding varices.
- Most tubes also contain an esophageal balloon to control esophageal bleeding. (See *Types of esophageal tubes*.)
- Gastric or esophageal balloons should be deflated within 24 hours.
- **⚡ WARNING** *If inflated longer than 24 hours, pressure necrosis can develop and cause further hemorrhage or perforation.*
- Irrigation with normal saline solution and drug therapy with a vasopressor may be used in conjunction for temporary control of acute variceal hemorrhage.

CONTRAINDICATIONS

- None known

Esophageal tube ◆ nasogastric (NG) tube (if using a Sengstaken-Blakemore tube) ◆ two suction sources ◆ basin of ice ◆ irrigation set ◆ 2 L of normal saline solution ◆ two 60-ml syringes ◆ water-soluble lubricant ◆ ½″ or 1″ adhesive tape ◆ stethoscope ◆ foam nose guard ◆ four rubber-shod clamps (two clamps and two plastic plugs for a Minnesota tube) ◆ anesthetic spray (as ordered) ◆ traction equipment (football helmet or a basic frame with traction rope, pulleys, and a 1-lb [0.5-kg] weight) ◆ mercury aneroid manometer ◆ Y-connector tube (for a Sengstaken-Blakemore or a Linton tube) ◆ basin of water ◆ cup of water with straw ◆ scissors ◆ gloves ◆ gown ◆ waterproof marking pen ◆ goggles ◆ sphygmomanometer

PREPARATION

- Keep the traction helmet at bedside or attach traction equipment to the bed, for availability after tube insertion.
- Keep suction machines nearby and plugged in.
- Open the irrigation set and fill the container with normal saline solution.
- Test the balloons on the esophageal tube for air leaks by inflating them and submerging them in the water. If no bubbles appear, remove and deflate.
- Clamp the tube lumens, so the balloons stay deflated during insertion.
- To prepare the Minnesota tube, connect the mercury manometer to the gastric pressure monitoring port. Note the pressure when the balloon fills with 100, 200, 300, 400, and 500 cc of air.
- Check the aspiration lumens for patency; make sure they're labeled. If they aren't identified, label them with the marking pen.
- Chill the tube in a basin of ice to stiffen it and facilitate insertion.

- Confirm the patient's identity using two patient identifiers according to facility policy.
- Explain the procedure and provide privacy.
- Wash your hands.
- Put on gloves, gown, and goggles to protect yourself from blood.
- Put the patient in semi-Fowler's position and turn him slightly to his left side. This position promotes stomach emptying and helps prevent aspiration.
- Explain to him that the physician will inspect his nostrils for patency.
- To determine tubing length, hold the balloon at the patient's xiphoid process, extend the tube to the patient's ear and forward to his nose. Using a waterproof pen, mark this point on the tubing.
- Lubricate the tip of the tube to reduce friction and facilitate insertion.
- The physician will pass the tube through the more patent nostril. He'll direct the patient to tilt his chin toward his chest and swallow when he senses the tip of the tube at the back of his throat.
- Swallowing helps advance the tube into the esophagus and prevents intubation of the trachea. (If introduced orally, the patient should swallow immediately.)
- As the patient swallows, the physician quickly advances the tube at least ½″ (1.3 cm) beyond the marked point on the tube.
- To confirm tube placement, the physician will aspirate stomach contents through the gastric port and auscultate the stomach with a stethoscope as he injects air.
- After partially inflating the gastric balloon with 50 to 100 cc of air, he'll order an X-ray to confirm correct balloon placement.

Types of esophageal tubes

When using an esophageal tube, consider the advantages of the most common types.

SENGSTAKEN-BLAKEMORE TUBE

A Sengstaken-Blakemore tube is a triple-lumen, double-balloon tube that has a gastric aspiration port, which allows drainage from below the gastric balloon and drug instillation.

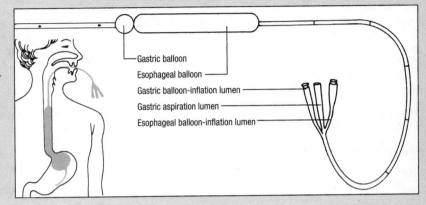

Gastric balloon
Esophageal balloon
Gastric balloon-inflation lumen
Gastric aspiration lumen
Esophageal balloon-inflation lumen

LINTON TUBE

A Linton tube is a triple-lumen, single-balloon tube that has ports for gastric aspiration and esophageal aspiration. This tube reduces risk of esophageal necrosis because it doesn't have an esophageal balloon.

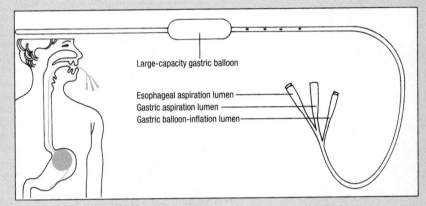

Large-capacity gastric balloon

Esophageal aspiration lumen
Gastric aspiration lumen
Gastric balloon-inflation lumen

MINNESOTA ESOPHAGOGASTRIC TAMPONADE TUBE

A Minnesota esophagogastric tamponade tube is an esophageal tube that has four lumens and two balloons. The device provides pressure-monitoring ports for both balloons without the need for Y connectors. One port is used for gastric suction, the other for esophageal suction.

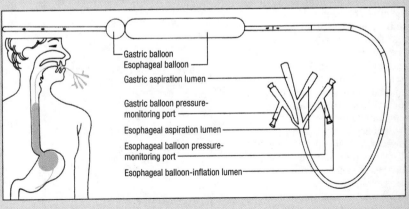

Gastric balloon
Esophageal balloon
Gastric aspiration lumen

Gastric balloon pressure-monitoring port
Esophageal aspiration lumen
Esophageal balloon pressure-monitoring port
Esophageal balloon-inflation lumen

(continued)

- Before fully inflating the balloon, he'll use the 60-ml syringe to irrigate the stomach with normal saline solution and empty the stomach as completely as possible. This helps the patient avoid regurgitating when the balloon inflates.
- After confirming tube placement, the physician fully inflates the gastric balloon (250 to 500 cc of air for the Sengstaken-Blakemore tube using rubber-shod clamps; 700 to 800 cc of air for the Linton tube) and clamps the tube.
- If using a Minnesota tube, the physician will connect the pressure-monitoring port for the gastric balloon lumen to the mercury manometer, then inflate the balloon in 100-cc increments until it fills with up to 500 cc of air.
- As he introduces air, he'll monitor intragastric balloon pressure to make sure the balloon stays inflated. Then he'll clamp the ports.
- For the Sengstaken-Blakemore or Minnesota tube, the physician will gently pull on the tube until he feels resistance, which indicates the gastric balloon is inflated and exerting pressure on the cardia of the stomach.
- When he senses the balloon is engaged, he'll place the foam nose guard where the tube emerges from the nostril.
- Tape the nose guard in place around the tube. This helps minimize pressure on the nostril from the traction and decreases the risk of necrosis.
- Traction can be applied to the tube with a traction rope and 1-lb weight, or the tube can be pulled gently and taped securely to the face guard of a football helmet. (See *Securing an esophageal tube.*)
- With pulley-and-weight traction, lower the head of the bed to about 25 degrees to produce countertraction.
- Lavage the stomach through the gastric aspiration lumen with normal saline solution until return fluid is clear. Vasoconstriction stops the hemorrhage; the lavage empties the stomach. Blood detected later indicates that bleeding is still uncontrolled.

- Attach one of the suction sources to the gastric aspiration lumen. This empties the stomach, helps prevent nausea and possible vomiting, and allows continuous observation of gastric contents for blood.
- If a Sengstaken-Blakemore or a Minnesota tube was used, the physician will inflate the esophageal balloon as he inflates the gastric balloon to compress the esophageal varices and control bleeding.
- With a Sengstaken-Blakemore tube, he'll attach the Y-connector tube to the esophageal lumen, then attach a sphygmomanometer inflation bulb to one end of the Y-connector and the manometer to the other end. Then he'll inflate the esophageal balloon until the pressure is between 30 and 40 mm Hg, and clamp the tube.
- With a Minnesota tube, he'll attach the mercury manometer directly to the esophageal pressure-monitoring outlet. Using the 60-ml syringe and pushing air slowly into the esophageal balloon port, he'll inflate the balloon until the pressure is between 35 and 45 mm Hg.

Securing an esophageal tube

One way to reduce risk of the gastric balloon slipping down or away from the cardia of the stomach is to secure it to a football helmet. Tape the tube to the face guard (as shown) and fasten the chin strap.

To remove the tube quickly, unfasten the chin strap and pull the helmet slightly forward. Cut the tape and the gastric balloon and esophageal balloon lumens. Be sure to hold onto the tube near the patient's nostril.

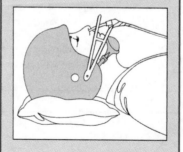

- Check balloon pressure every 2 hours.
- Set up esophageal suction to prevent accumulation of secretions that may cause vomiting and pulmonary aspiration; swallowed secretions can't pass into the stomach if the patient has an inflated esophageal balloon in place.
- If he has a Linton or a Minnesota tube, attach the suction source to the esophageal aspiration port.
- If he has a Sengstaken-Blakemore tube, advance an NG tube through the other nostril into the esophagus to the point where the esophageal balloon begins, and attach the suction source as ordered.

REMOVING THE TUBE
- The physician will deflate the esophageal balloon by aspirating the air with a syringe. (He may order that it be deflated at 5 mm Hg increments every 30 minutes for several hours.) If bleeding doesn't recur, he'll remove the traction from the gastric tube and deflate the gastric balloon (also by aspiration).
- The gastric balloon must be deflated before removing the tube because the balloon may ride up into the esophagus or pharynx and obstruct the airway, possibly causing asphyxia or rupture.
- After disconnecting all suction tubes, the physician will remove the tube. If he feels resistance, he'll aspirate the balloons again. (To remove a Minnesota tube, he'll grasp it near the patient's nostril and cut across all four lumens about 3″ [7.6 cm] below that point. This ensures deflation of all balloons.)
- After the tube has been removed, assist the patient with mouth care.

SPECIAL CONSIDERATIONS

◆ If the patient appears cyanotic, or other signs of airway obstruction develop during tube placement, remove the tube immediately; it may have entered the trachea instead of the esophagus.

◆ Keep scissors taped to the head of the bed.

⚡ **WARNING** *If respiratory distress occurs, cut across all lumens while holding the tube at the nares, and remove the tube quickly.*

◆ Unless contraindicated, the patient can sip water through a straw during intubation to facilitate tube advancement.

◆ Intraesophageal balloon pressure varies with respirations and esophageal contractions. Baseline pressure is the important pressure.

◆ The balloon on the Linton tube should stay inflated no longer than 24 hours; necrosis of the cardia may result.

◆ The physician usually removes the tube only after a trial period (lasting at least 12 hours) with the esophageal balloon deflated or with the gastric balloon tension released from the cardia to check for rebleeding.

◆ The physician may deflate the balloon for 5 to 10 minutes every hour to temporarily relieve pressure on the esophageal mucosa.

COMPLICATIONS

◆ Erosion and perforation of the esophagus and gastric mucosa from tension placed on these areas by balloons during traction

◆ Esophageal rupture, if the gastric balloon accidentally inflates in the esophagus

◆ Acute airway occlusion, if the balloon dislodges and moves upward into the trachea

◆ Other erosions

◆ Nasal tissue necrosis

◆ Aspiration of oral secretions

PATIENT TEACHING

◆ Explain the procedure and its purpose to the patient and his family.

◆ Tell the patient that the physician will spray his throat and nostrils with an anesthetic to minimize discomfort and gagging during intubation.

DOCUMENTATION

◆ Record the date and time of insertion and removal.

◆ Note the type of tube used.

◆ Document the name of the physician who performed the procedure.

◆ Record the intraesophageal balloon pressure for the Sengstaken-Blakemore and Minnesota tubes.

◆ Note the intragastric balloon pressure for the Minnesota tube.

◆ Record amount of air injected for the Sengstaken-Blakemore and Linton tubes.

◆ Note the amount of fluid used for gastric irrigation.

◆ Record the color, consistency, and amount of gastric returns, both before and after lavage.

SELECTED REFERENCES

Bair, A.E., et al. "An Assessment of a Tracheal Tube Introducer as an Endotracheal Tube Placement Confirmation Device," *American Journal of Emergency Medicine* 23(6):754-58, October 2005.

Chien, J.Y., Yu, C.J. "Images in Clinical Medicine. Malposition of a Sengstaken-Blakemore Tube," *New England Journal of Medicine* 352(8):e7, February 2005.

Chong, C.F. "Esophageal Rupture Due to Sengstaken-Blakemore Tube Misplacement," *World Journal of Gastroenterology* 11(41):6563-65, November 2005.

Gounot, E., et al. "Isolated Isoperistaltic Gastric Tube Interposition for Esophageal Replacement in Children," *Journal of Pediatric Surgery* 41(3):592-95, March 2006.

External fixation

DESCRIPTION

◆ External fixation is used to treat open, unstable fractures with extensive soft tissue damage; comminuted closed fractures; septic, nonunion fractures; and facilitate surgical immobilization of a joint.

◆ A physician inserts metal pins through skin and muscle layers into broken bones and affixes them to an adjustable external frame to maintain alignment. (See *Types of external fixation devices.*)

◆ Specialized external fixators may be used to lengthen leg bones or immobilize the cervical spine.

◆ External fixation stabilizes the fracture while allowing open wounds to be seen and accessed and enables earlier ambulation.

◆ The Ilizarov fixator is an external fixation device with a combination of rings and tensioned transosseous wires used primarily for limb lengthening, bone transport, and limb salvage. It provides gradual distraction resulting in good-quality bone formation.

CONTRAINDICATIONS

◆ None known

EQUIPMENT

Sterile cotton-tipped applicators ◆ antiseptic cleaning solution ◆ ice bag ◆ sterile gauze pads ◆ povidone-iodine solution ◆ analgesic or opioid ◆ antimicrobial ointment (optional)

PREPARATION

◆ Equipment varies with type of fixator and type and location of fracture; typically, sets of pins, stabilizing rods, and clips are available from manufacturers. Don't reuse pins.

◆ Make sure the external fixation set includes all necessary equipment and that it has been sterilized.

KEY STEPS

◆ Confirm the patient's identity using two patient identifiers according to facility policy.

◆ Explain the procedure to the patient to reduce his anxiety.

◆ After the fixation device is in place, perform neurovascular checks every 2 to 4 hours for 24 hours, then every 4 to 8 hours, as necessary.

◆ Assess color, motion, sensation, digital movement, edema, capillary refill, and pulses of the affected extremity, and compare with the unaffected side.

◆ Apply an ice bag to the surgical site, as ordered, to reduce swelling, relieve pain, and lessen bleeding.

◆ Administer analgesics or opioids, as ordered, before exercising or mobilizing the affected extremity to promote comfort. Instruct the patient in the use of the patient-controlled analgesia machine if applicable.

WARNING *Monitor for pain not relieved by analgesics or opioids and for burning, tingling, or numbness, which may indicate nerve damage or circulatory impairment.*

◆ Elevate the affected extremity, if appropriate, to minimize edema.

Types of external fixation devices

The physician's selection of an external fixation device depends on the severity of the patient's fracture and the type of bone alignment needed.

UNIVERSAL DAY FRAME

The universal day frame is used for simple tibial fractures. The frame allows the physician to readjust the position of bony fragments by angulation and rotation. The compression-distraction device allows compression and distraction of bony fragments.

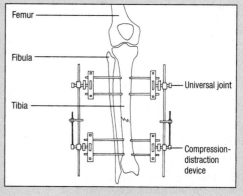

PORTSMOUTH EXTERNAL FIXATION BAR

The Portsmouth external fixation bar is used for complicated tibial fractures. The locking nut adjustment on the mobile carriage only allows bone compression, so the physician must accurately reduce bony fragments before applying the device.

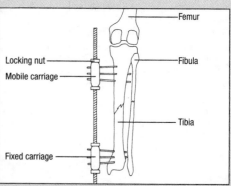

- Perform pin-site care, as ordered, to prevent infection:
  - Use sterile technique
  - Avoid digging at pin sites with the cotton-tipped applicator
  - If ordered, clean the pin site and surrounding skin with a cotton-tipped applicator dipped in ordered antiseptic solution
  - If ordered, apply antimicrobial ointment to pin sites
  - Apply a loose sterile dressing, or dress with sterile gauze pads soaked in povidone-iodine solution.
- Check for redness, tenting of skin, prolonged or purulent drainage from pin site, swelling, elevated body or pin-site temperature, and bowing or bending of pins, which may stress the skin.

SPECIAL CONSIDERATIONS

PATIENT WITH AN ILIZAROV FIXATOR

- When the device has been placed and preliminary calluses have begun to form at insertion sites (5 to 7 days), gentle distraction is initiated by turning the appropriate screws one-quarter turn (1 mm) every 4 to 6 hours as ordered.
- Don't administer nonsteroidal anti-inflammatory drugs to patients being treated with the Ilizarov fixator; they may decrease the necessary inflammation caused by the distraction, resulting in delayed bone formation.
- Pin sites are more prone to infection because of extended treatment period and the pins' movement to accomplish distraction. The small pins are also more likely to break because of their size; the large number of pins increases patient's risk of neurovascular compromise.

COMPLICATIONS

- Loosening of pins and loss of fracture stabilization
- Infection of the pin tract or wound
- Skin breakdown
- Nerve damage
- Muscle impingement

PATIENT TEACHING

- Before discharge, teach the patient and family members how to provide pin-site care using clean technique at home.
- Emphasize to the patient that he'll feel little pain after the fixation device is in place. Assure the patient that his feelings of anxiety are normal and that he'll be able to adjust to the apparatus.
- Tell the patient that he'll be able to move about with the apparatus in place, which may help him resume normal activities more quickly.
- Instruct the patient regarding his prescribed weight-bearing status.
- Teach the patient how to recognize signs of pin-site infection.
- Tell the patient to keep the affected limb elevated when sitting or lying down.

PATIENT WITH AN ILIZAROV FIXATOR

- Tell the patient he must be consistent in turning the screws every 4 to 6 hours around the clock. Make sure he understands he must be strongly committed to protocol compliance for the procedure to work.
- The treatment period may be prolonged (4 to 10 months); discuss with the patient and his family psychological effects of long-term care.

DOCUMENTATION

- Record the patient's reaction to the apparatus.
- Assess and document the condition of pin sites and skin.
- Document the patient's reaction to ambulation.
- Note understanding of patient teaching.

SELECTED REFERENCES

Capo, J.T., et al. "External Fixation Techniques for Distal Radius Fractures," *Clinical Orthopaedics and Related Research* 445:30-41, April 2006.

Haasper, C., et al. "Hinged External Fixation and Closed Reduction for Distal Humerus Fracture," *Archives of Orthopaedic and Trauma Surgery* 126(3): 188-91, April 2006.

Roukis, T.S., and Zgonis, T. "Minimally Invasive "Pinless" External Fixation for Foot and Ankle Reconstruction," *Orthopedics* 29(3):209-12, March 2006.

Sian, P.S., et al. "The Care of Pin Sites with External Fixation," *Journal of Bone and Joint Surgery* (British Volume) 88(4): 558, April 2006.

Yanmis, I., et al. "Application of Circular External Fixator under Arthroscopic Control in Comminuted Patella Fractures: Techniques and Early Results," *Journal of Trauma* 60(3):659-63, March 2006.

Eye compresses, hot and cold

DESCRIPTION

◆ Hot compresses relieve discomfort by increasing circulation, which enhances absorption and decreases inflammation.

◆ Hot compresses may promote drainage of superficial infections.

◆ Cold compresses can reduce swelling or bleeding and relieve itching.

◆ Cold compresses numb sensory fibers and may be ordered to ease periorbital discomfort between prescribed doses of pain drug.

◆ Hot and cold compresses should be applied for 20 minute periods, four to six times a day.

◆ To prevent ocular infection be sure to use aseptic technique.

CONTRAINDICATIONS

◆ Treatment of eye inflammation, such as keratitis or iritis, because capillary constriction inhibits delivery of nutrients to the cornea

HOT COMPRESSES

Prescribed solution, usually sterile water or normal saline solution ◆ sterile bowl ◆ sterile 4″ × 4″ gauze pads ◆ towel ◆ gloves

COLD COMPRESSES

Small plastic bag or glove filled with ice chips ◆ ½″ hypoallergenic tape ◆ sterile 4″ × 4″ gauze pads ◆ towel ◆ sterile water, normal saline solution, or prescribed ophthalmic irrigant ◆ gloves

PREPARATION

Hot compresses

◆ Place a capped bottle of sterile water or normal saline solution in a bowl of hot water or under a stream of hot tap water.

◆ Allow the solution to become warm, not hot (no warmer than 120° F [48.9° C]).

◆ Pour the warm water or normal saline solution into a sterile bowl.

◆ Place sterile gauze pads in the bowl.

Cold compresses

◆ Place ice chips in a plastic bag or glove to make an ice pack.

◆ Keep the ice pack small to avoid excessive pressure on the eye.

◆ Remove excess air from the bag or glove and knot, or close, the open end.

◆ Use hypoallergenic tape to secure the ice pack.

◆ Place all equipment on the bedside stand near the patient.

◆ Confirm the patient's identity using two patient identifiers according to facility policy.

◆ Explain the procedure to the patient.

◆ Make him comfortable and provide privacy.

◆ When applying hot compresses, have him sit, if possible.

◆ When applying cold compresses, have him lie supine. Support his head with a pillow, and turn his head slightly to the unaffected side. This position will help hold the compress in place.

◆ If he has an eye patch, remove it.

◆ Drape a towel around his shoulders to catch spills.

◆ Wash your hands and put on gloves.

APPLYING HOT COMPRESSES

◆ Take two 4″ × 4″ gauze pads from the basin and squeeze out excess solution.

◆ Instruct the patient to close his eyes.

◆ Apply the pads one on top of the other to the affected eye. If the patient complains that the compress is too hot, remove it immediately.

◆ Change the compress every few minutes, as necessary, for the prescribed length of time.

◆ After removing each compress, check the patient's skin for signs that the compress solution is too hot.

APPLYING COLD COMPRESSES

◆ Moisten the middle of one sterile 4″ × 4″ gauze pad with sterile water, normal saline solution, or ophthalmic irrigating solution. This conducts cold from the ice pack. Keep the edges dry so they can absorb excess moisture.

◆ Tell the patient to close his eyes; place the moist gauze pad over the affected eye.

◆ Place the ice pack on top of the gauze pad, and tape it in place. If he complains of pain, remove the ice pack. Some patients may have an adverse reaction to cold.

- After 15 to 20 minutes, remove the tape, ice pack, and gauze pad, and discard them.
- Use the remaining sterile 4″ × 4″ gauze pads to clean and dry the patient's face.
- If ordered, apply ophthalmic ointment or an eye patch. (See *Applying an eye patch*.)

(See *Applying an eye patch*.)

SPECIAL CONSIDERATIONS

- When applying hot compresses, change the prescribed solution frequently to maintain a constant temperature.
- If ordered to apply moist, cold compresses directly to the patient's eyelid, fill a bowl with ice and water and soak 4″ × 4″ gauze pads in it. Place a compress directly on the lid; change compresses every 2 to 3 minutes.

COMPLICATIONS
- None known

PATIENT TEACHING

- When teaching a patient to apply warm compresses at home, explain that he can substitute a clean bowl and washcloth for the sterile equipment.
- If both eyes are infected, emphasize importance of using separate equipment for each eye to keep from passing infection back and forth between eyes.
- Direct the patient to wash his hands thoroughly before and after treating each eye.

DOCUMENTATION

- Record the time and duration of the procedure.
- Describe the eye's appearance before and after treatment.
- Record ointments (and amounts) or dressings applied to the eye.
- Note the patient's tolerance of the procedure.

SELECTED REFERENCES
Boyd-Monk, H. "Bringing Common EYE Emergencies into Focus," *Nursing* 35(12):46-51, December 2005.
Colyar, M. "Stabilization after Eye Trauma," *Advance for Nurse Practitioners* 13(7):17, July 2005.
Wirbelauer, C. "Management of the Red Eye for the Primary Care Physician," *American Journal of Medicine* 119(4): 302-306, April 2006.

Applying an eye patch

You may apply an eye patch for a variety of reasons: to protect the eye after injury or surgery, to prevent accidental damage to an anesthetized eye, to promote healing, to absorb secretions, to protect the eye from drying when the patient is comatose or unable to close the eye (as in Bell's palsy), or to prevent the patient from touching or rubbing his eye.

A thicker patch, called a *pressure patch,* may be used to help corneal abrasions heal, compress postoperative edema, or control hemorrhage from traumatic injury. Application requires an ophthalmologist's prescription and supervision.

To apply a patch, choose an appropriate-sized gauze pad, place it gently over the closed eye (as shown) and secure it with tape. Extend the tape from mid-forehead across the eye to below the earlobe.

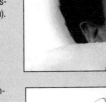

A pressure patch, which is thicker than a single-thickness gauze patch, exerts extra tension against the closed eye. After placing the initial gauze pad, you'll need to build it up with additional gauze pieces. Tape it firmly so the patch exerts even pressure over the closed eye (as shown).

For increased protection of an injured eye, place a plastic or metal shield (as shown) on top of the gauze pads and apply tape over the shield.

Occasionally, you may use a head dressing to secure a pressure patch. The dressing applies additional pressure; in burn patients, it holds the patch in place without tape.

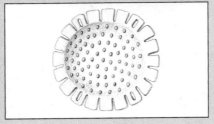

Eye drug application

DESCRIPTION

- Eye drugs (drops, ointments, disks) are used to lubricate the eye, treat eye conditions, protect vision of neonates, and lubricate the eye socket before insertion of a prosthetic eye.
- During eye examinations, eyedrops are used to anesthetize the eye, dilate the pupil to facilitate examination, and stain the cornea to identify corneal abrasions, scars, and other anomalies.
- Certain drugs may cause eye disorders or have serious ocular effects. For example, anticholinergics, commonly used during eye examinations, can precipitate acute glaucoma in patients predisposed to the disorder.

CONTRAINDICATIONS

- Conjunctivitis, keratitis, retinal detachment, and any condition that constricts the pupil (with drug disk)

EQUIPMENT

Prescribed eye drug ◆ patient's drug record and chart ◆ gloves ◆ warm water or normal saline solution ◆ sterile gauze pads ◆ facial tissues ◆ ocular dressing (optional)

PREPARATION

- Make sure drug is labeled for ophthalmic use and check expiration date.
- Date the container before using it. After it's opened, it may be used a maximum of 2 weeks to avoid contamination.
- Inspect solution for cloudiness, discoloration, and precipitation; some eye drugs are suspensions and normally appear cloudy.
- Don't use solution that appears abnormal.
- If the tip of an eye ointment tube has crusted, remove the crust with a sterile gauze pad.

KEY STEPS

- Verify the order on the patient's drug record by checking it against the prescriber's order.
- Wash your hands.
- Check the drug label against the patient's drug record.

  WARNING *Make sure you know which eye to treat because different drugs or doses may be ordered for each eye.*

- Confirm the patient's identity using two patient identifiers according to facility policy.
- If your facility uses a bar code scanning system, be sure to scan your ID badge, the patient's ID bracelet, and the medication's bar code.
- Explain the procedure, provide privacy, and put on gloves.
- If he's wearing an eye dressing, remove it by pulling down and away from his forehead. Don't contaminate your hands.
- Clean discharge from around the eye with sterile gauze pads moistened with warm water or normal saline solution. With his eye closed, clean from the inner to the outer canthus, using a fresh sterile gauze pad for each stroke.
- To remove crusted secretions, moisten a gauze pad with warm water or normal saline solution. Ask him to close the eye, and then place the gauze pad over it for 1 or 2 minutes.
- Remove the pad, then reapply moist sterile gauze pads, as necessary, until secretions are soft enough to be removed without traumatizing the mucosa.
- Have him sit or lie in the supine position. Tell him to tilt his head back and toward the side of the affected eye so excess drug can flow away from the tear duct, minimizing systemic absorption through the nasal mucosa.

INSTILLING EYEDROPS

- Remove the dropper cap and draw the drug into it. Don't contaminate the dropper tip or bottle top.
- Instruct the patient to look up and away to move the cornea away from the lower lid and minimize risk of touching the cornea with the dropper if he blinks.
- Rest the hand holding the dropper against his forehead. With your other hand, pull down the lower lid of the affected eye and instill drops in the conjunctival sac. (See *Instilling eye drugs.*)
- To prevent discomfort, avoid placing drops directly on the eyeball.
- Wait at least 5 minutes before instilling another prescribed agent.

APPLYING EYE OINTMENT

- Steady your hand by bracing it against the patient's forehead or cheek.
- Squeeze a small strip of drug on the edge of the conjunctival sac from the inner to the outer canthus; cut off the ribbon by turning the tube.
- Wait 10 minutes before applying additional prescribed drugs.

USING A DRUG DISK

- Press your fingertip against the disk so that it lies lengthwise across your fingertip.
- Lift the disk out of its packet.
- Gently pull the lower eyelid away from the eye and place the disk in the conjunctival sac.
- Pull the lower eyelid out, up, and over the disk.
- Tell the patient to blink several times.

AFTER INSTILLING EYEDROPS OR EYE OINTMENT

- For ointment, have the patient close his eyes, without squeezing the lids shut, and roll his eyes behind the closed lids.
- For drops, have him blink to distribute the drug.
- Use a clean tissue to remove excess solution or ointment leaking from the eye. Use a fresh tissue for each eye to prevent cross-contamination.
- Apply a new eye dressing, if necessary.
- Store drug according to label instructions.
- Wash your hands.

SPECIAL CONSIDERATIONS

◆ After giving an eye drug absorbed systemically, press your thumb on the inner canthus for 1 to 2 minutes (with patient's eyes closed). This helps prevent drug from flowing into the tear duct.
◆ Discard solution remaining in dropper before returning dropper to the bottle.
◆ Discard the dropper or bottle tip if contaminated.
◆ Don't use a container of eye drug for more than one patient.
◆ If both an ointment and drops have been ordered, administer drops first.
◆ A medication disk can release medication for up to 1 week before being replaced.

COMPLICATIONS

◆ Transient burning, itching, and redness
◆ Systemic effects (rare)

PATIENT TEACHING

◆ Teach the patient to instill eye drugs for treatment at home, if necessary.
◆ Review the procedure with the patient and ask him for a return demonstration.

DOCUMENTATION

◆ Record the drug instilled or applied.
◆ Note the eye or eyes treated.
◆ Document the date, time, and dose.
◆ Note adverse effects.
◆ Record the patient's response.

SELECTED REFERENCES

Abdollahi, M., et al. "Drug-Induced Toxic Reactions in the Eye: An Overview," *Journal of Infusion Nursing* 27(6):386-98, November-December 2004.
Marsden, J., and Shaw, M. "Correct Administration of Topical Eye Treatment," *Nursing Standard* 17(30):42-44, April 2003.
Sultana, Y., et al. "Review of Ocular Drug Delivery," *Current Drug Delivery* 3(2): 207-17, April 2006.

Instilling eye drugs

Eye drugs may be given either as eyedrops or ointment. To instill eyedrops, pull the lower eyelid down to expose the conjunctival sac. Have the patient look up and away, and then squeeze the prescribed number of drops into the sac (as shown). Release his eyelid, and have him blink to distribute the drug.

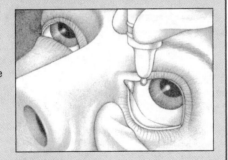

To apply ointment, lay a thin strip along the conjunctival sac from the inner canthus to the outer canthus (as shown). Don't touch the tube with the patient's eye. Release the eyelid and have him roll his eye behind closed lids to distribute the drug.

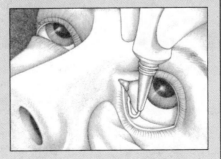

Eye irrigation

OVERVIEW

DESCRIPTION

- Irrigation flushes secretions, chemicals, and foreign bodies from the eye.
- It provides a way to administer drugs for corneal and conjunctival disorders.
- The amount of solution needed to irrigate the eye depends on the contaminant: secretions require a moderate volume and major chemical burns require a copious volume.
- An I.V. bottle or bag of normal saline solution (with I.V. tubing attached) usually supplies enough solution for continuous irrigation of a chemical burn. (See *Three devices for eye irrigation*.)

CONTRAINDICATIONS

- Noncompliant patient
- Possibility of orbital fracture

EQUIPMENT

Gloves ◆ goggles ◆ towels ◆ eyelid retractor ◆ sterile gauze pads ◆ I.V. pole ◆ commercially prepared bottles of sterile ophthalmic irrigant, as needed ◆ litmus paper, proparacaine topical anesthetic (optional)

MODERATE-VOLUME IRRIGATION

Prescribed sterile ophthalmic irrigant

COPIOUS IRRIGATION

One or more 1,000-ml bottles or bags of normal saline solution ◆ standard I.V. infusion set without needle

PREPARATION

- Wash your hands before setting up the equipment.
- Check the sterility, strength, and expiration date on the irrigant solution's label.
- Warm all solutions to body temperature.

Moderate-volume irrigation

- Remove the cap and keep the container within reach; keep the tip of the container sterile.

Copious irrigation

- Use sterile technique to set up I.V. tubing and bag or bottle of normal saline solution.
- Hang the container on an I.V. pole, fill the I.V. tubing with solution, and adjust the drip regulator valve to ensure adequate flow.

KEY STEPS

- Confirm the patient's identity using two patient identifiers according to facility policy.
- Explain the procedure to the patient (ease anxiety of a patient with a chemical burn by explaining that irrigation prevents further damage).
- Wear personal protective equipment throughout the procedure.
- Maintain asepsis throughout all procedures.
- **⚠ WARNING** *Identify type of irritant (if known) before irrigation; some irritants, such as alkali chemicals, are highly damaging to the eye and the patient should be referred for emergency or specialist care.*
- Put the patient in a supine position and turn his head slightly toward the affected side to prevent solution flowing over his nose and into the other eye.
- Place a towel under his head, and let him hold another towel against his affected side to catch excess solution.
- Separate his eyelids with your thumb and index finger.
- Instill ophthalmic anesthetic eyedrops, if ordered, as a comfort measure.
- **⚠ WARNING** *Use anesthetic drops only once; repeated use retards healing.*
- To irrigate the conjunctival cul-desac, continue separating the eyelids with your thumb and index finger.

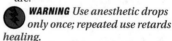

Three devices for eye irrigation

Depending on the type and extent of injury, the patient's eye may need to be irrigated using different devices.

SQUEEZE BOTTLE

For moderate-volume irrigation (to remove eye secretions, for example) apply sterile ophthalmic irrigant to the eye directly from the squeeze bottle container. Direct the stream at the inner canthus (as shown), and position the patient so that the stream washes across the cornea and exits at the outer canthus.

I.V. TUBE

For copious irrigation (to treat chemical burns, for example) set up an I.V. bag and tubing without a needle. Use the procedure described for moderate irrigation to flush the eye for at least 15 minutes (as shown).

MORGAN LENS

Connected to irrigation tubing, a Morgan lens permits continuous lavage and also delivers medication to the eye. Use an adapter to connect the lens to the I.V. tubing and the solution container. Begin irrigation at the prescribed flow rate. To insert the device, ask the patient to look down as you insert the lens under the upper eyelid (as shown). Then have him look up as you retract and release the lower eyelid over the lens.

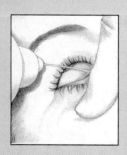

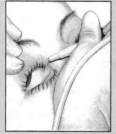

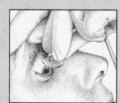

◆ To irrigate the upper eyelid (the superior fornix) use an eyelid retractor to keep eye open during irrigation; steady the hand holding the retractor by resting it on the patient's forehead.

USING MODERATE IRRIGATION
◆ Holding the bottle of sterile ophthalmic irrigant about 1" (2.5 cm) from the eye, direct a constant, stream at the inner canthus so the solution flows across the cornea to the outer canthus.

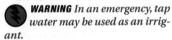 **WARNING** *In an emergency, tap water may be used as an irrigant.*

◆ Evert the lower eyelid, then the upper eyelid to inspect for retained foreign particles.
◆ Remove foreign particles by gently touching the conjunctiva with wet, sterile gauze pads, avoiding the cornea.
◆ Resume irrigating the eye until it's free from all visible foreign particles.

USING COPIOUS IRRIGATION
◆ Hold the control valve on the I.V. tubing about 1" above the eye, and direct a constant, gentle stream of normal saline solution at the inner canthus so that the solution flows across the cornea to the outer canthus.
◆ Ask the patient to rotate his eye periodically to help dislodge foreign particles while you continue the irrigation.
◆ Evert the lower eyelid and then the upper eyelid to inspect for retained foreign particles, especially when the patient has caustic lime in his eye.

AFTERCARE
◆ After irrigation, dry the eyelids with a sterile gauze pad, wiping from the inner to the outer canthus; use a new sterile gauze pad for each wipe.
◆ Remove and discard your gloves and goggles.
◆ When indicated, arrange for follow-up care.
◆ Wash your hands to avoid residual chemical contaminants.

SPECIAL CONSIDERATIONS

◆ When irrigating both eyes, have the patient tilt his head toward the side being irrigated to avoid cross-contamination.
◆ For chemical burns, irrigate each eye at least 15 minutes with normal saline solution to dilute and wash the harsh chemical.
◆ If the patient can't identify the specific chemical, use litmus paper to check if it's acidic or alkaline and to make sure the eye has been irrigated adequately.
◆ After irrigating any chemical, note the time, date, and chemical for your own reference in case you develop contact dermatitis.
◆ If an ophthalmic anesthetic agent was used, instruct the patient to not touch the eye before anesthetic has worn off; he might damage the cornea or conjunctiva.

COMPLICATIONS
◆ Trauma
◆ Infection

PATIENT TEACHING

◆ Tell the patient the purpose of the procedure and how it's performed.
◆ Explain to the patient that discomfort should be minimal and relief should be identified after the procedure or within a few hours.
◆ Advise the patient to keep the eye patch in place for 24 hours and avoid rubbing his eyes.
◆ Explain signs and symptoms (such as continued irritation, pain or discomfort, change in vision, or eye drainage) to report.
◆ Advise good hand-washing practices.
◆ Explain to the patient comfort measures such as applying cool, clean compresses.

DOCUMENTATION

◆ Record the date, time, duration of irrigation, and type and amount of solution.
◆ Note drainage characteristics.
◆ Document whether ophthalmic anesthetic was used and the amount.
◆ Note type of irritant seen, removed, or irrigated.
◆ Record litmus test findings.
◆ Document assessment of the patient's eye before and after irrigation.
◆ Note the patient's response to the procedure.
◆ Record patient teaching, such as what to expect during irrigation and care of the affected eye at home.

SELECTED REFERENCES
Hoyt, K.S., and Haley, R.J. "Innovations in Advanced Practice: Assessment and Management of Eye Emergencies," *Topics in Emergency Medicine* 27(2): 101-17, April-June 2005.
Kirkwood, B.J., et al. "Implementation and Evaluation of an Ophthalmic Nurse Practitioner Emergency Eye Clinic," *Clinical & Experimental Ophthalmology* 33(6):593-97, December 2005.
Sandiford, R. "How I Coped...With An Eyesplash," *Nursing Times* 101(31):24-25, August 2005.
Wilson, M.E. Jr., and Trivedi, R.H. "Low Molecular-Weight Heparin in the Intraocular Irrigating Solution in Pediatric Cataract and Intraocular Lens Surgery," *American Journal of Ophthalmology* 141(3):537-38, March 2006.

Fall prevention and management

DESCRIPTION

- Falls can occur because of poor lighting, slippery floors, throw rugs, unfamiliar surroundings, or physiologic factors, such as temporary muscle paralysis, vertigo, orthostatic hypotension, central nervous system lesions, dementia, failing eyesight, and decreased strength or coordination.
- With the elderly patient, fall injuries can cause psychological problems, loss of self-confidence, and hasten a move to a long-term care facility.

CONTRAINDICATIONS

- None known

EQUIPMENT

Stethoscope ◆ sphygmomanometer ◆ analgesics ◆ cold and warm compresses ◆ pillows ◆ blankets ◆ emergency resuscitation equipment (crash cart), if needed ◆ electrocardiograph (ECG) monitor, if needed

PREPARATION

- If helping a fallen patient, send someone for assessment or resuscitation equipment needed.

KEY STEPS

- Use patience and caution whether your care plan focuses on preventing falls or managing one in an elderly patient.

PREVENTING FALLS

- Assess the patient's fall risk at least once each shift (at least every 3 months if patient is in a long-term care facility). Your facility may require more frequent assessments. Note any changes in his condition that increase the risk of falling.
- If he's at risk, take steps to reduce danger.

- Correct potential dangers in his room.
- Position the call light so he can reach it.
- Provide adequate nighttime lighting.
- Place his personal belongings and care aids within easy reach.
- Instruct him to rise slowly from a supine position.
- Keep the bed in its lowest position so he can reach the floor when he gets out of bed.
- Lock the bed's wheels and place the bed against the wall, if possible.
- Frequently check side rails if they're to be raised.
- Advise him to wear nonskid footwear.
- Check him at least every 2 hours.
- Check a high-risk patient every 30 minutes.
- Alert other caregivers to his risk of falling and to interventions you've implemented.
- Encourage him to perform active range-of-motion exercises to improve flexibility and coordination.

MANAGING FALLS

- If you're with the patient as he falls, try to break his fall with your body.
- As you guide him to the floor, support his body — particularly his head and trunk.
- If possible, help him to a supine position.
- Try to maintain proper body alignment yourself to keep the center of gravity within your support base. Spread your feet to widen your support base.
- The wider the base, the better your balance will be. Bend your knees — not your back — to support the patient and avoid injuring yourself.
- Remain calm and stay with him to prevent further injury.
- Assess his airway, breathing, and circulation to see if the fall was caused by respiratory or cardiac arrest.

⚡ **WARNING** *If you don't detect respirations or a pulse, call a code and begin emergency resuscitation measures.*

- Note his level of consciousness (LOC); assess pupil size, equality, and reaction to light.
- Check for injuries, such as lacerations, abrasions, and obvious deformities.
- Note any deviations from the patient's baseline condition.
- If you weren't present during the fall, ask the patient or a witness what happened. Ask if he experienced pain or a change in LOC.
- Don't move him until you fully evaluate his status.
- Provide reassurance as needed, and observe for such signs and symptoms as confusion, tremor, weakness, pain, and dizziness.
- Assess his limb strength and motion.
- Alert the practitioner.

⚡ **WARNING** *If you suspect a disorder, don't move the patient until a practitioner examines him. Spinal cord injuries from falls are rare, but if one occurred, any movement may cause irreversible spinal damage.*

- While he lies on the floor awaiting the practitioner, offer pillows and blankets for comfort.

⚡ **WARNING** *If you suspect a spinal cord injury, don't place a pillow under his head.*

- If you don't detect problems, return the patient to his bed with the help of another staff member.

⚡ **WARNING** *Never try to lift a patient alone; you may injure yourself or the patient.*

- Take steps to control bleeding.
- Obtain an X-ray if you suspect a fracture.
- Provide first aid for minor injuries.
- Monitor his status for the next 24 hours.
- Even if he shows no signs of distress or has only minor injuries, monitor his vital signs every 15 minutes for one hour, every 30 minutes the next hour, then every hour for 2 hours or until his condition stabilizes. Notify the practitioner if you note change from the baseline.
- Perform necessary pain relief measures. Give analgesics as ordered; apply cold compresses the first 24 hours and warm compresses thereafter.

- Reassess the patient's environment and risk of falling. Discuss why he fell and how he thinks it could have been prevented.
- Check if drugs may have contributed to the fall. (See *Drugs associated with falls.*)
- Assess gait disturbances or improper use of canes, crutches, or walker.

Drugs associated with falls

Some classes of drugs commonly prescribed for older patients have possible adverse effects that may increase a patient's risk of falling.

DRUG CLASS	ADVERSE EFFECTS
Alcohol	Intoxication Motor incoordination Agitation Sedation Confusion
Antidiabetics	Acute hypoglycemia
Antihypertensives	Hypotension
Antipsychotics	Orthostatic hypotension Muscle rigidity Sedation
Benzodiazepines and antihistamines	Excessive sedation Confusion Paradoxical agitation Loss of balance
Diuretics	Hypovolemia Orthostatic hypotension Electrolyte imbalance Urinary incontinence
Hypnotics	Excessive sedation Ataxia Poor balance Confusion Paradoxical agitation
Opioids	Hypotension Sedation Motor incoordination Agitation
Tricyclic antidepressants	Orthostatic hypotension

SPECIAL CONSIDERATIONS

- After a fall, review the patient's medical history for other complications; if he hit his head, check whether he takes anticoagulants and is at greater risk for intracranial bleeding. Monitor him accordingly.
- Check if your facility has a fall prevention program.
- For a high-risk patient, in place of restraints, consider using a pressure pad or other alarm that warns when the patient gets out of the bed or the wheelchair.
- Place an "at risk" sign on the patient's door; put a red dot next to his room number on the call light console. Add appropriate notation to the Kardex and chart.
- Provide emotional support during prevention and management of a fall.
- Let the elderly patient know you recognize his limitations and acknowledge his fears. Point out measures that you'll take to provide a safe environment.

COMPLICATIONS
- None known

PATIENT TEACHING

- Teach the patient how to fall safely.
- If the patient uses a walker or a wheelchair, demonstrate how to cope with and recover from a fall.
- Instruct the patient to look for a low, sturdy, supportive piece of furniture to help himself up with; review the proper procedure for lifting himself and standing up with the walker or getting into the wheelchair.
- Before discharge, teach the patient and his family how to prevent accidental falls at home. Seek input from the patient and his family regarding potential safety hazards at home.
- As needed, refer the patient to the local visiting nurse association so nursing services can continue after discharge and during convalescence.

DOCUMENTATION

- Complete a detailed incident report after a fall in case of legal action.
- Note where and when the fall occurred, how the patient was found, and in what position.
- Record his vital signs.
- Document the events preceding the fall, names of witnesses, patient's reaction to the fall, and a detailed description of his condition, based on the assessment findings.
- Note the interventions taken and the names of staff members who helped care for the patient after the fall.
- Record the practitioner's name and date and time he was notified; include a copy of the practitioner's report.
- Note if the patient was given diagnostic tests or transferred to another unit.
- Note if the patient was monitored for a severe complication.
- This report is mainly for insurance purposes, not part of the patient's record. Send copies to the facility administrator, who may evaluate care given in the unit and propose safety policies as appropriate.

SELECTED REFERENCES
Hsu, S.S., et al. "Fall Risk Factors Assessment Tool: Enhancing Effectiveness in Falls Screening," *Journal of Nursing Research* 12(3):169-79, September 2004.

Lyons, S.S. "Evidence-Based Protocol: Fall Prevention for Older Adults," *Journal of Gerontological Nursing* 31(11):9-14, November 2005.

O'Hagan, C., and O'Connell, B. "The Relationship between Patient Blood Pathology Values and Patient Falls in an Acute-Care Setting: A Retrospective Analysis," *International Journal of Nursing Practice* 11(4):161-68, August 2005.

Vu, M.Q., et al. "Falls in the Nursing Home: Are They Preventable?" *Journal of the American Medical Directors Association* 7(Suppl 3):S53-58, March-April 2006.

Fecal impaction removal, digital

OVERVIEW

DESCRIPTION

- Fecal impaction is a large, hard, dry mass of stool in the folds of the rectum or sigmoid colon resulting from prolonged retention and accumulation of stool.
- Common causes are poor bowel habits, inactivity, dehydration, improper diet (inadequate fluid intake), constipation-inducing drugs, and incomplete bowel cleaning after a barium enema or barium swallow.
- As ordered, this procedure is used when oil retention and cleansing enemas, suppositories, and laxatives fail to clear the impaction.

CONTRAINDICATIONS

- Pregnancy
- After rectal, genitourinary, abdominal, perineal, or gynecologic reconstructive surgery
- Patients with myocardial infarction
- Coronary insufficiency
- Pulmonary embolus
- Heart failure
- Heart block
- Stokes-Adams syndrome (without pacemaker treatment)
- GI or vaginal bleeding
- Hemorrhoids
- Rectal polyps
- Blood dyscrasias

EQUIPMENT

Gloves (two pairs) ◆ linen-saver pad ◆ bedpan ◆ plastic disposal bag ◆ soap ◆ water-filled basin ◆ towel ◆ water-soluble lubricant ◆ washcloth ◆ bath blanket

Side-lying position

Use a draw sheet or bath blanket to place the patient in a side-lying position.

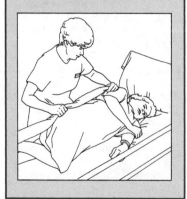

KEY STEPS

- Confirm the patient's identity using two patient identifiers according to facility policy.
- Explain the procedure to the patient and provide privacy.
- Position him on his left side and flex his knees to allow easier access to the sigmoid colon and rectum. (See *Side-lying position*.)
- Drape the patient with a bath blanket.
- Place a linen-saver pad beneath the buttocks to prevent soiling the bed linens.
- Put on gloves. Moisten an index finger with water-soluble lubricant to reduce friction during insertion and to avoid causing injury to sensitive tissue.
- Insert your lubricated index finger beyond the anal sphincter until you touch the impaction.
- Rotate the finger gently around the stool to dislodge and break it into small fragments.
- Work the fragments downward to the end of the rectum, and remove each one separately.
- Before removing your finger, gently stimulate the anal sphincter with a circular motion two or three times to increase peristalsis and encourage evacuation.
- Remove your finger and change your gloves.
- Clean the anal area with soap and water, and lightly pat dry with a towel.
- Offer the patient the bedpan or commode because digital manipulation stimulates the urge to defecate.
- Place disposable items in the plastic bag, and discard properly.
- If necessary, clean the bedpan and return it to the bedside stand.
- Wash your hands.

SPECIAL CONSIDERATIONS

⚡ **WARNING** *If the patient experiences pain, nausea, rectal bleeding, changes in pulse rate or skin color, diaphoresis, or syncope, stop the procedure immediately and notify the physician.*

COMPLICATIONS

◆ Vagus nerve stimulation—may decrease heart rate— causing syncope

PATIENT TEACHING

◆ To promote relaxation, instruct the patient to breathe deeply during the procedure.

DOCUMENTATION

◆ Record the time and date of the procedure.
◆ Note the patient's response.
◆ Document stool color, consistency, and odor.

SELECTED REFERENCES

Biggs, W.S., and Dery, W.H. "Evaluation and Treatment of Constipation in Infants and Children," *American Family Physician* 73(3):469-77, February 2006.

Kyle, G., et al. "A Procedure for the Digital Removal of Faeces," *Nursing Standard* 19(20):33-39, January-February 2005.

O'Donovan, E.J. and Bhuptani, S. "Manual Evacuation of the Rectum," *Annals of the Royal College of Surgeons of England* 87(3):213, May 2005.

Saddler, D. "A Literature Review of Fecal Impaction," *Gastroenterology Nursing* 28(1):49-50, January-February 2005.

Fecal occult blood tests

DESCRIPTION

- These tests determine the presence of occult blood (hidden GI bleeding) and distinguish between true melena and melena-like stools. Drugs such as iron supplements and bismuth compounds can darken stools so they resemble melena.
- Tests are easily performed on collected specimens or smears from digital rectal examination.
- Two common tests are:
- Hematest (an orthotolidine reagent tablet)
- Hemoccult slide (filter paper impregnated with guaiac)
- Both produce a blue reaction in a fecal smear if occult blood loss exceeds 5 ml in 24 hours.
- One positive test may not confirm GI bleeding or indicate colorectal cancer.
- The test should be repeated at least three times while the patient follows a special diet following manufacturer's recommendations for the particular test.
- A confirmed positive test indicates need for further diagnostic studies.
- GI bleeding can result from many causes including cancer, ulcers, colon polyps, and diverticula.

CONTRAINDICATIONS

- None known

EQUIPMENT

Test kit ◆ glass or porcelain plate ◆ tongue blade or other wooden applicator ◆ gloves

KEY STEPS

- Confirm the patient's identity using two patient identifiers according to facility policy.
- Put on gloves and collect a stool specimen.

HEMATEST REAGENT TABLET TEST

- Use a wooden applicator to smear a sample from a stool specimen on filter paper supplied with the test kit. Alternatively, after digital rectal examination, wipe the finger used on a square of the filter paper.
- Place the filter paper with the stool smear on a glass plate.
- Remove a reagent tablet from the bottle and immediately replace the cap tightly.
- Place the tablet in the center of the stool smear on the filter paper.
- Add one drop of water to the tablet, and allow it to soak for 5 to 10 seconds.
- Add a second drop, letting it run from the tablet onto the specimen and filter paper.
- If necessary, tap the plate gently to dislodge water from the top of the tablet.
- After 2 minutes, the filter paper will turn blue if the test is positive.
- Don't read the color that appears on the tablet itself or develops on the filter paper after the 2-minute period.
- Note the results, and discard the filter paper.
- Remove and discard your gloves, and wash your hands.

HEMOCCULT SLIDE TEST

- Open the flap on the slide packet; use a wooden applicator to apply a sample from the stool specimen to the guaiac-impregnated filter paper exposed in box A. Alternatively, after a digital rectal examination, wipe the finger used in the box A of the filter paper.
- Apply a second smear from another part of the specimen to the filter paper exposed in box B; some parts of the specimen may not contain blood.

- Allow the specimen to dry 3 to 5 minutes.
- Open the flap on the reverse side of the slide package; place two drops of Hemoccult developing solution on the paper over each smear.
- A blue reaction will appear in 30 to 60 seconds if the test is positive.
- Record the results and discard the slide package.
- Remove and discard your gloves, and wash your hands.

- Make sure stool specimens aren't contaminated with urine, soap solution, or toilet tissue; test them as soon as possible after collection.
- Menstrual or hemorrhoidal blood may contaminate the specimen. Ask the patient about menstrual status and presence of hemorrhoids.
- Test samples from different parts of the specimen; occult blood from the upper GI tract isn't always evenly dispersed throughout the stool. Blood from colorectal bleeding may occur mostly on the outer stool surface. If frank blood is observed, notify the physician immediately.
- Obtain the patient's medication history, noting drugs that may cause GI mucosal bleeding or alter results (such as nonsteroidal anti-inflammatory drugs and vitamin C).
- Check the condition of the reagent tablets and note their expiration date. Use only fresh tablets and discard outdated ones.
- Protect Hematest tablets from moisture, heat, and light.
- If repeat tests are needed after positive screening, explain this to the patient.
- Put him on a high-fiber diet; avoiding red meat, poultry, fish, turnips, and horseradish for 48 to 72 hours before and during the sample collection period.
- As ordered, have him discontinue use of iron preparations, bromides, iodides, rauwolfia derivatives, indomethacin, colchicine, salicylates, potassium, phenylbutazone, bismuth compounds, steroids, and ascorbic acid for 48 to 72 hours before and during the test to ensure accurate test results and to avoid possible bleeding.

COMPLICATIONS
- None known

- If the patient will be using the Hemoccult slide packet at home, advise him to complete the label on the slide packet before specimen collection.
- If the patient will be using a ColoCARE test packet, inform him that this test is a preliminary screen for occult blood in his stool. Tell him he won't have to obtain a stool specimen to perform the test but that he should follow your instructions carefully. (See *Home tests for fecal occult blood.*)

Home tests for fecal occult blood

Most fecal occult blood tests require the patient to collect a stool specimen and smear some of it on a slide. Newer tests such as as ColoCARE don't require the patient to handle stool, making the procedure safer and simpler.

If the patient will perform the ColoCARE test at home, tell him to avoid red meat and vitamin C supplements for 3 days before the test and check with his practitioner about discontinuing any drugs before the test. Drugs that may interfere with test results include aspirin, indomethacin, corticosteroids, phenylbutazone, reserpine, dietary supplements, anticancer drugs, and anticoagulants.

Tell him to flush the toilet twice just before the test to remove any toilet-cleaning chemicals from the tank. Tell him to defecate into the toilet but put no toilet paper into the bowl. Within 5 minutes, the test pad should be removed from its pouch and set to float printed side up on the water's surface. Tell him to watch the pad for 15 to 30 seconds for any evidence of blue or green color changes; have him record the result on the reply card.

Emphasize that he should perform this test with three consecutive bowel movements, then send the completed card to his physician. Have him call his practitioner immediately if he notes a positive color change in the first test.

- Record the date and time of the test.
- Note the result.
- Document unusual characteristics of the stool.
- Report positive results to the practitioner.

SELECTED REFERENCES

Bond, J.H. "The Place of Fecal Occult Blood Test in Colorectal Cancer Screening in 2006: The U.S. Perspective," *American Journal of Gastroenterology* 101(2):219-21, February 2006.

Greenwald, B. "A Comparison of Three Stool Tests for Colorectal Cancer Screening," *Medsurg Nursing* 14(5): 292-99, October 2005.

Pinheiro, J.M., et al. "A Critical Analysis of the Routine Testing of Newborn Stools for Occult Blood and Reducing Substances," *Advances in Neonatal Care* 3(3):133-38, June 2003.

Feeding tube insertion and removal

OVERVIEW

DESCRIPTION

- Nasal or oral insertion of a feeding tube into the stomach or duodenum allows the patient who can't or won't eat to receive nourishment.
- It permits supplemental feedings in the patient with high nutritional requirements.
- The procedure is commonly performed by a nurse.
- The preferred route is nasal; the oral route may be used for the patient with a deviated septum or nose injury.
- Duodenal feeding may be ordered when the patient can't tolerate gastric feeding or when gastric feeding may produce aspiration.
- Feeding tubes have small diameters and great flexibility, helping reduce oropharyngeal irritation, necrosis from pressure on the tracheoesophageal wall, distal esophageal irritation, and discomfort from swallowing.
- To facilitate passage, some feeding tubes are weighted with tungsten, and some need a guide wire to keep them from curling in the back of the throat. These small-bore tubes usually have radiopaque markings and a water-activated coating, which provides a lubricated surface.

CONTRAINDICATIONS

- Absence of bowel sounds
- Possible intestinal obstruction

EQUIPMENT

INSERTION

Feeding tube (#6 to #18 French, with or without guide) ◆ linen-saver pad ◆ gloves ◆ hypoallergenic tape ◆ water-soluble lubricant ◆ cotton-tipped applicators ◆ skin preparation (such as compound benzoin tincture) ◆ facial tissues ◆ penlight ◆ small cup of water with straw, or ice chips ◆ emesis basin ◆ 60-ml syringe ◆ pH test strip ◆ water

DURING USE

Mouthwash or normal saline solution ◆ toothbrush

REMOVAL

Linen-saver pad ◆ tube clamp ◆ bulb syringe

PREPARATION

- Have the proper size tube available; practitioner usually orders smallest-bore tube that will allow free passage of the liquid feeding formula.
- Read the package instructions; tube characteristics vary by manufacturer.
- Make sure the tube doesn't have any cracks, sharp edges, or other defects.
- Run water through the tube to check for patency, activate the coating, and facilitate removal of the guide.

KEY STEPS

- Confirm the patient's identity using two patient identifiers according to facility policy.
- Explain the procedure to the patient and show him the tube so he knows what to expect.
- Provide privacy, wash your hands, and put on gloves.
- Assist the patient into semi-Fowler's or high Fowler's position.
- Place a linen-saver pad across his chest to protect him from spills.
- To determine tube length needed to reach the stomach:
  - extend the tube's distal end from the tip of the patient's nose to his earlobe
  - coil this portion so the end stays curved until it's inserted
  - extend the uncoiled portion from the earlobe to the xiphoid process
  - use hypoallergenic tape to mark the total length of the two portions.

NASAL INSERTION

- Assess patient's history of nasal injury or surgery.
- Using the penlight, assess nasal patency. Inspect for a deviated septum, polyps, or other obstructions.
- Occlude one nostril, then the other, to determine which has better airflow.
- Lubricate the curved tip of the tube (and the feeding tube guide, as needed) with water-soluble lubricant to ease insertion and prevent injury.
- Have the patient hold the emesis basin and facial tissues in case he needs them.
- To advance the tube, insert the curved, lubricated tip into the nostril and direct it along the nasal passage toward the ear on the same side.
- When it passes the nasopharyngeal junction, turn the tube 180 degrees to aim it downward into the esophagus.
- Instruct the patient to lower his chin to his chest to close the trachea.
- Have him sip water with a straw to ease the tube's passage.
- Advance the tube as he swallows.

ORAL INSERTION

◆ Have the patient lower his chin to close his trachea.
◆ Have him open his mouth.
◆ Place the tip of the tube at the back of his tongue; give water, and instruct him to swallow.
◆ Remind him to not clamp his teeth down on the tube.
◆ Advance the tube as he swallows.

POSITIONING THE TUBE

◆ Keep passing the tube until the tape marker reaches his nostril or lips.
◆ To check tube placement, attach the syringe to the end of the tube and try to aspirate gastric secretions.
◆ If no gastric secretions return, the tube may be in the esophagus. Advance the tube or reinsert it before proceeding.
◆ Examine the aspirate and place a small amount on the pH test strip.
◆ Probability of gastric placement is increased if the aspirate has a typical gastric fluid appearance (grassy green, clear and colorless with mucous shreds, or brown) and the pH is 5.0 or less.
◆ After confirming proper tube placement, remove the marker tape.
◆ Tape the tube to the patient's nose and remove the guide wire.
◆ X-rays may be ordered to verify tube placement.
◆ To advance the tube to the duodenum, especially a tungsten-weighted tube, position the patient on his right side to let gravity assist tube passage through the pylorus. Move the tube forward 2″ to 3″ (5 to 7.5 cm) hourly.

⚡ **WARNING** *Confirm placement with an X-ray before feeding begins; duodenal feeding can cause nausea and vomiting if accidentally delivered to the stomach.*

◆ Apply a skin preparation to the patient's cheek before securing the tube with tape to help the tube adhere to the skin and prevent irritation.
◆ Tape the tube securely to avoid excessive pressure on the nostrils.

REMOVING THE TUBE

◆ Protect the patient's chest with a linen-saver pad.

◆ Flush the tube with air; then clamp or pinch it to prevent fluid aspiration and withdraw gently but quickly.
◆ Cover and discard the used tube.

SPECIAL CONSIDERATIONS

◆ Flush the feeding tube every 8 hours with up to 60 ml of normal saline solution or water to maintain patency.
◆ Retape the tube daily and as needed. Alternate taping areas to avoid constant pressure on the same area. Inspect the skin for redness and breakdown.
◆ Provide nasal hygiene daily using cotton-tipped applicators and water-soluble lubricant to remove crusted secretions.
◆ Help the patient brush his teeth, gums, and tongue with mouthwash or normal saline solution at least twice daily.
◆ If he can't swallow the feeding tube, use a guide to aid insertion.

⚡ **WARNING** *Precise feeding tube placement is important because small-bore feeding tubes may slide into the trachea without causing immediate signs or symptoms of respiratory distress; the patient will usually cough if the tube enters the larynx. To be sure the tube clears the larynx, ask the patient to speak. If he can't, the tube is in the larynx. Withdraw the tube at once and reinsert.*

◆ When aspirating gastric contents to check tube placement, pull gently on the syringe plunger to prevent trauma to the stomach lining or bowel.
◆ If you meet resistance during aspiration, stop the procedure; resistance may result from the tube lying against the stomach wall. If the tube coils above the stomach you won't be able to aspirate stomach contents; change patient's position or withdraw the tube a few inches, readvance it, and try to aspirate again.
◆ If the tube was inserted with a guide wire, don't use the guide wire to reposition the tube. The physician may reposition, using fluoroscopic guidance.

COMPLICATIONS

◆ Skin erosion at the nostril due to prolonged intubation
◆ Sinusitis
◆ Esophagitis
◆ Esophagotracheal fistula
◆ Gastric ulceration
◆ Pulmonary and oral infection

PATIENT TEACHING

◆ If the patient will use a feeding tube at home, make appropriate home care nursing referrals and teach him how to use and care for a feeding tube.
◆ Tell the patient how to get equipment, insert and remove the tube, and prepare and store feeding formula.
◆ Make sure the patient knows how to solve tube position and patency problems.

DOCUMENTATION

◆ Record the date, time, and tube type and size.
◆ Note the insertion site.
◆ Document the area of placement.
◆ Record confirmation of proper placement.
◆ Record the name of the person performing the procedure.
◆ For tube removal, record the date, time, and patient's tolerance of procedure.

SELECTED REFERENCES

Best, C. "Caring for the Patient with a Nasogastric Tube," *Nursing Standard* 20(3):59-65, September-October 2005.

Ellett, M.L., et al. "Predicting the Insertion Distance for Placing Gastric Tubes," *Clinical Nursing Research* 14(1):11-27, February 2005.

McKay, L. "Nasogastric Intubation," *Nursing Standard* 20(24):63, February 2006.

Rushing, J. "Inserting a Nasogastric Tube," *Nursing* 35(5):22, May 2005.

Sweeney, J. "How Do I Verify NG Tube Placement?" *Nursing* 35(8):25, August 2005.

Femoral compression

DESCRIPTION

- Femoral compression is used to maintain hemostasis at the arterial access site after such procedures as cardiac catheterization or angiography.
- A femoral compression device is used by a physician or specially trained nurse to apply direct pressure to the arterial access site.
- A nylon strap is placed under the patient's buttocks and attached to the device with an inflatable plastic dome.
- When the dome is positioned correctly over the puncture site, it's inflated to an individualized pressure (initially set approximately 20 mm Hg higher than the patient's systole pressure).

CONTRAINDICATIONS

- None known

EQUIPMENT

Femoral compression device strap ◆ compression arch with dome and three-way stopcock ◆ pressure inflation device ◆ sterile transparent dressing ◆ gloves (nonsterile and sterile) ◆ protective eyewear

KEY STEPS

- Confirm the patient's identity using two patient identifiers according to facility policy.

AFTER ARTERIAL ACCESS

- Obtain a practitioner's order for femoral compression device, including amount of pressure to be applied and length of time it should remain in place.
- Reinforce previous teaching about the device and possible complications of the procedure.
- Answer any questions the patient may have.
- Put the patient on a stretcher or bed; don't flex the involved extremity.
- Assess condition of the puncture site, obtain vital signs, perform neurovascular checks, and assess pain, according to facility policy.

APPLYING THE FEMORAL COMPRESSION DEVICE

- Put on nonsterile gloves and protective eyewear; place the device strap under the patient's hips before sheath removal (if a sheath is necessary).
- After achieving hemostasis, put on sterile gloves and apply a sterile transparent dressing over the puncture site, using sterile technique.
- With the assistance of another nurse, position the compression arch over the puncture site.
- Apply manual pressure over the dome area while the straps are secured to the arch.
- When the dome is properly positioned over the puncture site, connect the pressure inflation device to the stopcock.
- Turn the stopcock to the open position and inflate the dome with the pressure inflation device to the ordered pressure.
- Turn the stopcock off and remove the pressure-inflation device.
- Assess the puncture site for proper placement of the device and for signs of bleeding or hematoma.

- Assess distal pulses and neurovascular condition according to facility policy.
- Confirm distal pulses after adjustments of the device.

MAINTAINING THE DEVICE

- When the patient is transferred to the nursing unit, assess the distal pulses, the puncture site, and placement of the device; confirm the ordered amount of pressure. Make routine assessments according to facility policy.
- Deflate the device hourly and assess the puncture site for bleeding or hematoma. Assess for proper placement of the dome over the puncture site. Reposition the compression arch and dome as necessary; wear gloves and protective eyewear.
- Reinflate the device to the ordered pressure.

REMOVING THE DEVICE

- Explain the removal procedure to the patient.
- Put on nonsterile gloves and protective eyewear, remove the air from the dome, loosen the straps, and remove the device.
- Assess the puncture site for bleeding or hematoma.
- Change the sterile transparent dressing according to facility policy.
- Check the puncture site and distal pulses, and perform neurovascular assessments every 15 minutes the first half hour and every 30 minutes the next 2 hours. Your facility may require more frequent monitoring.
- Watch for signs of bleeding, hematoma, or infection.
- Dispose of the device and equipment according to facility policy.

SPECIAL CONSIDERATIONS

⚡ **WARNING** *If you note external bleeding or signs of internal bleeding, remove the device, apply manual pressure, and notify the physician.*

◆ Change the dressing at the puncture site every 24 to 48 hours, or according to facility policy.
◆ The sterile transparent dressing permits inspection of the site for bleeding, drainage, or hematoma.

COMPLICATIONS

⚡ **WARNING** *The Food and Drug Administration has issued warnings about adverse events that may occur with the use of femoral compression devices after arterial access for diagnostic and therapeutic procedures.*

◆ Bleeding
◆ Hematoma
◆ Retroperitoneal bleeding
◆ Pseudoaneurysm
◆ Infection
◆ Deep vein thrombosis
◆ Tissue damage from prolonged pressure

PATIENT TEACHING

◆ Advise the patient to use caution when moving in bed to avoid repositioning the device.
◆ Instruct the patient not to bend the involved extremity.

DOCUMENTATION

◆ Document the initial application of the device.
◆ Verify sheath removal.
◆ Note the patient's tolerance of the procedure.
◆ Document vital signs.
◆ Document the puncture site checks.
◆ Note distal pulses.
◆ Note neurovascular assessments.
◆ Note hourly deflation.
◆ Document repositioning of the device.
◆ Document the length of time the device was in place.
◆ Document when the device was removed.
◆ Document the patient and family teaching.
◆ Note complications.
◆ Note interventions.

SELECTED REFERENCES

Andersen, K., et al. "Haematoma after Coronary Angiography and Percutaneous Coronary Intervention via the Femoral Artery Frequency and Risk Factors," *European Journal of Cardiovascular Nursing* 4(2):123-27, June 2005.

Benson, L.M., et al. "Determining Best Practice: Comparison of Three Methods of Femoral Sheath Removal after Cardiac Interventional Procedures," *Heart & Lung* 34(2):115-21, March-April 2005.

Chlan, L.L., et al. "Effects of Three Groin Compression Methods on Patient Discomfort, Distress, and Vascular Complications Following a Percutaneous Coronary Intervention Procedure," *Nursing Research* 54(6):391-98, November-December 2005.

Jones, T., and McCutcheon, H. "A Randomised Controlled Trial Comparing the Use of Manual Versus Mechanical Compression to Obtain Haemostasis Following Coronary Angiography," *Intensive & Critical Care Nursing* 19(1): 11-20, February 2003.

Foot care

DESCRIPTION

◆ Daily foot baths and regular toenail trimming promotes cleanliness, prevents infection, stimulates peripheral circulation, and controls odor.

◆ Foot care is important for bedridden patients and those susceptible to foot infection.

◆ Peripheral vascular disease, diabetes mellitus (see *Foot care for the patient with diabetes*), poor nutritional status, arthritis, and conditions that impair peripheral circulation increase susceptibility to infection; proper foot care should include meticulous cleanliness and observation for signs of skin breakdown.

CONTRAINDICATIONS

◆ Toenail trimming in patients with the following (unless performed by a physician or podiatrist):
– Toe infections
– Diabetes mellitus
– Neurologic disorders
– Renal failure
– Peripheral vascular disease

⚡ **WARNING** *Some facilities prohibit nurses from trimming toenails. Check facility policy before performing the procedure.*

Bath blanket ◆ large basin ◆ soap ◆ water ◆ towel ◆ linen-saver pad ◆ pillow ◆ washcloth ◆ toenail clippers ◆ orangewood stick ◆ emery board ◆ 2″ × 2″ gauze pads ◆ cotton-tipped applicator ◆ cotton ◆ lotion ◆ water-absorbent powder ◆ bath thermometer ◆ gloves, if patient has open lesions ◆ heel protectors or protective boots (optional)

PREPARATION

◆ Fill the basin halfway with warm water.

⚡ **WARNING** *Test water temperature with a bath thermometer because patients with diminished peripheral sensation can burn their feet in excessively hot water (over 105° F [40.6° C]) without feeling pain.*

◆ If a bath thermometer isn't available, test the water by inserting your elbow. The water temperature should feel comfortably warm.

◆ Assemble equipment at the patient's bedside.

◆ Wash your hands and put on gloves if necessary.

◆ Tell him that you'll wash his feet and provide foot and toenail care.

◆ Cover him with a bath blanket. Fanfold the top linen to the foot of the bed.

◆ Place a linen-saver pad and towel under his feet to keep the bottom linen dry.

◆ Position the basin on the pad.

◆ Insert a pillow under his knee to provide support, and cushion the rim of the basin with the edge of the towel to prevent pressure on his leg.

◆ Immerse one foot in the basin.

◆ Wash it with soap, and then allow it to soak about 10 minutes. Soaking softens the skin and toenails, loosens debris under toenails, and comforts and refreshes the patient.

◆ After soaking the foot, rinse it with a washcloth, remove it from the basin, and place it on the towel.

◆ Dry the foot thoroughly, especially between the toes, to avoid skin breakdown.

◆ Blot gently to dry; harsh rubbing may damage the skin.

◆ Empty the basin, refill it with warm water, and clean and soak the other foot.

◆ While the second foot is soaking, give the first one a pedicure.

◆ Using the cotton-tipped applicator, carefully clean the toenails.

◆ Using an orangewood stick, gently remove dirt beneath the toenails; avoid injuring subungual skin.

◆ Consult a podiatrist if nails need trimming and if facility policy prevents you from trimming them.

◆ Rinse the foot that has been soaking, dry it thoroughly, and give it a pedicure.

◆ Apply lotion to moisten dry skin, or lightly dust water-absorbent powder between the toes to absorb moisture.

◆ Remove and clean all equipment and dispose of gloves.

◆ When providing foot care, observe the color, shape, and texture of the toenails.

WARNING *If you see redness, drying, cracking, blisters, discoloration, or other signs of traumatic injury, especially in patients with impaired peripheral circulation, notify the physician. Such patients are vulnerable to infection and gangrene and need prompt treatment.*

◆ If a patient's toenail grows inward at the corners, tuck cotton under it to relieve pressure on the toe.

◆ Unless contraindicated, when giving the bedridden patient foot care, perform range-of-motion exercises to stimulate circulation and prevent foot contractures or muscle atrophy.

◆ Tuck folded 2″ × 2″ gauze pads between overlapping toes to protect the skin from the toenails.

◆ Apply heel protectors or protective boots to prevent skin breakdown.

COMPLICATIONS
◆ None known

◆ Before discharge, teach the patient proper foot care techniques, particularly to patients with diabetes and patients with impaired peripheral circulation.

Foot care for the patient with diabetes

Because diabetes mellitus can reduce blood supply to the feet, minor foot injuries can lead to dangerous infection. Use these foot care guidelines for the patient with diabetes:

◆ Exercise the feet daily to improve circulation. While the patient sits on the edge of the bed, have him point his toes up and down 10 times, then make a circle with each foot 10 times.

◆ Make sure shoes fit properly. Instruct the patient to break in new shoes by wearing them 30 minutes longer each day. Tell him to check older shoes frequently for rough spots in the lining.

◆ Tell him to wear clean socks daily and avoid socks with holes, darned spots, or rough, irritating seams.

◆ Advise him to see a practitioner if he has corns or calluses.

◆ Tell him to wear warm socks or slippers and use extra blankets to avoid cold feet. He shouldn't use heating pads and hot water bottles; they may cause burns.

◆ Tell him to regularly check his feet for cuts, cracks, blisters, or red, swollen areas, and consult a practitioner about even slight cuts on his feet. If there's a cut, tell him to wash the wound thoroughly and apply a mild antiseptic. Urge him to avoid harsh antiseptics, such as iodine; they can damage tissue.

◆ Advise him to avoid tight-fitting garments or activities that decrease circulation. He should especially avoid elastic garters, crossing the knees, picking at sores or rough spots on his feet, walking barefoot, or applying adhesive tape.

◆ Record the date and time of bathing and toenail trimming.

◆ Record and report abnormal findings and nursing actions taken.

SELECTED REFERENCES
Martinez, N.C., and Tripp-Reimer, T. "Diabetes Nurse Educators' Prioritized Elder Foot Care Behaviors," *Diabetes Educator* 31(6):858-68, November-December 2005.

Seidel, K.W. "Ingrown Toenail. End the Cryptosis Cycle," *Advance for Nurse Practitioners* 13(8):45-6, 48, 50, August 2005.

Sieggreen, M.Y. "Stepping up Care for Diabetic Foot Ulcers," *Nursing* 35(10):36-41, October 2005.

Woodrow, P., et al. "Foot Care for Non-Diabetic Older People," *Nursing Older People* 17(8):31-32, November 2005.

Functional assessment

DESCRIPTION

- Functional assessment is used to evaluate the older adult's overall well-being and self-care abilities.
- It helps you identify individual needs and care deficits, develop a care plan to enhance abilities of the older adult with disease and chronic illness, and provide feedback about treatment and rehabilitation.
- You can use the information to help the older patient maintain independence by matching his needs with housekeeping, home health care, and daycare services.

CONTRAINDICATIONS

- None known

EQUIPMENT

Your facility's functional assessment tool

KEY STEPS

- Review the patient's health history to obtain subjective data about problem areas and subtle physical changes.
- Obtain the patient's name, age, birth date, and other vital information, if not already provided.
- Administer the functional assessment tool.
- If the patient is unable to answer, have his caregiver provide answers.

USING THE KATZ INDEX

- The Katz Index of Activities of Daily Living is widely used for evaluating a person's ability to perform six daily personal care activities: bathing, dressing, toileting, transfer, continence, and feeding.
- It describes his functional level at a specific point in time and scores his performance on a 3-point scale.

USING THE LAWTON SCALE

- The Lawton Scale for Instrumental Activities of Daily Living is used to evaluate more complex personal care activities, such as the ability to use the telephone, cook, shop, do laundry, manage finances, take drugs, and prepare meals.
- Activities are rated on a 3-point scale, ranging from independence to needing some help to complete disability. (See *Lawton Scale for Instrumental Activities of Daily Living*.)

USING THE BARTHEL INDEX AND SCALE

- The Barthel Index evaluates 10 self-care functions: feeding, moving from wheelchair to bed and returning, getting on and off the toilet, bathing, walking on a level surface or propelling a wheelchair, going up and down stairs, dressing and undressing, maintaining bowel continence, and controlling the bladder.
- Each item is scored according to degree of help needed; over time, results reveal improvement or decline.

- The Barthel Self-Care Rating Scale is a more detailed evaluation of function.
- Both tools provide information to help you determine assistance needed.

USING THE MINIMUM DATA SET

- To improve quality of care in extended care facilities, the federal government developed a standardized assessment tool called the Minimum Data Set to make patient assessments more consistent and reliable nationally.
- This method is required in all extended care facilities that receive federal funding.

USING OASIS-B1

- The Outcome and Assessment Information Set (OASIS), now known as OASIS-B1, is a comprehensive assessment of home care that patients receive; it's required by the government for Medicare-certified agencies.
- Using this instrument, you'll collect data to measure changes in health status over time. Typically, you'll collect OASIS data when a patient starts home care, at the 60-day recertification point, and when the patient is discharged or transferred to another facility, such as a hospital or subacute care facility.

- In a long-term care facility the physical assessment and care plan should be completed by a licensed nurse within 24 hours of a patient's admission.

- Functional assessment should be done after a 7- to 14-day assessment period.
- A comprehensive care plan should be developed within 21 days.
- When using the Lawton scale, evaluate the patient in terms of safety. For example, a person may be able to cook a meal, but forget to turn off the burner.

- The Barthel Index and Self-Care Rating Scale are used more often in rehabilitation and long-term care settings as tools to document improvement in a patient's abilities.

COMPLICATIONS
- None known

PATIENT TEACHING

- Explain the test to the patient; tell him whether it will take place in the hospital room or treatment room.

DOCUMENTATION

- Document all assessment findings according to facility policy.

SELECTED REFERENCES

Clifford, P.A., et al. "Assessing Resistance to Activities of Daily Living in Long-Term Care," *Journal of the American Medical Directors Association* 4(6):313-19, November-December 2003.

Houlden, H., et al. "Use of the Barthel Index and the Functional Independence Measure During Early Inpatient Rehabilitation After Single Incident Brain Injury," *Clinical Rehabilitation* 20(2):153-59, February 2006.

Josman, N., and Katz, N. "Relationships of Categorization on Tests and Daily Tasks in Patients with Schizophrenia, Post-Stroke Patients and Healthy Controls," *Psychiatry Research* 141(1):15-28, January 2006.

King, J.T. Jr., et al. "The Physical Performance Test and the Evaluation of Functional Status in Patients with Cerebral Aneurysms," *Journal of Neurosurgery* 104(4):525-30, April 2006.

Lawton Scale for Instrumental Activities of Daily Living

The Lawton scale evaluates more sophisticated functions than the Katz Index of Activities of Daily Living. Patients or caregivers can complete the form in a few minutes. The first answer (3) in each case (except for 8a) indicates independence; the second (2) indicates capability with assistance; and the third (1), dependence. In this version the maximum score is 29, although scores have meaning only for a particular patient, as when declining scores over time reveal deterioration.

Questions 4 to 7 tend to be gender specific; modify them as necessary.

Name _Mary Stevens_ Rated by _Joan Masterson, RN_ Date _August 4, 2001_

1. Can you use the telephone?
without help	③
with some help	2
completely unable	1

2. Can you get to places beyond walking distance?
without help	③
with some help	2
not without special arrangements	1

3. Can you go shopping for groceries?
without help	③
with some help	2
completely unable	1

4. Can you prepare your own meals?
without help	③
with some help	2
completely unable	1

5. Can you do your own housework?
without help	3
with some help	②
completely unable	1

6. Can you do your own handyman work?
without help	3
with some help	②
completely unable	1

7. Can you do your own laundry?
without help	③
with some help	2
completely unable	1

8a. Do you take medicines or use any medications?
Yes (If yes, answer Question 8b.)	
No (If no, answer Question 8c.)	

8b. Do you take your own medicine?
without help (in the right doses at the right times)	③
with some help (if someone prepares it for you and/or reminds you to take it)	2
completely unable	1

8c. If you had to take medicine, could you do it?
without help (in the right doses at the right time)	3
with some help (if someone prepared it for you and reminded you to take it)	2
completely unable	1

9. Can you manage your own money?
without help	③
with some help	2
completely unable	1

Adapted with permission from Lawton, M.P., and Brody, E.M. "Assessment of Older People: Self-Maintaining and Instrumental Activities of Daily Living," *The Gerontologist* 9(3):179-186, Autumn 1969. Copyright ©The Gerontological Society of America. Reproduced by permission of the publisher.

Gastric lavage

OVERVIEW

DESCRIPTION

- After poisoning or drug overdose, lavage flushes the stomach and removes ingested substances through a tube; it's useful in patients who have central nervous system depression or an inadequate gag reflex.
- Lavage can be continuous or intermittent; it's usually done in the emergency room or intensive care unit by a physician, gastroenterologist, or nurse.
- Lavage is used to empty the stomach before an endoscopic examination.

CONTRAINDICATIONS

- After ingestion of corrosive substances (such as lye, petroleum distillates, ammonia, alkalis, or mineral acids), the lavage tube may perforate the already compromised esophagus

EQUIPMENT

Lavage setup (two graduated containers for drainage, three pieces of large-lumen rubber tubing, Y-connector, and clamp or hemostat) ◆ 2 to 3 L of normal saline solution, tap water, or appropriate antidote, as ordered ◆ Ewald tube or any large-lumen gastric tube, typically #36 to #40 French ◆ I.V. pole ◆ water-soluble lubricant or anesthetic ointment ◆ stethoscope ◆ ½" hypoallergenic tape ◆ 50-ml bulb or catheter-tip syringe ◆ gloves ◆ face shield ◆ linen-saver pad or towel ◆ Yankauer or tonsil-tip suction device ◆ suction apparatus ◆ labeled specimen container ◆ laboratory request form ◆ norepinephrine ◆ basin of ice, if ordered ◆ patient restraints, charcoal tablets (optional)

PREPARATION

⚡ **WARNING** *A prepackaged, syringe-type irrigation kit may be used for intermittent lavage. For poisoning or drug overdose the continuous lavage setup is faster and more effective for diluting and removing the harmful substance.*

- Connect one of the three pieces of large-lumen tubing to the irrigant container. (See *Using wide-bore gastric tubes.*)
- Insert the Y-connector stem in the other end of the tubing.
- Connect the remaining two pieces of tubing to the free ends of the Y-connector.
- Place the unattached end of one of the tubes into one of the drainage containers. (Later, you'll connect the other piece of tubing to the patient's gastric tube.)
- Clamp the tube leading to the irrigant.
- Suspend the entire setup from the I.V. pole, hanging the irrigant container at the highest level.
- If iced lavage is ordered, chill the ordered irrigant in a basin of ice.
- Lubricate the end of the lavage tube with water-soluble lubricant or anesthetic ointment.

KEY STEPS

- Confirm the patient's identity using two patient identifiers according to facility policy.
- Provide privacy.
- Wash your hands and put on gloves and a face shield.
- Drape the towel or linen-saver pad over the patient's chest to protect from spills.
- The physician inserts the lavage tube nasally and advances it slowly; forceful insertion may injure tissues and cause epistaxis. Tube placement is checked by injecting about 30 cc of air with the bulb syringe, then auscultating the patient's abdomen with a stethoscope.

⚡ **WARNING** *The patient may vomit when the lavage tube reaches the posterior pharynx; be prepared to suction the airway immediately.*

Using wide-bore gastric tubes

To deliver a large volume of fluid rapidly through a gastric tube (for such conditions as profuse gastric bleeding or poisoning), a wide-bore gastric tube works best. Typically inserted orally, the tube remains in place long enough to complete the lavage and evacuate stomach contents.

EWALD TUBE

In an emergency, using the Ewald tube — a single-lumen tube with several openings at the distal end — allows you to aspirate large amounts of gastric contents quickly.

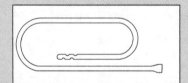

LEVACUATOR TUBE

The Levacuator tube has two lumens. Use the larger lumen for evacuating gastric contents; the smaller, for instilling an irrigant.

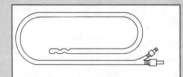

EDLICH TUBE

The Edlich tube is a single-lumen tube that has four openings near the closed distal tip. A funnel or syringe may be connected at the proximal end. Like the Ewald tube, the Edlich tube lets you withdraw large quantities of gastric contents quickly.

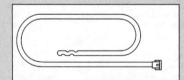

- After the tube passes the posterior pharynx, put the patient in Trendelenburg's position and turn him to his left in a three-quarter prone posture to minimize passage of gastric contents into the duodenum and prevent the patient from aspirating vomitus.
- After securing the tube with tape and making sure the irrigant inflow tube on the lavage setup is clamped, connect the unattached end of the irrigant inflow tube to the lavage tube.
- Allow stomach contents to empty into the drainage container before instilling irrigant. This confirms proper tube placement and decreases risk of overfilling the stomach with irrigant and inducing vomiting.
- If using a syringe irrigation set, aspirate stomach contents with a 50-ml bulb or catheter-tip syringe before instilling irrigant.
- After you confirm proper tube placement, begin gastric lavage by instilling about 250 ml of irrigant to assess patient's tolerance and prevent vomiting.
- If using a syringe, instill about 50 ml of solution at a time until you've instilled between 250 and 500 ml. Clamp the inflow tube and unclamp the outflow tube to allow irrigant to flow out.
- If using the syringe irrigation kit, aspirate the irrigant with the syringe and empty into a calibrated container. Measure outflow to make sure it at least equals the amount of irrigant instilled. This prevents stomach distention and vomiting.
- If drainage amount is significantly less than instilled amount, reposition the tube until sufficient solution flows out. Gently massage the abdomen over the stomach to promote outflow.
- Repeat the inflow-outflow cycle until returned fluids appear clear, signaling that the stomach no longer contains harmful substances or bleeding has stopped.
- Assess vital signs, urine output, and level of consciousness (LOC) every 15 minutes. Notify the physician of changes.
- If ordered, remove the lavage tube.

SPECIAL CONSIDERATIONS

- To control GI bleeding, the physician may order continuous stomach irrigation including a vasoconstrictor. The drug is delivered directly to the liver via the portal septum, thus preventing systemic circulation that can cause a hypertensive response.
- Alternatively, the outflow tube can be clamped for a prescribed period after instilling irrigant and vasoconstrictive drug and before withdrawing it. This allows the mucosa time to absorb the drug.
- Never leave a patient alone during gastric lavage. Watch for changes in LOC and monitor vital signs frequently; the vagal response to intubation can depress the patient's heart rate.
- If you need to restrain the patient, secure restraints on one side of the bed or stretcher so you can free them quickly.
- Keep tracheal suctioning equipment nearby; watch closely for airway obstruction caused by vomiting or excess oral secretions.
- Suction the oral cavity often to ensure an open airway and prevent aspiration.
- If the patient doesn't have an adequate gag reflex, he may need an endotracheal tube before the procedure.
- When aspirating the stomach for ingested poisons or drugs, save the contents in a labeled container for laboratory analysis.
- If ordered, after lavage to remove poisons or drugs, mix charcoal tablets with the irrigant and administer the mixture through the tube.
- When lavage is done to stop bleeding, keep precise intake and output records to determine amount of bleeding. When large volumes of fluid are instilled and withdrawn, serum electrolyte and arterial blood gas levels may be measured during or after lavage.

COMPLICATIONS

- Vomiting and aspiration
- Bradyarrhythmias
- After iced lavage, body temperature may drop, triggering cardiac arrhythmias

PATIENT TEACHING

- Explain the procedure to the patient.

DOCUMENTATION

- Record the date and time of lavage.
- Note the size and type of NG tube used.
- Document the volume and type of irrigant.
- Record the amount of drained gastric contents.
- Record information on intake and output record sheet.
- Note the color and consistency of drainage.
- Keep precise records of patient's vital signs and LOC.
- Document drugs instilled through the tube.
- Note the time the tube was removed.
- Record the patient's tolerance of the procedure.

SELECTED REFERENCES

Bartlett, D. "Acetaminophen Toxicity," *Journal of Emergency Nursing* 30(3): 281-83, June 2004.

Heard, K. "Gastrointestinal Decontamination," *Medical Clinics of North America* 89(6):1067-78, November 2005.

Madden, M.A. "Pediatric Poisonings: Recognition, Assessment, and Management," *Critical Care Nursing Clinics of North America* 17(4):395-404, xi, December 2005.

Gastrostomy feeding button care

OVERVIEW

DESCRIPTION

- A gastrostomy feeding button is used as an alternative feeding device for an ambulatory patient receiving long-term enteral feedings.
- It's approved for 6-month implantation and can replace gastrostomy tubes.
- The button is inserted into an established stoma (takes less than 15 minutes) and lies almost flush with skin; only the top of safety plug is visible.
- Advantages over ordinary feeding tubes include cosmetic appeal, ease of maintenance, reduced skin irritation and breakdown, and less chance of being dislodged or migrating.
- The button has a one-way antireflux valve inside a mushroom dome that prevents leakage of gastric contents; it's usually replaced after 3 to 4 months, typically because the antireflux valve wears out.

CONTRAINDICATIONS

- Intestinal obstruction that prohibits use of the bowel
- Diffuse peritonitis
- Intractable vomiting
- Paralytic ileus
- Severe diarrhea that makes metabolic management difficult

EQUIPMENT

Gastrostomy feeding button of correct size (all three sizes, if correct one isn't known) ◆ obturator ◆ water-soluble lubricant ◆ gloves ◆ feeding accessories, including adapter, feeding catheter, food syringe or bag, and formula ◆ catheter clamp ◆ cleaning equipment, including water, a syringe, cotton-tipped applicator, pipe cleaner, and mild soap or povidone-iodine solution ◆ I.V. pole, pump to provide continuous infusion over several hours (optional)

KEY STEPS

- Confirm the patient's identity using two patient identifiers according to facility policy.
- Explain the insertion, reinsertion, and feeding procedure to the patient. (See *How to reinsert a gastrostomy feeding button.*)
- Tell the patient the physician will perform initial insertion.
- Make sure signed consent has been obtained.
- Wash your hands and put on gloves.
- Attach the adapter and feeding catheter to the syringe or feeding bag.
- Clamp the catheter and fill the syringe or bag and catheter with formula.
- Open the safety plug and attach the adapter and feeding catheter to the button.

How to reinsert a gastrostomy feeding button

If a gastrostomy feeding button pops out, follow these procedures to reinsert the device.

PREPARE EQUIPMENT

- Collect the feeding button (shown below); wash it with soap and water; rinse thoroughly and dry. Also obtain an obturator and water-soluble lubricant.

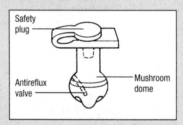

INSERT THE BUTTON

- Check the depth of the patient's stoma to make sure you have a feeding button of the correct size; clean around the stoma.
- Lubricate the obturator with water-soluble lubricant and distend the button several times to ensure the patency of the antireflux valve within the button.
- Lubricate the mushroom dome and stoma. Push the button through the stoma into the stomach (as shown).

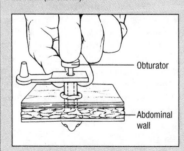

- Remove the obturator by rotating it as you withdraw it, to keep the antireflux valve from adhering to it. If the valve sticks, push the obturator back into the button until the valve closes.
- After removing the obturator, make sure the valve is closed.
- Close the flexible safety plug, which should be relatively flush with the skin surface (as shown).

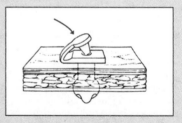

- If you need to give a feeding right away, open the safety plug and attach the feeding adapter and feeding tube (as shown). Deliver feeding as ordered.

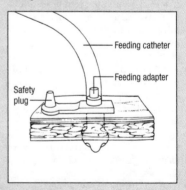

- Elevate the syringe or feeding bag above stomach level, and gravity-feed the formula for 15 to 30 minutes, varying height as needed to alter flow rate.
- Use a pump for continuous infusion or for feedings lasting several hours.
- Refill the syringe before it's empty to prevent air from entering the stomach and distending the abdomen.
- After feeding, flush the button with 10 ml of water.
- Lower the syringe or bag below stomach level to allow burping.
- Remove the adapter and feeding catheter; the antireflux valve should prevent gastric reflux.
- Snap the safety plug in place to keep the lumen clean and prevent leakage if the antireflux valve fails.
- If the patient feels nauseated or vomits after the feeding, vent the button with the adapter and feeding catheter to control emesis.
- Wash the catheter and syringe or feeding bag in warm, soapy water and rinse thoroughly.
- Clean the catheter and adapter with a pipe cleaner.
- Rinse well before using for the next feeding.
- Soak equipment weekly, or according to manufacturer's recommendations.

SPECIAL CONSIDERATIONS

- If the button pops out while feeding, reinsert it, estimate the formula already delivered, and resume feeding.
- Clean the peristomal skin with mild soap and water or povidone-iodine once daily, and let the skin air-dry for 20 minutes, to avoid skin irritation.
- Clean the peristomal site whenever spillage from the feeding bag occurs.

COMPLICATIONS
- Nausea and vomiting
- Abdominal distention
- Exit-site infection
- Exit-site leakage
- Peritonitis

PATIENT TEACHING

- Explain to the patient how the gastrostomy feeding button is inserted and cared for.
- Tell the patient how to use the button for feedings.
- Advise the patient how to clean the equipment.
- Explain to the patient peristomal skin care.
- Tell the patient when and whom to call for questions.

DOCUMENTATION

- Note the date, time, and duration of feeding.
- Record the amount and type of feeding formula used.
- Document the patient's tolerance of the procedure.
- Note intake and output.
- Record the appearance of the stoma and surrounding skin.
- Document skin care.

SELECTED REFERENCES

Chang, P.F., et al. "Percutaneous Endoscopic Gastrostomy to Set up a Long-Term Enteral Feeding Route in Children: An Encouraging Result," *Pediatric Surgery International* 19(4): 283-85, June 2003.

Gopalan, S., and Khanna, S. "Enteral Nutrition Delivery Technique," *Current Opinion in Clinical Nutrition and Metabolic Care* 6(3):313-17, May 2003.

Michaud, L., et al. "Longevity of Balloon-Sized Skin-Level Gastrostomy Device," *Journal of Pediatric Gastroenterology and Nutrition* 38(4):426-29, April 2004.

Halo-vest traction

DESCRIPTION

◆ A halo-vest immobilizes the head and neck after traumatic injury to the cervical vertebrae (most common spinal injury) to prevent further spinal cord injury.

◆ Application of the device is done by an orthopedic surgeon, with nursing assistance, in the emergency room, a specially equipped room, or operating room after surgical reduction of vertebral injuries.

◆ The device consists of a metal ring that fits over the patient's head and metal bars that connect the ring to a plastic vest that distributes the weight of the entire apparatus around the chest. (See *Comparing halo-vest traction devices.*)

◆ The halo-vest allows greater mobility than traction with skull tongs, and has less infection risk because it doesn't require skin incisions and drill holes to position skull pins.

CONTRAINDICATIONS

◆ None known

Halo-vest traction unit ◆ halo ring ◆ cervical collar or sandbags (if needed) ◆ plastic vest board or padded headrest ◆ tape measure ◆ halo ring conversion chart ◆ scissors and razor ◆ $4'' \times 4''$ gauze pads ◆ povidone-iodine solution ◆ sterile gloves ◆ Allen wrench ◆ four positioning pins ◆ multiple-dose vial of 1% lidocaine (with or without epinephrine) ◆ alcohol pads ◆ 3-ml syringe ◆ 25G needles ◆ five sterile skull pins (one more than needed) ◆ torque screwdriver ◆ sheepskin liners ◆ cotton-tipped applicators ◆ ordered cleaning solution ◆ medicated powder or cornstarch ◆ sterile water or normal saline solution ◆ hair dryer, analgesic (optional)

PREPARATION

◆ Packaged units that include software (jacket and sheepskin liners), hardware (halo, head pins, upright bars, and screws), and tools (torque screwdriver, two conventional wrenches, Allen wrench, and screws and bolts) are commonly used.

◆ Obtain a halo-vest traction unit with halo rings and plastic vests in several sizes. Vest sizes are based on patient's chest and head measurements.

◆ Check for sterility and expiration date of the prepackaged tray.

◆ Assemble equipment at the patient's bedside.

◆ Check support applied to patient's neck on the way to the hospital. As needed, apply cervical collar or immobilize the head and neck with sandbags.

⚡ **WARNING** *Keep the cervical collar or sandbags in place until halo is applied; then remove to facilitate application of the vest.*

◆ Because the patient is likely to be frightened, try to reassure him.

◆ Remove the headboard and any furniture near the head of the bed to provide ample working space.

◆ Carefully place the patient's head on a board or padded headrest that extends beyond the edge of the bed.

⚡ **WARNING** *To avoid further spinal cord injury, don't put the patient's head on a pillow before applying the halo.*

◆ Elevate the bed so the physician has access to the front and back of the halo unit.

◆ Stand at the head of the bed, and see if the patient's chin lines up with his midsternum, indicating proper alignment.

◆ If ordered, support the patient's head in your hands and rotate the neck into alignment without flexing or extending it.

ASSISTING WITH HALO APPLICATION

◆ Explain the procedure to the patient, wash your hands, and provide privacy.

◆ Have an assisting nurse hold the patient's head and neck stable while the physician removes the cervical collar or sandbags. Maintain support until the halo is secure — while you assist with pin insertion.

◆ The physician measures the patient's head with a tape measure and refers to the halo ring conversion chart to determine correct ring size.

◆ The ring should clear the head by ⅝" (1.6 cm) and fit ½" (1.3 cm) above the bridge of the nose.

Comparing halo-vest traction devices

TYPE	DESCRIPTION		ADVANTAGES
Low profile (standard)	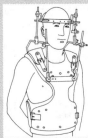	◆ Traction and compression are produced by threaded support rods on either side of halo ring. ◆ Flexion and extension are obtained by moving the swivel arm to an anterior or posterior position, depending on location of skull pins.	◆ Immobilizes cervical spine fractures while allowing patient mobility ◆ Facilitates surgery of cervical spine and permits flexion and extension ◆ Allows airway intubation without losing skeletal traction ◆ Facilitates necessary alignment by adjustment at the junction of the threaded support rods and horizontal frame
Mark II (type of low profile)	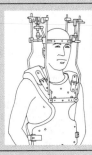	◆ Traction and compression are produced by threaded support rods on either side of halo ring. ◆ Flexion and extension are obtained by swivel clamps that allow the bars to intersect and hold at any angle.	◆ Enables physicians to assemble metal framework more quickly ◆ Allows unobstructed access for anteroposterior and lateral X-rays of cervical spine ◆ Allows patient to wear his usual clothing because uprights are closer to the body
Mark III (update of Mark II)	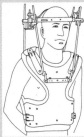	◆ Traction and compression are produced by threaded support rods on either side of halo ring. ◆ Flexion and extension are accommodated by a serrated split articulation coupling attached to the halo ring, which can be adjusted in 4-degree increments.	◆ Simplifies application while promoting patient comfort ◆ Eliminates shoulder pressure and discomfort by using a flexible padded strap instead of the vest's solid plastic shoulder ◆ Accommodates the tall patient with modified hardware and shorter uprights ◆ Allows unobstructed access for medial and lateral X-rays
Trippi-Wells tongs	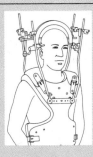	◆ Traction is produced by four pins that compress the skull. ◆ Flexion and extension are obtained by adjusting the midline vertical plate.	◆ Makes it possible to change from mobile to stationary traction without interrupting traction ◆ Adjusts to three planes for mobile and stationary traction ◆ Allows unobstructed access for medial and lateral X-rays

(continued)

- The physician selects four pin sites: ½″ above the lateral one-third of each eyebrow and ½″ above the top of each ear in the occipital area.
- The physician also considers the degree and type of correction needed to provide proper cervical alignment.
- Trim and shave hair at the pin sites to facilitate subsequent care and help prevent infection, and then put on gloves.
- Use 4″ × 4″ gauze pads soaked in povidone-iodine solution to clean sites.
- Open the halo-vest unit using sterile technique to avoid contamination.
- The physician puts on sterile gloves, and then removes the halo and Allen wrench.
- The physician places the halo over the patient's head and inserts the four positioning pins to hold the halo in place temporarily.
- Help the physician prepare anesthetic. Clean the injection port of the multidose vial of lidocaine with an alcohol pad. Invert the vial so the physician can insert a 25G needle attached to the 3-ml syringe and withdraw the anesthetic.
- The physician injects the anesthetic at the four pin sites; he may change needles on the syringe after each injection.
- The physician removes four of the five skull pins from the sterile setup and firmly screws in each pin at a 90-degree angle to the skull.
- When the pins are in place, he removes the positioning pins.
- The physician tightens the skull pins with the torque screwdriver.

APPLYING THE VEST
- After the physician measures the patient's chest and abdomen, he selects an appropriate sized vest.
- Place sheepskin liners inside the front and back of the vest for comfort and to help prevent pressure ulcers.
- Help the physician carefully raise the patient while another nurse supports the head and neck; slide the back of the vest under the patient and gently lay him down.

- The physician fastens the front of the vest on the patient's chest using Velcro straps and attaches the metal bars to the halo and vest. He tightens each bolt in turn, avoiding tightening completely, which causes maladjusted tension.

⚡ **WARNING** *When halo-vest traction is in place, X-rays should be taken to check depth of skull pins and verify proper alignment.*

CARING FOR THE PATIENT
- Take routine and neurologic vital signs at least every 2 hours for 24 hours (preferably every hour for 48 hours), then every 4 hours until stable.

⚡ **WARNING** *Notify physician immediately of any loss of motor function or decreased sensation from baseline, which could indicate spinal cord trauma.*

- Put on gloves and clean the pin sites every 4 hours with cotton-tipped applicators dipped in cleaning solution.
- Rinse the sites with sterile water or normal saline solution to remove any excess cleaning solution.
- Clean pin sites with povidone-iodine or other ordered solution to prevent infection and remove debris that might block drainage and cause abscesses.
- Watch for signs of infection — a loose pin, swelling or redness, purulent drainage, pain at the site — and notify the physician if signs develop.
- The physician retightens the skull pins with the torque screwdriver 24 and 48 hours after the halo is applied.
- If the patient complains of headache after pins are tightened, obtain an order for an analgesic.

⚡ **WARNING** *If pain occurs with jaw movement, notify physician; this may indicate that pins have slipped onto the thin temporal plate.*

- Examine the halo-vest every shift to make sure everything is secure and the patient's head is centered.

- If the vest fits correctly, you should be able to insert one or two fingers under the jacket at the shoulder and chest when the patient is in a supine position.
- Wash the patient's chest and back daily. Place him on his back, loosening the bottom Velcro straps so you can get to the chest and back.
- Turn the patient on his side (less than 45 degrees) to wash his back. Then close the vest.

⚡ **WARNING** *Don't put stress on the apparatus, which could knock it out of alignment and lead to subluxation of the cervical spine.*

- Check for tender areas or pressure spots that may develop into ulcers.
- If necessary, use a hair dryer to dry damp sheepskin; moisture predisposes the skin to pressure ulcer formation.
- Dust the skin with medicated powder or cornstarch to prevent itching. If itching persists, check to see if patient is allergic to sheepskin or if any drug he's taking might cause skin rash.
- Change the vest lining as necessary, per facility policy.

SPECIAL CONSIDERATIONS

⚡ **WARNING** *Keep two wrenches available. They may be taped to the halo vest on the chest area. If cardiac arrest occurs, you'll need them to remove the distal anterior bolts. Pull the two upright bars outward, unfasten straps, and remove front of vest. Use back of the vest as a board for cardiopulmonary resuscitation (CPR); some vests have a hinged front. To prevent subluxating the cervical injury, start CPR with the jaw-thrust maneuver, to avoid hyperextending the neck. Pull his mandible forward, while maintaining proper head and neck alignment. This pulls the tongue forward to open the airway.*

⚡ **WARNING** *Always be aware of what type of vest your patient is wearing so that in an emergency, CPR can be performed quickly and effectively.*

⚡ **WARNING** *Never lift the patient up by the vertical bars. This could strain or tear the skin at the pin sites or misalign the traction.*

◆ To prevent falls, walk with the ambulatory patient. He may have trouble seeing objects at or near his feet, and the weight of the halo-vest unit (about 10 lb [4.5 kg]) may throw him off balance.
◆ If he's in a wheelchair, lower the leg rests to prevent the chair from tipping backward.
◆ The vest limits chest expansion; routinely assess pulmonary function, especially in a patient with pulmonary disease.

COMPLICATIONS
◆ Subluxation of the spinal cord or a bone fragment pushed into the spinal cord, possibly causing paralysis below the break due to manipulating the patient's neck during application of halo-vest traction
◆ Puncturing of the skull and dura mater, causing loss of cerebrospinal fluid and central nervous system infection, due to inaccurate skull pin positioning

◆ Infection at pin sites due to nonsterile technique during application or inadequate pin-site care

PATIENT TEACHING

◆ Teach the patient about pin-site care and shampooing and hair care.
◆ Teach the patient to turn slowly and incrementally to avoid losing balance.
◆ Remind the patient to avoid bending forward; the extra weight of the apparatus may cause him to fall. Teach him to bend at the knees, not the waist.
◆ Have a physical therapist teach the patient how to use assistive devices to extend his reach and help him put on socks and shoes.
◆ Suggest to the patient that he wear large shirts that button in front to accommodate the halo-vest.

DOCUMENTATION

◆ Record the date and time halo-vest traction was applied.
◆ Note the length of the procedure and the patient's response.
◆ After application, record routine and neurologic vital signs.
◆ Document pin-site care and note signs of infection.

SELECTED REFERENCES
Betz, R.R., et al. "Acute Evaluation and Management of Pediatric Spinal Cord Injury," *The Journal of Spinal Cord Medicine* 27(Suppl 1):S11-15, 2004.

Caird, J., and Bolger, C. "Preoperative Cervical Traction in Cases of Cranial Settling with Halo Ring and Mayfield Skull Clamp," *British Journal of Neurosurgery* 19(6):488-89, December 2005.

Hayes, V.M., et al. "Complications of Halo Fixation of the Cervical Spine," *American Journal of Orthopedics* 34(6):271-76, June 2005.

Patterson, M.M. "Multicenter Pin Care Study," *Orthopaedic Nursing* 24(5):349-60, September-October 2005.

Hand hygiene

OVERVIEW

DESCRIPTION
◆ Hand hygiene is important for preventing infection. Clean hands with intact skin, short fingernails, and no rings minimize risk of contamination.
◆ To protect patients from health care-associated infections, hand hygiene must be performed routinely and thoroughly.
◆ Artificial nails can trap microorganisms and shouldn't be worn.
◆ Rough or chapped hands may also trap microorganisms.

CONTRAINDICATIONS
◆ None known

EQUIPMENT

HANDWASHING
Soap or detergent ◆ warm running water ◆ paper towels ◆ antiseptic cleaning agent, fingernail brush, disposable sponge brush or plastic cuticle stick (optional)

HAND-SANITIZING
◆ Alcohol-based hand rub

KEY STEPS

HANDWASHING
◆ Remove rings as facility policy dictates. Remove your watch or wear it well above the wrist.
◆ Artificial fingernails shouldn't be worn. Nail polish, if permitted, must be kept in good repair to minimize potential to harbor microorganisms; refer to your facility's policy pertaining to nail polish.
◆ Wet your hands and wrists with warm water and apply soap from a dispenser. Don't use bar soap; it allows cross-contamination.
◆ Hold your hands below elbow level to prevent water from running up your arms and back down, thus contaminating clean areas. (See *Proper hand-washing technique*.)
◆ Work up a generous lather and rub hands together vigorously for at least 15 seconds. Soap and warm water loosen surface microorganisms, which wash away in lather.
◆ Pay special attention to areas under fingernails and around cuticles and to the thumbs, knuckles, and sides of the fingers and hands; microorganisms thrive in these protected or overlooked areas.
◆ If you don't remove a ring, slide it up and down your finger to clean beneath it.
◆ Avoid splashing water on yourself or the floor; microorganisms spread more easily on wet surfaces and slippery floors are dangerous.
◆ Don't touch the sink or faucets; they're considered contaminated.
◆ Rinse hands and wrists well under running water to flush suds, soil, and microorganisms away.
◆ Pat hands and wrists dry with paper towels. Avoid rubbing, which can cause abrasion and chapping.
◆ If the sink isn't equipped with knee or foot controls, turn off faucets by gripping them with a dry paper towel to avoid recontaminating your hands.

Proper hand-washing technique

To minimize spread of infection, practice proper hand washing. With your hands downward under the faucet, adjust water temperature until it's comfortably warm.

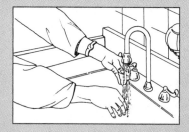

Add soap and work up a generous lather, scrubbing vigorously for at least 15 seconds. Clean under your fingernails, around knuckles, and along the sides of your fingers and hands.

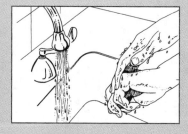

Rinse completely to wash away suds and microorganisms. Pat your hands dry with paper towels. To prevent recontamination from faucet handles, cover each one with a dry paper towel when turning off the water.

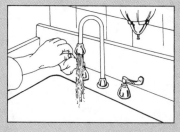

HAND-SANITIZING

◆ Apply a small amount of alcohol-based hand rub to all hand surfaces.
◆ Rub hands together until all of the product has dried (usually 30 seconds).

SPECIAL CONSIDERATIONS

◆ Before sterile procedures, wash forearms, clean under fingernails and around cuticles with a disposable fingernail brush, sponge brush, or plastic cuticle stick.
◆ Follow facility policy on when to wash with soap and when to use an antiseptic cleaning agent. Generally, wash with soap:
– before coming on duty
– before and after direct or indirect patient contact
– before and after performing any bodily functions, such as blowing your nose or using the bathroom
– before preparing or serving food
– before preparing or administering drugs
– after direct or indirect contact with excretions, secretions, or blood
– after completing your shift.
◆ Use an antiseptic cleaning agent before invasive procedures, wound care, dressing changes, and after contamination.
◆ Antiseptic cleaning is recommended before working in isolation rooms and neonate nurseries and before caring for highly susceptible patients.
◆ If your hands aren't visibly soiled, an alcohol-based hand rub can be used for routine decontamination.
◆ Wash your hands before and after performing patient care or procedures or having contact with contaminated objects, even though you may have worn gloves.
◆ Always wash your hands after removing gloves.
◆ If you're providing care in the patient's home, bring your own supply of soap and disposable paper towels.
◆ If there's no running water, disinfect your hands with an antiseptic cleaning agent.

COMPLICATIONS

◆ Dryness, cracking, and irritation from excessive hand washing, which strips the skin of natural oils (The effects are more common after repeated antiseptic cleansing.)
◆ Irritation — to minimize, rinse your hands thoroughly
◆ Chapping — to prevent, apply an emollient hand cream after washing (make sure hand cream or lotion won't cause gloves to deteriorate)
◆ Dermatitis (have your employee health care provider determine whether you should work with patients until condition resolves)

PATIENT TEACHING

◆ Teach the patient proper hand washing when he'll provide self-care.
◆ Tell the patient that cleaning agents will be supplied by your facility and not to use lotions from home.

DOCUMENTATION

◆ Document proper hand washing as it pertains to specific patient care.

SELECTED REFERENCES

Allen, G. "Hand Hygiene, An Essential Process in the OR," *AORN Journal* 82(4):561-62, October 2005.

Bissett, L., and Craig, K. "Hand Inspection Cabinets as an Aid to Washing Technique," *Nursing Times* 101(31):38-40, August 2005.

Fry, D.A. "Hand Hygiene Compliance: Step Up, Reach Out," *Nursing Management* (Suppl):12-15, November 2005.

Lam, B.C., et al. "Hand Hygiene Practices in a Neonatal Intensive Care Unit: A Multimodal Intervention and Impact on Nosocomial Infection," *Pediatrics* 114(5):e565-71, November 2004.

Petty, C. "Hand Washing: Essential in the PACU," *Journal of Perianesthesia Nursing* 19(4):261-62, August 2004.

Wakefield, A. "Hand Washing — Rituals and Regimes in Practice," *Nursing New Zealand* 9(11):16-17, December 2003-January 2004.

Heat application

DESCRIPTION

- Heat raises tissue temperature and enhances inflammatory process by causing vasodilation and increasing local circulation, promoting leukocytosis, suppuration, drainage, and healing.
- It increases tissue metabolism, reduces pain caused by muscle spasm, and decreases congestion in deep visceral organs.
- Dry heat can be delivered at higher temperatures and longer times than moist heat.
- Moist heat softens crusts and exudates, penetrates deeper than dry heat, is less drying to skin, produces less perspiration, and is more comfortable.

CONTRAINDICATIONS

- Hemorrhage or risk for hemorrhage
- Acute sprain
- Acute inflammation

   ❀ **AGE FACTOR** *Heat should be applied cautiously to pediatric and elderly patients.*

EQUIPMENT

Thermometer ◆ towel ◆ adhesive tape or roller gauze ◆ absorbent, protective cloth covering ◆ gloves, if patient has an open lesion ◆ hot tap water ◆ pitcher ◆ bath thermometer ◆ absorbent, protective cloth covering for electric heating pad ◆ K pad ◆ distilled water ◆ temperature-adjustment key ◆ chemical hot pack (disposable) ◆ compress material (flannel, 4″ × 4″ gauze pads) or pack material (absorbent towels, large absorbent pads) ◆ cotton-tipped applicators ◆ bowl or basin ◆ waterproof covering ◆ dressings ◆ forceps (optional)

PREPARATION
Hot-water bottle

- Wash your hands before all procedures.

- Fill the bottle with hot tap water to detect leaks and warm the bottle, and then empty it.
- Run hot tap water into a pitcher and measure temperature with the bath thermometer.
- Adjust temperature as ordered, usually 115° to 125° F (46.1° to 51.7° C) for adults.

   ❀ **AGE FACTOR** *Adjust water temperature to 105° to 115° F (40.6° to 46.1° C) for a child younger than age 2, an elderly patient, or when preparing an eye compress.*

- Pour hot water into bottle, filling it one-half to two-thirds full to keep it lightweight and flexible.
- Squeeze the bottle until water reaches the neck to expel air.
- Fasten the top and cover the bag with an absorbent cloth.
- Secure the cover with tape or roller gauze.

Electric heating pad

- Check the cord for frayed or damaged insulation.
- Plug in the pad and adjust the control switch to desired setting.
- Wrap the pad in a protective cloth covering, and secure the cover with tape or roller gauze.

K pad

- Check the cord for safety and fill the control unit two-thirds full with distilled water according to manufacturer's directions.
- Check for leaks, then tilt the unit in several directions to clear tubing of air.
- Tighten the cap, and then loosen it a quarter turn to allow heat expansion within the unit.
- Place the unit on the bedside table, slightly above the patient, so gravity can assist water flow.
- Use the temperature-adjustment key provided to set the temperature on the control unit to 105° F (40.6° C), or as ordered.
- Place the pad in a protective cloth covering and secure it with tape or roller gauze.
- Plug in the unit, turn it on, and allow the pad to warm for 2 minutes.

Chemical hot pack

- Select a pack of the correct size.
- Follow the manufacturer's directions to activate the heat-producing chemicals.
- Place the pack in a protective cloth covering and secure it with tape or roller gauze.

Sterile warm compress or pack

- Warm the container of sterile water or solution by setting it in a sink or basin of hot water.
- Measure its temperature with a sterile bath thermometer.
- If a sterile thermometer isn't available, pour some solution into a container, check temperature with a regular bath thermometer, then discard the test solution.
- Adjust the temperature by adding hot or cold water to the sink or basin until the solution reaches 131° F (55° C) for adults.
- Pour heated solution into a sterile bowl or basin.
- Using sterile technique, soak the compress or pack in the heated solution.
- If necessary, prepare a hot-water bottle, K pad, or chemical hot pack to keep the compress or pack warm.

Nonsterile warm compress or pack

- Fill a bowl or basin with hot tap water or other solution and measure the temperature of the fluid with a bath thermometer.
- Adjust temperature as ordered, usually to 131° F (55° C) for adults.
- Soak the compress or pack in the hot liquid.
- If necessary, prepare a hot-water bottle, K pad, or chemical hot pack to keep the compress or pack warm.

- Check the practitioner's order and assess patient's condition.
- Confirm the patient's identity using two patient identifiers according to facility policy.
- Explain the procedure to the patient.
- Provide privacy and make sure the room is warm and free from drafts.
- Take the patient's vital signs as a baseline.
- If heat is being applied to raise body temperature, monitor vital signs.

⚡ **WARNING** *Monitor a patient with cardiovascular disease for dizziness and hypotension.*

- Expose only the treatment area because vasodilation will make the patient feel chilly.

APPLYING A HOT-WATER BOTTLE, ELECTRIC HEATING PAD, K PAD, OR CHEMICAL HOT PACK

- Before applying the heating device, check heat distribution. If it heats unevenly, obtain a new device.
- Apply the device to the treatment area; if necessary, secure with tape or roller gauze.
- Time the application.
- Assess patient's skin condition frequently; remove the device if you see increased swelling or excessive redness, blistering, maceration, or pallor, or if patient reports discomfort.
- Refill the hot-water bottle as necessary to maintain correct temperature.
- Remove the device after 20 to 30 minutes or as ordered.
- Dry patient's skin with a towel and redress site, as needed.
- Take vital signs for comparison with baseline.

APPLYING A WARM COMPRESS OR PACK

- Place a linen-saver pad under the site.
- Remove the warm compress or pack from the bowl or basin, using sterile forceps, if needed.
- Wring excess solution from the compress or pack.

- Apply the compress gently to the affected site.
- After a few seconds, lift the compress and check skin for excessive redness, maceration, or blistering.
- When you're sure the compress isn't causing a burn, mold it firmly to the skin to keep out air, which reduces effectiveness.
- Apply a waterproof covering (sterile, if necessary) to the compress and secure it with tape or roller gauze to prevent slippage.
- Place a hot-water bottle, K pad, or chemical hot pack over the compress and waterproof covering to maintain correct temperature.
- Time the application.
- Check the patient's skin every 5 minutes and remove the device if the skin shows excessive redness, maceration, blistering, or pain.
- Change the compress as needed to maintain correct temperature.
- After 15 or 20 minutes, or as ordered, remove the compress.
- Dry the patient's skin with a towel (sterile, if necessary).
- Note the condition of the skin and redress the area, if necessary.
- Take vital signs for comparison with baseline.

SPECIAL CONSIDERATIONS

- If the patient is unconscious, anesthetized, irrational, neurologically impaired, or insensitive to heat, stay with him throughout the treatment.

COMPLICATIONS

- Tissue damage
- Hypotension

PATIENT TEACHING

- Tell the patient the reason for the heat treatment.
- Advise the patient that he needs to avoid leaning or lying directly on the heating unit.
- Explain the importance of not adjusting the temperature of the heating device or adding hot water to a hot-water bottle.
- Tell the patient he needs to report pain immediately and remove the device, if necessary.
- Explain to the patient how to perform heat treatment at home, if necessary.

DOCUMENTATION

- Record the date, time, and duration of heat application.
- Note the type of heat treatment.
- Document the temperature or heat setting.
- Record the site of application.
- Note the patient's vital signs and skin condition before, during, and after treatment.
- Document signs of complications.
- Record the patient's tolerance of treatment.
- Note patient teaching.

SELECTED REFERENCES

Beyerman, K.L., et al. "Efficacy of Treating Low Back Pain and Dysfunction Secondary to Osteoarthritis: Chiropractic Care Compared with Moist Heat Alone," *Journal of Manipulative and Physiological Therapeutics* 29(2):107-14, February 2006.

"Hot and Cold Treatments. Relieving Aches and Pains," *Mayo Clinic Health Letter* 23(8):7, August 2005.

Masuda, A., et al. "The Effects of Repeated Thermal Therapy for Patients with Chronic Pain," *Psychotherapy and Psycosomatics* 74(5):288-94, 2005.

Sherman, K.J., et al. "The Diagnosis and Treatment of Chronic Back Pain by Acupuncturists, Chiropractors, and Massage Therapists," *Clinical Journal of Pain* 22(3):227-34, March-April 2006.

Height and weight measurement

DESCRIPTION

◆ Accurate record of height and weight is essential for calculating dosages of drugs, anesthetics, and contrast agents; assessing the patient's nutritional status; and determining height-weight ratio.
◆ Weight provides the best overall picture of fluid status; daily monitoring is important for patients receiving sodium-retaining or diuretic medications.
◆ Rapid weight gain may signal fluid retention; rapid weight loss may indicate diuresis.
◆ Weight can be measured with a standing scale, chair scale, or bed scale; height can be measured with the measuring bar on a standing scale or with a tape measure for a supine patient.

CONTRAINDICATIONS

◆ None known

EQUIPMENT

Standing scale (with measuring bar) or chair or bed scale ◆ wheelchair (if needed to transport patient) ◆ tape measure, if needed ◆ drawsheet (optional)

PREPARATION

◆ Select the appropriate scale, usually a standing scale for an ambulatory patient or a chair or bed scale for an acutely ill or debilitated patient.
◆ Check to make sure the scale is balanced.

KEY STEPS

◆ Confirm the patient's identity using two patient identifiers according to facility policy.
◆ Explain the procedure to the patient.

USING A STANDING SCALE

◆ Place a paper towel on the scale's platform.
◆ Have the patient remove his robe and slippers or shoes.
◆ If the scale has wheels, lock them. Help the patient onto the scale and remain close to prevent falls.
◆ If using an upright balance (gravity) scale, slide the lower rider to the groove representing the largest increment below his actual weight.
◆ Slide the small upper rider until the beam balances.
◆ Add the upper and lower rider figures to determine weight.
◆ If using a multiple-weight scale, move appropriate ratio weights onto the weight holder to balance the scale; ratio weights are labeled 50, 100, and 200 lbs.
◆ Add ratio weights until the next weight causes the main beam to fall.
◆ Adjust the main beam poise until the scale balances.
◆ To obtain the weight, add the sum of the ratio weights to the figure on the main beam.
◆ Return ratio weights to their rack and the weight holder to its proper place.
◆ If you're using a digital scale, make sure the display reads "0" before use.
◆ Read the display with the patient standing as still as possible.

MEASURING HEIGHT

◆ Tell the patient to stand erect on the platform of the scale.
◆ Raise the measuring bar above his head, extend the horizontal arm, and lower the bar until it touches the top of his head.
◆ Read the patient's height.
◆ Help him off the scale, and give him his robe and slippers or shoes.
◆ Return the measuring bar to its initial position.

USING A CHAIR SCALE

◆ Take the patient to the weighing area or the scale to the patient's bedside.
◆ Lock the scale in place to prevent it from moving.
◆ If using a scale with a swing-away chair arm, unlock the arm. When unlocked, the arm swings back 180 degrees to permit easy access.
◆ Position the scale beside his bed or wheelchair with the chair arm open.
◆ Transfer him onto the scale, swing the chair arm to the front of the scale, and lock it in place.
◆ Weigh him by adding ratio weights and adjusting the main beam poise.
◆ Unlock the swing-away chair arm as before, and transfer him back to his bed or wheelchair.
◆ Lock the main beam to avoid damaging the scale during transport.

USING A MULTIPLE-WEIGHT BED SCALE

◆ Provide privacy; tell the patient you're going to weigh him on a special bed scale.
◆ Position the scale next to his bed and lock the scale's wheels.
◆ Turn him on his side, facing away from the scale.
◆ Release the stretcher frame to the horizontal position, and pump the hand lever until the stretcher is positioned over the mattress.
◆ Lower the stretcher onto the mattress, and roll him onto the stretcher.
◆ Raise the stretcher 2″ (5.1 cm) above the mattress.
◆ Add ratio weights and adjust the main beam poise as for the standing and chair scales.
◆ After weighing the patient, lower the stretcher onto the mattress, turn the patient on his side, and remove the stretcher.

USING A DIGITAL BED SCALE

◆ Provide privacy, and tell the patient you're going to weigh him on a special bed scale.
◆ Release the stretcher to the horizontal position; then lock it in place.
◆ Turn the patient on his side, facing away from the scale.

- Roll the base of the scale under his bed. Adjust the lever to widen the base of the scale, providing stability. Lock the scale's wheels.
- Center the stretcher above the bed, lower it onto the mattress, and roll the patient onto the stretcher.
- Position the circular weighing arms of the scale over him, and attach them securely to the stretcher bars.
- Pump the handle with slow strokes to raise him a few inches off the bed.

⚡ **WARNING** *Make sure that the patient doesn't lean on or touch the bed or any equipment; this will affect weight measurement.*

- Press the operate button, and read his weight on the digital display panel.
- Press in the scale's handle to lower the patient.
- Detach the circular weighing arms from the stretcher bars, roll the patient off the stretcher and remove it, and position him comfortably in bed.
- Release the wheel lock and withdraw the scale. Return the stretcher to its vertical position.

SPECIAL CONSIDERATIONS

- Reassure and steady a patient at risk for losing his balance on a scale.
- Weigh the patient at the same time each day (usually before breakfast), in similar clothing, using the same scale.
- If he uses crutches, weigh him with the crutches, then weigh the crutches and subtract their weight from the total to determine his weight.
- Before using a bed scale, cover its stretcher with a drawsheet. Balance the scale with the drawsheet in place to ensure accurate weighing.

- When rolling the patient onto the stretcher, be careful not to dislodge I.V. lines, indwelling catheters, and other supportive equipment.

COMPLICATIONS
- None known

PATIENT TEACHING

- Refer the patient to a chart of suggested healthy weight ranges to determine norms for his height and weight. (See *Suggested weights for adults.*)
- Teach the patient the correct method for weighing himself at home.

DOCUMENTATION

- Record the patient's height and weight on the nursing assessment form and other records as required.

SELECTED REFERENCES

Brown, I. "Nurses' Attitudes Towards Adult Patients Who Are Obese: Literature Review," *Journal of Advanced Nursing* 53(2):221-32, January 2006.

Gance-Cleveland, B., and Bushmiaer, M. "Arkansas School Nurses' Role in Statewide Assessment of Body Mass Index to Screen for Overweight Children and Adolescents," *Journal of School Nursing* 21(2):64-69, April 2005.

McKey, A., and Huntington, A. "Obesity in Pre-School Children: Issues and Challenges for Community Based Child Health Nurses," *Contemporary Nurse* 18(1-2):145-51, December 2004-January 2005.

Thornton, M.J., et al. "Height Change and Bone Mineral Density: Revisited," *Orthopaedic Nursing* 23(5):315-20, September-October 2004.

Suggested weights for adults

This table is a guide for determining healthy weights. Higher weights in each category typically apply to men, who on average have more muscle and bone; lower weights usually apply to women, who on average have less muscle and bone. Height is measured without shoes; weight is measured without clothes. The health risks of excess weight appear to apply to older and younger adults alike.

HEIGHT	WEIGHT (IN LB)
4'10"	91 to 119
4'11"	92 to 124
5'0"	97 to 128
5'1"	101 to 132
5'2"	104 to 137
5'3"	107 to 141
5'4"	111 to 146
5'5"	114 to 150
5'6"	118 to 155
5'7"	121 to 160
5'8"	125 to 164
5'9"	129 to 169
5'10"	132 to 174
5'11"	136 to 179
6'0"	140 to 184
6'1"	144 to 189
6'2"	148 to 195
6'3"	152 to 200
6'4"	156 to 205
6'5"	160 to 211
6'6"	164 to 216

Hemodialysis

DESCRIPTION

◆ Hemodialysis is used for regular long-term treatment of patients with chronic end-stage renal disease, temporary support for patients with acute reversible renal failure, and, less commonly, acute poisoning.

◆ Procedure extracts toxic wastes from the blood of patients in renal failure by removing blood from the body, circulating it through a purifying dialyzer, then returning it to the body.

◆ For long-term treatment, various access sites, including arteriovenous (AV) fistula, are used. (See *Hemodialysis access sites.*)

◆ Hemodialysis restores or maintains balance of the body's buffer system and electrolyte level, promoting rapid return to normal serum values and preventing complications associated with uremia.

◆ Special hemodialysis units are available for home use.

CONTRAINDICATIONS

◆ Hypotension
◆ Active bleeding

EQUIPMENT

MACHINE PREPARATION

Hemodialysis machine with appropriate dialyzer ◆ I.V. solution, administration sets, lines, and related equipment ◆ dialysate ◆ heparin, 3-ml syringe with needle, medication label, hemostats (optional)

HEMODIALYSIS WITH A DOUBLE-LUMEN CATHETER

Povidone-iodine pads ◆ two sterile 4″×4″ gauze pads ◆ two 3-ml and two 5-ml syringes ◆ tape ◆ heparin bolus syringe ◆ clean gloves ◆ sterile labels ◆ sterile marker

HEMODIALYSIS WITH AN AV FISTULA

Two winged fistula needles (each attached to a 10-ml syringe filled with heparin flush solution) ◆ linen-saver pad ◆ povidone-iodine pads ◆ sterile 4″×4″ gauze pads ◆ tourniquet ◆ clean gloves ◆ adhesive tape ◆ sterile labels ◆ sterile marker

HEMODIALYSIS WITH AN AV SHUNT

Alcohol pads ◆ povidone-iodine pads ◆ sterile gloves ◆ two sterile shunt adapters ◆ sterile Teflon connector ◆ two bulldog clamps ◆ two 10-ml syringes ◆ normal saline solution ◆ four short strips of adhesive tape ◆ sterile shunt spreader, sterile labels, sterile marker (optional)

DISCONTINUING HEMODIALYSIS WITH A DOUBLE-LUMEN CATHETER

Sterile 4″×4″ gauze pads ◆ povidone-iodine pads ◆ precut gauze dressing ◆ clean gloves ◆ sterile gloves ◆ normal saline solution ◆ alcohol pads ◆ heparin flush solution ◆ luer-lock injection caps ◆ transparent occlusive dressing, skin barrier preparation, tape, materials for culturing drainage ◆ sterile labels ◆ sterile marker (optional)

DISCONTINUING HEMODIALYSIS WITH AN AV FISTULA

Clean gloves ◆ sterile 4″×4″ gauze pads ◆ two adhesive bandages ◆ hemostats ◆ sterile absorbable gelatin sponges: Gelfoam, topical thrombin solution (optional)

PREPARATION

◆ Prepare hemodialysis equipment following manufacturer's instructions and facility protocol.

◆ Test the dialyzer and dialysis machine for residual disinfectant after rinsing, and test all alarms.

KEY STEPS

◆ Confirm the patient's identity using two patient identifiers according to facility policy.

◆ Wash your hands before procedure.

◆ If the patient is undergoing hemodialysis for the first time, explain the procedure.

◆ Maintain strict sterile technique to prevent introducing pathogens into the patient's bloodstream.

◆ Wear appropriate personal protective equipment, as necessary, throughout all procedures.

◆ Weigh patient and compare before-weight to his weight after the last dialysis and his target-weight to determine ultrafiltration requirements.

◆ Record baseline vital signs, taking blood pressure while he's sitting and standing; auscultate the heart for rate, rhythm, and abnormalities; assess for edema; observe respiratory rate, rhythm, and quality; and check his mental status.

◆ Assess the condition and patency of the access site.

◆ Check for problems since last dialysis; evaluate previous laboratory data.

◆ Help the patient into a comfortable position (supine or sitting in recliner chair with feet elevated).

◆ Support the access site and rest it on a clean drape.

◆ Label all medications, medication containers, and other solutions on and off the sterile field.

BEGINNING HEMODIALYSIS WITH A DOUBLE-LUMEN CATHETER

◆ If extension tubing isn't already clamped, clamp it to prevent air from entering the catheter.

◆ Clean each catheter extension tube, clamp, and luer-lock injection cap with povidone-iodine pads to remove contaminants.

◆ Place a sterile 4″×4″ gauze pad under the extension tubing, and place two 5-ml syringes and two sterile gauze pads on the drape.

◆ Prepare the anticoagulant regimen.

◆ Identify arterial and venous blood lines, and place them near the drape.

◆ To remove clots and ensure catheter patency, remove catheter caps, attach syringes to each catheter port, open the clamp, aspirate 1.5 to 3 ml of blood, close the clamp, and flush each port with 5 ml of heparin flush solution.

- To gain patient access, remove the syringe from the arterial port and attach the line to it; administer heparin according to protocol to prevent clotting in the extracorporeal circuit.
- Grasp the venous blood line and attach it to the venous port; open the clamps on the extension tubing and secure the tubing to the patient's extremity with tape to reduce tension on the tube and minimize trauma at insertion site.
- Begin hemodialysis according to facility protocol.

Hemodialysis access sites

Hemodialysis requires vascular access. The site and type of access depends on expected duration of dialysis, surgeon's preference, and patient's condition.

SUBCLAVIAN VEIN CATHETERIZATION

Using the Seldinger technique, the surgeon inserts an introducer needle into the subclavian vein. He then inserts a guide wire through the introducer needle and removes the needle. Using the guide wire, he threads a 5″ to 12″ (12.5- to 30.5-cm) plastic or Teflon catheter (with a Y-hub) into the patient's vein.

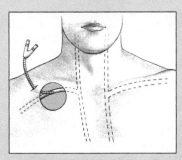

FEMORAL VEIN CATHETERIZATION

Using the Seldinger technique, the surgeon inserts an introducer needle into the left or right femoral vein. He then inserts a guide wire through the introducer needle and removes the needle. Using the guide wire, he threads a 5″ to 12″ plastic or Teflon catheter with a Y-hub or two catheters, one for inflow and the other placed about ½″ (1.3 cm) distal to the first for outflow.

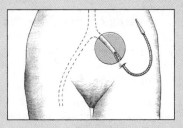

ARTERIOVENOUS FISTULA

To create a fistula, the surgeon makes an incision in the patient's lower forearm, then a small incision in the side of an artery, and another in the side of a vein. He sutures the edges of the incisions together to make a common opening ⅛″ to ¼″ (3 to 6 mm) long.

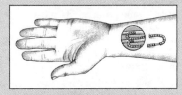

ARTERIOVENOUS SHUNT

To create a shunt, the surgeon makes an incision in the patient's lower forearm or (rarely) ankle. He inserts a 6″ to 10″ (15- to 25-cm) transparent Silastic cannula into an artery and another into a vein. Finally, he tunnels the cannulas out through stab wounds and joins them with a piece of Teflon tubing.

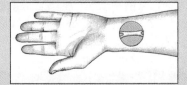

ARTERIOVENOUS GRAFT

To create a graft, the surgeon makes an incision in the patient's forearm, upper arm, or thigh. He then tunnels a natural or synthetic graft under the skin and sutures the distal end to an artery and the proximal end to a vein.

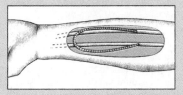

BEGINNING HEMODIALYSIS WITH AN AV FISTULA

- Flush the fistula needles, using attached syringes containing heparinized saline solution, and set them aside.
- Place a linen-saver pad under the patient's arm.
- Using sterile technique, clean a 3″ × 10″ (7.5 × 25 cm) area of skin over the fistula with povidone-iodine pads. If the patient is sensitive to iodine, use chlorhexidine gluconate or alcohol instead.
- Discard each pad after one wipe.
- Apply a tourniquet above the fistula to distend the veins and facilitate venipuncture; avoid occluding the fistula.
- Put on clean gloves.
- Remove the fistula needle guard and squeeze the wing tips firmly together.
- Insert the arterial needle at least 1″ (2.5 cm) above the anastomosis, being careful not to puncture the fistula.
- Release the tourniquet and flush the needle with heparin flush solution to prevent clotting.
- Clamp the arterial needle tubing with a hemostat, and secure the wing tips of the needle to the skin with adhesive tape to prevent it from dislodging.
- Perform another venipuncture with the venous needle a few inches above the arterial needle.
- Flush the venous needle with heparin flush solution.
- Clamp the venous needle tubing, and secure the wing tips of the venous needle and secure with tape.
- Remove the syringe from the end of the arterial tubing, uncap the arterial line from the hemodialysis machine, and connect the two lines.
- Tape the connection securely to prevent separation during the procedure.
- Remove the syringe from the end of the venous tubing, uncap the venous line from the hemodialysis machine, and connect the two lines.
- Tape the connection securely.
- Release the hemostats and start hemodialysis.

(continued)

BEGINNING HEMODIALYSIS WITH AN AV SHUNT

♦ Remove the bulldog clamps and place them within easy reach of the sterile field.
♦ Remove the shunt dressing, and use sterile technique to clean the shunt.
♦ Assemble the shunt adapters according to the manufacturer's instructions.
♦ Clean the arterial and venous shunt connection with povidone-iodine pads. Use a separate pad for each tube, and wipe in one direction only, from the insertion site to the connection site.
♦ Allow the tubing to air dry.
♦ Put on sterile gloves.
♦ Clamp the arterial and venous sides with bulldog clamps.
♦ Open the shunt by separating its sides with your fingers or with a sterile shunt spreaders, if available. Both sides of the shunt should be exposed.
♦ Inspect the Teflon connector on one side of the shunt to see if it's damaged or bent. If necessary, replace it before proceeding. Note which side contains the connector so you can use the new one to close the shunt after treatment.
♦ Attach a shunt adapter and 10-ml syringe filled with about 8 ml of normal saline to the side of the shunt containing the Teflon connector.
♦ Attach the new Teflon connector to the other side of the shunt with the second adapter. Attach the second 10-ml syringe filled with about 8 ml of normal saline solution to the same side.
♦ Flush the shunt's arterial tubing by releasing its clamp and gently aspirating it with the normal saline solution-filled syringe.
♦ Flush the tubing slowly while observing it for sings of fibrin buildup. Repeat the procedure on the venous side of the shunt.
♦ Secure the shunt to the adapter connection with adhesive tape.
♦ Connect the arterial and venous lines to the adapters and secure the connections with tape. Tape each line to the patient's arm.
♦ Begin hemodialysis according to facility policy.

DISCONTINUING HEMODIALYSIS WITH A DOUBLE-LUMEN CATHETER

♦ Clamp the extension tubing to prevent air from entering the catheter.
♦ Clean all connection points on all lines and clamps to reduce risk of infections.
♦ Place a clean drape under the catheter, and place two sterile povidone-iodine soaked 4″ × 4″ gauze pads on the drape beneath the catheter lines.
♦ Prepare the catheter flush solution with normal saline or heparin flush solution, as ordered.
♦ Put on clean gloves.
♦ Grasp each blood line with a gauze pad and disconnect each line from the catheter.
♦ Flush each port with saline solution to clear extension tubing and catheter of blood.
♦ Administer additional heparin flush solution as ordered to ensure catheter patency. Attach luer-lock injection caps to prevent air entry or loss of blood.
♦ Clamp the extension tubing.
♦ Redress catheter insertion site; also redress if it's occluded, soiled, or wet.
♦ During dressing change, put patient in a supine position with his face turned from the insertion site so he doesn't contaminate the site by breathing on it.
♦ After washing your hands, put on gloves and remove the outer occlusive dressing.
♦ Put on sterile gloves, remove the old inner dressing, and discard the gloves and the dressing.
♦ Set up a sterile field, and observe site for drainage; obtain a drainage sample for culture if necessary.
♦ Notify the physician if the suture appears to be missing.
♦ Put on sterile gloves and clean the insertion site with an alcohol pad.
♦ Clean the site with a povidone-iodine pad and allow it to air-dry.
♦ Place a precut gauze dressing under the catheter, and another gauze dressing over the catheter.
♦ Apply a skin barrier preparation to the skin surrounding the gauze dressing and cover the gauze and catheter with a transparent occlusive dressing.

♦ Apply a 4″ to 5″ (10 to 12.5 cm) piece of 2″ tape over the cut edge of the dressing to reinforce the lower edge.

DISCONTINUING HEMODIALYSIS WITH AN AV FISTULA

♦ Turn the blood pump on the hemodialysis machine to 50 to 100 ml/minute.
♦ Put on clean gloves and remove tape from the connection site of arterial lines.
♦ Clamp the needle tubing with the hemostat and disconnect the lines. The blood in the machine's arterial line will continue to flow toward the dialyzer, followed by a column of air. Just before the blood reaches the point where the normal saline solution enters the line, clamp the blood line with another hemostat.
♦ Unclamp the normal saline solution to allow a small amount to flow through the line.
♦ Unclamp the hemostat on the machine line to allow all blood to flow into the dialyzer where it passes through the filter and back to the patient through the venous line.
♦ After the blood is retransfused, clamp the venous needle tubing and the machine's venous line with hemostats and turn off the blood pump.
♦ Remove tape from connection site of the venous lines and disconnect the lines.
♦ Remove the venipuncture needle and apply pressure to the site with a folded 4″ × 4″ gauze pad until all bleeding stops, usually within 10 minutes.
♦ Apply an adhesive bandage.
♦ Repeat procedure on the arterial line.
♦ Disinfect and rinse the delivery system according to manufacturer's instructions.

DISCONTINUING HEMODIALYSIS WITH AN AV SHUNT

♦ Wash your hands.
♦ Turn the blood pump on the hemodialysis machine to 50 to 100 ml/minute.
♦ Put on sterile gloves.
♦ Remove the tape from the connection site of the arterial line.

- Clamp the arterial cannula with a bulldog clamp, and then disconnect the lines. Just before the blood reaches the point where the normal saline solution enters the line, clamp the blood line with a hemostat.
- Unclamp the normal saline solution to allow a small amount to flow through the line.
- Reclamp the normal saline solution line and unclamp the hemostat on the machine line.
- Just before the last volume of blood enters the patient, clamp the venous cannula with a bulldog clamp and the machine's venous line with a hemostat.
- Remove the tape from the connection site of the venous lines.
- Turn off the blood pump and disconnect the lines.
- Reconnect the shunt cannula. Remove the older of the two Teflon connectors and discard it. Connect the shunt, positioning the Teflon connector equally between the two cannulas.
- Remove the bulldog clamp.
- Secure the shunt connection with plasticized or hypoallergenic tape.
- Clean the shunt and its site with the gauze pads soaked with povidone-iodine solution.
- When the cleaning procedure is finished, remove the povidone-iodine with alcohol pads.
- Make sure that blood flows through the shunt adequately.
- Apply a dressing to the shunt site and wrap it securely (but not too tightly) with elastic gauze bandages.
- Attach the bulldog clamps to the outside dressing.
- When hemodialysis is complete, assess the patient's weight, vital signs, and mental status. Compare your findings with your predialysis assessment data.
- Document your findings.
- Disinfect and rinse the delivery system according to the manufacturer's instructions.

SPECIAL CONSIDERATIONS

- Obtain blood samples from the patient as ordered, usually before beginning hemodialysis.

WARNING *To avoid pyrogenic reactions and bacteremia with septicemia, use strict sterile technique while preparing machine.*

- Immediately report any machine malfunction or equipment defect.
- Avoid unnecessary handling of hemodialysis tubing.
- Assess the catheter insertion site for signs of infection, such as purulent drainage, inflammation, and tenderness.

WARNING *Complete each step of dialysis correctly to avoid unnecessary blood loss or inefficient treatment from poor clearances or inadequate fluid removal. Failure to perform hemodialysis properly can lead to patient injury and death.*

- If bleeding continues after you remove the needle, apply pressure with a sterile, absorbable gelatin sponge or topical thrombin solution.
- Monitor vital signs throughout hemodialysis at least hourly or as often as every 15 minutes.
- After dialysis, assess the patient's weight, vital signs, and mental status; compare findings with your predialysis assessment.
- Perform periodic tests for clotting time on patient's blood samples and samples from the dialyzer.
- The patient may have a light meal during treatment.
- Give necessary drugs during dialysis unless the drug would be removed in the dialysate.

COMPLICATIONS

- Fever
- Dialysis disequilibrium syndrome
- Hypovolemia
- Hypotension
- Hyperglycemia
- Hypernatremia
- Hyperosmolarity
- Cardiac arrhythmias
- Angina
- Air embolism
- Hemolysis
- Hyperthermia
- Exsanguination
- Thrombosis of AV fistula
- Stenosis of AV fistula

PATIENT TEACHING

- Teach the patient how to care for the vascular access site at home.
- Advise the patient, as needed, how to perform hemodialysis at home — usually a complex process requiring 2 to 3 months to feel comfortable and be competent.
- Provide the telephone number of the dialysis center.
- Provide emotional support.

DOCUMENTATION

- Note the time treatment began and ended.
- Record problems with treatment.
- Document vital signs and weight before, during, and after treatment.
- Note time blood specimens were taken for testing, test results, and treatment for complications.
- Document his response to treatment.
- Note the condition of vascular access site and site care.

SELECTED REFERENCES

Cleary, J., and Drennan, J. "Quality of Life of Patients on Haemodialysis for End-Stage Renal Disease," *Journal of Advanced Nursing* 51(6):577-86, September 2005.

Desmet, C., et al. "Falls in Hemodialysis Patients: Prospective Study of Incidence, Risk Factors, and Complications," *American Journal of Kidney Diseases* 45(1):148-53, January 2005.

Harwood, L., et al. "Preparing for Hemodialysis: Patient Stressors and Responses," *Nephrology Nursing Journal* 32(3):295-302, May-June 2005.

Holley, J.L., et al. "Managing Homeless Dialysis Patients," *Nephrology News & Issues* 20(1):49-50, 52-53, January 2006.

Priester-Coary, A. "Creating a Successful Daily Home Hemodialysis Program," *Nephrology Nursing Journal* 31(6):677-79, November-December 2004.

Hip-spica cast care

DESCRIPTION

- After orthopedic surgery to correct a fracture or deformity, the patient may need a hip-spica cast to immobilize both legs.
- Occasionally, the physician may apply a hip-spica cast to treat an orthopedic deformity that doesn't require surgery.
- Caring for the patient in a hip-spica cast poses several challenges, including protecting the cast from urine and feces, keeping the cast dry, ensuring proper blood supply to the legs, and teaching the patient and his parents how to care for the cast at home.
- Infants usually adapt more easily to the cast than do older children, but both need encouragement, support, and diversionary activity during their prolonged immobilization.

CONTRAINDICATIONS

- None known

EQUIPMENT

Waterproof adhesive tape ◆ moleskin or plastic petals ◆ cast cutter or saw ◆ scissors ◆ nonabrasive cleaner ◆ hair dryer ◆ disposable diaper or perineal pad (optional)

KEY STEPS

- Before the physician applies the cast, describe the procedure to the patient and his parents. For patients ages 3 to 12, illustrate your explanation. Draw a picture, present a diagram, or use a doll with a cast or an elastic gauze dressing wrapped around its trunk and limbs.
- Once the physician constructs the cast, keep all but the perineal area uncovered.
- Provide privacy by draping a small cover over this opening.
- Turn the patient every 1 to 2 hours to speed drying time. Be sure to turn the patient to his unaffected side to prevent adding pressure to the affected side. If the patient is an infant, you can turn him by yourself. If the patient is an older child or an adolescent, seek assistance before attempting to turn him.

  WARNING *When turning the patient, don't use the stabilizer bar between his legs for leverage. Excessive pressure on this bar may disrupt the cast.*

  WARNING *Handle a damp cast only with your palms to avoid misshaping the cast material.*

- After the cast dries, inspect the inside edges of the cast for stray pieces of casting material that can irritate the skin. (A traditional hip-spica cast requires 24 to 48 hours to dry. However, a hip-spica cast made from newer, quick-drying substances takes only 8 to 10 hours to dry. If made of fiberglass, it will dry in less than 1 hour.)

- Cut several petal-shaped pieces of moleskin and place them, overlapping, around the open edges of the cast to protect the patient's skin. Use waterproof adhesive tape around the perineal area.
- Bathe the patient to remove any cast fragments from his skin.
- Assess the patient's legs for coldness, swelling, cyanosis, or mottling. Also assess pulse strength, toe movement, sensation (numbness, tingling, or burning), and capillary refill. Perform these circulatory assessments every 1 to 2 hours while the cast is wet and every 2 to 4 hours after the cast dries.
- If the cast is applied after surgery, remember that the most accurate way to assess for bleeding is to monitor vital signs.

  WARNING *A visible blood spot on the cast can be misleading: One drop of blood can produce a circle 3" (7.6 cm) in diameter.*

- Check the patient's exposed skin for redness or irritation, and observe the patient for pain or discomfort caused by hot spots (pressure-sensitive areas under the cast). Also be alert for a foul odor. These signs and symptoms suggest a pressure ulcer or infection.
- To relieve itching, set a handheld hair dryer on "cool." Then blow air under the cast.
- Warn the patient and his parents not to insert any object (such as a ruler, coat hanger, or knitting needle) into the cast to relieve itching by scratching because these objects could disrupt the suture line, break adjacent skin, and introduce infection. Also, be vigilant in ensuring that small objects or food particles don't become lodged under the cast and cause skin breakdown and infection.
- Encourage the patient's family to visit and participate in his care and recreation. This increases the patient's sense of security and enhances the parents' sense of participation and control.

SPECIAL CONSIDERATIONS

◆ If the patient is incontinent (or not toilet-trained), protect the cast from soiling. Tuck a folded disposable diaper or perineal pad around the perineal edges of the cast. Then apply a second diaper to the patient, over the top of the cast, to hold the first diaper in place. Also tuck plastic petals into the cast to channel urine and feces into a bedpan.

■ **TROUBLESHOOTER** *If the cast still becomes soiled, wipe it with a nonabrasive cleaner and a damp sponge or cloth. Then air-dry it with a hair dryer set on "cool."*

◆ Keep a cast cutter or saw available at all times to remove the cast quickly in case of an emergency.

◆ During mealtimes, position older children on their abdomens to promote safer eating and swallowing.

◆ Before removing the cast, reassure the parents and the patient that the noisy sawing process is painless. If necessary, explain how the saw works.

COMPLICATIONS

◆ Constipation, urinary stasis, kidney stones, skin breakdown, respiratory compromise, and contractures due to immobility (Frequent turnings, range-of-motion exercises, incentive spirometry, and adequate hydration and nutrition can minimize complications.)

PATIENT TEACHING

◆ Before discharge, teach the parents how to care for the cast, and give them an opportunity to demonstrate their understanding.

◆ Include instructions for checking circulatory status, recognizing signs of circulatory impairment, and notifying the physician.

◆ Also demonstrate to the parents how to turn the patient, apply moleskin, clean the cast, and ensure adequate nourishment.

◆ Teach the parents to treat dry, scaly skin around the cast by washing the patient's skin frequently. After the cast is removed, they may apply baby oil or other lotion to soothe the skin. Urge them to schedule and keep all follow-up medical appointments.

◆ Teach the parents how to use a car restraint device, such as the E-Z-ON Vest, because the child won't be able to use a conventional car seat.

DOCUMENTATION

◆ Record the date and time of cast care.

◆ Describe circulatory status in the patient's legs, and record measurements of any bleeding or drainage.

◆ Note the condition of the cast and the patient's skin.

◆ Describe all skin care given.

◆ Record findings of bowel and bladder assessments.

◆ Note patient and family tolerance of the cast.

◆ Document patient- and family-teaching topics discussed as well.

SELECTED REFERENCES

Flynn, J.M. "Early Application of Hip Spica Led to Higher Malunion Rates in Pediatric Femoral Fracture," *Journal of Bone and Joint Surgery* (American Volume) 87(8):1891, August 2005.

Kiter, E., et al. "A New Technique for Creating an Abdominal Window in a Hip Spica Cast," *Journal of Orthopaedic Trauma* 17(6):442-43, July 2003.

Rebello, G., et al. "Connecting Bar for Hip Spica Reinforcement: Does it Help?" *Journal of Pediatric Orthopaedics B* 13(5):345-46, September 2004.

Song, K.S., and Kim, H.K. "Femoral Neck Fracture in a Child with Autosomal-Dominant Osteopetrosis: Failure of Spica Cast Treatment and Successful Outcome by Internal Fixation," *Journal of Orthopaedic Trauma* 19(7):494-97, August 2005.

Wright, J.G., et al. "Treatments for Paediatric Femoral Fractures: A Randomised Trial," *Lancet* 365(9465):1153-58, March-April 2005.

Humidifiers

DESCRIPTION

- Humidifiers prevent drying and irritation of an inflamed upper airway, such as with croup or when secretions are thick and tenacious.
- Some humidifiers heat the water vapor, which raises the moisture-carrying capacity of gas and increases the amount of humidity delivered to the patient.
- Room humidifiers add humidity to an entire room, while humidifiers added to gas lines humidify only air being delivered to the patient.

CONTRAINDICATIONS

- None known

EQUIPMENT

Humidifier ◆ sterile distilled water, or tap water if unit has a demineralizing capability container for waste water ◆ bleach ◆ white vinegar

PREPARATION

Bedside humidifier

- Open the reservoir and add sterile distilled water to the fill line, and then close the reservoir.
- Keep all windows and doors closed to maintain adequate humidification.
- Plug the unit into the electrical outlet. Steam should soon rise.

Heated vaporizer

- Remove the top and fill the reservoir to the fill line with tap water.
- Replace the top securely.
- Place the vaporizer about 4' (1.1 m) from the patient, directing the steam toward but not directly onto the patient.
- To avoid hot water burns, place unit in a spot where it can't be overturned.

   AGE FACTOR *Making sure the unit is stable is especially important if children will be in the room.*

- Close all windows and doors to maintain adequate humidification.
- Plug the unit into an electrical outlet. Steam should soon rise.

Diffusion head humidifier

- Unscrew the humidifier reservoir; add sterile distilled water to proper level.
- If using a disposable unit, screw the cap with the extension onto the top of the unit. Screw the reservoir back onto the humidifier and attach the flowmeter to the oxygen source.
- Screw the humidifier onto the flowmeter until the seal is tight. Set the flowmeter at 2 L/minute and check for bubbling.
- Check the positive-pressure release valve by occluding the end valve on the humidifier. Pressure should back up into the humidifier, signaled by a high-pitched whistle. If this doesn't occur, tighten all connections and try again.

Cascade bubble diffusion humidifier

- Unscrew the cascade reservoir and add sterile distilled water to the fill line.
- Screw the top back onto the reservoir.
- Plug in the heater unit, and set the temperature between 95° and 100.4° F (35° and 38° C).

- Make sure the humidifier or vaporizer has been prepared properly.

BEDSIDE HUMIDIFIER

- Direct the humidifier unit's nozzle away from the patient's face (but toward the patient) for effective treatment.
- Check for mist emission from the nozzle, which indicates proper operation.
- Check the unit every 4 hours for proper operation; check water level every 8 hours.
- When refilling, unplug the unit, discard any old water, wipe with a disinfectant, rinse the reservoir container, and refill with sterile distilled water as necessary.
- Keep the unit cleaned and refilled with sterile water to reduce risk of bacterial growth.
- Replace the unit every 7 days; send used units for proper decontamination.

HEATED VAPORIZER

- Check unit every 4 hours for proper functioning.
- If steam production seems insufficient, unplug the unit, discard water, and refill with half distilled water and half tap water or clean the unit well.
- Check the water level every 8 hours.
- To refill, unplug the unit, discard old water, wipe with a disinfectant, rinse the reservoir container, and refill with tap water.

DIFFUSION HEAD HUMIDIFIER

- Attach the oxygen delivery device to the humidifier, and then to the patient.
- Adjust the flowmeter to the appropriate oxygen flow rate.
- Check the reservoir every 4 hours.
- If the water level drops too low, empty the remaining water, rinse the jar, and refill with sterile water.
- As the water level decreases, evaporation of water in the gas decreases, reducing humidification of delivered gas.

- Change the humidification system regularly to prevent bacterial growth.
- Periodically check patient's sputum; if it's too thick, it can hinder mobilization and expectoration. If this occurs, the patient needs a device that can provide higher humidity.

CASCADE BUBBLE DIFFUSION HUMIDIFIER

- Check the temperature of inspired gas near the patient's airway every 2 hours when used in critical care; every 4 hours when used in general patient care.
- If the cascade becomes too hot, drain water and replace.

⚡ **WARNING** *Overheated water vapor can cause respiratory tract burns.*

- Check the water level every 2 to 4 hours, and fill as necessary.
- If water level falls below the minimum water level mark, humidity will decrease to that of room air.
- Be alert for condensation buildup in the tubing, which can result from high humidification produced by the cascade.
- Check tubing frequently and empty condensate as necessary so it can't drain into the patient's respiratory tract, encourage growth of microorganisms, or obstruct dependent sections of tubing. To do so, disconnect tubing, drain condensate into a container, and dispose properly.
- Never drain the condensate into the humidification system.
- Change the cascade regularly according to facility policy.

SPECIAL CONSIDERATIONS

- Because it creates a humidity level comparable to ambient air, the diffusion head humidifier is only used for oxygen flow rates greater than 4 L/minute.
- The bedside humidifier doesn't deliver a precise amount of humidification; assess patient regularly to determine effectiveness of therapy. Ask him if he feels any improvement and evaluate his sputum.
- The heated vaporizer doesn't deliver a precise amount of humidification; assess patient regularly by asking if he feels better and checking his sputum.
- An unclean humidifier can cause or aggravate respiratory problems, especially for people allergic to molds.
- Refer to facility policy for changing and disposing of equipment.

COMPLICATIONS

- Aspiration of tubal condensation (with cascade humidifiers)
- Pulmonary burns if air is heated

PATIENT TEACHING

- Make sure the patient and his family understand the reason for using a humidifier and know how to use the equipment.
- Give the patient specific, written guidelines on home care.
- Instruct the patient using a bedside humidifier at home to fill it with plain tap water and periodically use distilled water to prevent mineral buildup.
- Advise the patient to run white vinegar through a bedside humidifier or heated vaporizer to clean the unit, prevent bacterial buildup, and dissolve deposits.

DOCUMENTATION

- Record the date and time humidification started and stopped.
- Note the type of humidifier.
- Document flow rate (of a gas system).
- Note thermometer readings (if heated).
- Record complications and nursing action taken.
- Document the patient's reaction to humidification.

SELECTED REFERENCES

Moran, I., et al. "Heat and Moisture Exchanges and Heated Humidifiers in Acute Lung Injury/Acute Respiratory Distress Syndrome Patients. Effects on Respiratory Mechanics and Gas Exchange," *Intensive Care Medicine* 32(4):524-31, April 2006.

Scolnik, D., et al. "Controlled Delivery of High vs. Low Humidity vs. Mist Tent Therapy for Croup In Emergency Departments: A Randomized Controlled Trial," *JAMA* 295(11):1274-80, March 2006.

Hydrotherapy

OVERVIEW

DESCRIPTION

- Hydrotherapy is commonly used to debride serious burns, hasten healing, and promote circulation and comfort in patients with peripheral vascular disease and musculoskeletal disorders.
- It usually involves immersing the patient in a tub of water ("tubbing"). Showers or other water-spray techniques are used in some hospitals and burn centers. (See *Positioning the patient for hydrotherapy*.)
- The nurse or physical therapist assists the patient into the tub or shower area if he's ambulatory. If he isn't ambulatory, he can be put in the water using a stretcher or hoist device.

CONTRAINDICATIONS

- Fever
- Electrolyte or fluid imbalance
- Unstable vital signs

EQUIPMENT

Water tank or tub or shower table ◆ plastic tub liner ◆ chemical additives, as ordered ◆ plinth (padded table for patient to sit or lie on) ◆ stretcher ◆ headrest ◆ hydraulic hoist ◆ gown ◆ cap ◆ mask ◆ gloves (for removing dressings) ◆ shoulder-length gloves (for tubbing) ◆ apron ◆ debridement instruments ◆ razor, shaving cream, mild soap, shampoo, and washcloth (for general cleaning) ◆ fluffed gauze pads ◆ cotton-tipped applicators ◆ sterile sheets ◆ warm, sterile bath blankets ◆ analgesic (optional)

PREPARATION

- Barriers, sheets, and bath blankets may be sterile or clean, depending on patient's condition and facility infection-control policies.
- Thoroughly clean and disinfect the tub or shower, its equipment, and the tub or shower room before each treatment to prevent cross-contamination.
- After cleaning, place the tub liner in the tub and fill the tub with warm water (98° to 104° F [36.7° to 40° C]).
- Attach the headrest to sides of the tub. Add prescribed chemicals to water to maintain normal isotonic level and prevent dialysis and tissue irritation.
- Add potassium chloride to prevent potassium loss and calcium hypochlorite detergent, as ordered.
- Warm the bath blankets and ensure that the room is warm enough to prevent chills.

KEY STEPS

- Confirm the patient's identity using two patient identifiers according to facility policy.
- As necessary, administer an analgesic 20 minutes before the procedure.
- Check the patient's vital signs.
- If he's receiving an I.V. infusion, make sure there's enough solution to last through the procedure.
- Transfer him to a stretcher and transport him to the therapy room or, if he's ambulatory and the room is nearby, assist him in walking.
- Wash your hands and put on gown, gloves, mask, and surgical cap.
- Remove outer dressings and dispose of them properly before immersing the patient.
- Leave inner gauze layers on wounds unless they can be easily removed.
- If he's ambulatory, position him on the plinth for transfer to the tub, or assist him into the tub and situate him on the already-lowered plinth.
- If he isn't ambulatory, attach the stretcher to the overhead hydraulic hoist.
- Ensure that the hoist hooks are fastened securely. Use the hoist to transfer the patient to and from the tub.
- Lower the patient into the tub.
- Position him so that the headrest supports his head.
- Allow him to soak for 3 to 5 minutes.
- Remove your gloves, wash your hands, and put on the shoulder-length tubbing gloves and apron.
- Remove any remaining gauze dressings from the patient's wounds.
- If ordered, place the tub's agitator into the water and turn it on.

    WARNING *The motor may burn out if it's turned on out of the water. Some tubs have aerators to agitate the water.*

- Clean all unburned areas first. Encourage the patient to do this if he can.
- Wash unburned skin, and clip or shave hair near the wound.
- Shave facial hair, shampoo the scalp, and give mouth care, as appropriate.

- Provide perineal care, and clean inside the patient's nose and the folds of the ears and eyes with cotton-tipped applicators.
- Gently scrub burned areas with fluffed gauze pads to remove topical agents, exudates, necrotic tissue, and other debris.
- Debride the wound after turning off the agitator.
- Exercise the patient's extremities with active or passive range of motion, depending on his condition and tolerance. You may have the physical therapist exercise the patient.
- After treatment, use the hoist to raise the patient above the water.
- With the patient still suspended over the water, spray-rinse his body to remove debris from shaving, cleaning, and debridement.
- Transfer him to a stretcher covered with a clean sheet and bath blanket, and cover him with a warm sterile sheet (a blanket may be added for warmth).
- Pat unburned areas dry to prevent chilling.
- Remove the wet or damp sheets, and cover the patient with dry sheets.
- Remove your gown, gloves, and mask before transporting the patient to the dressing area for further debridement, if needed, and new sterile dressings.
- Have the tub drained, cleaned, and disinfected according to facility policy.

WARNING *Remain with the patient at all times to prevent an accident in the tub.*
- Limit hydrotherapy to 20 or 30 minutes.
- Watch the patient closely for adverse reactions.
- A patient with an endotracheal tube may receive hydrotherapy. Spray his wounds while he's suspended over the tub on a plinth.
- Immerse a patient with a long-standing tracheostomy only with a physician's order.
- If needed, weigh the patient during hydrotherapy to assess nutritional status and fluid shifts. Use a hoist that has a table scale.
- Whirlpool treatments should be discontinued when wounds are assessed as clean; the whirlpool's agitating water may cause trauma to regenerating tissue.

COMPLICATIONS
- Infection due to incomplete disinfection of tub, drains, and faucets or cross-contamination from members of the tubbing team
- Chills from decreased resistance to temperature changes
- Fluid and electrolyte imbalance from a chemical imbalance between the patient and the tub solution

- Before the patient's first hydrotherapy session, explain the procedure to allay fears and promote cooperation.

- Record the date and time of procedures.
- Note the patient's reaction.
- Note the patient's condition (vital signs and wound appearance).
- Document wound infection or bleeding.
- Note treatments given, such as debridement and dressing changes.
- Record special treatments in the care plan.

SELECTED REFERENCES
Fiscus, K.A., et al. "Changes in Lower-Leg Blood Flow During Warm-, Cold-, and Contrast-Water Therapy," *Archives of Physical Medicine and Rehabilitation* 86(7):1404-10, July 2005.

Lazarov, A., et al. "Self-Reported Skin Disease in Hydrotherapists Working in Swimming Pools," *Contact Dermatitis* 53(6):327-31, December 2005.

Taylor, S. "The Ventilated Patient Undergoing Hydrotherapy: A Case Study," *Australian Critical Care* 16(3):111-15, August 2003.

Vitorino, D.F., et al. "Hydrotherapy and Conventional Physiotherapy Improve Total Sleep Time and Quality of Life of Fibromyalgia Patients: Randomized Clinical Trial," *Sleep Medicine* 7(3):293-96, April 2006.

Positioning the patient for hydrotherapy

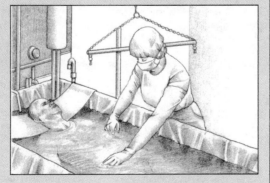

Immerse the patient in a tub or Hubbard tank (as shown). Alternatively, you may spray his wounds with water as he lies on a special shower table. Hydrotherapy is traumatic and painful for the burn patient. Provide continual support and encouragement.

Hyperthermia-hypothermia blanket

OVERVIEW

DESCRIPTION

- The procedure is used to raise, lower, or maintain body temperature through conductive heat or cold transfer between the blanket and the patient.
- Used manually, the temperature on the unit is set and the blanket reaches and maintains a temperature independent of the patient's temperature.
- For automatic use, the patient's temperature is monitored by thermistor probe (rectal, skin, or esophageal) and the unit alternates heating and cooling to achieve and maintain desired body temperature.
- The procedure is used most often to reduce high fever when baths, ice packs, and antipyretics are unsuccessful.
- The procedure is also used to maintain normal temperature during surgery or shock; induce hypothermia during surgery to decrease metabolic activity and thereby reduce oxygen requirements; reduce intracranial pressure; control bleeding and intractable pain in patients with amputations, burns, or cancer; and provide warmth in cases of severe hypothermia.

CONTRAINDICATIONS

- None known

EQUIPMENT

Hyperthermia-hypothermia control unit ◆ operation manual ◆ fluid for control unit (distilled water with or without 20% ethyl alcohol) ◆ thermistor probe (rectal, skin, or esophageal) ◆ patient thermometer ◆ one or two hyperthermia-hypothermia blankets ◆ one or two disposable blanket covers, sheets, or bath blankets ◆ lanolin or a mixture of lanolin and cold cream ◆ adhesive tape ◆ towel ◆ sphygmomanometer ◆ gloves and gowns, if necessary ◆ protective wraps for the patient's hands and feet (optional)

PREPARATION

- Read the operation manual.
- Wash your hands.
- Inspect the control unit and blankets for leaks and the plugs and connecting wires for broken prongs, kinks, or fraying.
- Disposable hyperthermia-hypothermia blankets are available for single-patient use.

WARNING *If you detect or suspect malfunction, don't use equipment.*

- Prepare one or two blankets by covering them with disposable covers (or use a sheet or bath blanket when positioning the blanket on the patient) to absorb perspiration and condensation and prevent tissue breakdown.
- Connect the blanket to the control unit and set controls for manual or automatic operation and for ordered blanket or body temperature.
- Make sure the machine is properly grounded before plugging it in.
- Turn on the machine; add liquid to the unit reservoir, if necessary, as fluid fills the blanket.
- Allow blanket to preheat or precool so patient receives immediate thermal benefit.

KEY STEPS

- Confirm the patient's identity using two patient identifiers according to facility policy.
- Explain the procedure.
- Make sure signed consent has been obtained.
- Make sure room is warm and free from drafts.
- Help the patient into a hospital gown with cloth ties.
- Take vital signs and assess level of consciousness, pupil reaction, limb strength, and skin condition.
- Keeping the bottom sheet in place and patient recumbent, roll him to one side; slide the blanket halfway underneath him so its top edge aligns with his neck.
- Roll him back, and pull and flatten the blanket across the bed.
- Place a pillow under his head.
- Make sure his head doesn't lie directly on the blanket; its rigid surface may be uncomfortable and cause tissue breakdown.
- Use a sheet or bath blanket as insulation between the patient and blanket, as needed.
- Apply lanolin or cold cream to his skin where it touches the blanket to help protect the skin from heat or cold sensation.
- In automatic operation, insert the thermistor probe in his rectum and tape it in place.
- If rectal insertion is contraindicated, tuck a skin probe deep into the axilla, and secure with tape.
- If he's comatose or anesthetized, an esophageal probe may be inserted.
- Plug the other end of the probe into the unit's control panel.
- Place a sheet or, if ordered, the second hyperthermia-hypothermia blanket over the patient, increasing thermal benefit by trapping cooled or heated air.
- Wrap his hands and feet to minimize chilling and promote comfort.
- Monitor vital signs and neurologic activity every 5 minutes until desired body temperature is reached, then every 15 minutes until temperature is stable.
- Check fluid intake and output hourly or as ordered.
- Watch for color changes in skin, lips, and nail beds and for edema, induration, inflammation, pain, or sensory impairment; if these occur, discontinue the procedure and notify the physician.
- Reposition the patient every 30 minutes to 1 hour, unless contraindicated.
- Keep his skin, bedclothes, and blanket cover free from perspiration and condensation.
- Some units must remain plugged in for at least 30 minutes after use to allow the condenser fan to remove water vapor from the mechanism; follow the manufacturer's guidelines.
- Continue to monitor his temperature until it stabilizes; body temperature can fall as much as 5° F (2.8° C) after this procedure.

- Remove equipment.
- Dry the patient and make him comfortable.
- Supply a fresh gown, if needed, and cover him lightly.
- Continue checking neurologic function, vital signs, fluid intake and output, and general condition every 30 minutes for 2 hours, then hourly or as ordered.
- Return equipment to central supply for cleaning, servicing, and storage.

SPECIAL CONSIDERATIONS

- If the patient shivers excessively during treatment, discontinue and notify the practitioner immediately.

Using a warming system

Shivering, the compensatory response to falling body temperature, may use more oxygen than the body can supply, especially in a surgical patient. In the past, the caregiver would cover the patient with blankets to warm his body. Now, hospitals may supply a warming system such as the Bair Hugger patient-warming system.

This system helps to gradually increase body temperature. Like a large hair dryer, the warming unit draws air through a filter, warms the air to the desired temperature, and circulates it through a hose to a warming blanket placed over the patient.

When using the warming system, be sure to:
- use a bath blanket in a single layer over the warming blanket to minimize heat loss
- place the warming blanket directly over the patient with the paper side facing down and the clear tubular side facing up
- make sure the connection hose is at the foot of the bed
- take the patient's temperature during the first 15 to 30 minutes and at least every 30 minutes while the warming blanket is in use
- obtain guidelines from the patient's physician for discontinuing use of the warming blanket.

⚠ **WARNING** *Shivering increases tissue oxygen demand and may lead to mixed venous desaturation, lactic acidosis, and ischemia of vital organs.*

✿ **AGE FACTOR** *Elderly patients who have diminished cardiopulmonary reserves are particularly at risk for complications related to shivering.*

- Avoid lowering the temperature more than 1° F (0.6° C) every 15 minutes to prevent premature ventricular contractions.
- To prevent punctures, don't use pins to secure catheters, tubes, or blanket covers.
- With hyperthermia or hypothermia therapy a secondary defense reaction may occur, causing body temperature to rebound and negate the treatment.
- If patient requires isolation, use a disposable blanket or put a nondisposable blanket, blanket cover, and probe in a plastic bag marked with the type of isolation so central supply can give it special handling.
- To avoid bacterial growth in the reservoir or blankets, use sterile distilled water and change it monthly.
- Check if facility policy calls for adding a bacteriostatic agent to the water.
- Avoid using deionized water; it can corrode the system.
- To gradually increase body temperature, especially in postoperative patients, the physician may order a disposable blanket warming system. (See *Using a warming system.*)
- The control unit is equipped with an alarm to warn of abnormal temperature fluctuations and a circuit breaker that protects against current overload.

COMPLICATIONS

- Shivering
- Marked changes in vital signs
- Increased intracranial pressure
- Respiratory distress or arrest
- Cardiac arrest
- Oliguria; anuria
- Increased tissue oxygen demand

PATIENT TEACHING

- Explain to the patient the reason for procedure and what to expect.
- Tell the patient signs and symptoms to report.
- Explain to the patient the need for frequent monitoring and position changes.

DOCUMENTATION

- Record the date, time, and duration of treatment.
- Note type of hyperthermia-hypothermia unit used.
- Document control settings (manual or automatic and temperature settings).
- Note the patient's tolerance.
- Note complications and actions taken.
- Document pulse, respirations, blood pressure, neurologic signs, fluid intake and output, and skin condition.
- Note frequency of position changes.
- Record the patient's and blanket's temperature every 30 minutes.

SELECTED REFERENCES

"A Reusable, Custom-Made Warming Blanket Prevents Core Hypothermia During Major Neonatal Surgery," *Survey of Anesthesiology* 47(3):157-58, June 2003.

Loke, A.Y., et al. "Comparing the Effectiveness of Two Types of Cooling Blankets for Febrile Patients," *Nursing in Critical Care* 10(5):247-54, September-October 2005.

Mayer, S.A., et al. "Clinical Trial of a Novel Surface Cooling System for Fever Control in Neurocritical Care Patients," *Critical Care Medicine* 32(12):2508-15, December 2004.

Singer, A.J., et al. "The Effect of a Commercially Available Burn-Cooling Blanket on Core Body Temperatures in Volunteers," *Academic Emergency Medicine* 13(6):686-90, June 2006.

Impaired swallowing and aspiration precautions

OVERVIEW

DESCRIPTION
- Impaired swallowing and aspiration may result from several problems.
- Oropharyngeal dysphagia carries high risk of aspiration.
- Aspiration can occur with esophageal dysphagia.
- Impaired swallowing can occur with tracheostomy or ventilation support.

CONTRAINDICATIONS
- None known

EQUIPMENT

Meal tray ◆ call bell ◆ wall suction or portable suction apparatus suction kit ◆ gloves ◆ protective eyewear ◆ pulse oximeter

KEY STEPS

- Confirm the patient's identity using two patient identifiers according to facility policy.
- Explain the procedure to the patient and his family.
- Wash your hands and put on gloves and protective eyewear before suctioning the patient or providing mouth care.
- Set up meal tray, and position the patient properly for eating.
- For all procedures, monitor the patient for signs and symptoms of aspiration.

MANAGING IMPAIRED SWALLOWING DUE TO OROPHARYNGEAL DYSPHAGIA
- Assist with a bedside swallow evaluation (usually conducted by a speech-language pathologist).
- Develop a management plan that includes common swallowing strategies, nutritional status, and supervision.

USING COMMON SWALLOWING STRATEGIES
- Have suction equipment available at the bedside.
- Position the patient at 90-degree angle during meals to decrease aspiration risk.
- Have the patient sit up for 30 minutes after meals.
- Provide oral care before and after meals; be sure to check for food residue.
- Crush drugs, as appropriate, and mix in applesauce.
- Avoid mixed consistencies, such as combining soft food with solid food.
- Avoid straws. Encourage small sips.
- If applicable, make sure that the temperature, consistency, and amount of foods and liquids are appropriate. Water should be chilled; avoid tepid liquids or food.
- Minimize distractions when the patient is eating and drinking.
- If applicable, make sure that dentures are in place and fit well.
- If one side of the patient's face is paralyzed, place food on the unaffected side. Check the affected side of the mouth for food that may lodge in the cheek during meals. If appropriate, teach him to perform a finger-sweep.
- If fatigue impairs swallowing, provide rest periods before and during meals.
- Assess swallowing between bites by feeling the rise and fall of the larynx.
- Use cold or sour foods and massage the cheeks or throat to stimulate swallowing.

USING ONE-ON-ONE SUPERVISION
- Make sure that someone remains with the patient throughout every meal.
- Provide feeding assistance or cueing for feeding and swallowing strategies during the entire meal. Encourage the patient to take 30 to 45 minutes to eat; patients with dysphagia need to eat slowly.

USING CLOSE SUPERVISION
- Check on the patient often during meals; remind him to use swallowing strategies.

- Encourage the patient to increase intake, if needed, and provide other options to maximize safety and nutritional intake.
- Keep the call bell within the patient's reach.

USING DISTANT SUPERVISION
- Provide initial cueing to start swallowing strategies.
- Check on the patient frequently.
- Assess the patient's progress at least two to three times during meals.
- Keep the call bell within the patient's reach.

MANAGING IMPAIRED SWALLOWING DUE TO ESOPHAGEAL DYSPHAGIA
- Monitor for reflux and aspiration risks related to esophageal dysphagia.
- Perform a bedside swallow evaluation to assist with a differential diagnosis of oropharyngeal versus esophageal dysphagia.
- Consult with a speech-language pathologist in determining alternative nutrition.

  WARNING Monitor respiratory rate, depth, and lung sounds for cough, dyspnea, cyanosis, crackles, or wheezes that may indicate aspiration and airway obstruction.
- Monitor bowel sounds and assess for abdominal distention.

  WARNING Absence of bowel sounds and increasing abdominal distention may indicate an ileus or bowel obstruction with resulting vomiting and risk of aspiration.
- Monitor the patient's intake and output, and daily weight. Weight loss may indicate an esophageal problem.
- Implement strategies for oral intake.
- Position the patient at a 90-degree angle during oral feeding; maintain this position for 45 to 60 minutes after a meal to decrease reflux, regurgitation, and aspiration.
- Offer thin liquids and pureed and moist foods that may be easier to swallow if esophageal dysmotility exists.

- Feed the patient slowly; allow adequate time for esophageal emptying.
- If the patient feels full quickly, offer small, frequent meals of high-calorie foods.
- Alternate liquids and solids to improve esophageal emptying of solids.
- Avoid spicy and acidic foods and lessen caffeine use to decrease reflux.
- Tell the patient to avoid eating before bed, and keep the head of his bed elevated above a 30-degree angle at night.

MANAGING THE PATIENT WITH A FEEDING TUBE

- Initiate a dietary consult.
- Provide oral care for the patient who's on nothing-by-mouth status to decrease bacteria in the mouth if he's at risk for secretion aspiration.
- Ensure accurate placement of a feeding tube by X-ray.
- Assess placement of the feeding tube before feeding and every 4 hours for a patient with a continuous feeding.
- Aspirate contents from the tube; examine the aspirate and place a small amount on a pH test strip. The probability of gastric placement is increased if the aspirate has a typical gastric fluid appearance (grassy-green, clear and colorless with mucus shreds, or brown) and the pH is less than or equal to 5.
- If assessment indicates the possibility of feeding solution in mucus coughed or suctioned from trachea, test the mucus for glucose. A positive result may indicate tube displacement and aspiration of feeding solution.
- Assess gastric residual amounts before feedings and at least every 4 hours for the patient with continuous feeding.

  WARNING *If the amount aspirated is greater than 100 ml, follow facility policy for withholding feeding. Retained feeding solution can increase intragastric pressure and risk for regurgitation and aspiration.*

- Keep the patient in semi-Fowler's position (at least 30 degrees) during feedings and for 30 to 45 minutes afterward.

MANAGING IMPAIRED SWALLOWING CAUSED BY TRACHEOSTOMIES OR ENDOTRACHEAL TUBES

- Request a referral for a speech-language pathologist for a bedside swallow evaluation before beginning feeding if risk of aspiration is likely.
- Suction the patient every 2 hours or as needed to maintain a patent airway.
- Get a practitioner's order for speaking valve trials and blue dye testing, as appropriate.
- Follow speech therapy and practitioner recommendations on cuff inflation versus deflation for oral intake. The patient may still be able to aspirate around an inflated cuff.

CONDUCTING THE BLUE DYE TEST

- Suction the patient after the speech-language pathologist has given him a once-daily food or fluid tinged with blue dye.
- Note the presence or absence of blue dye around the tracheostomy or in the suction catheter immediately after oral intake and throughout the day.
- Absence of blue dye indicates the patient may be ready for a modified barium swallow test preceding oral intake. The blue dye test is accurate only to test for gross aspiration.

SPECIAL CONSIDERATIONS

- Airway obstruction and aspiration may occur more often during meals.

COMPLICATIONS

- Pneumonitis or pneumonia due to aspiration
- Decreased oral intake, leading to dehydration and malnutrition due to difficulty swallowing

PATIENT TEACHING

- Train and supervise the patient's family to feed the patient as needed.
- Encourage slow intake with adequate chewing.
- Teach the patient's family how to perform the abdominal thrust maneuver and how to use suction equipment as needed.
- Praise the patient for achieving nutritional goals.

DOCUMENTATION

- Record the amount of intake.
- Note the patient's food preferences.
- Document the patient's progress with meals.
- Record techniques effective in helping swallowing.
- Document the effectiveness of family teaching.
- Note complications and interventions taken.

SELECTED REFERENCES

Brookes, J.T., et al. "Prospective Randomized Trial Comparing the Effect of Early Suturing of Tracheostomy Sites on Postoperative Patient Swallowing and Rehabilitation," *Journal of Otolaryngology* 35(2):77-82, April 2006.

Ramsey, D., et al. "Silent Aspiration: What Do We Know?" *Dysphagia* 20(3):218-25, Summer 2005.

Smith Hammond, C.A., and Goldstein, L.B. "Cough and Aspiration of Food and Liquids Due to Oral-Pharyngeal Dysphagia: ACCP Evidence-Based Clinical Practice Guidelines," *Chest* 129(Suppl 1):154S-68S, January 2006.

Terre, R., and Mearin, F. "Oropharyngeal Dysphagia after the Acute Phase of Stroke: Predictors of Aspiration," *Neurogastroenterology and Motility* 18(3):200-205, March 2006.

Yoshikawa, M., et al. "Influence of Aging and Denture Use on Liquid Swallowing in Healthy Dentulous and Edentulous Older People," *Journal of the American Geriatrics Society* 54(3):444-49, March 2006.

Incentive spirometry

DESCRIPTION

♦ Incentive spirometry encourages deep breathing by providing visual feedback to the patient while measuring respiratory flow or volume.
♦ The procedure increases lung volume, boosts alveolar inflation, and promotes venous return. It hyperinflates the alveoli, preventing and reversing alveolar collapse that causes atelectasis and pneumonitis.
♦ The procedure is used for patients at low risk for developing atelectasis. Patients at high risk need a volume incentive spirometer, which measures lung inflation more precisely.
♦ The procedure benefits a patient on prolonged bed rest, especially a postoperative patient who may regain normal respiration slowly due to abdominal or thoracic surgery, advanced age, inactivity, obesity, smoking, and decreased ability to cough effectively and expel lung secretions.
♦ Presence of an open tracheal stoma requires the adaptation of a spirometer.

CONTRAINDICATIONS

♦ Patients unable to cooperate or properly use the device
♦ Patients unable to deep-breathe effectively

Flow or volume incentive spirometer, as indicated, with sterile disposable tube and mouthpiece (the tube and mouthpiece are sterile on first use and clean on subsequent uses) ♦ stethoscope ♦ watch ♦ pencil ♦ paper

PREPARATION

♦ Wash your hands.
♦ Assemble equipment at the patient's bedside.
♦ Attach the sterile flow tube and mouthpiece to the device.
♦ Set the flow rate or volume goal as determined by the practitioner and based on the patient's preoperative performance.

♦ Confirm the patient's identity using two patient identifiers according to facility policy.
♦ Assess the patient's condition.
♦ Explain the procedure to the patient.
♦ Help the patient into a comfortable sitting or semi-Fowler's position to promote optimal lung expansion.

⚡ **WARNING** *Tilting a flow incentive spirometer decreases the required patient effort and reduces the exercise's effectiveness.*

♦ Auscultate the patient's lungs to provide a baseline for comparison with posttreatment auscultation.
♦ Instruct the patient to insert the mouthpiece and close his lips tightly around it.
♦ Tell the patient to exhale normally, then inhale as slowly and deeply as possible.
♦ Ask the patient to retain the entire volume of air he inhaled for 3 seconds or, if using a device with a light indicator, until the light turns off.
♦ Note the tidal volume.
♦ Tell the patient to remove the mouthpiece and exhale normally.
♦ Allow the patient to relax and take several normal breaths before attempting another breath with the spirometer.
♦ Repeat this sequence 5 to 10 times during every waking hour.
♦ Encourage the patient to cough after each effort because deep lung inflation may loosen secretions and facilitate their removal. Observe expectorated secretions.
♦ Auscultate the patient's lungs, and compare findings with the first auscultation.
♦ Instruct the patient to remove the mouthpiece, wash it in warm water, and shake it dry.
♦ Place the mouthpiece in a plastic storage bag between exercises, and label it and the spirometer with the patient's name.
♦ After completing the exercise, compute the volume by multiplying the setting by the duration the patient kept the ball (or balls) suspended.

- When using a volume incentive spirometer, take the volume reading directly from the spirometer. For example, record 1,000 cc × 5 breaths.

SPECIAL CONSIDERATIONS

- If the patient is scheduled for surgery, make a preoperative assessment of his respiratory pattern and capability to ensure development of appropriate postoperative goals.
- Teach the patient how to use the spirometer preoperatively so he can concentrate on your instructions and practice the exercise.
- To prevent nausea, avoid exercising the patient at mealtime.
- Provide paper and pencil so the patient can note exercise times and volumes.
- Immediately after surgery, encourage the patient to use the exercise frequently to ensure compliance and enable assessment of his achievement.

COMPLICATIONS
- Hyperventilation
- Increased surgical pain
- Nausea
- Barotrauma (emphysematous lungs)
- Hypoxemia secondary to interruption of prescribed oxygen therapy
- Exacerbation of bronchospasm
- Fatigue

PATIENT TEACHING

- Explain the purpose of incentive spirometry and how to use the device.
- Explain the importance of recording exercise times and volumes, so the patient can see improvement.
- Explain the importance of performing exercise regularly to maintain alveolar inflation.

DOCUMENTATION

- Note preoperative teaching.
- Document preoperative flow or volume levels.
- Record the date and time of procedure, type of spirometer, flow or volume levels achieved, and number of breaths taken.
- Note the patient's condition before and after the procedure, his tolerance of the procedure, and results of both auscultations.

SELECTED REFERENCES
Basoglu, O.K., et al. "The Efficacy of Incentive Spirometry in Patients with COPD," *Respirology* 10(3):349-53, June 2005.

Hsu, L.L., et al. "Positive Expiratory Pressure Device Acceptance by Hospitalized Children with Sickle Cell Disease is Comparable to Incentive Spirometry," *Respiratory Care* 50(5):624-27, May 2005.

Ong, G.L. "Incentive Spirometry for Children with Sickle Cell Disorder," *Nursing Times* 101(42):55-57, October 2005.

Reardon, C.C., et al. "Intrapulmonary Percussive Ventilation vs. Incentive Spirometry for Children with Neuromuscular Disease," *Archives of Pediatrics & Adolescent Medicine* 159(6):526-31, June 2005.

Incontinence management

DESCRIPTION

◆ Treatment for urinary and fecal incontinence usually aims to control the condition through bladder or bowel retraining or behavior management techniques, diet modification, drug therapy, and possibly surgery.

URINARY INCONTINENCE

◆ Urinary incontinence results from confusion, dehydration, fecal impaction, restricted mobility, or urethral sphincter damage after prostatectomy or from drugs including diuretics, hypnotics, sedatives, anticholinergics, antihypertensives, and alpha antagonists.

◆ The condition may indicate prostatic hyperplasia, bladder calculus, bladder cancer, urinary tract infection (UTI), stroke, diabetic neuropathy, Guillain-Barré syndrome, multiple sclerosis, prostatic cancer, prostatitis, spinal cord injury, or urethral stricture.

◆ Chronic urinary incontinence includes four types: stress, caused by strain; overflow, from urine retention; urge, marked by uncontrollable impulse; and functional, which occurs despite a normally functioning bladder and urethra usually as result of mental impairment or lack of appropriate or timely care.

◆ Corrective surgery includes transurethral resection of prostate, repair of anterior vaginal wall or retropelvic suspension of the bladder, urethral sling, and bladder augmentation.

FECAL INCONTINENCE

◆ Fecal incontinence may occur gradually (as with dementia) or suddenly (as with spinal cord injury) because of fecal stasis and impaction with reduced activity, inappropriate diet, or untreated painful anal conditions.

◆ The condition also results from chronic laxative use; reduced fluid intake; neurologic deficit; pelvic, prostatic, or rectal surgery; and certain drugs, including antihistamines, psychotropics, and iron preparations.

CONTRAINDICATIONS

◆ None known

Bladder retraining record sheet ◆ gloves ◆ stethoscope (to assess bowel sounds) ◆ lubricant ◆ moisture barrier cream ◆ incontinence pads ◆ bedpan ◆ specimen container ◆ label ◆ laboratory request form ◆ stool collection kit, urinary catheter (optional)

◆ Confirm the patient's identity using two patient identifiers according to facility policy.

◆ For urinary or fecal incontinence, perform initial and continuing assessments to plan interventions.

◆ Protect the patient's bed with an incontinence pad.

URINARY INCONTINENCE

◆ Ask the patient when leakage started and if it began suddenly or gradually.

◆ Have the patient describe his typical urinary pattern and whether incontinence usually occurs at night or day.

◆ Have the patient rate his urinary control from moderate to no control.

◆ Evaluate related problems, such as urinary hesitancy, frequency, urgency, nocturia, and decreased force or interrupted urine stream.

◆ Have the patient describe previous treatment or self-treatment for incontinence.

◆ Ask about drugs the patient takes, including nonprescription drugs.

◆ Assess the patient's environment. Is a toilet or commode readily available and how long does it take to reach it?

◆ Assess the patient's manual dexterity in unbuttoning or unzipping.

◆ Evaluate the patient's mental status and cognitive function.

◆ Quantify the patient's normal daily fluid intake.

◆ Review the patient's history for drugs and foods that affect digestion and elimination.

◆ Review the patient's medical history, noting number and route of births, incidence of UTI, prostate disorders, spinal injury or tumor, stroke, and bladder, prostate, or pelvic surgery.

◆ Assess the patient for such disorders as delirium, dehydration, urine retention, restricted mobility, fecal impaction, infection, inflammation, or polyuria.

◆ Inspect the urethral meatus for inflammation or anatomic defects.

◆ Have a female patient bear down while you note urine leakage.

◆ Palpate the abdomen for bladder distention, which signals urine retention. If needed, have the patient examined by a urologist.

◆ Obtain urine specimens for laboratory tests.

◆ Label the specimen containers and send to the laboratory with a request form.

◆ Begin incontinence management by starting a bladder retraining program.

◆ To manage stress incontinence, start an exercise regimen to help strengthen the pelvic floor muscles. (See *Strengthening pelvic floor muscles*.)

◆ To manage functional incontinence, frequently assess the patient's mental and functional status.

◆ Regularly remind the patient to void.

◆ Respond to the patient's calls promptly, and help the patient get to the bathroom quickly.

◆ Provide positive reinforcement.

◆ To ensure hydration and prevent UTI, make sure the patient maintains adequate daily fluid intake.

◆ Restrict fluid intake after 6 p.m.

FECAL INCONTINENCE

◆ Ask the patient to identify onset, duration, severity, and pattern.

◆ Focus history on GI, neurologic, and psychological disorders.

- Note frequency, consistency, and volume of stool passed in last 24 hours.
- Obtain a stool specimen, if ordered.
- Assess for chronic constipation, GI and neurologic disorders, and laxative abuse.
- Inspect the patient's abdomen for distention and auscultate for bowel sounds.
- If not contraindicated, check for fecal impaction, using proper technique.
- Assess the patient's drug regimen.
- Check for use of drugs that may affect bowel activity.
- For the neurologically capable patient with chronic incontinence, provide bowel retraining.

SPECIAL CONSIDERATIONS

- The patient with urinary or fecal incontinence should be carefully assessed for underlying disorders.
- To rid the bladder of residual urine, teach the patient Valsalva's or Credé's maneuver or institute clean intermittent catheterization.
- Avoid using an indwelling urinary catheter because of the risk of UTI.
- For fecal incontinence, maintain effective hygienic care to increase comfort, prevent skin breakdown and infection, and control odors.
- Clean the perineal area frequently, and apply a moisture barrier cream.

COMPLICATIONS

- Skin breakdown and infection due to incontinence
- Psychological problems including social isolation, loss of independence, lowered self-esteem, and depression due to incontinence

PATIENT TEACHING

- Provide encouragement and support to help ease psychological distress.
- Advise the patient to consume a fiber-rich diet, with raw, leafy vegetables, unpeeled fruits, and whole grains.
- If the patient has a lactase deficiency, suggest calcium supplements to replace calcium lost by eliminating dairy products from the diet.
- Encourage adequate fluid intake.

Strengthening pelvic floor muscles

Stress incontinence, the most common kind of urinary incontinence in women, usually results from weakening of the urethral sphincter. In men, it may sometimes occur after a radical prostatectomy.

You can help a patient prevent or minimize stress incontinence by teaching the patient pelvic floor (Kegel) exercises to strengthen the pubococcygeal muscles.

LEARNING KEGEL EXERCISES

First, explain how to locate the muscles of the pelvic floor. Instruct the patient to tense the muscles around the anus, as if to retain stool.

Next, teach the patient to tighten the muscles of the pelvic floor to stop the flow of urine while urinating and then to release the muscles to restart the flow. Once learned, these exercises can be done anywhere at any time.

ESTABLISHING A REGIMEN

Explain to the patient that contraction and relaxation exercises are essential to muscle retraining. Suggest starting out by contracting the pelvic floor muscles for 10 seconds, and then relax for 10 seconds before slowly tightening the muscles and then releasing them. Typically, the patient starts with 15 contractions in the morning and afternoon and 20 at night. Alternatively, the patient may exercise for 10 minutes three times per day, working up to 25 contractions at a time as strength improves.

Advise the patient not to use stomach, leg, or buttock muscles, and discourage leg crossing or breath holding during these exercises.

- Promote exercise. Explain how it helps regulate bowel motility. Even a nonambulatory patient can exercise while sitting or lying in bed.

AGE FACTOR *Teach the elderly patient to gradually eliminate laxative use. Using laxatives to promote regular bowel movement may eventually lead to constipation or incontinence.*

- Suggest natural laxatives, such as prunes and prune juice.

DOCUMENTATION

- Record bladder and bowel retraining efforts.
- Note scheduled bathroom times.
- Document food and fluid intake.
- Note elimination amounts.
- Record duration of continent periods.
- Note complications, including emotional problems.
- Document signs of skin breakdown.
- Note infection.
- Record treatments given for complications.

SELECTED REFERENCES

Berry, A. "Helping Children with Dysfunctional Voiding," *Urologic Nursing* 25(3):193-200, June 2005.

Gray, M. "Assessment and Management of Urinary Incontinence," *The Nurse Practitioner* 30(7):32-33, 36-43, July 2005.

Jansen, L., and Forbes, D. "The Psychometric Testing of a Urinary Incontinence Nursing Assessment Instrument," *Journal of Wound, Ostomy & Continence Nursing* 33(1):69-76, January-February 2006.

Karon, S. "A Team Approach to Bladder Retraining: A Pilot Study," *Urologic Nursing* 25(4):269-76, August 2005.

Milne, J.L., and Moore, K.N. "Factors Impacting Self-Care for Urinary Incontinence," *Urologic Nursing* 26(1):41-51, February 2006.

Intermittent infusion device, drug administration

OVERVIEW

DESCRIPTION
- Device allows drug to be given intermittently by infusion, I.V. bolus, or I.V. push injection methods.
- It eliminates the need for multiple venipunctures or for maintaining venous access with a continuous I.V. infusion (saline lock).

CONTRAINDICATIONS
- None known

EQUIPMENT

Patient's drug record and chart ♦ gloves ♦ alcohol pads ♦ three 3-ml syringes with needleless adapter ♦ normal saline solution ♦ extra intermittent infusion device ♦ prescribed drug in an I.V. container with administration set and needle (for infusion) or in a syringe with needle (for I.V. bolus or push) ♦ tourniquet ♦ T-connector, sterile bacteriostatic water (optional)

PREPARATION
- Check the order on the patient's drug record against the practitioner's order.
- Wash your hands, and then wipe the tops of the normal saline solution, heparin flush solution, and drug containers with alcohol pads.
- Fill two of the 3-ml syringes (bearing 22G needles) with normal saline solution; draw 1 ml of heparin flush solution into the third syringe, according to facility policy.
- If you'll be infusing the drug, insert the administration set spike into the I.V. container, attach the needleless adapter, and prime the line.
- If you'll be injecting the drug I.V., fill a syringe with the prescribed drug.

KEY STEPS

- Confirm the patient's identity using two patient identifiers according to facility policy.
- If your facility uses a bar code scanning system, be sure to scan your ID badge, the patient's ID bracelet, and the medication's bar code.
- Explain the procedure to the patient.
- Put on gloves.
- Wipe the injection port of the intermittent infusion device with an alcohol pad, and insert the needleless adapter of a saline-filled syringe.
- Aspirate the syringe to verify the patency of the device. If no blood appears during aspiration, apply a tourniquet slightly above the site, keep it in place for about 1 minute, and then aspirate again. If blood still doesn't appear, remove the tourniquet and inject the normal saline solution slowly.

WARNING *Stop the injection immediately if you feel resistance because this may mean the device is occluded. If you feel resistance, remove the device and insert a new saline lock.*

- If you feel no resistance, watch for signs of infiltration (puffiness or pain at the site) as you slowly inject the saline solution. If these signs occur, insert a new intermittent infusion device.
- If blood is aspirated, slowly inject the saline solution and observe for signs of infiltration.
- Withdraw the saline syringe and needleless adapter.
- Flush with dilute normal saline solution to prevent clotting in the device.

GIVING I.V. BOLUS OR PUSH INJECTIONS
- Insert the needleless adapter and syringe with the drug for the I.V. bolus or push injection into the injection port of the device.
- Inject the drug at the required rate.
- Remove the needleless adapter and syringe from the injection port.

- Insert the needleless adapter of the remaining saline-filled syringe into the injection port, and slowly inject the normal saline solution to flush all of the drug through the device.
- Remove the needleless adapter and syringe, and insert and inject the heparin (or saline) flush solution to prevent clotting in the device.

GIVING AN INFUSION
- Insert and secure the needleless adapter attached to the administration set.
- Open the infusion line and adjust the flow rate as needed.
- To give fluids and drugs simultaneously or to give a drug incompatible with the primary I.V. solution, use a T-connector or needleless adapter.
- Infuse the drug for the prescribed period; then flush the device with normal saline solution to prevent clotting in the device.

SPECIAL CONSIDERATIONS

- In the last step, to avoid clotting in the device, flush with bacteriostatic water if the drug you're injecting (such as diazepam) is incompatible with normal saline solution.
- Change intermittent infusion devices every 48 to 72 hours, according to standard precaution guidelines and facility policy.
- Before administering an injectable drug, make sure you know the prescribed infusion period.

COMPLICATIONS
- Infiltration
- Specific reaction to infused drug

PATIENT TEACHING

- Explain the reason for the medication and possible adverse effects.

DOCUMENTATION

- Record the type, amount, and times of drug given.
- Document I.V. solutions used to dilute the drug and flush the line on the intake record.
- If you can't rotate injection sites because the patient has fragile veins, document this fact.
- Note the use of normal saline solution.

SELECTED REFERENCES
Menyhay, S.Z., and Maki, D.G. "Disinfection of Needleless Catheter Connectors and Access Ports with Alcohol May Not Prevent Microbial Entry: The Promise of a Novel Antiseptic-Barrier Cap," *Infection Control and Hospital Epidemiology* 27(1):23-27, January 2006.

Paparella, S. "Avoiding Disastrous Outcomes with Rapid Intravenous Push Medications," *Journal of Emergency Nursing* 30(5):478-80, October 2004.

Porter, J.J., and Lopez, T.C. "Maximum Intravenous Morphine Push Rate: Discrepancies between the Primary and Tertiary Literature," *Journal of Pain & Palliative Care Pharmacotherapy* 19(1):67-68, 2005.

Intermittent infusion device insertion

OVERVIEW

DESCRIPTION
- Device consists of a cannula with an attached injection cap (also called a *saline lock*).
- Filled with normal saline solution to prevent clotting, the device maintains venous access in patients receiving I.V. drugs regularly or intermittently, but who don't require continuous infusion.
- Device minimizes risk of fluid overload and electrolyte imbalance better than slow infusion with an I.V.
- Device cuts costs, reduces contamination risk by eliminating I.V. solution containers and equipment, increases patient comfort and mobility, reduces anxiety, and allows multiple blood sample collection without repeated venipuncture.

CONTRAINDICATIONS
- None known

EQUIPMENT

Intermittent infusion device ◆ needleless system device ◆ 1 ml of dilute heparin solution in a 3-ml syringe ◆ normal saline solution ◆ tourniquet ◆ alcohol pad or other approved antimicrobial solution, such as tincture of iodine 2% or 10% povidone-iodine ◆ venipuncture equipment ◆ transparent semipermeable dressing ◆ tape ◆ prefilled saline cartridges (available for use in a syringe cartridge holder)

Converting an I.V. line to an intermittent infusion device

The male adapter plug (shown below) allows you to convert an existing I.V. line into an intermittent infusion device. Follow these steps:
- Prime the adapter cap with dilute heparin or normal saline solution, as appropriate.
- Clamp the I.V. tubing and remove the administration set from the cannula hub.
- Insert the male adapter cap.
- Inject the remaining dilute heparin or normal saline solution to fill the line and to prevent clot formation.

This short luer-lock adapter cap twists into place.

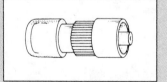

KEY STEPS

- Confirm the patient's identity using two patient identifiers according to facility policy.
- Wash your hands.
- Explain the procedure and describe the purpose of the intermittent infusion device.
- Remove set from packaging, wipe port with an alcohol pad, and inject normal saline solution to fill the tubing and needleless system. This removes air, preventing an air embolus.
- Select a venipuncture site.
- Put on gloves.
- Apply a tourniquet 2″ (5 cm) proximal to the chosen area.
- Clean the venipuncture site with alcohol or other antimicrobial solution, wiping outward from the site.
- Perform the venipuncture and ensure correct needle placement in the vein.
- Release the tourniquet.
- Tape the set in place.
- Loop the tubing, if applicable, so the injection port is accessible.
- Flush the catheter with saline solution.
- Apply a transparent semipermeable dressing.
- Initial the dressing label, write time and date, and put it on the dressing.
- Remove and discard gloves.
- Inject normal saline solution according to facility policy, to maintain the patency of the intermittent infusion device.
- Inject saline slowly to prevent stinging.

SPECIAL CONSIDERATIONS

◆ When accessing an intermittent infusion device, be sure to stabilize it to prevent dislodging from the vein.

◆ If the patient feels a burning sensation during the injection of saline, stop the injection and check cannula placement.

◆ If the cannula is in the vein, inject the saline slower to minimize irritation. If the needle isn't in the vein, remove and discard it. Then redo the procedure.

◆ Change the intermittent infusion administration set every 48 to 72 hours, according to facility policy.

◆ You may use a transparent semipermeable dressing, which allows the patient greater freedom and better observation of the injection site.

◆ If the practitioner orders an I.V. infusion stopped and an intermittent infusion device inserted, convert the existing line by disconnecting the I.V. tubing and inserting a male adapter plug into the device. (See *Converting an I.V. line to an intermittent infusion device.*)

◆ Most health organizations require use of luer-lock systems on all infusion cannulas and lines.

COMPLICATIONS

◆ Same potential complications as a peripheral I.V. line

PATIENT TEACHING

◆ If you're caring for a patient who's going home with a peripheral line, teach him how to care for the I.V. site and how to identify complications.

◆ Discuss movement restrictions that may have been ordered.

◆ If the patient has drug delivery equipment different from the type used in the facility, demonstrate its use and have the patient give a return demonstration.

◆ Have the patient notify the nurse if the dressing becomes moist, if blood appears in the tubing, or if redness, swelling, or discomfort develops.

◆ Tell the patient to report problems with the I.V. line — if the solution stops infusing or an alarm goes off on the infusion pump controller.

◆ Explain to the patient that the I.V. site will be changed regularly by a home care nurse.

◆ Teach the patient or caregiver how and when to flush the device.

◆ Teach the patient to document daily whether the I.V. site is free from pain, swelling, and redness.

DOCUMENTATION

◆ Record the date and time of insertion.

◆ Note the type, brand, and gauge of needle.

◆ Document the length of the cannula.

◆ Record the anatomic location of the insertion site.

◆ Note the patient's tolerance of the procedure.

◆ Document the date and time of each saline flush.

SELECTED REFERENCES

Eakle, M., et al. "Luer-lock Misconnects Can Be Deadly," *Nursing* 35(9):73, September 2005.

Holmes, K., and Snow, D. "More Problems with Luer-lock Connections," *Anaesthesia* 61(1):73, January 2006.

Niesen, K.M., et al. "The Effects of Heparin versus Normal Saline for Maintenance of Peripheral Intravenous Locks in Pregnant Women,"*Journal of Obstetric, Gynecologic, and Neonatal Nursing* 32(4):503-508, July-August 2003.

Vorweg, M., et al. "The 'Heparin Lock': Cause for Iatrogenic Coagulopathy," *European Journal of Anaesthesiology* 23(1):50-53, January 2006.

Intermittent positive-pressure breathing

OVERVIEW

DESCRIPTION

◆ Intermittent positive-pressure breathing (IPPB) delivers room air or oxygen to the lungs at a pressure higher than atmospheric pressure; delivery stops when pressure in the mouth or breathing circuit tube increases to a predetermined airway pressure.

◆ The procedure has been used extensively in pulmonary therapy because it delivers aerosolized drugs deeper into the lungs, decreases the work of breathing, and helps mobilize secretions.

◆ Respiratory therapy department personnel deliver the treatments.

CONTRAINDICATIONS

◆ Untreated tension pneumothorax

EQUIPMENT

IPPB machine ◆ breathing circuit tubing ◆ other necessary tubing (usually one or two sections) ◆ mouthpiece or mask ◆ source of pressurized gas at 50 psi, if needed ◆ prescribed drug and normal saline solution ◆ 3-ml syringe with needle ◆ sphygmomanometer ◆ stethoscope ◆ facial tissues and waste bag or specimen cup ◆ warm, soapy water ◆ nose clips, oxygen, glutaraldehyde solution, suction equipment (optional)

PREPARATION

◆ Follow the manufacturer's instructions to set up the equipment properly.

KEY STEPS

◆ Confirm the patient's identity using two patient identifiers according to facility policy.

◆ Explain the procedure to the patient to ensure his cooperation.

◆ Tell the patient to sit erect in a chair, if possible, to allow for optimal lung expansion. Alternatively, place him in semi-Fowler's position.

◆ Wash your hands.

◆ Assess baseline blood pressure and heart rate, especially if a bronchodilator will be given, and listen to breath sounds for posttreatment comparisons.

◆ Instruct the patient to breathe deeply and slowly through his mouth as if sucking on a straw.

◆ Encourage the patient to let the machine do the work.

◆ During treatment, instruct the patient to hold his breath for a few seconds after full inspiration to allow for greater distribution of gas and drug.

◆ Instruct the patient to exhale normally.

◆ During treatment, take the patient's blood pressure and heart rate.

⚡ **WARNING** *IPPB treatment increases intrathoracic pressure and may temporarily decrease cardiac output and venous return, resulting in tachycardia, hypotension, or headache. Monitoring also detects reactions to the bronchodilator. If you find a sudden change in blood pressure or increase in heart rate by 20 or more beats per minute, stop the treatment and notify the practitioner.*

◆ If the patient is tolerating the treatment, continue until the drug in the nebulizer is exhausted, usually about 10 minutes.

◆ After treatment, or as needed, have the patient expectorate into tissues and discard in a waste bag, expectorate in a specimen cup, or suction him as needed.

◆ Listen to the patient's breath sounds, and compare them with the pretreatment assessment.

◆ Shake excess moisture from the nebulizer and the mouthpiece or mask.

- After 24 hours of use, either discard the equipment or clean it with warm, soapy water.
- After washing, rinse with warm water and immerse in glutaraldehyde solution (Control III) for 10 minutes. Then remove the equipment, rinse in warm water, and air-dry.
- Store in a clean plastic bag.

SPECIAL CONSIDERATIONS

- If possible, avoid giving IPPB treatment right before or after a meal because the treatment may induce nausea and a full stomach reduces lung expansion.

  WARNING *Never give IPPB treatment without a drug in the nebulizer because this could dry the patient's airways and make secretions more difficult to mobilize.*
- If the purpose of treatment is to mobilize secretions, use a specimen cup to measure the secretions obtained.
- If the patient wears dentures, leave them in place to ensure a proper seal, but remove them if they slide out of position.
- If the patient has an artificial airway, use a special adapter, such as mechanical ventilation tubing, to give the treatments.
- When using a mask to give treatments, allow the patient frequent rest periods and observe for gastric distention, which is more likely to occur when a mask is used.
- If the patient's blood pressure is stable during the first treatment, you may not need to check it during subsequent treatments unless he has a history of cardiovascular disease, hypotension, or sensitivity to any drug delivered in the treatment.

COMPLICATIONS
- Gastric insufflation from swallowed air; occurs more commonly in patient with a mask than with a mouthpiece
- Dizziness, from hyperventilation
- Difficulty breathing, especially in an uncomfortable or frightened patient
- Decreased blood pressure from decreased venous return, especially in the patient with hypovolemia or cardiovascular disease
- Increased intracranial pressure from impeded venous return from the brain
- Spontaneous pneumothorax (rare), from increased intrathoracic pressure; most likely in patients with emphysematous blebs

PATIENT TEACHING

- If the patient will continue IPPB treatments at home, have him demonstrate the proper setup, use, and cleaning of the equipment before discharge. Tell the patient that he shouldn't change the pressure settings without checking with his practitioner.
- Suggest to the patient that he avoid using IPPB immediately before or after a meal because of possible nausea and reduced lung expansion. Instruct the patient to discontinue treatment and call his practitioner if he experiences dizziness.

DOCUMENTATION

- Record the date, time, and duration of treatment.
- Document the drug given.
- Record the pressure used.
- Note vital signs.
- Document breath sounds before and after treatment.
- Note the amount of sputum produced.
- Record complications and nursing actions taken and the patient's tolerance of the procedure.

SELECTED REFERENCES
Capasso, L., et al. "A Randomized Trial Comparing Oxygen Delivery on Intermittent Positive Pressure with Nasal Cannulae versus Facial Mask in Neonatal Primary Resuscitation," *Acta Paediatrica* 94(2):197-200, February 2005.

D'Angio, C.T., et al. "Pressure-regulated Volume Control Ventilation vs. Synchronized Intermittent Mandatory Ventilation for Very Low-Birth-Weight Infants: A Randomized Controlled Trial," *Archives of Pediatrics & Adolescent Medicine* 159(9):868-75, September 2005.

Dohna-Schwake, C., et al. "IPPB-assisted Coughing in Neuromuscular Disorders," *Pediatric Pulmonology* 41(6):551-57, June 2006.

Internal fixation

DESCRIPTION

- The procedure involves using an implanted fixation device (consisting of nails, screws, pins, wires, or rods, possibly used with metal plates) to stabilize a fracture (also known as *surgical reduction* or *open reduction-internal fixation*).
- The device may remain in the body indefinitely unless the patient has adverse reactions after the healing process is complete. (See *Reviewing internal fixation devices*.)
- The device is used to treat fractures of the face and jaw, spine, bones of the arms and legs, and joints (usually hip).
- The procedure permits earlier mobilization and shorter hospitalization, particularly needed in elderly patients with hip fractures.

CONTRAINDICATIONS

- Infection

Ice bag ◆ analgesic or opioid ◆ incentive spirometer ◆ elastic stockings ◆ overhead frame with trapeze ◆ pressure-relief mattress crutches or walker or abductor pillow (optional for leg fracture or hip fracture patients)

PREPARATION

- Collect and prepare equipment in the operating room.

- Explain the procedure to the patient.
- Tell the patient what to expect during postoperative assessment and monitoring, teach him how to use an incentive spirometer, and prepare him for proposed exercise and progressive ambulation regimens if needed.
- Instruct the patient to report pain to the practitioner.
- After the procedure, monitor the patient's vital signs every 2 to 4 hours for 24 hours, then every 4 to 8 hours, according to facility protocol.

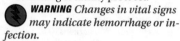 **WARNING** *Changes in vital signs may indicate hemorrhage or infection.*

- Monitor fluid intake and output every 4 to 8 hours.

Reviewing internal fixation devices

The choice of a specific internal fixation device depends on the location, type, and configuration of the fracture.

In trochanteric or subtrochanteric fractures, the surgeon may use a hip pin or nail, with or without a screw plate. A pin or plate with extra nails stabilizes the fracture by impacting the bone ends at the fracture site.

In an uncomplicated fracture of the femoral shaft, the surgeon may use an intramedullary rod to permit early ambulation with partial weight bearing.

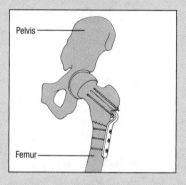

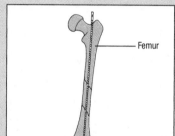

Another choice for fixation of a long-bone fracture is a screw plate, shown below on the tibia.

In an arm fracture, the surgeon may fix the involved bones with a plate, rod, or nail. Most radial and ulnar fractures may be fixed with plates, whereas humeral fractures are commonly fixed with rods.

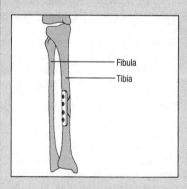

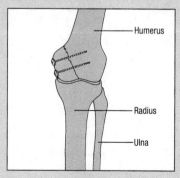

- Perform neurovascular checks every 2 to 4 hours for 24 hours, then every 4 to 8 hours as appropriate. Assess color, motion, sensation, digital movement, edema, capillary refill, and pulses of the affected area.
- Compare findings with the unaffected side.
- Apply an ice bag to the operative site to reduce swelling, relieve pain, and lessen bleeding.
- Give analgesics or opioids before exercising or mobilizing the affected area. If the patient is using patient-controlled analgesia, instruct him to give himself a dose before exercising or mobilizing.
- Monitor the patient for pain unrelieved by analgesics or opioids and for burning, tingling, or numbness, which may indicate infection or impaired circulation.
- Elevate the affected limb on a pillow, if appropriate, to minimize edema.
- Check surgical dressings for excessive drainage or bleeding.
- Check the incision site for signs of infection (erythema, drainage, edema, unusual pain).
- Help the patient perform range-of-motion and other muscle-strengthening exercises to promote circulation, improve muscle tone, and maintain joint function.
- Gradually and progressively teach the patient to move and walk, helped by use of an overhead frame with trapeze, crutches, or a walker.

SPECIAL CONSIDERATIONS

- To avoid the complications of immobility after surgery, have the patient use an incentive spirometer.
- Apply elastic stockings and sequential compression device, as appropriate.
- The patient may also require a pressure-relief mattress.

COMPLICATIONS

- Wound infection, especially involving metal fixation device (may require reopening the incision, draining the suture line, and removing the fixation device)
- Malunion
- Nonunion
- Fat or pulmonary embolism
- Neurovascular impairment
- Comaprtment syndrome

PATIENT TEACHING

- Before discharge, teach the patient and his family how to care for the incisional site.
- Explain to the patient signs and symptoms of wound infection.
- Teach the patient and his family about giving pain drugs.
- Advise the patient about practicing an exercise regimen as appropriate.
- Teach the patient how to use crutches or a walker as appropriate.

DOCUMENTATION

- Document perioperative findings on cardiovascular, respiratory, and neurovascular status in the patient record.
- Name the pain-management techniques used.
- Describe wound appearance and alignment of the affected bone.
- Document the patient's response to teaching about appropriate exercise.
- Note care of the insertion site.
- Record use of assistive devices (if appropriate).
- Document symptoms that should be reported to the practitioner.

SELECTED REFERENCES
Beaty, J.H. "Fractures of the Hip in Children," *Orthopedic Clinics of North America* 37(2):223-32, April 2006.
Brooks, K.R., et al. "Internal Fixation of Distal Radius Fractures with Novel Intramedullary Implants," *Clinical Orthopaedics & Related Research* 445:42-50, April 2006.
Horn, E.M., et al. "Innovative Internal Fixation for Cervical Spine Fractures," *Clinical Neurosurgery* 52:311-14, 2005.
Ramsey, M.L., et al. "Open Reduction and Internal Fixation of Distal Humerus Fractures," *Techniques in Shoulder & Elbow Surgery* 7(1):44-51, March 2006.

Intra-aortic balloon counterpulsation

OVERVIEW

DESCRIPTION

◆ Intra-aortic balloon counterpulsation temporarily supports the heart's left ventricle by mechanically displacing blood by an intra-aortic balloon attached to an external pump console.

◆ The device is usually inserted through the common femoral artery and positioned with its tip just distal to the left subclavian artery. (See *Interpreting intra-aortic balloon waveforms*.)

◆ The procedure is used to monitor myocardial perfusion and the effects of drugs on myocardial function and perfusion.

◆ It increases the supply of oxygen-rich blood to the myocardium and decreases myocardial oxygen demand.

◆ It's used for refractory angina, ventricular arrhythmia from ischemia, pump failure caused by cardiogenic shock, intraoperative myocardial infarction (MI), low cardiac output after bypass surgery, and for low cardiac output from acute mechanical defects after MI, such as ventricular septal defect, papillary muscle rupture, and left ventricular aneurysm.

◆ It's used perioperatively to support and stabilize patients with a suspected high-grade lesion undergoing angioplasty, thrombolytic therapy, cardiac surgery, and cardiac catheterization.

CONTRAINDICATIONS

◆ Severe aortic insufficiency
◆ Aortic aneurysm
◆ Severe peripheral vascular disease

EQUIPMENT

Intra-aortic balloon counterpulsation (IABC) console and balloon catheters ◆ insertion kit ◆ Dacron graft (for surgically inserted balloon) ◆ electrocardiogram (ECG) monitor and electrodes ◆ sedative, analgesic ◆ pulmonary artery catheter setup ◆ temporary pacemaker setup ◆ 18G angiography needle ◆ sterile drape ◆ sterile gloves ◆ gown ◆ mask ◆ sutures ◆ povidone-iodine swabs ◆ suction setup ◆ defibrillator and emergency drugs ◆ fluoroscope ◆ indwelling catheter ◆ urinometer ◆ arterial blood gas (ABG) kits and tubes for laboratory studies ◆ 4″ × 4″ gauze pads ◆ hair clipping supplies ◆ I.V. heparin ◆ oxygen setup and ventilator (optional)

PREPARATION

◆ Depending on facility policy, you or a perfusionist must balance the pressure transducer in the external pump console and calibrate the oscilloscope monitor to ensure accuracy.

KEY STEPS

◆ Confirm the patient's identity using two patient identifiers according to facility policy.

◆ Tell the patient that the physician will place a special balloon catheter in his aorta to help his heart pump more easily.

◆ Explain the insertion procedure; mention that the catheter will be connected to a large console next to the patient's bed.

◆ Tell the patient that the balloon will temporarily reduce his heart's workload, to ease healing.

◆ Let the patient know the balloon will be removed after his heart can resume an adequate workload.

PREPARING FOR INTRA-AORTIC BALLOON INSERTION

◆ Make sure the patient or a family member understands the procedure and signs a consent form. Verify that the form is attached to his chart.

◆ Record the patient's baseline vital signs, including pulmonary artery pressure (PAP).

◆ Connect the patient to an ECG machine for continuous monitoring.

◆ Apply chest electrodes in a standard lead II position (or whatever position produces the largest R wave) because the R wave triggers balloon inflation and deflation.

◆ Obtain a baseline ECG.

◆ Attach another set of ECG electrodes to the patient, unless the ECG pattern is being transmitted from the patient's bedside monitor to the balloon pump monitor through a phone cable.

◆ Give oxygen as needed.

◆ Make sure the patient has an arterial line for withdrawing blood samples, monitoring blood pressure, and assessing the timing and effectiveness of therapy; a pulmonary artery line to measure PAP, aspirate blood samples, and perform cardiac output studies (increased PAP indicates increased myocardial workload and ineffective balloon pumping); and a peripheral I.V. line in place.

- Cardiac output studies are usually performed with and without the balloon to check the patient's progress. The central lumen of the intra-aortic balloon monitors central aortic pressure, lets you check for proper timing of the inflation-deflation cycle, and demonstrates the effects of counterpulsation, elevated diastolic pressure, and reduced end-diastolic and systolic pressures.
- Insert an indwelling urinary catheter with a urinometer to evaluate the patient's urine output, fluid balance, and renal function.
- To reduce the risk of infection, clip hair bilaterally from the lower abdomen to the lower thigh, including the pubic area. Clip hair at the insertion site, if needed.
- Monitor the patient's peripheral leg pulse and document sensation, movement, color, and temperature of the legs.
- Give the patient a sedative.

⚡ **WARNING** *Have a defibrillator, suction and temporary pacemaker setups, and emergency drugs readily available in case the patient develops complications during insertion, such as an arrhythmia.*

- Before the physician inserts the balloon, he puts on sterile gloves, gown, and mask, cleans the site with povidone-iodine solution, and covers the area with a sterile drape.

INSERTING THE INTRA-AORTIC BALLOON PERCUTANEOUSLY

- The physician may insert the balloon percutaneously through the femoral artery into the descending thoracic aorta, using a modified Seldinger technique.
- He accesses the vessel with an 18G angiography needle, removes the inner stylet, and then passes the guide wire through the needle and removes the needle.
- He passes an introducer (dilator and sheath assembly) over the guide wire into the vessel until 1″ (2.5 cm) remains above the insertion site.
- He removes the inner dilator, leaving the introducer sheath and guide wire in place.

(continued)

Interpreting intra-aortic balloon waveforms

During intra-aortic balloon counterpulsation, you can use electrocardiogram and arterial pressure waveforms to determine whether the balloon pump is functioning properly.

NORMAL INFLATION-DEFLATION TIMING

Balloon inflation occurs after aortic valve closure; deflation, during isovolumetric contraction, occurs just before the aortic valve opens. In a properly timed waveform such as the one shown at right, the inflation point lies at or slightly above the dicrotic notch. Both inflation and deflation cause a sharp V. Peak diastolic pressure exceeds peak systolic pressure; peak systolic pressure exceeds assisted peak systolic pressure.

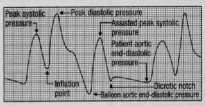

EARLY INFLATION

With early inflation, the inflation point lies before the dicrotic notch. Early inflation dangerously increases myocardial stress and decreases cardiac output.

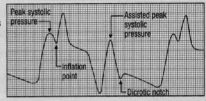

EARLY DEFLATION

With early deflation, a U shape appears and peak systolic pressure is less than or equal to assisted peak systolic pressure. This won't decrease afterload or myocardial oxygen consumption.

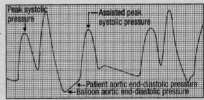

LATE INFLATION

With late inflation, the dicrotic notch precedes the inflation point, and the notch and the inflation point create a W shape. This can lead to a reduction in peak diastolic pressure, coronary and systemic perfusion augmentation time, and augmented coronary perfusion pressure.

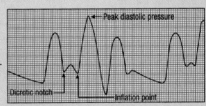

LATE DEFLATION

With late deflation, peak systolic pressure exceeds assisted peak systolic pressure. This threatens the patient by increasing afterload, myocardial oxygen consumption, cardiac workload, and preload. It occurs when the balloon has been inflated for too long.

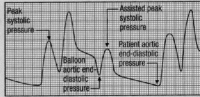

- After passing the balloon over the guide wire into the introducer sheath, the physician advances the catheter into position, ⅜" to ¾" (1 to 2 cm) distal to the left subclavian artery under fluoroscopic guidance.
- The physician attaches the balloon to the control system to start counterpulsation; the balloon catheter then unfurls.

INSERTING THE INTRA-AORTIC BALLOON SURGICALLY

- The physician may decide to insert the catheter through a femoral arteriotomy.
- After making an incision and isolating the femoral artery, the physician attaches a Dacron graft to a small opening in the arterial wall and passes the catheter through this graft.
- Using fluoroscopic guidance, the physician advances the catheter up the descending thoracic aorta and positions the catheter tip between the left subclavian and renal arteries.
- The physician sews the Dacron graft around the catheter at the insertion point and connects the other end of the catheter to the pump console.
- If the balloon can't be inserted through the femoral artery, the physician may use the transthoracic method and insert it in an antegrade direction through the anterior wall of the ascending aorta.
- The physician positions it ⅜" to ¾" beyond the left subclavian artery and brings the catheter out through the chest wall.

MONITORING THE PATIENT AFTER BALLOON INSERTION

⚫ *WARNING If the control system malfunctions or becomes inoperable, don't let the balloon catheter remain dormant for more than 30 minutes. Get another control system and attach it to the balloon; then resume pumping. In the meantime, inflate the balloon manually, using a 60-cc syringe and room air a minimum of once every 5 minutes, to prevent thrombus formation in the catheter.*

- The physician will clean the insertion site with povidone-iodine swabs and apply a sterile dressing.
- Verify correct balloon placement with chest X-ray.
- Assess and record pedal and posterior tibial pulses as well as color, sensation, and temperature in the affected limb every 15 minutes for 1 hour and then hourly.

⚫ *WARNING Notify the physician immediately if you detect circulatory changes; the balloon may need to be removed.*

- Monitor the patient's baseline arm pulses, arm sensation and movement, and arm color and temperature every 15 minutes for 1 hour after balloon insertion; repeat every 2 hours while the balloon is in place.

⚫ *WARNING Loss of left arm pulses may indicate upward balloon displacement. Notify the physician of left-arm pulse changes.*

- Monitor the patient's urine output every hour. Note baseline blood urea nitrogen (BUN) and creatinine levels; monitor these levels daily.
- Changes in urine output, BUN, and creatinine levels may signal reduced renal perfusion from downward balloon displacement.
- Auscultate and record bowel sounds every 4 hours. Check for abdominal distention and tenderness and elimination-pattern changes.
- Take the patient's temperature every 1 to 4 hours; if it's elevated, get blood samples for a culture, send them to the laboratory immediately, and notify the physician. Culture drainage at the insertion site.
- Monitor the patient's hematologic status. Watch for bleeding gums, blood in the urine or stools, petechiae, and bleeding at the insertion site. Monitor his platelet count, hemoglobin level, and hematocrit daily.
- If the platelet count drops, expect to give blood products to maintain hematocrit at 30%.

- Monitor partial thromboplastin time (PTT) every 6 hours while the I.V. heparin dose is adjusted to maintain PTT at 1.5 to 2 times the normal value; repeat every 12 to 24 hours while the balloon remains in place.
- Measure PAP and pulmonary artery wedge pressure (PAWP) every 1 to 2 hours.

⚫ *WARNING A rising PAWP reflects preload, signaling increased ventricular pressure and workload; notify the physician if this occurs. Some patients require I.V. nitroprusside (Nitropress) during IABC to reduce preload and afterload.*

- Obtain a sample for ABG analysis.
- Monitor electrolyte levels (especially sodium and potassium) to assess the patient's fluid and electrolyte balance and to help prevent arrhythmias.

⚫ *WARNING Notify the physician immediately if you notice signs and symptoms of a dissecting aortic aneurysm: difference between blood pressure readings in left and right arms, elevated blood pressure, syncope, pallor, diaphoresis, dyspnea, throbbing abdominal mass, decreased red blood cell count with increased white blood cell count, and pain in the chest, abdomen, or back.*

WEANING THE PATIENT FROM IABC

- Assess the cardiac index, systemic blood pressure, and PAWP to help the physician evaluate the patient's readiness for weaning — usually about 24 hours after balloon insertion. The patient's hemodynamic status should be stable on minimal doses of inotropic agents, such as dopamine or dobutamine.
- To begin weaning, gradually decrease the frequency of balloon augmentation to 1:2 and 1:4, as ordered.
- Assist frequency is usually maintained for 1 hour or longer, depending on facility policy. If the patient's hemodynamic indices remain stable during this time, weaning may continue.

WARNING *Don't leave the patient on a low augmentation setting for more than 2 hours, to prevent embolus formation.*

◆ Assess the patient's tolerance of weaning.

WARNING *Notify the physician immediately if you notice signs and symptoms of poor tolerance: confusion and disorientation, urine output below 30 ml/hour, cold and clammy skin, chest pain, arrhythmias, ischemic ECG changes, and elevated PAP.*

REMOVING THE INTRA-AORTIC BALLOON

◆ The balloon is removed when the patient's hemodynamic status remains stable after the frequency of balloon augmentation is decreased.

◆ The control system is turned off and the connective tubing disconnected from the catheter to ensure balloon deflation.

◆ The physician withdraws the balloon until the proximal end of the catheter contacts the distal end of the introducer sheath.

◆ He then applies pressure below the puncture site and removes the balloon and introducer sheath as a unit, allowing a few seconds of free bleeding to prevent thrombus formation.

◆ To promote distal bleed-back, he applies pressure above the puncture site.

◆ Apply direct pressure to the site for 30 minutes or until bleeding stops, if facility policy permits. (Sometimes this is the physician's responsibility.)

◆ If the balloon was inserted surgically, the physician closes the Dacron graft and sutures the insertion site. If the balloon was inserted percutaneously, the cardiologist usually removes the catheter.

◆ After balloon removal, provide wound care according to facility policy.

◆ Record the patient's pedal and posterior tibial pulses and the color, temperature, and sensation of the affected limb.

◆ Enforce bed rest, usually for 24 hours.

SPECIAL CONSIDERATIONS

◆ Before using the IABC control system, make sure you know what the alarms and messages mean and how to respond to them.

WARNING *Respond immediately to alarms and messages.*

◆ Change the dressing at the balloon insertion site every 24 hours or as needed, using strict sterile technique. Don't let povidone-iodine solution contact the catheter.

◆ Make sure the head of the bed is elevated no more than 30 degrees.

TROUBLESHOOTER *Pump interruptions may result from loose ECG electrodes or leadwires, static or 60 cycle interference, catheter kinking, or improper body alignment.*

◆ Make sure PTT is within normal limits before the balloon is removed to prevent hemorrhage at the insertion site.

COMPLICATIONS

◆ Arterial embolism from clot formation on the balloon surface

◆ Extension or rupture of an aortic aneurysm

◆ Femoral or iliac artery perforation

◆ Femoral artery occlusion

◆ Sepsis

◆ Bleeding at the insertion site that may become aggravated by pump-induced thrombocytopenia caused by platelet aggregation around the balloon

PATIENT TEACHING

◆ Teach the patient and his family about the procedure and the reason for the pump, and tell him who will insert it.

DOCUMENTATION

◆ Document all aspects of patient assessment and management.

◆ Note the patient's response to therapy.

◆ Document routine checks, problems, and troubleshooting measures if you're responsible for the IABC device.

◆ If a technician is responsible for the IABC device, record only when and why the technician was notified as well as the result of his actions on the patient, if any.

◆ Document teaching of the patient and his family as well as their responses.

SELECTED REFERENCES

Davies, A.N., et al. "Extra-Ascending Aortic versus Intra-Descending Aortic Balloon Counterpulsation-Effect on Coronary Artery Blood Flow," *Heart, Lung & Circulation* 14(3):178-86, September 2005.

Reid, M.B., and Cottrell, D. "Nursing Care of Patients Receiving: Intra-Aortic Balloon Counterpulsation," *Critical Care Nurse* 25(5):40-44, 46-49, October 2005.

Santa-Cruz, R.A., et al. "Aortic Counterpulsation: A Review of the Hemodynamic Effects and Indications for Use," *Catheterization and Cardiovascular Interventions* 67(1):68-77, January 2006.

Trost, J.C., and Hillis, L.D. "Intra-Aortic Balloon Counterpulsation," *American Journal of Cardiology* 97(9):1391-98, May 2006.

Intracranial pressure monitoring

DESCRIPTION

- Intracranial pressure monitoring is performed on patients with head trauma with bleeding or edema, overproduction or insufficient absorption of cerebrospinal fluid (CSF), cerebral hemorrhage, and space-occupying brain lesions.
- The procedure measures pressure exerted by the brain, blood, and CSF against the inside of the skull and detects elevated intracranial pressure (ICP).
- There are four basic ICP monitoring systems: intraventricular catheter, subarachnoid bolt, epidural sensor, and intraparenchymal pressure monitoring.
- The procedure is typically performed by a neurosurgeon in the operating room, emergency department, or intensive care unit.

CONTRAINDICATIONS

- For intraventricular catheter monitoring:
  - stenotic cerebral ventricles
  - cerebral aneurysms in path of catheter placement
  - suspected vascular lesions.

EQUIPMENT

Monitoring unit and transducers ✦ 16 to 20 sterile 4″ × 4″ gauze pads ✦ linen-saver pads ✦ hair scissors ✦ sterile drapes ✦ chlorhexidine solution ✦ sterile gown ✦ surgical mask ✦ sterile gloves ✦ head-dressing supplies (two rolls of 4″ elastic gauze dressing, one roll of 4″ roller gauze, adhesive tape) ✦ ✦ sterile marker ✦ sterile labels ✦ suction apparatus, I.V. pole, and yardstick (optional)

PREPARATION

- Set up monitoring units according to facility policy.

- Various types of preassembled ICP monitoring units are available, each with its own setup protocols designed to reduce the risk of infection by eliminating the need for multiple stopcocks, manometers, and transducer dome assemblies.

⚡ **WARNING** *Inserting an ICP monitoring device and setting up equipment for the monitoring system require strict sterile technique to reduce risk of central nervous system (CNS) infection.*

KEY STEPS

- Confirm the patient's identity using two patient identifiers according to facility policy.
- Explain the procedure to the patient or his family.
- Make sure the patient or a responsible family member has signed an appropriate consent form.
- Wash your hands thoroughly.
- Wear appropriate personal protection equipment throughout all procedures.
- Obtain baseline routine and neurologic vital signs.
- Place the patient in a supine position and elevate the head of the bed 30 degrees (or as ordered).
- Document the number of bed crank rotations, or hang a yardstick on an I.V. pole and mark the exact elevation.
- Place linen-saver pads under the patient's head. Clip his hair at the insertion site to decrease the risk of infection.
- Cover the patient with sterile drapes.
- Scrub the insertion site for 2 minutes with chlorhexidine solution.
- The physician puts on the sterile gown, mask, and gloves and opens the interior wrap of the sterile supply tray and proceeds with insertion of the catheter or bolt.
- Label all medications, medication containers, and other solutions on and off the sterile field.

- To facilitate placement of the device, hold the patient's head in your hands or attach a long strip of 4″ roller gauze to one side rail and bring it across the patient's forehead to the opposite rail.
- Reassure the conscious patient to help ease his anxiety.
- Talk to the patient frequently to assess his level of consciousness (LOC) and detect signs of deterioration.
- Watch for cardiac arrhythmias and abnormal respiratory patterns.
- After insertion, put on sterile gloves and apply chlorhexidine solution and a sterile dressing to the site.
- If not done by the physician, connect the catheter to the appropriate monitoring device, depending on the system used.
- If the physician has set up a ventriculostomy drainage system, attach the drip chamber to the headboard or bedside I.V. pole.

🔲 **TROUBLESHOOTER** *Positioning the drip chamber too high can increase ICP; positioning it too low can cause excessive CSF drainage.*

- Inspect the insertion site at least every 24 hours (or according to facility policy) for redness, swelling, and drainage.
- Clean the insertion site, apply chlorhexidine solution, and apply a fresh sterile dressing.
- Assess the patient's status, evaluating routine and neurologic vital signs every hour or as ordered.
- Obtain orders for waveforms and pressure parameters.
- Calculate cerebral perfusion pressure (CPP) hourly, using the equation: CPP = mean arterial pressure × ICP.
- Observe digital ICP readings and waves.

⚡ **WARNING** *The pattern of ICP readings is more significant than any single reading. Notify the physician immediately if you observe continually elevated ICP readings that last several minutes.*

- Record and describe CSF drainage.

SPECIAL CONSIDERATIONS

AGE FACTOR *In infants, ICP can be monitored externally, without scalp penetration at the fontanel, using a photoelectric transducer with a pressure-sensitive membrane taped to the anterior fontanel.*

◆ Osmotic diuretics, such as I.V. mannitol, reduce cerebral edema by shrinking intracranial contents by drawing water from tissues into plasma.

◆ When giving mannitol, monitor electrolyte levels and osmolality readings closely to avoid dehydration.

◆ To avoid rebound increased ICP after giving mannitol, give 50 ml of albumin with the mannitol bolus, monitoring for a residual rise in ICP before it decreases.

WARNING *Monitor the patient with heart failure or severe renal dysfunction for problems adapting to the increased intravascular volumes.*

◆ Fluid restriction, usually 1,200 to 1,500 ml/day, prevents cerebral edema from developing or worsening.

◆ Steroid therapy, although controversial, may be used to lower elevated ICP by reducing sodium and water levels in the brain.

WARNING *Give steroids with antacids and histamine-2 receptor antagonists to reduce the risk of peptic ulcers and monitor for GI bleeding and hyperglycemia.*

◆ Barbiturate-induced coma reduces the brain's metabolic demand, which reduces cerebral blood flow and ICP.

◆ Hyperventilation with oxygen from a handheld resuscitation bag or ventilator eliminates excess carbon dioxide, constricting cerebral vessels and reducing cerebral blood volume and ICP.

WARNING *Hyperventilation with a handheld resuscitation bag or a ventilator should be performed with care because hyperventilation may cause ischemia in areas of marginally perfused brain.*

◆ Before tracheal suctioning, hyperventilate the patient with 100% oxygen and suction for no more than 15 seconds to avoid inducing hypoxia and increasing cerebral blood flow.

◆ Because fever raises brain metabolism, which increases cerebral blood flow and ICP, reduce fever by giving acetaminophen, sponge baths, or a hypothermia blanket.

WARNING *Rebound increases in ICP and brain edema may occur if rapid rewarming takes place after hypothermia or if cooling induces shivering.*

◆ Withdrawal of CSF through the drainage system reduces CSF volume and thus reduces ICP.

◆ Watch for signs of decompensation: pupillary dilation (unilateral or bilateral); decreased pupillary response to light; decreasing LOC; rising systolic blood pressure and widening pulse pressure; bradycardia; slowed, irregular respirations; and, in late decompensation, decerebrate posturing.

COMPLICATIONS

◆ Hemorrhage
◆ CNS infection
◆ Seizure activity

WARNING *Excessive CSF loss, from faulty stopcock placement or a drip chamber that's too low, can decompress the cranial contents and damage cortical veins, leading to hematoma formation, rupture of hematomas or aneurysms, and hemorrhage.*

PATIENT TEACHING

◆ Explain to the patient the ICP monitor and its nursing care.

◆ Advise the patient of the importance of proper body positioning to reduce ICP.

◆ Explain to the patient that he must avoid Valsalva's maneuver and isometric muscle contractions and remain calm and quiet.

◆ Review the indications for removing the monitor and how it will be performed.

DOCUMENTATION

◆ Note the time and date of the insertion procedure.
◆ Record the name of the physician performing the procedure.
◆ Document the patient's response to the procedure.
◆ Note the insertion site and type of monitoring system used.
◆ Record hourly ICP digital readings, waveforms, and CPP.
◆ Document factors that affect ICP.
◆ Note routine and neurologic vital signs hourly.
◆ Record neurologic assessment findings.
◆ Document the amount, character, and frequency of any CSF drainage; record ICP after CSF drainage.
◆ Note patient teaching and emotional support given.

SELECTED REFERENCES

Cremer, O.L., et al. "Need for Intracranial Pressure Monitoring Following Severe Traumatic Brain Injury," *Critical Care Medicine* 34(5):1583-84, May 2006.

Kuo, J.R., et al. "Intraoperative Applications of Intracranial Pressure Monitoring in Patients with Severe Head Injury," *Journal of Clinical Neuroscience* 13(2):218-23, February 2006.

March, K. "Intracranial Pressure Monitoring: Why Monitor?" *AACN Clinical Issues* 16(4):456-75, October-December 2005.

Marcoux, K.K. "Management of Increased Intracranial Pressure in the Critically Ill Child with an Acute Neurological Injury," *AACN Clinical Issues* 16(2):212-31, April-June 2005.

Intradermal injection

DESCRIPTION

◆ Intradermal injections are used to produce a local effect, as in allergy or tuberculin testing, because little of an intradermally injected drug is systemically absorbed.

◆ Injections are given in small volumes — usually 0.5 ml or less — into the outer layers of the skin.

◆ The ventral forearm is the most commonly used site for intradermal injection because of its easy accessibility and lack of hair.

◆ In extensive allergy testing, the outer aspect of the upper arms may be used as well as the area of the back located between the scapulae. (See *Intradermal injection sites.*)

CONTRAINDICATIONS

◆ None known

Patient's drug record and chart ◆ tuberculin syringe with a 26G or 27G ½" to ⅜" needle ◆ prescribed drug ◆ gloves ◆ alcohol pads

PREPARATION

◆ Verify the order on the patient's drug record by checking it against the practitioner's orders.

◆ Inspect the drug to make sure it isn't abnormally discolored or cloudy and doesn't contain precipitates.

◆ Wash your hands.

◆ Choose equipment appropriate to the prescribed drug and injection site and make sure it works properly.

◆ Check the drug label against the patient's drug record.

◆ Read the label again as you draw up the drug for injection.

◆ Confirm the patient's identity using two patient identifiers according to facility policy.

◆ Tell the patient where you'll be giving the injection.

◆ Instruct the patient to sit up and to extend her arm and support it on a flat surface, with the ventral forearm exposed.

◆ Put on gloves.

◆ With an alcohol pad, clean the surface of the ventral forearm about two or three fingerbreadths distal to the antecubital space. Be sure the test site you've chosen is free of hair or blemishes.

◆ Allow the skin to dry completely before giving the injection.

◆ While holding the patient's forearm in your hand, stretch the skin taut with your thumb.

◆ With your free hand, hold the needle at a 10- to 15-degree angle to the patient's arm, with its bevel up.

◆ Insert the needle about ⅛" (0.3 cm) below the epidermis at sites 2" (5 cm) apart.

◆ Stop when the needle's bevel tip is under the skin, and inject the antigen slowly.

◆ You should feel some resistance as you do this, and a wheal should form as you inject the antigen. (See *Giving an intradermal injection.*)

◆ If no wheal forms, you've injected the antigen too deeply; withdraw the needle at the same angle at which it was inserted, and give another test dose at least 2" from the first site.

Intradermal injection sites

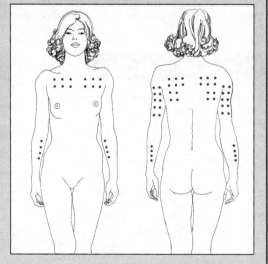

The most common intradermal injection site is the ventral forearm. Other sites (indicated by dotted areas) include the upper chest, upper arm, and shoulder blades. Skin in these areas is usually lightly pigmented, thinly keratinized, and relatively hairless, facilitating detection of adverse reactions

⚡ **WARNING** *Don't rub the injection site. This could irritate the underlying tissue, which may affect test results.*

◆ Circle each test site with a marking pen, and label each site according to the recall antigen given.
◆ Instruct the patient to refrain from washing off the circles until the test is completed.
◆ Dispose of needles and syringes according to facility policy.
◆ Remove and discard your gloves and wash your hands.
◆ Assess the patient's response to the skin testing in 24 to 48 hours.

SPECIAL CONSIDERATIONS

◆ A patient hypersensitive to the test antigens can have a severe anaphylactic response, requiring immediate epinephrine injection and other emergency resuscitation procedures.
◆ Be especially alert after giving a test dose of penicillin or tetanus antitoxin.

COMPLICATIONS
◆ None known

PATIENT TEACHING

◆ Tell the patient the reason for the injection.
◆ Explain to the patient that she may feel burning or itching.
◆ Tell the patient not to wash the circled injection site until after results are determined

DOCUMENTATION

◆ Document on the type and amount of drug given.
◆ Note the time the injection was given.
◆ Record the injection site.
◆ Document skin and other adverse reactions.

SELECTED REFERENCES
Laurent, P.E., et al. "Evaluating New Hypodermic and Intradermal Injection Devices," *Medical Device Technology* 17(2):16-19, March 2006.

Notman, M.J., et al. "Clindamycin Skin Testing has Limited Diagnostic Potential," *Contact Dermatitis* 53(6):335-38, December 2005.

Shirtcliffe, P.M., et al. "Effect of Repeated Intradermal Injections of Heat-Inactivated Mycobacterium Bovis Bacillus Calmette-Guerin in Adult Asthma," *Clinical and Experimental Allergy* 34(2):207-12, February 2004.

Tarnow, K., and King, N. "Intradermal Injections: Traditional Bevel Up Versus Bevel Down," *Applied Nursing Research* 17(4):275-82, November 2004.

Giving an intradermal injection

Secure the forearm. Insert the needle at a 10- to 15-degree angle so that it just punctures the skin's surface. The antigen should raise a small wheal as it's injected.

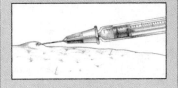

Intramuscular injection

DESCRIPTION

◆ I.M. injections deposit drug deep into muscle and provide rapid systemic action and absorption of up to 5 ml in certain sites.

◆ I.M. injection is used when the patient can't take drug orally, I.V. administration is inappropriate, or the drug can be altered by digestive juices.

◆ Because muscle tissue has few sensory nerves, irritating drugs can be given least painfully by this route.

◆ Injection site choice depends on the patient's physical status and purpose of the injection. The site shouldn't be inflamed, edematous, or irritated or contain mole, birthmark, scar tissue, or other lesions.

◆ Needle length depends on the injection site, the patient's size, and the amount of subcutaneous fat covering the muscle.

◆ The needle gauge for I.M. injections should be larger to accommodate viscous solutions and suspensions.

CONTRAINDICATIONS

◆ Coagulation problems
◆ Occlusive peripheral vascular disease
◆ Edema
◆ Shock
◆ After thrombolytic therapy
◆ During acute myocardial infarction (MI)

EQUIPMENT

Patient's drug record and chart ◆ prescribed drug ◆ 3- or 5-ml syringe 20G to 25G 1″ to 3″ needle ◆ gloves ◆ alcohol pads ◆ diluent or filter needle, gauze pad, 1″ tape, ice (optional)

PREPARATION

◆ Verify the order on the patient's drug record by checking it against the practitioner's order.
◆ Note if the patient has any allergies.
◆ Check the prescribed drug for color and clarity.
◆ Note the expiration date of the drug.

WARNING *Never use the drug if it's cloudy, discolored, or contains a precipitate, unless the manufacturer's instructions allow it. For some drugs (such as suspensions), the presence of particles is normal.*

◆ Observe for abnormal changes. If in doubt, check with the pharmacist.
◆ Choose equipment appropriate to the prescribed drug and injection site.
◆ The needle should be straight, smooth, and free of burrs.

Single-dose ampules

◆ Wrap an alcohol sponge around the ampule's neck and snap off the top, directing the force away from your body.
◆ Attach a filter to the needle and withdraw the drug, keeping the needle's bevel tip below the level of the solution.
◆ Tap the syringe to clear air from it.
◆ Cover the needle with the needle sheath.
◆ Before discarding the ampule, check the drug label against the patient's drug record. Discard the filter needle and the ampule.
◆ Attach the appropriate needle to the syringe.

Single-dose or multidose vials

◆ Reconstitute powdered drugs according to instructions; make sure all crystals dissolve.
◆ Warm the vial by rolling it between your palms to help the drug dissolve faster.
◆ Wipe the stopper of the drug vial with an alcohol pad, and then draw up the prescribed amount of drug.
◆ Read the drug label as you select the drug, as you draw it up, and after you have drawn it up to verify the correct dosage.
◆ Don't use an air bubble in the syringe.
◆ Gather all needed equipment and proceed to the patient's room.

◆ Confirm the patient's identity using two patient identifiers according to facility policy.
◆ If your facility utilizes a bar code scanning system, be sure to scan your ID badge, the patient's ID bracelet, and the medication's bar code.
◆ Provide privacy, explain the procedure to the patient, and wash your hands.
◆ Select an appropriate injection site.

AGE FACTOR *The gluteal muscles (gluteus medius and minimus and the upper outer corner of the gluteus maximus) are used most commonly for healthy adults, although the deltoid muscle may be used for a small-volume injection (2 ml or less).*

◆ Remember to always rotate injection sites for patients who require repeated injections.

AGE FACTOR *For infants and children, the vastus lateralis muscle of the thigh is used most often because it's usually the best developed and contains no large nerves or blood vessels, minimizing the risk of serious injury. The rectus femoris muscle may also be used in infants but is usually contraindicated in adults.*

◆ Position and drape the patient appropriately.
◆ Loosen the protective needle sheath, but don't remove it.
◆ After selecting the injection site, gently tap it to stimulate the nerve endings and minimize pain.
◆ Clean the skin at the site with an alcohol pad. Move the pad outward in a motion to about 2″ (5 cm) from the injection site, and allow the skin to dry.
◆ Keep the alcohol pad for later use.
◆ Put on gloves.
◆ With the thumb and index finger of your nondominant hand, gently stretch the skin of the injection site taut.
◆ While you hold the syringe in your dominant hand, remove the needle sheath by slipping it between the free fingers of your nondominant hand and then drawing back the syringe.

- Position the syringe at a 90-degree angle to the skin surface, with the needle a few inches from the skin.
- Tell the patient that he'll feel a prick as you insert the needle.
- Quickly and firmly thrust the needle through the skin and subcutaneous tissue, deep into the muscle.
- Support the syringe with your non-dominant hand, if desired.
- Pull back slightly on the plunger with your dominant hand to aspirate for blood. If no blood appears, slowly inject the drug into the muscle.

⚡ **WARNING** *If blood appears in the syringe on aspiration, the needle is in a blood vessel. If this occurs, stop the injection, withdraw the needle, prepare another injection with new equipment, and inject another site. Don't inject the bloody solution.*

- A slow, steady injection rate allows the muscle to distend gradually and accept the drug under minimal pressure. You should feel little or no resistance against the force of the injection.
- After the injection, gently but quickly remove the needle at a 90-degree angle.
- Cover the injection site immediately with the used alcohol pad, apply gentle pressure, and unless contraindicated, massage the relaxed muscle to help distribute the drug.
- Remove the alcohol pad and inspect the injection site for signs of active bleeding or bruising. If bleeding continues, apply pressure to the site; if bruising occurs, you may apply ice.
- Watch for adverse reactions at the site for 10 to 30 minutes after the injection.

✿ *AGE FACTOR An elderly patient will probably bleed or ooze from the site after the injection because of decreased tissue elasticity. Applying a small pressure bandage may be helpful.*

- Discard equipment according to standard precautions and facility policy.
- Don't recap needles; dispose of them in an appropriate sharps container to avoid needle-stick injuries.

SPECIAL CONSIDERATIONS

- To slow their absorption, some drugs for I.M. administration are dissolved in oil or other special solutions. Mix these preparations well before drawing them into the syringe.

✿ *AGE FACTOR The gluteal muscles can be used as the injection site only after a toddler has been walking for about 1 year.*

- Never inject into sensitive muscles, especially those that twitch or tremble when you assess site landmarks and tissue depth.
- For repeated injections, keep a rotation record that lists all available injection sites, divided into various body areas, for patients who require repeated injections. Rotate from a site in the first area to a site in each of the other areas. Then return to a site in the first area that is at least 1″ (2.5 cm) away from the previous injection site in that area.
- If the patient has experienced pain or emotional trauma from repeated injections, consider numbing the area before cleaning it by holding ice on it for several seconds.
- If you must inject more than 5 ml of solution, divide the solution and inject it at two separate sites.
- Encourage the patient to relax the muscle you'll be injecting because injections into tense muscles are more painful and may bleed more readily.
- I.M. injections can damage local muscle cells, causing elevations in enzyme levels (creatine kinase) that can be confused with elevations resulting from damage to cardiac muscle, as in MI.
- Dosage adjustments are usually needed when changing from the I.M. route to the oral route.

COMPLICATIONS
- Sterile abscesses due to accidental injection of concentrated or irritating drugs into subcutaneous tissue, or other areas where they can't be fully absorbed

- Deposits of unabsorbed drugs due to failure to rotate sites in patients who require repeated injections

✿ *AGE FACTOR Elderly patients have decreased muscle mass, so I.M. drugs can be absorbed more quickly than expected.*

PATIENT TEACHING

- Explain to the patient the need for the injection.
- Tell the patient he will feel a needle prick.
- Advise the patient to report adverse effects if they occur.
- Tell the patient when he can expect to feel the effects from the medicine.

DOCUMENTATION

- Document the drug given.
- Note the dose, date, and time.
- Record the route of administration and injection site.
- Note the patient's tolerance of injection and the injection's effects, including adverse effects.

SELECTED REFERENCES
Donaldson, C., and Green, J. "Using the Ventrogluteal Site for Intramuscular Injections," *Nursing Times* 101(16):36-38, April 2005.

Prettyman, J. "Subcutaneous or Intramuscular? Confronting a Parenteral Administration Dilemma," *Medsurg Nursing* 14(2):93-98, April 2005.

Pullen, R.L., Jr. "Administering Medication by the Z-Track Method," *Nursing* 35(7):24, July 2005.

Wynaden, D., et al. "Establishing Best Practice Guidelines for Administration of Intramuscular Injections in the Adult: A Systematic Review of the Literature," *Contemporary Nurse* 20(2):267-77, December 2005.

Intraosseous infusion

OVERVIEW

DESCRIPTION

- Intraosseous infusion allows delivery of fluids, drugs, or whole blood into the bone marrow when rapid venous infusion is difficult or impossible.
- The procedure is performed on infants and children in such emergencies as cardiopulmonary arrest or circulatory collapse, hypokalemia from traumatic injury or dehydration, status epilepticus, status asthmaticus, burns, near-drowning, and overwhelming sepsis.
- Any drug that can be given I.V. can be given by intraosseous infusion with comparable absorption and effectiveness. Intraosseous infusion has been used as an acceptable alternative for infants and children.
- The procedure is commonly undertaken at the anterior surface of the tibia; alternative sites include the iliac crest, spinous process and, rarely, the upper anterior portion of the sternum.
- It should be performed only by trained personnel; usually, a nurse assists. (See *Understanding intraosseous infusion.*)

CONTRAINDICATIONS

- Osteogenesis imperfecta
- Osteopetrosis
- Ipsilateral fracture
- Infusion through an area with cellulitis or an infected burn increases the risk of infection
- Osteomyelitis

EQUIPMENT

Bone marrow biopsy needle or specially designed intraosseous infusion needle (cannula and obturator) ◆ povidone-iodine pads ◆ sterile gauze pads ◆ sterile gloves ◆ sterile drape ◆ heparin or flush solution ◆ I.V. fluids and tubing ◆ 1% lidocaine ◆ 3- to 5-ml syringe ◆ tape ◆ sterile marker ◆ sterile labels ◆ sedative (optional)

PREPARATION

- Prepare I.V. fluids and tubing.

Understanding intraosseous infusion

During intraosseous infusion, the bone marrow serves as a noncollapsible vein; thus, fluid infused into the marrow cavity rapidly enters the circulation by way of an extensive network of venous sinusoids. Here, the needle is shown positioned in the patient's tibia.

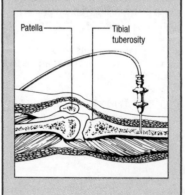

Patella — Tibial tuberosity

KEY STEPS

- Confirm the patient's identity using two patient identifiers according to facility policy.
- Make sure that the patient or a responsible family member understands the procedure and signs a consent form.
- Check the patient's history for hypersensitivity to the local anesthetic.
- Wash your hands.
- Provide a sedative, if ordered, before the procedure.
- Position the patient based on the selected puncture site.
- Using sterile technique, the physician cleans the puncture site with a povidone-iodine sponge and allows it to dry.
- The physician then covers the area with a sterile drape.
- Label all medications, medication containers, and other solutions on and off the sterile field.
- Using sterile technique, hand the physician the 3- or 5-ml syringe with 1% lidocaine so that he can anesthetize the infusion site.
- The physician inserts the infusion needle through the skin and into the bone at an angle of 10 to 15 degrees from vertical.
- He advances it with a forward and backward rotary motion through the periosteum until the needle penetrates the marrow cavity. The needle should "give" suddenly as it enters the marrow and should stand erect when released.
- Then the physician removes the obturator from the needle and attaches a 5-ml syringe.
- He aspirates some bone marrow to confirm needle placement.
- The physician replaces this syringe with a syringe containing 5 ml of heparin flush solution and flushes the cannula to confirm needle placement and clear the cannula of clots or bone particles.
- Next, the physician removes the syringe of flush solution and attaches I.V. tubing to the cannula to allow infusion of drugs and I.V. fluids.

- Put on sterile gloves.
- Clean the infusion site with povidone-iodine pads; then secure the site with tape and a sterile gauze dressing.
- Monitor vital signs and check the infusion site for bleeding and extravasation.

- Stop intraosseous infusion as soon as conventional vascular access is established (within 2 to 4 hours, if possible). Prolonged infusion significantly increases the risk of infection.
- After the needle has been removed, place a sterile dressing over the injection site, and apply firm pressure to the site for 5 minutes.
- Intraosseous flow rates are determined by needle size and flow through the bone marrow.
- Fluids should flow freely if needle placement is correct. Normal saline solution has been given intraosseously at a rate of 600 ml/minute and up to 2,500 ml/hour when delivered under pressure of 300 mm Hg through a 13G needle.

COMPLICATIONS

- Extravasation of fluid into subcutaneous tissue, resulting from incorrect needle placement
- Subperiosteal effusion, resulting from failure of fluid to enter the marrow space
- Clotting in the needle, resulting from delayed infusion or failure to flush the needle after placement
- Subcutaneous abscess
- Osteomyelitis
- Epiphyseal injury

- If the patient is conscious, explain the procedure to allay his fears and promote his cooperation.
- If the patient isn't an infant, tell him which bone site will be infused.
- Inform the patient that he'll receive a local anesthetic and will feel pressure from needle insertion.

- Record the time, date, and location.
- Note the patient's tolerance of the procedure.
- Document the amount of fluid infused on the input and output record.

SELECTED REFERENCES

DeBoer, S., et al. "Intraosseous Infusion: Not Just for Kids Anymore," *Emergency Medical Service* 34(3):54, 56-63, March 2005.

Fiorito, B.A., et al. "Intraosseous Access in the Setting of Pediatric Critical Care Transport," *Pediatric Critical Care Medicine* 6(1):50-53, January 2005.

Koschel, M.J. "Sternal Intraosseous Infusions: Emergency Vascular Access in Adults," *AJN* 105(1):66-68, January 2005.

Smith, R., et al. "The Utilisation of Intraosseous Infusion in the Resuscitation of Paediatric Major Trauma Patients," *Injury* 36(9):1034-1038, September 2005.

Intrapleural administration

DESCRIPTION

- Drug is injected through the chest wall into the pleural space or instilled through a chest tube placed intrapleurally for drainage to promote analgesia, treat spontaneous pneumothorax, resolve pleural effusions, and give chemotherapy.
- Intrapleurally given drugs diffuse across the parietal pleura and innermost intercostal muscles to affect the intercostal nerves.
- Common intrapleurally given drugs include tetracycline, streptokinase, anesthetics, and chemotherapeutic agents (to treat malignant pleural effusion or lung adenocarcinoma).

CONTRAINDICATIONS

- Pleural fibrosis
- Adhesions
- Pleural inflammation
- Sepsis
- Infection at the puncture site
- Bullous emphysema
- Those receiving respiratory therapy using positive end-expiratory pressure

EQUIPMENT

INTRAPLEURAL CATHETER INSERTION

Gloves ◆ gauze ◆ antiseptic solution, such as povidone-iodine ◆ drape ◆ local anesthetic, such as 1% lidocaine ◆ 3- or 5-ml syringe with 22G 1″ and 25G ⅝″ needles ◆ 18G needle or scalpel ◆ saline-lubricated glass syringe ◆ dressings ◆ sutures ◆ tape

CHEST TUBE INSERTION

Towels ◆ gloves ◆ gauze ◆ antiseptic solution, such as povidone-iodine ◆ 3- to 5-ml syringe ◆ local anesthetic, such as 1% lidocaine ◆ 18G needle or scalpel ◆ chest tube with or without trocar (#16 to #20 catheter for air or serous fluid, #28 to #40 for blood, pus, or thick fluid) ◆ two rubber-tipped clamps ◆ sutures ◆ drain ◆ dressings ◆ sterile marker

◆ sterile labels ◆ tape ◆ thoracic drainage system and tubing

DRUG ADMINISTRATION

Sterile gloves ◆ sterile gauze pads ◆ antiseptic solution, such as povidone-iodine solution ◆ prescribed drug ◆ appropriate-sized needles and syringes ◆ dressings ◆ tape ◆ 1% lidocaine (optional)

KEY STEPS

INSERTING AN INTRAPLEURAL CATHETER

- Confirm the patient's identity using two patient identifiers according to facility policy.
- Assist the physician as he inserts the intrapleural catheter at the patient's bedside.
- Position the patient on his side with the affected side up.
- Label all medications, medication containers, and other solutions on and off the sterile field.
- The physician will insert the catheter into the fourth to eighth intercostal space, 3″ to 4″ (7.5 to 10 cm) from the posterior midline.
- The physician puts on sterile gloves, cleans around the puncture site with antiseptic-soaked gauze, and then covers the area with a sterile drape.
- He fills the 3- to 5-ml syringe with local anesthetic and injects it into the skin and deep tissues.
- The physician punctures the skin with the 18G needle or scalpel, which helps the blunt-tipped intrapleural needle penetrate the skin over the superior edge of the lower rib in the chosen interspace.
- Keeping the bevel tilted upward, he directs the needle medially at a 30- to 40-degree angle to the skin.
- When the needle tip punctures the posterior intercostal membrane, the physician removes the stylet and attaches a saline-lubricated glass syringe containing 2 to 4 cc of air to the needle hub.
- During puncture, tell the patient to hold his breath (or momentarily disconnect him from mechanical venti-

lation) until the needle is removed. This helps prevent the needle from injuring lung tissue.
- The physician advances the needle slowly.
- When the needle punctures the parietal pleura, negative intrapleural pressure moves the plunger outward.
- The physician then removes the syringe from the needle and threads the intrapleural catheter through the needle until he has advanced it about 2″ (5 cm) into the pleural space.
- Without removing the catheter, he carefully withdraws the needle.
- Tell the patient that he can breathe again (or reconnect mechanical ventilation).
- After inserting the catheter, the physician coils it to prevent kinking and then sutures it securely to the patient's skin. He confirms placement by aspirating the catheter.
- The physician orders a chest X-ray to detect pneumothorax.
- Apply a sterile dressing over the insertion site to prevent catheter dislodgment.
- Evaluate and record the patient's vital signs every 15 minutes for the first hour after the procedure and then as needed.

INSERTING A CHEST TUBE

- The physician inserts the chest tube with the nurse assisting.
- First, position the patient with the affected side up, and drape him with sterile towels.
- Label all medications, medication containers, and other solutions on and off the sterile field
- The physician puts on gloves and cleans the appropriate site with antiseptic-soaked gauze.
- If the patient has a pneumothorax, the physician uses the second intercostal space as the access site because air rises to the top of the pleural space.
- If the patient has a hemothorax or pleural effusion, the physician uses the sixth to eighth intercostal space because fluid settles to the bottom of the pleural space.

- The physician fills the syringe with a local anesthetic and injects the site.
- He makes a small incision with the 18G needle or scalpel, inserts the appropriate-sized chest tube, and immediately connects it to the thoracic drainage system or clamps it close to the patient's chest.
- He then sutures the tube to the patient's skin.
- Tape the chest tube to the patient's chest distal to the insertion site to help prevent accidental dislodgment.
- Tape the junction of the chest tube and drainage tube to prevent their separation.
- Apply sterile drain dressings, and tape them to the site.
- After insertion, the physician checks tube placement with an X-ray.
- Check the patient's vital signs every 15 minutes for 1 hour and then as needed.
- Auscultate his lungs at least every 4 hours to assess air exchange in the affected lung.

🔔 **WARNING** *Diminished or absent breath sounds mean that the lung hasn't reexpanded.*

GIVING THE DRUG

- The physician injects the drug through the intrapleural catheter or chest tube.
- If the patient will receive chemotherapy, expect to give an antiemetic at least 30 minutes before.
- Position the patient with the affected side up.
- Help the physician move the dressing away from the intrapleural catheter or chest tube and clamp the drainage tube, if present.
- The physician disinfects the access port of the catheter or chest tube with antiseptic-soaked gauze.
- Draw up the appropriate drug dose, and hand it to the physician with the vial for verification.
- The physician injects the drug.
- If it's an anesthetic, he gives a bolus or loading dose initially and then a continuous infusion. For tetracycline, he mixes it with an anesthetic such as lidocaine to alleviate pain during injection.

- Reapply the dressings around the catheter.
- Monitor the patient closely during and after drug administration.

SPECIAL CONSIDERATIONS

- Make sure the patient has signed a consent form.
- Before catheter insertion, ask the patient to urinate to reduce the risk of bladder perforation and promote comfort.
- If the patient is receiving a continuous infusion, label the solution bag clearly.
- Cover all injection ports so that other drugs aren't injected into the pleural space accidentally.
- If the chest tube dislodges, cover the site at once with a sterile gauze pad and tape it in place.

🔔 **WARNING** *Stay with the patient, monitor his vital signs, and observe carefully for signs and symptoms of tension pneumothorax: hypotension, jugular vein distention, absent breath sounds, tracheal shift, hypoxemia, dyspnea, tachypnea, diaphoresis, chest pain, and a weak, rapid pulse. Have another nurse call the physician and gather the equipment for reinsertion.*

- Keep rubber-tipped clamps at the bedside in case a commercial chest tube system cracks or a tube disconnects.
- Wrap a piece of petroleum gauze around the chest tube at the insertion site to make an airtight seal; then apply the sterile dressing.
- After the chest tube is removed, dress the wound with petroleum gauze; then cover it with a new piece of sterile gauze.
- After the catheter is removed, inspect the skin at the entry site for signs of infection and then cover the wound with a sterile dressing.

COMPLICATIONS

- Bleeding
- Pneumothorax or tension pneumothorax

- Respiratory distress caused by accidental catheter placement in the lung
- Increased drug effect caused by catheter placement within a vessel
- Lung puncture with catheter fracture
- Local anesthetic toxicity can lead to tinnitus, metallic taste, light-headedness, somnolence, visual and auditory disturbances, restlessness, delirium, slurred speech, nystagmus, muscle tremor, seizures, arrhythmias, and cardiovascular collapse
- Tachycardia and hypertension caused by a local anesthetic containing epinephrine
- Irritation of the pleura chemically causing such systemic effects as neutropenia and thrombocytopenia from intrapleural chemotherapeutic drugs
- Infection at the insertion site

PATIENT TEACHING

- Encourage the patient to follow instructions.

DOCUMENTATION

- Document the drug given.
- Note the drug dosage.
- Record the patient's response to treatment.
- Note the condition of the catheter insertion site.

SELECTED REFERENCES

Bouros, D., et al. "Intrapleural Streptokinase for Pleural Infection," *British Medical Journal* 332(7534):133-34, January 2006.

Ishida, T., et al. "Intrapleural Cisplatin and OK432 Therapy for Malignant Pleural Effusion Caused by Non-Small Cell Lung Cancer," *Respirology* 11(1): 90-97, January 2006.

Jankovic, Z., et al. "Chronic Intrapleural Effusion Drainage Using an Epidural Catheter," *Anesthesia & Analgesia* 101(4):1242, October 2005.

Skeete, D.A., et al. "Intrapleural Tissue Plasminogen Activator for Complicated Pleural Effusions," *Journal of Trauma-Injury Infection & Critical Care* 57(6):1178-83, December 2004.

Iontophoresis

DESCRIPTION

- Iontophoresis delivers dermal analgesia quickly (in 10 to 20 minutes) with minimal discomfort and without distorting the tissue.
- The procedure is performed with an iontophoretic drug-delivery system— a handheld battery-powered device with two electrodes that delivers ions of lidocaine 2% and epinephrine 1:100,000 solution into the skin.
- It acts quickly and is an excellent choice for numbing an I.V. injection site, especially in children.

CONTRAINDICATIONS

- Implanted pacemaker or other implanted device sensitive to electricity
- Allergy or sensitivity to lidocaine or epinephrine
- Scarred skin

Dose-control device with battery ◆ drug-delivery electrode kit ◆ lidocaine 2% with epinephrine 1:100,000 solution ◆ alcohol pads ◆ syringe with needle ◆ gloves ◆ tongue blade

PREPARATION

- Thoroughly wash your hands before preparing the equipment.
- Gather the equipment at the bedside.
- Turn on the dose-control device and check that the battery has a charge.

- Confirm the patient's identity using two patient identifiers according to facility policy.
- Ask the patient if he has any allergies or sensitivity to drugs.

    AGE FACTOR *If the patient is a child, ask the parents if he has allergies or sensitivities to lidocaine or epinephrine.*

- Explain the procedure to the patient and tell him that he may feel tingling or warmth under the electrode pads while they're on the skin.
- Examine the patient's skin and select intact electrode placement sites, avoiding areas with pimples, unhealed wounds, or ingrown hairs.

    WARNING *Avoid placing electrodes over bony prominences and damaged, denuded, or recently scarred skin, which could impede electrical conduction.*

- With alcohol pads, briskly rub an area slightly larger than the electrode at each site.
- Remove the paper flap from the back of the drug-delivery electrode.
- Draw up the lidocaine with epinephrine in a syringe according to the amount indicated on the electrode pad (about 1 ml for a standard-sized pad and about 2.5 ml for a large pad).
- Remove the needle from the syringe and saturate the drug pad with the lidocaine and epinephrine solution (as shown below).

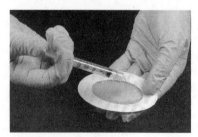

- Remove the remaining backing from the drug-delivery pad and apply the pad to the selected I.V. site.
- Remove the backing from the grounding electrode and apply it to the second prepared site about 4″ to 6″ (10 to 15 cm) away.

- Connect the lead clips: red (positive charge) to the drug-delivery electrode and black (negative charge) to the grounding electrode.
- Turn on the device. (See *Using an iontophoresis delivery device.*)
- After the dose has been delivered, remove the electrodes.
- Assess the skin at the drug-delivery site for numbness by touching it with a blunt object such as a tongue blade.
- Promptly prepare the site and perform the venipuncture because the numbness may last only a few minutes.
- Discard gloves and wash your hands.

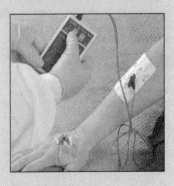
SPECIAL CONSIDERATIONS

- To avoid interfering with energy emission, don't tape or compress the electrodes.
- If you need to stop the treatment for any reason, press the OFF button and hold it until the device beeps and turns off.

  WARNING *When turning the device off, don't disconnect the lead clips or the electrodes until all signals have stopped because the device is still transmitting energy until it turns off.*

COMPLICATIONS
- Allergic reaction
- Prolonged redness at site

PATIENT TEACHING

- Tell the patient the purpose of the procedure.
- Explain the equipment to be used.
- Explain to the patient the feelings and sensations he may experience during the procedure.
- Tell the patient how long it takes for analgesia to occur (about 10 to 20 minutes).
- Instruct the patient to report any tingling sensation during the procedure.

DOCUMENTATION

- Record the date and time of treatment.
- Document sites used.
- Note if analgesia was achieved.
- Note if an allergic response occurred and the resulting treatment if needed.

SELECTED REFERENCES
Brown, M.B., et al. "Dermal and Transdermal Drug Delivery Systems: Current and Future Prospects," *Drug Delivery* 13(3):175-87, May-June 2006.

Pasero, C. "Lidocaine Iontophoresis for Dermal Procedure Analgesia," *Journal of Perianesthesia Nursing* 21(1):48-52, February 2006.

Strout, T.D., et al. "Reducing Pain in ED Patients During Lumbar Puncture: The Efficacy and Feasibility of Iontophoresis, Collaborative Approach," *Journal of Emergency Nursing* 30(5):423-30, October 2004.

Isolation equipment use

DESCRIPTION

- Use of isolation equipment prevents spread of infection from patient to patient, patient to health care worker, or health care worker to patient.
- Its use reduces risk of infection in immunocompromised patients.
- Proper equipment must be selected and those who use it must be adequately trained.

CONTRAINDICATIONS

- None known

Putting on a face mask

To avoid spreading airborne particles, wear a face mask — sterile or nonsterile, as indicated. Position the mask to cover your nose and mouth, and secure it high enough to ensure stability. Tie the top strings at the back of your head above the ears. Then tie the bottom strings at the base of your neck.

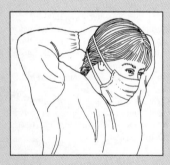

Adjust the metal nose strip if the mask has one.

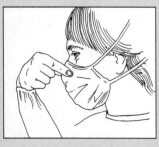

EQUIPMENT

Door card announcing isolation precautions ◆ gowns ◆ gloves ◆ goggles ◆ masks ◆ specially marked laundry bags ◆ plastic trash bags ◆ isolation cart, water-soluble laundry bags (optional)

PREPARATION

- An isolation cart may be used when the patient's room has no anteroom. It should include a work area (such as a pullout shelf), drawers or a cabinet area for holding isolation supplies and, possibly, a pole on which to hang coats or jackets.
- Remove the cover from the isolation cart, if needed, and set up the work area.
- Check the cart or anteroom to ensure that correct and sufficient supplies are in place for the designated isolation category.

KEY STEPS

- Remove your watch (or push it well up your arm) and any rings, according to facility policy, to prevent the growth of microorganisms under jewelry.
- Wash your hands with an antiseptic cleaning agent to prevent the growth of microorganisms under gloves.

PUTTING ON ISOLATION GARB

- Put on the gown and wrap it around the back of your uniform.
- Tie the strings or fasten the snaps or pressure-sensitive tabs at the neck.
- Make sure your uniform is completely covered, and secure the gown at the waist.
- Place the mask snugly over your nose and mouth.
- Secure ear loops around your ears or tie the strings behind your head high enough so the mask won't slip off.
- If the mask has a metal strip, squeeze it to fit your nose firmly but comfortably. (See *Putting on a face mask*.)
- If you wear glasses, tuck the mask under their lower edge.
- Put on the gloves.

- Pull the gloves over the gown cuffs to cover the edges of the sleeves.

REMOVING ISOLATION GARB

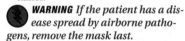 **WARNING** *The outside surfaces of your barrier clothes are contaminated.*

- Wearing gloves, untie the gown's waist strings.
- With your gloved left hand, remove the right glove by pulling on the cuff, turning the glove inside out as you pull. Don't touch any skin with the outside of either glove. (See *Removing contaminated gloves*.)
- Remove the left glove by wedging one or two fingers of your right hand inside the glove and pulling it off, turning it inside out as you remove it.
- Discard the gloves in the trash container that contains a plastic trash bag.
- Untie your mask, holding it only by the strings.
- Discard the mask in the trash container.

WARNING *If the patient has a disease spread by airborne pathogens, remove the mask last.*

- Untie the neck straps of your gown.
- Grasp the outside of the gown at the back of the shoulders and pull the gown down over your arms, turning it inside out as you remove it to contain the pathogens.
- Holding the gown well away from your uniform, fold it inside out.
- Discard it in the specially marked laundry bags or trash container, as needed.
- If the sink is inside the patient's room, wash your hands and forearms with soap or antiseptic before leaving the room.
- Turn off the faucet using a paper towel, and discard the towel in the room.
- Grasp the door handle with a clean paper towel to open it; discard the towel in a trash container inside the room.
- Close the door from the outside with your bare hand.
- If the sink is in an anteroom, wash your hands and forearms with soap or antiseptic after leaving the room.

◆ Use the gown, gloves, goggles, and mask only once; discard in the appropriate container before leaving a contaminated area.

◆ If your mask is reusable, undamaged, and not damp, keep it for future use.

WARNING *Isolation garb loses its effectiveness when wet because moisture lets organisms seep through the material. Change masks and gowns as soon as moisture is noticeable or according to the manufacturer's recommendations or facility policy.*

◆ At the end of your shift restock used items for the next person.
◆ After patient transfer or discharge, return the isolation cart to the appropriate area for cleaning and restocking of supplies.
◆ An isolation room or other room prepared for isolation purposes must be thoroughly cleaned and disinfected before use by another patient.

COMPLICATIONS

◆ None known

PATIENT TEACHING

◆ Explain to the patient the need for isolation precautions.
◆ Explain that anyone entering the room must wear a gown, gloves, and a mask.

DOCUMENTATION

◆ Document that isolation precautions were initiated.

SELECTED REFERENCES

Bissett, L. "Reducing the Risk of Acquiring Antimicrobial-Resistant Bacteria," *British Journal of Nursing* 15(2):68-71, January-February 2006.

Girou, E., et al. "Misuse of Gloves: The Foundation for Poor Compliance with Hand Hygiene and Potential for Microbial Transmission?" *Journal of Hospital Infection* 57(2):162-69, June 2004.

Jeanes, A. "Putting on Gloves," *Nursing Times* 101(29):28-29, July 2005.

Trick, W.E., et al. "Comparison of Routine Glove Use and Contact-Isolation Precautions to Prevent Transmission of Multidrug-Resistant Bacteria in a Long-term Care Facility," *Journal of the American Geriatrics Society* 52(12): 2003-2009, December 2004.

Removing contaminated gloves

Proper removal techniques are essential for preventing the spread of pathogens from gloves to your skin surface. Follow these steps:

1. Using your left hand, pinch the right glove near the top. Avoid allowing the glove's outer surface to buckle inward against your wrist.

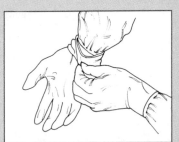

3. Now insert the first two fingers of your ungloved right hand under the edge of the left glove. Avoid touching the glove's outer surface or folding it against your left wrist.

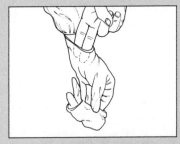

2. Pull downward, allowing the glove to turn inside out as it comes off. Keep the right glove in your left hand after removing it.

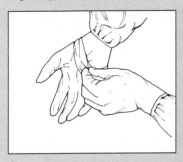

4. Pull downward so the glove turns inside out as it comes off. Continue pulling until the left glove completely encloses the right and its uncontaminated inner surface is facing out.

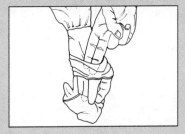

I.V. bolus injection

DESCRIPTION

◆ I.V. bolus injection is used to allow rapid drug administration in an emergency — to provide immediate drug effect; to give drugs that can't be given I.M.; to achieve peak drug levels in the bloodstream; and to deliver drugs that can't be diluted.
◆ "Bolus" refers to the concentration or amount of a drug.
◆ The drug usually takes effect quickly; the patient must be monitored for adverse reactions such as cardiac arrhythmia and anaphylaxis.
◆ Some facilities permit only specially trained nurses to give bolus injections.

CONTRAINDICATIONS

◆ Rapid drug administration possibly causing life-threatening complications

Patient's drug record and chart ◆ gloves ◆ prescribed drug ◆ 20G needle and syringe ◆ povidone-iodine or alcohol pad ◆ noncoring needle if used with a venous access port ◆ diluent (optional)

PREPARATION

◆ One useful dosage form is the ready injectable. (See *Using a ready injectable*.)
◆ Verify the order on the patient's drug record by checking against the practitioner's order.
◆ Know the actions, adverse effects, and administration rate of the drug to be injected.
◆ Draw up the prescribed drug in the syringe and dilute it if needed.

◆ Confirm the patient's identity using two patient identifiers according to facility policy.
◆ Wash your hands, put on gloves, and explain the procedure.
◆ If your facility utilizes a bar code scanning system, be sure to scan your ID badge, the patient's ID bracelet, and the medication's bar code.

Using a ready injectable

The ready injectable is a commercially premeasured medication packaged with a syringe and needle that allows for rapid drug administration in an emergency. Preparing a ready injectable usually takes only 15 to 20 seconds. Other advantages include the reduced risk of breaking sterile technique during administration and the easy identification of drug and dose.

When using a commercially prefilled syringe, be sure to give the precise dose prescribed. For example, if a 50 mg/ml cartridge is supplied but the patient's prescribed dose is 25 mg, you must administer only 0.5 ml — half of the volume contained in the cartridge. Be alert for potential errors whenever dispensing drugs in premeasured dosage forms.

GIVING INJECTIONS THROUGH AN EXISTING I.V. LINE

- Check the compatibility of the drug with the I.V. solution.
- Close the flow clamp, wipe the injection port with an alcohol pad, and inject the drug as you would a direct injection.
- Some I.V. lines have a secondary injection port or T-connector; others have a latex cap at the end of I.V. tubing where the needle is attached.
- Open the flow clamp and readjust the flow rate.
- If the drug isn't compatible with the I.V. solution, flush the line with normal saline solution before and after injection.

GIVING A BOLUS INJECTION THROUGH A VENOUS ACCESS PORT

- Wash your hands, put on gloves, and clean injection site with an alcohol or povidone-iodine pad starting at center of the port and working outward in a circular motion over a 4″ to 5″ (10- to 12.5-cm) diameter. Do this three times.
- Palpate the area over the port to locate the port septum.
- Anchor the port between your thumb and first two fingers.
- Insert a noncoring needle into the appropriate area of the device and deliver the injection.

SPECIAL CONSIDERATIONS

- Drugs given by I.V. bolus or push injections are delivered directly to the circulatory system; acute allergic reaction or anaphylaxis can develop rapidly.

  WARNING *If signs of anaphylaxis occur, notify the practitioner immediately and begin emergency procedures, as needed.*
- Watch for extravasation, redness, or swelling. If extravasation occurs, stop the injection, estimate the amount of infiltration, and notify the practitioner.
- If giving diazepam or chlordiazepoxide hydrochloride through an I.V. line, flush with normal saline solution to prevent drug precipitation resulting from incompatibility.

COMPLICATIONS

- Excessively rapid drug administration causing adverse effects, depending on drug given

PATIENT TEACHING

- Explain the reason for the medication and possible adverse effects.

DOCUMENTATION

- Record the amount and type of drug given.
- Note the time of injection.
- Document appearance of the site.
- Record duration of administration.
- Note the patient's tolerance of the procedure.
- Document the drug's effect.
- Note adverse reactions.

SELECTED REFERENCES

Bidlingmaier, C., et al. "Continuous Infusion of Factor Concentrates in Children with Haemophilia A in Comparison with Bolus Injections," *Haemophilia* 12(3):212-17, May 2006.

Papadakos, P.J. "The Long and Short of Sedation Practices: Daily Interruption or Bolus Dosing?" *Critical Care Medicine* 34(5):1544-45, May 2006.

Sheth, A., et al. "Bolus Thrombolytic Infusion during Prolonged Refractory Cardiac Arrest of Undiagnosed Cause," *Emergency Medicine Journal* 23(3):e19, March 2006.

Stewart, A., et al. "Long-term Metabolic Control on Analogue Insulin and Glargine Basal: Bolus Regime," *Diabetic Medicine* 23(Suppl 2):86, March 2006.

I.V. flow rate calculation and manual control

OVERVIEW

DESCRIPTION
- Calculated from a practitioner's orders, flow rate is expressed as total volume of I.V. solution infused over a prescribed interval or as total volume given in milliliters per hour.
- Many devices are used to regulate flow of I.V. solution, including clamps, controllers, the flow regulator (or rate minder), and the volumetric pump.
- When regulated by a clamp or controller, flow rate is usually measured in drops per minute; by a volumetric pump, in milliliters per hour.
- Flow regulators can be set to deliver desired amount of solution, also in milliliters per hour; they're less accurate than infusion pumps or controllers and are most reliable when used with inactive adult patients.
- Flow rate can be monitored by using a time tape, which indicates the prescribed solution level at hourly intervals.

CONTRAINDICATIONS
- None known

EQUIPMENT

I.V. administration set with clamp ◆ 1″ paper or adhesive tape (or premarked time tape) ◆ infusion pump and controller (if infusing medication) ◆ watch with second hand ◆ drip rate chart, as needed ◆ pen

PREPARATION
- A standard macrodrip set delivers from 10 to 20 drops/ml, depending on manufacturer; a microdrip set delivers 60 drops/ml; and a blood transfusion set delivers 10 drops/ml.
- An adapter can convert a macrodrip set to a microdrip system.

KEY STEPS

- Flow rate requires close monitoring and correction; factors such as venous spasm, venous pressure changes, patient movement or manipulation of the clamp, and bent or kinked tubing can cause rate to vary.

CALCULATING AND SETTING THE DRIP RATE
- Follow the steps in calculating flow rates to determine the proper drip rate, or use your unit's drip rate chart.
- After calculating the desired drip rate, hold your watch next to the drip chamber of the I.V. set and time the drops.
- Release the clamp to the approximate drip rate, then count drops for 1 minute, to account for flow irregularities.
- Adjust the clamp as needed and count drops for another minute. Continue to adjust the clamp and count drops until the correct rate is achieved.

MAKING A TIME TAPE
- Calculate the number of milliliters to be infused per hour. Place a piece of tape vertically on the container alongside the volume-increment markers.
- Starting at current solution level, move down the number of milliliters to be infused in 1 hour; mark the time and a horizontal line on the tape at this level. Mark 1-hour intervals until you get to the bottom of the container.
- Check flow rate every 15 minutes until stable, then recheck every hour, or according to facility policy, and adjust as needed.
- With each check, inspect the I.V. site for complications and assess patient's response to therapy.

SPECIAL CONSIDERATIONS

- If infusion rate slows significantly, a slight rate increase may be needed. If the rate must be increased more than 30%, consult the physician.
- Use an I.V. pump or controller to avoid flow rate inaccuracies when possible; always use pump or controller to infuse solutions by central line.
- Large-volume solution containers have about 10% more fluid than amount indicated on the bag, to allow for tubing purges.

COMPLICATIONS
- A too-slow flow rate (may cause insufficient intake of fluids, drugs, and nutrients)
- A too-rapid flow rate (may cause circulatory overload, which could lead to heart failure, pulmonary edema, and drug adverse effects). (See *Managing I.V. flow rate deviations.*)

Managing I.V. flow rate deviations

PROBLEM	CAUSE	INTERVENTION
Flow rate too slow	◆ Venous spasm after insertion	◆ Apply warm soaks over site.
	◆ Venous obstruction from bending arm	◆ Secure with an arm board, if necessary.
	◆ Pressure change (decreasing fluid in bottle causes solution to run slower due to decreasing pressure)	◆ Readjust the flow rate.
	◆ Elevated blood pressure	◆ Readjust the flow rate. Use an infusion pump or a controller to ensure correct flow rate.
	◆ Cold solution	◆ Allow the solution to warm to room temperature before hanging.
	◆ Change in solution viscosity from medication added	◆ Readjust the flow rate.
	◆ I.V. container too low or patient's arm or leg too high	◆ Hang the container higher or remind the patient to keep his arm below heart level.
	◆ Bevel against vein wall (positional cannulation)	◆ Withdraw the needle slightly, or place a folded 2″ × 2″ gauze pad over or under the catheter hub to change the angle.
	◆ Excess tubing dangling below insertion site	◆ Replace the tubing with a shorter piece or tape the excess tubing to the I.V. pole below the flow clamp (make sure the tubing isn't kinked).
	◆ Cannula too small	◆ Remove the cannula in use and insert a larger-bore cannula or use an infusion pump.
	◆ Infiltration or clotted cannula	◆ Remove the cannula in use and insert a new cannula.
	◆ Kinked tubing	◆ Check the tubing over its entire length and unkink it.
	◆ Clogged filter	◆ Remove the filter and replace it with a new one.
Flow rate too fast	◆ Patient or visitor manipulates the clamp	◆ Instruct the patient not to touch the clamp, and place tape over it.
	◆ Tubing disconnected from the catheter	◆ Restrain the patient or administer the I.V. solution with an infusion pump or a controller, if necessary.
	◆ Change in patient position	◆ Wipe the distal end of the tubing with alcohol, reinsert firmly into the catheter hub, and tape at the connection site. Consider using tubing with luer-lock connections.
	◆ Bevel against vein wall (positional cannulation)	◆ Administer the I.V. solution with an infusion pump or a controller to ensure the correct flow rate.
	◆ Flow clamp drifting as a result of patient movement	◆ Place tape below the clamp.

PATIENT TEACHING

◆ Advise the patient to inform you if he notices a change in flow rate.

DOCUMENTATION

◆ Record the original flow rate when setting up a peripheral line.
◆ If you adjust the rate, record the change, and date and time.

SELECTED REFERENCES

Jayanthi, N.V., and Dabke, H.V. "The Effect of I.V. Cannula Length on the Rate of Infusion," *Injury* 37(1):41-45, January 2006.

Prot, S., et al. "Drug Administration Errors and Their Determinants in Pediatric In-Patients," *International Journal for Quality in Health Care* 17(5):381-89, October 2005.

Schumacher, D.L. "Teaching Tips: Do Your CATS PRrr?: A Mnemonic Device to Teach Safety Checks for Administering Intravenous Medications," *Journal of Continuing Education in Nursing* 36(3):104-106, May-June 2005.

I.V. pumps

DESCRIPTION
- Various types of pumps electronically regulate flow of I.V. solutions or drugs. (See *Infusion pumps.*)
- Volumetric pumps are used for high-pressure drug infusion and highly accurate delivery of fluids or drugs. Systems include:
- Portable syringe pump: delivers small amounts of fluid over a long period, gives fluids to infants, and delivers intra-arterial drugs.
- Peristaltic pump: applies pressure to I.V. tubing to force solution. (Not all peristaltic pumps are volumetric; some count drops.)
- Piston-cylinder pump: pushes solution through disposable cassettes at high pressure, delivering from 1 to 999 ml/hour with 98% accuracy.
- Other specialized devices include the controlled-release infusion system, secondary syringe converter, and patient-controlled analgesia device.
- Pumps have detectors and alarms that signal completion of infusion, air in line, low battery power, and occlusion or inability to deliver at set rate.

CONTRAINDICATIONS
- None known

Pump ◆ I.V. pole ◆ I.V. solution ◆ sterile administration set ◆ sterile peristaltic tubing or cassette, if needed ◆ alcohol pads ◆ adhesive tape

PREPARATION
- Attach the pump to the I.V. pole.
- Swab the I.V. container port with alcohol, insert the administration set spike, and fill the drip chamber to prevent air bubbles from entering the tubing.
- Prime the tubing and close the clamp.
- Follow manufacturer's instructions for tubing placement.

- Position the pump on the same side of the bed as the I.V. or anticipated venipuncture site to avoid crossing I.V. lines over the patient.
- If necessary, perform the venipuncture.
- Plug in the machine and attach its tubing to the needle or catheter hub.
- Depending on the machine, turn it on and press the START button.
- Set the appropriate dials on the front panel to the desired infusion rate and volume.
- Set the volume dial at 50 ml less than prescribed volume or 50 ml less than container volume so you can hang a new container before the old one empties.
- Check the patency of the I.V. line and watch for infiltration.
- Tape all connections.
- Turn on alarm switches.
- Explain the alarm system to the patient to prevent anxiety when a change in infusion activates the alarm.

SPECIAL CONSIDERATIONS

◆ Monitor the pump and patient frequently to ensure correct operation and flow rate and to detect infiltration and such complications as infection and air embolism.
◆ If electrical power fails, pumps automatically switch to battery power.
◆ Check manufacturer's recommendations before giving opaque fluids, such as blood; some pumps fail to detect opaque fluids and others may cause hemolysis of infused blood.
◆ Change the tubing and cassette every 48 hours, or according to facility policy.
◆ Remove I.V. solutions from the refrigerator 1 hour before infusing them to help release gas bubbles. Small bubbles in the solution can join to form larger bubbles, which can activate the pump's air-in-line alarm.

COMPLICATIONS

◆ Same as those associated with peripheral lines
◆ Infiltration developing rapidly with infusion by a volumetric pump (because increased subcutaneous pressure won't slow infusion until significant edema occurs)

PATIENT TEACHING

◆ Explain the use and purpose of the pump to the patient and his family. If necessary, demonstrate how the device works.
◆ Show the patient how to maintain the system until you're confident that he and his family can use it safely. Have them repeat the demonstration.
◆ Discuss with the patient possible complications and actions that should be taken.
◆ Schedule a teaching session with the patient or his family before discharge so you can answer any questions.

DOCUMENTATION

◆ Document the I.V. infusion.
◆ Record use of a pump on the I.V. record and in your notes.

SELECTED REFERENCES

Dulak, S.B. "Smart I.V. Pumps," *RN* 68(12): 38-43, December 2005.
Husch, M, et al. "Insights from the Sharp End of Intravenous Medication Errors: Implications for Infusion Pump Technology," *Quality & Safety in Health Care* 14(2):80-86, April 2005.
Sofer, D. "PCA Pumps: An Illusion of Safety?" *AJN* 105(2):22, February 2005.
Steingass, S.K. "Beyond Pumps: Smarter Infusion Systems," *Nursing Management* 35(Suppl 5):10, October 2004.
Sumrall, C.D., et al. "Getting Pumped: Continuous Insulin Infusion Therapy," *Advance for Nurse Practitioners* 13(12):41-42, 44-46, December 2005.

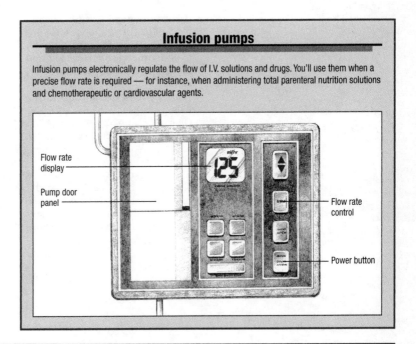

Infusion pumps

Infusion pumps electronically regulate the flow of I.V. solutions and drugs. You'll use them when a precise flow rate is required — for instance, when administering total parenteral nutrition solutions and chemotherapeutic or cardiovascular agents.

Flow rate display

Pump door panel

Flow rate control

Power button

I.V. therapy, pediatric

DESCRIPTION

◆ I.V. therapy may be prescribed to administer medications or to correct a fluid deficit, improve serum electrolyte balance, or provide nourishment.

◆ Primary nursing concerns related to pediatric I.V. therapy include correlating the I.V. site and equipment with the reason for therapy and the patient's age, size, and activity level. For example, a scalp vein is a typical I.V. site for an infant, whereas a peripheral hand, wrist, or foot vein may suit older children.

◆ During I.V. therapy, the nurse must continually assess the patient and the infusion to prevent fluid overload and other complications.

CONTRAINDICATIONS

◆ Vary based on medication administered

EQUIPMENT

Prescribed I.V. fluid ◆ volume-control set with microdrip tubing ◆ infusion pump ◆ I.V. pole ◆ normal saline solution or sterile dextrose 5% in water (D_5W) for injection ◆ povidone-iodine solution ◆ alcohol pads ◆ 3-ml syringe ◆ child-sized butterfly needle or I.V. catheter ◆ tourniquet ◆ ½" or 1" sterile tape ◆ gloves ◆ transparent semipermeable dressing ◆ optional: armboard, insulated foam or medicine cup

PREPARATION

◆ Gather the I.V. equipment, and take it to the patient's bedside.

◆ Check the expiration date on the I.V. fluid and inspect the I.V. container (an I.V. bag for leakage, a bottle for cracks). Examine the I.V. tubing for defects or cracks. Make sure that the packaging surrounding the I.V. catheter or needle remains intact.

◆ Open the wrappings on the I.V. solution and the volume-control tubing set.

◆ Close all clamps on the tubing set; then insert the tip of the tubing set into the entry port of the I.V. bag or bottle.

◆ If you're using an I.V. bag, be sure to hold the bag upright when attaching the tubing. This will keep the sterile air inside the bag from escaping and making the fluid level difficult to read.

◆ Hang the bottle or bag from the I.V. pole.

◆ Open the clamp between the bag and the volume-control set and allow 30 to 50 ml of solution to flow into the calibrated chamber.

◆ Close the clamp.

◆ Squeeze the drip chamber located below the calibrated chamber or volume-control set to create a vacuum.

◆ Release the drip chamber and allow it to fill halfway with solution.

◆ Then release the clamp below the drip chamber so that fluid flows into the remaining tubing, removing any air.

◆ After the tubing fills, close the clamp.

◆ If you're using an infusion pump, attach the I.V. tubing to the infusion cassette, and insert the cassette into the infusion pump.

◆ Prime the cassette tubing according to the manufacturer's instructions.

◆ If you're using an air eliminator I.V. filter, attach the filter to the end of the cassette tubing.

◆ To prevent any air bubbles from entering the patient's circulatory system, place the filter as close to the patient as possible.

◆ To minimize the risk of infection, maintain sterility at the tip of the I.V. tubing until you connect it to the I.V. needle.

◆ Cut as many strips of ½" or 1" tape as you'll need to secure the I.V. line.

◆ Prepare a syringe with 3 ml of flush solution — either the normal saline solution or D_5W.

- Confirm the patient's identity using two patient identifiers according to facility policy.
- Ask the patient (or his parents) whether he's allergic to povidone-iodine solution or to any type of tape.
- Explain the reason for the I.V. therapy. Reassure the parents, and enlist their assistance in explaining the procedure to the patient in terms he can understand.
- Have a staff member available to assist you. Inform the parents that the staff member will help the patient remain still, if necessary, during the procedure.

- Wash your hands and put on gloves.
- Select the insertion site for the butterfly needle or catheter. (See *Common pediatric I.V. sites.*)
- Aim for the most distal site possible, and avoid placing the I.V. line in the patient's dominant arm or in areas of flexion if possible. Avoid previously used or sclerotic veins.
- To locate an appropriate scalp vein, carefully palpate the site for arterial pulsations. If you feel these pulsations, select another site. Then, before inserting the I.V. line, prepare the selected site as ordered.
- To find an appropriate peripheral site, apply a tourniquet to the patient's arm or leg and palpate a suitable vein.

- If you're inserting a butterfly needle, flush the tubing connected to the butterfly with D_5W or normal saline solution.
- Clean the insertion site. Unless contraindicated, use a povidone-iodine pad. If contraindicated, use an alcohol pad. Wipe with a circular motion from the insertion site's center to the outer rim. Let the solution dry.
- Insert the I.V. needle into the vein.
- Watch for blood to flow backward through the catheter or butterfly tubing, which confirms that the needle is in the vein.
- Loosen the tourniquet, and attach the I.V. tubing to the hub of the needle or catheter.
- Begin the infusion.
- Secure the device by applying a piece of ½″ tape over the hub.
- Next, place a piece of tape, adhesive side up, underneath and perpendicular to the device.
- Lift the ends of the tape and crisscross them over the device; then cover the insertion site and device with a transparent semipermeable dressing.
- Further secure and protect the I.V. line as needed. (See *Protecting an I.V. site,* page 290.)

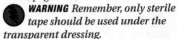 **WARNING** *Remember, only sterile tape should be used under the transparent dressing.*

- Adjust the infusional flow, as ordered, by using the clamp on the I.V. voume-control tubing or by setting the infusion rate on the infusion pump.
- Add solution hourly (or as needed) from the I.V. bag to the volume-control set.
- Assess the I.V. site frequently for signs of infiltration, and check the I.V. bottle or bag for the amount of solution infused.
- Change the I.V. dressing every 48 hours (or per facility policy) to prevent infection.
- Also change the I.V. tubing every 72 hours and the I.V. solution bottle or bag every 24 hours (or per facility policy).
- Label the I.V. bottle or bag, tubing, and volume control set with the time and date of change.

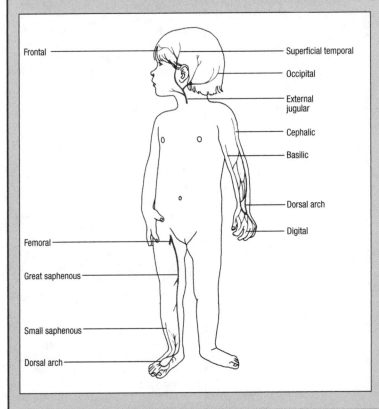

Common pediatric I.V. sites

Here are the most common sites for I.V. therapy in infants and children. Peripheral hand, wrist, or foot veins are typically used with older children, whereas scalp veins are used with infants.

Frontal
Superficial temporal
Occipital
External jugular
Cephalic
Basilic
Dorsal arch
Digital
Femoral
Great saphenous
Small saphenous
Dorsal arch

(continued)

- Change the I.V. insertion site every 72 hours (or per facility policy) to minimize the risk of infection.

- If you inserted the I.V. line without proper skin preparation (during an emergency, for example), change the site sooner.

Protecting an I.V. site

Protecting a child's I.V. site can be a challenge. An active child can easily dislodge an I.V. line, which will necessitate your reinserting it — thus causing him further discomfort. A child may also injure himself by dislodging the I.V. line.

To prevent a child from dislodging an I.V. line, first secure the needle or catheter carefully. Tape the I.V. site as you would for an adult, so that the skin over the tip of the venipuncture device is easily visible. However, avoid overtaping the site because doing so makes it harder to inspect the site and the surrounding tissue.

If the child is old enough to understand, warn him not to play with or jostle the equipment, and teach him how to walk with an I.V. pole to minimize tension on the line. If necessary, you can restrain the extremity.

You should also create a protective barrier between the I.V. site and the environment using one of the following methods.

PAPER CUP

Consider using a small paper cup to protect a scalp site. First, cut off the cup's bottom. (Make sure there are no sharp edges that could damage the child's skin.)

Next, cut a small slot through the top rim to accommodate the I.V. tubing. Place the cup upside down over the insertion site, so the I.V. tubing extends through the slot. Then, secure the cup with strips of tape (shown at right). The opening you cut in the cup allows you to examine the site.

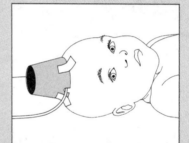

STOCKINETTE

Cut a piece of 4″ (10.2-cm) stockinette the same length as the patient's arm. Slip the stockinette over the patient's arm, and lay the arm on an arm board. Then grasp the stockinette at both sides of the arm, and stretch it under the arm board. Securely tape the stockinette beneath the arm board (shown at right).

Note: You may also protect a scalp site by placing a stockinette on the patient's head, leaving a hole to allow access to the site.

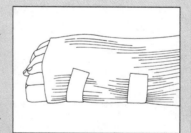

I.V. SHIELD

Peel off the strips covering the adhesive backing on the bottom of the shield. Position the shield over the site so that the I.V. tubing runs through one of the shield's two slots. Then firmly press the shield's adhesive backing against the patient's skin. The shield's clear plastic composition allows you to see the I.V. site clearly.

If the shield is too large to fit securely over the site, just cut off the shield's narrow end below the two air holes. Now you can easily shape the device to the patient's arm.

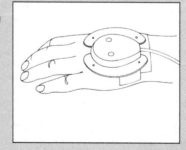

SPECIAL CONSIDERATIONS

- When selecting an I.V. site, try not to use a site that impairs the patient's ability to seek comfort. For example, if an infant typically sucks the thumb or fingers on his right hand, avoid placing the I.V. needle or catheter in his right arm.

- Forewarn parents if you'll start the I.V. infusion in a scalp vein. Also tell them that you may have to clip hair from a small section of the infant's head.

- Ask an older child to participate in selecting the I.V. site, if possible, to give him a sense of control.

- For a mobile patient, aim for an I.V. site on the upper extremity so that he can still get out of bed.

- Avoid starting the I.V. in the same arm as the patient's identification band, unless you first remove the band and replace it on the other arm, to prevent potential circulatory impairment.

- Evaluate the need for restraints after inserting the I.V. line. Apply them only if I.V. needle displacement seems imminent. If you must use restraints, follow facility policy. Assess the patient's skin integrity and provide hourly skin care to prevent skin breakdown. Remove the restraints at frequent intervals to let the patient move freely. Encourage the parents to hold and comfort the patient when he's unrestrained.

- For precise regulation of the I.V. infusion, use a volumetric infusion pump. These pumps infuse fluids at a predetermined rate regardless of temperature fluctuations, vessel variations, or fluid volume changes. Before using an infusion pump, review the operator's manual.

- After inserting the I.V. needle or catheter, reward preschool and school-age patients. Popular rewards are colorful stickers to wear on clothes or on the I.V. dressing.

- You may apply an antimicrobial ointment over the I.V. site to prevent infection.

PATIENT TEACHING

◆ Pediatric patients requiring long-term I.V. medications or nourishment may continue receiving I.V. therapy at home. Assess conditions that promote successful home I.V. therapy — first and foremost, a patient and parent (or other caregiver) who can and want to participate in home I.V. therapy. Other factors include the availability of relief caregivers to provide occasional assistance (especially in an emergency), and a conducive home environment with electricity, running water, a telephone, refrigeration, storage space for supplies, and an area set up for solution and tubing changes and I.V. site care. Additionally, a hospital should be accessible should the patient need emergency assistance or routine reinsertion of an I.V. line.

◆ Teach the parents (and the patient, if appropriate) how to identify and manage complications, such as site infiltration and clotting in the I.V. needle. Show them how to operate equipment such as the infusion pump. Supplement verbal instructions with written patient-teaching materials for later reference. Before discharge, watch the parents operate the infusion pump for 24 hours so that you can evaluate areas for further instruction and identify skills needing refinement.

◆ At discharge, arrange for a home health nurse to visit the patient daily for 2 to 3 days to support and guide initial home therapy. Inform the parents that after her daily visits, the home health nurse will probably visit every 2 to 3 days to assess the I.V. site, provide care, and answer questions.

COMPLICATIONS

◆ Infection
◆ Fluid overload
◆ Electrolyte imbalance
◆ Infiltration
◆ Circulatory impairment

DOCUMENTATION

◆ Record the date and time of the I.V. infusion, the insertion site, and the type and size of I.V. needle or catheter.
◆ Note the patient's tolerance of the procedure.
◆ Describe patient- and parent-teaching activities.
◆ Document the condition of the I.V. site according to facility policy.
◆ If infiltration affects the I.V. site, document the condition of the site at every shift change until the condition resolves.

SELECTED REFERENCES

Black, K.J., et al. "Pediatric Intravenous Insertion in the Emergency Department: Bevel Up or Bevel Down?" *Pediatric Emergency Care* 21(11):707-11, November 2005.

Fein, J.A., and Gorelick, M.H. "The Decision to Use Topical Anesthetic for Intravenous Insertion in the Pediatric Emergency Department," *Academic Emergency Medicine* 13(3):264-68, March 2006.

Lininger, R.A. "Pediatric Peripheral I.V. Insertion Success Rates," *Pediatric Nursing* 29(5):351-54, September-October 2003.

Luhmann, J., et al. "A Comparison of Buffered Lidocaine versus ELA-Max before Peripheral Intravenous Catheter Insertions in Children," *Pediatrics* 113(3 Pt 1):e217-20, March 2004.

I.V. therapy preparation

DESCRIPTION

- Appropriate equipment selection and preparation are essential for accurate delivery of I.V. solution; selection depends on rate and type of infusion desired and type of solution container used.
- Macrodrip set delivers a large amount of solution quickly.
- Microdrip set delivers smaller quantity of solution; it's used for pediatric patients and adults requiring small or closely regulated amounts of solution.
- Tubing with a secondary injection port permits separate or simultaneous infusion of two solutions.
- Tubing with a piggyback port and backcheck valve permits intermittent infusion of a secondary solution and return to infusion of the primary solution.
- Vented I.V. tubing is used for solutions in nonvented bottles.
- Nonvented tubing is used for solutions in bags or vented bottles.

CONTRAINDICATIONS

- None known

I.V. solution ◆ 2:1 chlorhexidine swabs ◆ I.V. administration set ◆ in-line filter, if needed ◆ I.V. pole ◆ drug and label, if needed

PREPARATION

- Verify type, volume, and expiration date of I.V. solution.
- For solutions in a glass bottle, inspect for chips and cracks; for solutions in a plastic bag, squeeze the bag to detect leaks.
- Examine I.V. solution for particles, abnormal discoloration, or cloudiness.

WARNING *If particles, abnormal discoloration, or cloudiness are present, discard the solution and notify the pharmacy.*

- If ordered, add drug to the solution and place a completed drug-added label on the container.
- Remove the administration set from its box and check for cracks, holes, and missing clamps.

- Wash your hands to prevent contamination.
- Slide the flow clamp of the administration set tubing down to the drip chamber or injection port, and close the clamp.

PREPARING A BAG

- Place the bag on a flat, stable surface.
- Remove the protective cap or tear the tab from the tubing insertion port.
- Remove the protective cap from the administration set spike.
- Holding the port firmly with one hand, insert the spike with your other hand.
- Hang the bag on the I.V. pole and squeeze the drip chamber until it's one-half full.

PREPARING A NONVENTED BOTTLE

- Remove the bottle's metal cap and inner disk, if present.

When to use an in-line filter

An in-line filter removes pathogens and particles from I.V. solutions, helping to reduce the risk of infusion phlebitis. Because in-line filters are expensive and their installation cumbersome and time-consuming, they aren't used routinely. Many facilities require that a filter be used only when administering an admixture. If you're unsure of whether to use a filter, check facility policy or follow this list of do's and don'ts.

DO'S

- Use an in-line filter:
- when giving solutions to an immunodeficient patient
- when administering total parenteral nutrition
- when infusing intraspinal infusions (0.2 micron filter)
- when using additives that include many separate particles, such as antibiotics requiring reconstitution
- when using rubber injection ports or plastic diaphragms repeatedly

- when phlebitis is likely to occur.
- Change the in-line filter according to the manufacturer's recommendations (blood and blood by-product filters every 4 hours or to coincide with blood administration set changes). If you don't, bacteria trapped in the filter releases endotoxin, a pyrogen small enough to pass through the filter into the bloodstream.
- Use an add-on filter of larger pore size (1.2 microns) when infusing albumin mixed with nutritional solutions and amphotericin B.

DON'TS

- Don't use an in-line filter:
- when administering solutions with large particles that will clog a filter and stop I.V. flow, such as suspensions, lipid emulsions, and high-molecular-volume plasma expanders
- when administering a drug dose of 5 mg or less (because the filter may absorb it).

- Place the bottle on a stable surface and wipe the rubber stopper with a chlorhexidine pad.
- Remove the protective cap from the administration set spike, and push the spike through the center of the bottle's rubber stopper.

   WARNING *Avoid twisting or angling the spike to prevent pieces of the stopper from breaking off and falling into the solution.*

- Invert the bottle. If its vacuum is intact, you'll hear a hissing sound and see air bubbles rise (this may not occur if you've already added drug).
- If the vacuum isn't intact, discard the bottle and begin again.
- Hang the bottle on the I.V. pole and squeeze the drip chamber until it's one-half full.

PREPARING A VENTED BOTTLE

- Remove the bottle's metal cap and latex diaphragm to release the vacuum. If the vacuum isn't intact (except after drug has been added), discard the bottle and begin again.
- Place the bottle on a stable surface and wipe the rubber stopper with a chlorhexidine pad.
- Remove the protective cap from the administration set spike and push the spike through the insertion port next to the air vent tube opening.
- Hang the bottle on the I.V. pole, and squeeze the drip chamber until it's one-half full.

PRIMING THE I.V. TUBING

- If necessary, attach a filter to the opposite end of the I.V. tubing, and follow manufacturer's instructions for filling and priming.
- Purge the tubing before attaching the filter to avoid forcing air into the filter and clogging filter channels.
- Most filters are positioned with the distal end of the tubing facing upward so the solution completely wets the filter membrane and all air bubbles are eliminated from the line. (See *When to use an in-line filter.*)
- If you aren't using a filter, aim the distal end of the tubing over a wastebasket or sink and slowly open the flow clamp.

- Most distal tube coverings allow the solution to flow without having to remove the protective cover.
- Leave the clamp open until the I.V. solution flows through the entire length of tubing to release trapped air bubbles and force out all the air.
- Invert all Y-ports and backcheck valves and tap them, if needed, to fill them with solution.
- After priming the tubing, close the clamp.
- Loop the tubing over the I.V. pole.
- Label the container with patient's name and room number, date and time, container number, ordered rate and duration of infusion, and your initials.

SPECIAL CONSIDERATIONS

- Always use aseptic technique when preparing I.V. solutions.
- You can use vented tubing with a vented bottle. If doing so, don't remove the latex diaphragm. Instead, insert the spike into the larger indentation in the diaphragm.
- Change I.V. tubing every 48 or 72 hours, according to facility policy, or more frequently if you suspect contamination.
- Change filter according to the manufacturer's recommendations or sooner if it becomes clogged.

COMPLICATIONS
- None known

PATIENT TEACHING

- Before starting I.V. therapy, explain to the patient what he can expect.
- Tell the patient that a plastic catheter or needle will be placed in his vein.
- Tell the patient about how long the catheter or needle will stay in place.
- Explain to the patient that the physician will decide what fluids he needs.
- Tell the patient that I.V. fluid may feel cold at first but the feeling will subside.
- Tell the patient to report any discomfort.
- Explain any activity restrictions.
- Teach the patient how to care for the I.V. line.
- Instruct the patient to call a nurse if the flow rate suddenly slows down or speeds up.

DOCUMENTATION

- Document the date, time, and venipuncture site.
- Note the type of equipment used.
- Record how the patient tolerated the procedure.
- Document patient and family teaching.
- Note changes of insertion site, venipuncture device, or I.V. tubing.
- Document reasons for changing the I.V. site, such as extravasation, phlebitis, occlusion, patient removal, or routine policy adherence.

SELECTED REFERENCES

Hicks, R.W., and Becker, S.C. "An Overview of Intravenous-related Medication Administration Errors as Reported to MEDMARX, a National Medication Error-Reporting Program," *Journal of Infusion Nursing* 29(1):20-27, January-February 2006.

Morris, R. "Intravenous Drug Administration: A Skill for Student Nurses?" *Paediatric Nursing* 18(3):35-38, April 2006.

van der Hoogen, A., et al. "In-Line Filters in Central Venous Catheters in a Neonatal Intensive Care Unit," *Journal of Perinatal Medicine* 34(1):71-74, 2006.

Jugular venous oxygen saturation monitoring

DESCRIPTION

- The procedure measures venous oxygenation saturation of blood as it leaves the brain, reflecting oxygen saturation of blood after cerebral perfusion has taken place. (See *Common causes of desaturation*.)
- It helps determine if blood flow to the brain matches the brain's metabolic demand.
- The normal range is 55% to 70%; values higher than 70% indicate hyperperfusion. Values between 40% and 54% indicate relative hypoperfusion; values lower than 40% indicate ischemia.
- Criteria for monitoring include any neurologic injury where ischemia is a threat and may include intraoperative monitoring, subarachnoid hemorrhage, and post-acute head injury with increased intracranial pressure (ICP).

CONTRAINDICATIONS

- None known

EQUIPMENT

INSERTION OF SJVO$_2$ CATHETER

Sterile towels ◆ sterile drapes ◆ surgical caps ◆ gowns ◆ sterile gloves ◆ masks ◆ antiseptic scrub ◆ chlorhexidine solution ◆ central venous catheter insertion kit ◆ 1% or 2% lidocaine without epinephrine ◆ 5- or 10-cc syringe, with an 18G and 23G needle ◆ 5 French percutaneous introducer ◆ 4 French fiber-optic SjvO$_2$ catheter ◆ oximetric monitor with cable ◆ 500 ml 0.9% sodium chloride solution (heparinized or non-heparinized based on facility policy) ◆ pressure tubing with continuous flush device ◆ pressure bag or device ◆ sterile occlusive dressing ◆ sterile marker ◆ sterile labels

REMOVAL OF SJVO$_2$ CATHETER

Sterile gloves ◆ suture removal set ◆ sterile hemostat ◆ sterile scissors ◆ chlorhexidine solution ◆ sterile occlusive dressing

KEY STEPS

- Confirm the patient's identity using two patient identifiers according to facility policy.
- Explain the procedure and provide privacy.
- Wash your hands and put on sterile gloves.
- Using aseptic technique, prime the pressure tubing system, removing all air bubbles and maintaining sterility.
- Follow manufacturer's instructions for in vitro calibration of catheter before insertion.
- Position the patient with his head elevated at 30 to 45 degrees and his neck in a neutral position. Document baseline ICP; note any subsequent changes.
- Turn his head laterally, away from the site chosen for catheter insertion.
- Follow dressing procedure guidelines for insertion of central lines.
- Put on new sterile gloves.
- Using sterile technique, open and prepare the central venous pressure insertion tray, and add a 5 French sterile introducer and a 4 French fiber-optic SjvO$_2$ catheter.
- Label all medications, medication containers, and other solutions containers on and off the sterile field.
- The physician will scrub the insertion site with antiseptic scrub solution and position sterile drapes, exposing only the insertion site.

INSERTING OF SJVO$_2$ CATHETER

- Assist the physician during insertion, as needed.
- Monitor neurologic status, vital signs, ICP, and pain during insertion.
- After the line is in place, attach pressure tubing and confirm patency of both jugular catheter lumens by aspirating and flushing.
- Clean the insertion site with chlorhexidine solution and apply sterile occlusive dressing.
- Obtain a lateral cervical spine or lateral skull X-ray to confirm catheter placement at the level of the jugular bulb.

WARNING *Optimum placement of the SjvO$_2$ catheter tip is at the level of the jugular bulb of the internal jugular vein. The tip of the catheter should be viewed at the upper border of the second cervical vertebra.*

- Draw a jugular venous blood gas sample and perform in vivo calibration according to manufacturer's guidelines.
- Assess neurologic status, vital signs, and ICP immediately after insertion.

WARNING *The catheter in the jugular bulb can inhibit venous*

Common causes of desaturation

CAUSES	INTERVENTIONS
Systemic hypoxemia (one of the most common causes of cerebral hypoxia)	If the oxygen saturation (Sao$_2$) is less than 90%, increase the oxygen percentage or fraction of inspired oxygen and adjust the ventilator settings, as ordered.
Anemia (hemoglobin less than 90 g/L)	Report abnormal results and administer a blood transfusion, if ordered.
Systemic hypotension (mean blood pressure less than 70 mm Hg)	Report abnormal results to the practitioner, and administer a fluid challenge or vasopressors, if ordered.
Increased intracranial pressure (more than 20 mm Hg)	Elevate the head of the bed 30 degrees, decrease external stimuli, administer prescribed osmotic diuretics, such as mannitol, and adjust ventilator settings to produce mild hyperventilation, as ordered. Other measures may include drainage of cerebrospinal fluid and methods to reduce cerebral oxygen demand, such as sedation, neuromuscular blockade, or barbiturate coma.

outflow; sustained ICP greater than 5 mm Hg over preinsertion baseline may require catheter removal.

- Record baseline measurements for continuously monitored $SjvO_2$. Calculate $AvjDO_2$, CeO_2, and O_2ER as a baseline.

● **WARNING** *Repeated patterns of desaturation are reliable indicators of poor outcomes in patients with severe head injury.*

- Continuously monitor $SjvO_2$.
- Verify accuracy of reading by drawing $SjvO_2$ every 8 to 12 hours; blood sample reading should be within 4% of reading shown on monitor.
- Record $SjvO_2$ and ICP values hourly and note trends. Assess ICP in relation to $SjvO_2$. Notify practitioner of any deviations.
- Calculate CeO_2 and O_2ER as indicated.
- Maintain a safe environment during monitoring to prevent catheter dislodgment.
- Use sedation or analgesia as indicated.
- Perform in vivo calibration with jugular blood gas sample as recommended (usually each shift).
- Change dressing using aseptic technique if it becomes soiled or loosened.
- Change I.V. solution and tubing for catheter according to facility policy for central lines.
- Replace an $SjvO_2$ catheter with low light intensity.
- Check the fiber-optic catheter for obstruction or occlusion. Aspirate the catheter until blood can be freely sampled and normal light intensity is displayed.

● **WARNING** *Low light intensity may indicate catheter occlusion or damage to fiber optics. High light intensity indicates vessel wall artifact.*

- For an $SjvO_2$ catheter with high light intensity, adjust the patient's head to ensure neutral neck position.
- To prevent catheter coiling, identify rhythmic fluctuations in $SvjO_2$ trends.
- Rhythmic fluctuations of trends that are unrelated to changes in ICP, cerebral perfusion pressure, or systemic

blood pressure signify coiling of the catheter.
- Obtain a lateral cervical spine or lateral skull X-ray to assess catheter position in the external jugular vein. If coiling is confirmed, replace catheter.
- Identify $SjvO_2$ desaturations and notify the practitioner.
- Assess for ICP changes. In patients with brain injury, increased ICP is a common cause of desaturation.

● **WARNING** *Desaturations are emergent events requiring immediate interventions to restore cerebral blood flow and oxygen delivery.*

- Confirm the $SjvO_2$ data by obtaining a jugular venous blood gas sample.
- Perform in vivo calibration.

● **WARNING** *To avoid reading sample errors, aspirate blood slowly during the sampling procedure (1 ml/minute).*

REMOVING AN $SJVO_2$ CATHETER

- Explain the procedure and provide privacy.
- Wash your hands and prepare equipment.
- Deactivate alarms.
- Turn stopcocks off, position the patient properly, monitor vital signs, put on sterile gloves, and assist physician with catheter removal as needed.
- Apply direct pressure to the site until there are no signs of active bleeding.
- Put on new sterile gloves.
- Apply chlorhexidine solution and sterile occlusive dressing to catheter site.
- Assess the site for signs of bleeding every 15 minutes for 1 hour, then every 30 minutes the next hour, then 1 hour later.

SPECIAL CONSIDERATIONS

- Complications associated with $SvjO_2$ monitoring are similar to those that can occur with any central line; line sepsis is most common.

COMPLICATIONS

- Pneumothorax

- Carotid artery puncture
- Internal jugular thrombosis
- Excessive bleeding
- Impaired cerebral venous drainage
- Increased ICP

PATIENT TEACHING

- Explain the procedure to the patient and his family.

DOCUMENTATION

- Document difficulties encountered during insertion.
- Note the depth (in centimeters) of the catheter.
- Record the patient's tolerance of the procedure.
- Document the ICP reading during insertion.
- Record the baseline $SjvO_2$ reading.
- Note the initial CeO_2 and $AvjDO_2$ calculations.
- Record $SjvO_2$ and ICP hourly.
- Record CeO_2, $AvjDO_2$, and O_2ER when indicated.
- Document assessments of the insertion site.
- Record expected and unexpected outcomes and interventions taken.
- Note patient and family education provided.

SELECTED REFERENCES

Alten, J., and Mariscalco, M.M. "Critical Appraisal of Perez et al.: Jugular Venous Oxygen Saturation or Arteriovenous Difference of Lactate Content and Outcome in Children with Severe Traumatic Brain Injury," *Pediatric Critical Care Medicine* 6(4):480-82, July 2005.

Dunn, I.F., et al. "Neuromonitoring in Neurological Critical Care," *Neurocritical Care* 4(1):83-92, 2006.

Stevens, W.J. "Multimodal Monitoring: Head Injury Management Using $SjvO_2$ and LICOX," *Journal of Neuroscience Nursing* 36(6):332-39, December 2004.

Tobias, J.D. "Cerebral Oxygenation Monitoring: Near-Infrared Spectroscopy," *Expert Review of Medical Devices* 3(2):235-43, March 2006.

Knee extension therapy

OVERVIEW

DESCRIPTION

◆ Knee extension therapy is used in treatment of a patient with joint stiffness and limited range of motion (ROM) from fractures, dislocations, ligament and tendon repairs, joint arthroplasty, burns, total knee replacement, hemophilia, spinal cord injuries, rheumatoid arthritis, tendon release, cerebral palsy, multiple sclerosis, and other traumatic and nontraumatic disorders.

◆ Therapy involves application of low-load, prolonged-duration stretching force to knee joint.

◆ It restores functional ROM to limbs stiffened by immobility and possibly contractures or adhesions and helps patient regain ROM by applying dynamic stress continuously while he's sleeping or resting.

◆ It provides support to upper and lower limbs by struts fitted with tension rods that apply firm force to coax muscles and connective tissues to stretch.

CONTRAINDICATIONS

◆ Unhealed or unstable fracture
◆ Septic joints
◆ Acute thrombophlebitis
◆ Severe arthritic joint inflammation
◆ Recent trauma with possible hidden fractures or internal injuries
   Use cautiously in patients with:
◆ Osteoporosis, spasticity, edema, gross ligament instability, and circulatory impairment

EQUIPMENT

Knee extension system ◆ knee extension system and tension adjustment tool ◆ pillow, adhesive tape, marking pen (optional)

PREPARATION

◆ Hold the knee extension system so that the adjustment scale is visible on one of the struts.

◆ To read the tension, look at the number on the tension scale lined up with the flat top of the tension spacer inside the strut. The tension spacer is visible in the window next to the tension scale.

◆ If the top of the tension spacer isn't lined up with the "0" on the tension scale with each strut, adjust the tension screw in the top of each spacer with the tension adjustment tool until they're lined up.

KEY STEPS

◆ Confirm the patient's identity using two patient identifiers according to facility policy.
◆ Wash your hands.
◆ Explain the procedure to the patient.

ADJUSTING STRUT LENGTH

◆ To shorten or lengthen the distal strut, first remove the ⅛″ screw or screws located near the cam, using the tension adjustment tool.

◆ Slide the smaller tube in or out of the larger tube to obtain correct strut length.

◆ Line up the screw holes, replace and tighten the screw or screws.

◆ Repeat this adjustment on each strut as necessary.

◆ Open the front-of-thigh, shin, and over-the-knee straps, pull them out of the D-wire that's attached to the strut, and fold the strap's Velcro closure onto itself.

◆ Loosen the back-of-thigh and calf cuffs to widen the splint to accommodate the patient's calf and thigh dimensions.

◆ Place the system under his leg.

◆ Position the distal struts, which are the larger tubes with the tension adjusters, beneath the calf.

◆ Pull the proximal and distal struts up with both hands until the struts are even with the midlines of the sides of the thigh and calf.

◆ Align the cams across the knee axis, making sure they're in a straight line.

◆ With the cams aligned, close the over-the-knee straps making sure that you can slide one finger under the upper and lower edges of each strap.

◆ Close the front-of-thigh cuffs and shin cuffs.

◆ Adjust and close the back-of-thigh cuffs and calf cuffs.

◆ If necessary, adjust strut length so that cuffs are positioned on the bulk of the muscle mass at midthigh and midcalf.

AGE FACTOR *Elderly patients are at increased risk of skin breakdown; assess for pressure ulcer development while using a knee extension system.*

SETTING SPLINT TENSION

◆ Insert the tension adjustment tool into the open end of the lower strut.
◆ Increase the tension by turning the tool clockwise; reduce the tension by turning it counterclockwise.
◆ Make sure the cams are aligned across the knee axis, struts are placed on the medial and lateral axes of the leg, and cuffs are evenly contoured across the leg.
◆ Mark the backs of both cuffs to keep the patient from changing the fitting.
◆ Mark a reference line with a pen on the over-the-knee straps and the front-of-thigh and shin cuffs so the patient knows where to close them.
◆ Make sure he practices applying and removing the splint.

SPECIAL CONSIDERATIONS

◆ The system is custom-fitted and tension is adjusted to patient's tolerance; worn at the optimal tolerable tension for the longest time (8 to 10 hours), preferably at night.
◆ When applied early in treatment program, duration of rehabilitation is greatly reduced.

COMPLICATIONS

◆ Pain
◆ Stiffness
◆ Alterations in skin integrity

PATIENT TEACHING

◆ Explain the reasons for knee extension therapy.
◆ Tell the patient how to apply the equipment.
◆ Advise the patient about length of time for each session.
◆ Explain to the patient how to adjust tension settings.
◆ Inform the patient about signs and symptoms to report.

DOCUMENTATION

◆ Note the date and time of the procedure.
◆ Record the tension ordered by the practitioner, length of time the patient can tolerate tension, increases or decreases in tension, and reasons for tension changes.
◆ Document the patient's tolerance of the procedure.
◆ Record patient teaching.

SELECTED REFERENCES

Hertel, J., et al. "Combining Isometric Knee Extension Exercises with Hip Adduction Does Not Increase Quadriceps EMG Activity," *British Journal of Sports Medicine* 38(2):210-13, April 2004.

Petrella, J.K., et al. "Resistance Training Improves Knee Extension Power, Contractile Velocity, and Fatigue Resistance in Older Men and Women," *Medicine & Science in Sports & Exercise* 37(5) Suppl:S130, May 2005.

Roelants, M., et al. "Whole-Body-Vibration Training Increases Knee-Extension Strength and Speed of Movement in Older Women," *Journal of the American Geriatrics Society* 52(6):901-908, June 2004.

Townsend, D., et al. "The Influence of Adipose Tissue Thickness on Near-Infrared Spectrometry During Intra-Contraction Knee Extension Exercise," *Medicine & Science in Sports & Exercise* 36(5) Suppl: S23, May 2004.

Laser therapy

OVERVIEW

DESCRIPTION

- Laser surgical equipment is used by surgeons to treat various skin lesions. It offers precise control, spares normal tissue, speeds healing, and deters infection by sterilizing the operative site.
- The procedure leaves a nearly bloodless operative field because it seals blood vessels as it vaporizes tissue.
- It can be performed on an outpatient basis.
- The most commonly used lasers are vascular, pigment, and carbon dioxide (CO_2) lasers. (See *Understanding types of laser therapy*.)

CONTRAINDICATIONS

- None known

EQUIPMENT

Laser ◆ filtration face masks ◆ protective eyewear ◆ laser vacuum ◆ extra vacuum filters ◆ surgical drape ◆ prescribed cleaning solution ◆ sterile gauze ◆ nonadherent dressings ◆ surgical tap ◆ cotton-tipped applicators ◆ nonreflective surgical instruments ◆ gowns ◆ sterile gloves

PREPARATION

- Prepare the tray including a local anesthetic, as ordered, and dry and wet gauze.
- Gauze is used to control bleeding, protect healthy tissue, and abrade and remove any eschar, which would otherwise inhibit laser absorption.
- Prepare nonreflective surgical instruments as needed.

KEY STEPS

- Confirm the patient's identity using two patient identifiers according to facility policy.
- Explain how the laser works and describe its benefits. Explain the equipment and outline the procedure to help allay the patient's concerns.
- Put on gown, filtration face mask, and protective eyewear.
- Before the surgeon begins, position the patient comfortably, drape him, and place protective gauze, if needed, around the operative site.
- **WARNING** *Confirm that everyone in the room — including the patient — has protective eyewear on to filter laser light.*
- Lock the door to the surgical suite to keep unprotected persons from entering the room.
- After the surgeon administers the anesthetic and it takes effect, activate the laser vacuum.
- The CO_2 laser has a vacuum hose attached to a separate apparatus; use this to clean the surgical site. The vacuum has a filter that traps and collects most of the vaporized tissue. Change the filter whenever suction decreases; follow facility guidelines for filter disposal.
- After the procedure, put on sterile gloves and apply direct pressure with a sterile gauze pad to any bleeding wound for 20 minutes. If wound continues to bleed, notify the physician.
- When bleeding is controlled, use aseptic technique to clean the area with a cotton-tipped applicator dipped in prescribed cleaning solution.
- Size and cut a nonadherent dressing.
- Secure the dressing with surgical tape.
- Vascular and pigment lasers won't result in a wound; only superficial skin changes will occur.

Understanding types of laser therapy

Laser therapy is an essential tool for treating many types of skin lesions. The types of lasers used in dermatology keep increasing, and each has specific applications. It's important to be familiar with the various lasers and the indications for each use.

LASERS FOR VASCULAR LESIONS

The laser most commonly used for vascular lesions is the flashlamp-pumped dye laser (FLPDL). Other lasers used for vascular lesions include copper vapor, argon, potassium titanyl phosphate (KTP), krypton, frequency-doubled Q-switched, and Nd:YAG lasers. The choice of laser depends on the specific vascular lesion. Port-wine stains, hemangiomas, venous lake, rosacea, telangiectasia, and the skin symptoms of Kaposi's sarcoma are examples of vascular lesions that are appropriate for laser therapy with these instruments.

LASERS FOR PIGMENTED LESIONS

Lasers that are effective in removing tattoos and dermal and epidermal pigmented lesions include Q-switched ruby, Q-switched Nd:YAG, Q-switched alexandrite, FLPDL, copper vapor, krypton, and KTP. Pigmented lesions that are appropriate for these laser treatments include tattoos, nevi of Ota, melasma, solar lentigo, café au lait spots, Becker's nevi, and epidermal nevi.

CARBON DIOXIDE LASER

The carbon dioxide laser is one of the oldest lasers; it's used less frequently since the advent of lasers that work on the principle of selective photothermolysis. This laser causes thermal injury, resulting in ablation in the defocused mode; it cuts tissue in the focused mode. It's used to treat actinic cheilitis, rhinophyma, warts, keloids, and other lesions.

LASERS FOR HAIR REMOVAL

Lasers used to eliminate unwanted hair include ruby, diode, alexandrite, and Nd:YAG. Laser treatment is only effective in removing dark-colored hair; it isn't effective for removing blonde, red, white, or gray hair.

SPECIAL CONSIDERATIONS

◆ The surgeon uses the laser beam like a scalpel to excise lesions.
◆ The nurse must have knowledge of how each laser operates and of laser safety considerations for the patient and health care providers.
◆ Laser surgery is generally safe, although bleeding and scarring can result.
◆ The most significant hazard to patients and staff is eye damage or other injury caused by unintended laser beam reflection. All patients and surgical staff must wear special goggles to filter laser light.
◆ Special nonreflective instruments must be used during the procedure.
◆ Access to the room must be controlled; all windows must be covered.

COMPLICATIONS
◆ Bleeding
◆ Scarring
◆ Infection

PATIENT TEACHING

◆ Explain to the patient that the laser causes a burnlike wound that can be deep.
◆ Inform the patient that the wound will appear charred. Tell him that some of the eschar will be removed during initial postoperative cleaning and more will gradually dislodge at home.
◆ Tell the patient to expect a burning odor and smoke during the procedure. A smoke evacuator machine will clear it away.
◆ Advise the patient that he may sense heat from the laser. Urge him to tell the physician at once if pain occurs.
◆ Teach the patient how to dress his wound and care for his skin as ordered by the surgeon.
◆ Tell the patient that he can take showers, but to promote wound healing and prevent infection, he should not immerse the wound site in water.
◆ If the wound bleeds while the patient is at home, demonstrate how to apply direct pressure with clean gauze or a washcloth for 20 minutes. If pressure doesn't control bleeding, tell him to call his physician.
◆ If the patient's foot or leg was operated on, urge him to keep the extremity elevated and to use it as little as possible because pressure can inhibit healing.
◆ Warn the patient to protect the treated area from exposure to the sun to avoid changes in pigmentation.
◆ Tell the patient to call the physician if a fever of 100° F (37.8° C) or higher persists longer than 1 day.

DOCUMENTATION

◆ Note the patient's skin condition before and after the procedure.
◆ Document any bleeding.
◆ Record type of dressing applied.
◆ Note if the patient complained of pain.
◆ Note whether the patient comprehends home care instructions.

SELECTED REFERENCES
Chandu, A., and Smith, A.C. "The Use of CO_2 Laser in the Treatment of Oral White Patches: Outcomes and Factors Affecting Recurrence," *International Journal of Oral and Maxillofacial Surgery* 34(4):396-400, June 2005.
Inzeo, D., and Haughney, A. "Laser Therapy in the Management of Lung Cancer," *Clinical Journal of Oncology Nursing* 8(1):94-95, February 2004.
Kontoes, P., et al. "Hair Induction after Laser-Assisted Hair Removal and its Treatment," *Journal of the American Academy of Dermatology* 54(1):64-67, January 2006.
Moise, K.J., Jr. "Neurodevelopmental Outcome after Laser Therapy for Twin-Twin Transfusion Syndrome," *American Journal of Obstetrics and Gynecology* 194(5):1208-210, May 2006.

Latex allergy protocol

OVERVIEW

DESCRIPTION

◆ People at risk for latex allergy include those who undergo multiple surgical procedures, health care workers, latex product manufacturers, and those with a genetic predisposition to latex allergy.

◆ Symptoms include generalized itching, irritated eyes, sneezing and coughing, rash, hives, bronchial asthma, scratchy throat, difficulty breathing, anaphylaxis, and edema of face, hands, or neck. (See *Latex allergy screening*.)

◆ There are three categories of latex sensitivity:

– History of anaphylaxis or systemic reaction when exposed to a natural latex product

– History of nonsystemic allergic reaction

– No history of latex hypersensitivity but high risk because of associated medical condition, occupation, or allergy.

⚡ **WARNING** *Due to the risk of life-threatening hypersensitivity reaction, a patient with latex sensitivity shouldn't have contact with any latex products; keep a cart with latex-free equipment in the patient's room.*

CONTRAINDICATIONS

◆ None known

EQUIPMENT

Latex allergy patient identification wristband ◆ latex-free equipment, including room contents ◆ anaphylaxis kit ◆ latex allergy sign (optional)

PREPARATION

◆ After you've determined the patient is sensitive to latex, place him in a private room.

◆ If a private room isn't available, make the room latex-free to prevent spread of airborne particles from latex products used on the other patient.

Latex allergy screening

To determine if your patient has a latex sensitivity or allergy, ask these screening questions:

◆ What's your occupation?

◆ Have you experienced an allergic reaction, local sensitivity, or itching following exposure to any latex products, such as balloons or condoms?

◆ Do you have shortness of breath or wheezing after blowing up balloons or after a dental visit? Do you have itching in or around your mouth after eating a banana?

If your patient answers yes to any of these questions, proceed with the following questions:

◆ Do you have a history of allergies, dermatitis, or asthma? If so, what type of reaction do you have?

◆ Do you have congenital abnormalities? If yes, explain.

◆ Do you have food allergies? If so, what specific allergies do you have? Describe your reaction.

◆ If you experience shortness of breath or wheezing when blowing up latex balloons, describe your reaction.

◆ Have you had previous surgical procedures? Did you experience associated complications? If so, describe them.

◆ Have you had previous dental procedures? Did complications result? If so, describe them.

◆ Are you exposed to latex in your occupation? Do you experience a reaction to latex products at work? If so, describe your reaction.

KEY STEPS

◆ Assess for latex allergy in all patients, including those admitted to the delivery room or short-procedure unit or those having a surgical procedure.

◆ If the patient has a confirmed latex allergy, bring a cart with latex-free supplies into his room.

◆ Document that he has a latex allergy on his chart.

◆ Place a latex allergy identification bracelet on the patient, if required by facility policy.

◆ If he will be receiving anesthesia, make sure that "latex allergy" is clearly visible on the front of his chart.

◆ Notify the circulating nurse in the surgical unit, the postanesthesia care unit nurses, and any other team members that the patient has a latex allergy. (See *Anesthesia induction and latex allergy*.)

◆ If the patient is transported to another area, have the latex-free cart accompany him and have all staff who come in contact with him wear latex-free gloves.

◆ Place a mask with cloth ties on the patient when he leaves his room to protect him from inhaling airborne latex particles.

◆ Make sure I.V. access is accomplished using all latex-free products.

◆ Post a "latex allergy" sign on the I.V. tubing to prevent access of the line using latex products.

◆ Flush I.V. tubing with 50 ml of I.V. solution to rinse the tubing out because of latex ports in the I.V. tubing.

◆ Place a warning label on I.V. bags that says, "Do not use latex injection ports."

◆ Use a latex-free tourniquet or a latex tourniquet over clothing, if none are available.

◆ Remove the vial stopper to mix and draw up drugs.

◆ Use latex-free oxygen administration equipment; remove the elastic and tie equipment on with gauze.

◆ Wrap your stethoscope with a latex-free product to protect the patient.

- Wrap Tegaderm over patient's finger before using pulse oximetry.
- Use latex-free syringes when administering drug.
- Have an anaphylaxis kit available. If he has an allergic reaction, you must act immediately.

⚡ **WARNING** *Be prepared to treat life-threatening hypersensitivity with antihistamines, epinephrine, corticosteroids, I.V. fluids, oxygen, intubation, and mechanical ventilation, if necessary.*

SPECIAL CONSIDERATIONS

- Signs and symptoms of latex allergy usually occur within 30 minutes of anesthesia induction, but can occur up to 5 hours later.
- If you suspect that you're sensitive to latex, contact employee health services concerning facility protocol for latex-sensitive employees.
- Use latex-free products as often as possible to reduce your exposure to latex.
- Remember that people allergic to certain "cross-reactive" foods (apricots, cherries, grapes, kiwis, passion fruit, bananas, avocados, chestnuts, tomatoes, and peaches) may be allergic to latex.

⚡ **WARNING** *Latex doesn't always look like rubber. It's found in much equipment, including electrocardiograph leads, oral and nasal airway tubing, tourniquets, nerve stimulation pads, temperature strips, and blood pressure cuffs.*

COMPLICATIONS

- Asthma (increased risk for developing worsening symptoms from airborne latex)
- Anaphylactic reaction

PATIENT TEACHING

- Explain latex allergy to the patient.
- Discuss signs and symptoms of latex allergy.
- Inform the patient about the importance of wearing latex allergy identification.
- Explain the importance of informing all health care workers of the patient's latex allergy.
- Explain to the patient what to do if hypersensitivity reaction occurs.
- Teach the patient measures to reduce latex exposure.

DOCUMENTATION

- Note patient history of allergies, including reactions to latex.
- Record signs and symptoms observed or reported by the patient.
- Document notification of other departments of the patient's latex allergy.
- Note the allergy identification placed on wrist.
- Record the latex allergy alert placed on the medical record and in the patient's room.
- Document that a cart with latex-free items was placed in the patient's room.
- Record measures taken to prevent latex exposure.
- Note patient teaching.

SELECTED REFERENCES

Beckford-Ball, J. "Tackling Latex Allergies in Patients and Nursing Staff," *Nursing Times* 101(24):26-27, June 2005.

Chiu, A.M., and Kelly, K.J. "Anaphylaxis: Drug Allergy, Insect Stings, and Latex," *Immunology and Allergy Clinics of North America* 25(2):389-405, viii, May 2005.

Kimata, H. "Latex Allergy in Infants Younger than 1 Year," *Clinical and Experimental Allergy* 34(12):1910-915, December 2004.

Noble, K.A. "The Patient with Latex Allergy," *Journal of Perianesthesia Nursing* 20(4):285-88, August 2005.

Anesthesia induction and latex allergy

Latex allergy can cause signs and symptoms in conscious and anesthetized patients.

CAUSES OF AN INTRAOPERATIVE REACTION	SIGNS AND SYMPTOMS IN A CONSCIOUS PATIENT	SIGNS AND SYMPTOMS IN AN ANESTHETIZED PATIENT
◆ Latex contact with mucous membrane	◆ Abnormal cramping	◆ Bronchospasm
◆ Latex contact with intraperitoneal serosal lining	◆ Anxiety	◆ Cardiopulmonary arrest
◆ Inhalation of airborne latex particles during anesthesia	◆ Bronchoconstriction	◆ Facial edema
◆ Injection of antibiotics and anesthetic agents through latex ports	◆ Diarrhea	◆ Flushing
	◆ Feeling of faintness	◆ Hypotension
	◆ Generalized pruritus	◆ Laryngeal edema
	◆ Itchy eyes	◆ Tachycardia
	◆ Nausea	◆ Urticaria
	◆ Shortness of breath	◆ Wheezing
	◆ Swelling of soft tissue (hands, face, tongue)	
	◆ Vomiting	
	◆ Wheezing	

Lipid emulsion administration

DESCRIPTION

◆ Lipid emulsion is a source of calories and essential fatty acids typically given as a separate solution in conjunction with parenteral nutrition.

◆ Essential fatty acids deficiency can hinder wound healing, adversely affect production of red blood cells, and impair prostaglandin synthesis.

◆ It may be given alone or administered through either a peripheral or a central venous line.

CONTRAINDICATIONS

◆ Conditions that disrupt normal fat metabolism, such as pathologic hyperlipidemia, lipid nephrosis, or acute pancreatitis

EQUIPMENT

Lipid emulsion ◆ I.V. administration set with vented spike (separate adapter may be used if administration set with vented spike isn't available) ◆ access pin with reflux valve ◆ tape ◆ time tape ◆ alcohol pads

⚡ **WARNING** *If administering lipid emulsion as part of a 3-in-1 solution, also obtain a filter that's 1.2 microns or greater because lipids will clog a smaller filter.*

PREPARATION

◆ Inspect the lipid emulsion for opacity and consistency of color and texture.

◆ If the emulsion looks frothy or oily or contains particles, or if you think its stability or sterility is questionable, return the bottle to the pharmacy.

◆ To prevent aggregation of fat globules, don't shake the lipid container excessively.

◆ Protect the emulsion from freezing, and never add anything to it.

◆ Make sure you have the correct lipid emulsion; verify the physician's order and patient's name.

KEY STEPS

◆ Confirm the patient's identity using two patient identifiers according to facility policy.

◆ Explain the procedure to promote cooperation.

CONNECTING THE TUBING

◆ Connect the I.V. tubing to the access pin. Access pins with reflux valves take the place of needles when connecting piggyback tubing to primary tubing.

◆ Close the flow clamp on the I.V. tubing.

⚡ **WARNING** *If the tubing doesn't contain luer-lock connections, tape all connections securely to prevent accidental separation, which can lead to air embolism, exsanguination, or sepsis.*

◆ Using aseptic technique, remove the protective cap from the lipid emulsion bottle and wipe the rubber stopper with an alcohol pad.

◆ Hold the bottle upright and, using strict aseptic technique, insert the vented spike through the inner circle of the rubber stopper.

◆ Invert the bottle and squeeze the drip chamber until it fills to the level indicated in the tubing package instructions.

◆ Open the flow clamp and prime the tubing.

◆ Tap the tubing to dislodge air bubbles trapped in the Y-ports.

◆ If necessary, attach a time tape to the lipid emulsion container to allow accurate measurement of fluid intake.

◆ Label the tubing, noting the date and time it was hung.

STARTING THE INFUSION

◆ If this is the patient's first lipid infusion, administer a test dose at the rate of 1 ml/minute for 30 minutes.

⚡ **WARNING** *Monitor vital signs. Watch for symptoms of adverse reaction, such as fever; flushing, sweating, or chills; pressure sensation over eyes; nausea; vomiting; headache; chest and back pain; tachycardia; dyspnea; and cyanosis. Allergic reaction is usually due either to the source of lipids or to eggs, which occur in the emulsion as egg phospholipids, an emulsifying agent.*

◆ If the patient has no adverse reactions to the test dose, begin infusion at prescribed rate.

◆ Use an infusion pump if you'll be infusing the lipids at less than 20 ml/hour.

◆ The maximum infusion rate is 125 ml/hour for a 10% lipid emulsion and 60 ml/hour for a 20% lipid emulsion.

SPECIAL CONSIDERATIONS

◆ Always maintain strict aseptic technique while preparing and handling equipment.
◆ Observe the patient's reaction to lipid emulsion. Most patients report feeling full, and some complain of an unpleasant metallic taste.
◆ Change I.V. tubing and lipid emulsion container every 24 hours.
◆ Monitor the patient for hair or skin changes; monitor his lipid tolerance rate.
◆ Cloudy plasma in a centrifuged sample of citrated blood indicates that lipids haven't been cleared from patient's bloodstream.
◆ Lipid emulsion may clear from the blood at an accelerated rate in patients with full-thickness burns, multiple traumatic injuries, or metabolic imbalance.
◆ Obtain weekly laboratory tests, as ordered. Usual tests include liver function, prothrombin time, platelet count, and serum triglyceride levels.
◆ If possible, draw blood for triglyceride levels at least 6 hours after completion of lipid emulsion infusion to avoid falsely elevated results.
◆ Lipid emulsion is a medium for bacterial growth; never rehang a partially empty bottle of emulsion.

COMPLICATIONS

◆ Immediate or early adverse reactions (occurring in fewer than 1% of patients):
– Fever
– Dyspnea
– Cyanosis
– Nausea and vomiting
– Headache
– Flushing
– Diaphoresis
– Lethargy
– Syncope
– Chest and back pain
– Slight pressure over eyes
– Irritation at infusion site
– Hyperlipidemia
– Hypercoagulability
– Thrombocytopenia

AGE FACTOR *Thrombocytopenia has been reported in infants receiving a 20% I.V. lipid emulsion.*
◆ Delayed but uncommon complications associated with prolonged administration include:
– hepatomegaly
– splenomegaly
– jaundice secondary to central lobular cholestasis
– blood dyscrasias (such as thrombocytopenia, leukopenia, and transient increases in liver function studies)
– dry or scaly skin, thinning hair, abnormal liver function studies, and thrombocytopenia, which may indicate a deficiency of essential fatty acids
– brown pigmentation in the reticuloendothelial system.

AGE FACTOR *In premature or low-birth-weight infants, peripheral parenteral nutrition with a lipid emulsion may cause lipids to accumulate in an infant's lungs.*

WARNING *Report adverse reactions to the patient's physician so he can change the parenteral nutrition regimen as needed.*

PATIENT TEACHING

◆ Explain to the patient the need for the infusion.
◆ Advise the patient to report adverse reactions.

DOCUMENTATION

◆ Record the times of all dressing and solution changes.
◆ Note the condition of the catheter insertion site.
◆ Document the patient's condition.
◆ Record complications and actions taken.

SELECTED REFERENCES

Krohn, K., and Koletzko, B. "Parenteral Lipid Emulsions in Paediatrics," *Current Opinion in Clinical Nutrition and Metabolic Care* 9(3):319-23, May 2006.
Picard, J., and Meek, T. "Lipid Emulsion to Treat Overdose of Local Anaesthetic: The Gift of the Glob," *Anaesthesia* 61(2):107-109, February 2006.
Song, D., et al. "The Pharmacodynamic Effects of a Lower-Lipid Emulsion of Propofol: A Comparison with the Standard Propofol Emulsion," *Anesthesia & Analgesia* 98(3):687-91, March 2004.
Wanten, G. "An Update on Parenteral Lipids and Immune Function: Only Smoke, or is There any Fire?" *Current Opinion in Clinical Nutrition and Metabolic Care* 9(2):79-83, March 2006.

Lumbar puncture

OVERVIEW

DESCRIPTION

- Lumbar puncture involves insertion of a sterile needle into the subarachnoid space of the spinal canal, usually between the third and fourth lumbar vertebrae.
- It's used to determine the presence of blood in cerebrospinal fluid (CSF), to obtain CSF specimens for laboratory analysis, to inject dyes for contrast in radiologic studies, to administer drugs or anesthetics, and to relieve increased intracranial pressure (ICP).

CONTRAINDICATIONS

- ICP
- Lumbar deformity
- Infection at the puncture site

⚡ **WARNING** *Lumbar puncture isn't recommended for patients with increased ICP. Rapid reduction in pressure that follows withdrawal of CSF can cause tonsillar herniation and medullary compression.*

EQUIPMENT

Overbed table ◆ two or three pairs of sterile gloves ◆ povidone-iodine solution ◆ sterile gauze pads ◆ alcohol pads ◆ sterile fenestrated drape ◆ 3-ml syringe for local anesthetic ◆ 25G ¾" sterile needle for injecting anesthetic ◆ local anesthetic (usually 1% lidocaine) ◆ 18G or 20G 3½" spinal needle with stylet (22G needle for children) ◆ three-way stopcock manometer ◆ small adhesive bandage ◆ three sterile collection tubes with stoppers ◆ sterile marker ◆ sterile labels ◆ laboratory request forms ◆ labels ◆ patient-care reminder ◆ light source (optional)

PREPARATION

- Gather the equipment and take it to the patient's bedside.

KEY STEPS

- Confirm the patient's identity using two patient identifiers according to facility policy.
- Explain the procedure to the patient to ease anxiety and ensure cooperation.
- Make sure a consent form has been signed.
- Provide privacy and instruct the patient to void immediately before the procedure.
- Wash your hands.
- Open the equipment tray on an overbed table, being careful not to contaminate the sterile field.
- Label all medications, medication containers, and other solutions containers on and off the sterile field.
- Provide adequate lighting at the puncture site.
- Adjust the bed height for physician comfort.
- Position the patient and reemphasize the importance of remaining as still as possible to minimize discomfort and trauma. (See *Positioning for lumbar puncture.*)
- Before the physician injects the anesthetic, tell the patient he'll experience a burning sensation and local pain. Ask him to report any other persistent pain or sensations because this may indicate irritation or puncture of a nerve root, requiring repositioning of the needle.
- The puncture site is cleaned with sterile gauze pads soaked in povidone-iodine solution, wiping in a circular motion away from the puncture site.
- The physician uses three different pads to prevent contamination of spinal tissues by the body's normal skin flora.
- The area is draped with the fenestrated drape to provide a sterile field. (If the physician uses povidone-iodine pads instead of sterile gauze pads, he may replace his sterile gloves to avoid introducing povidone-iodine into the subarachnoid space with the lumbar puncture needle.)

Positioning for lumbar puncture

PATIENT POSITIONING

Position the patient on his side at the edge of the bed, with his chin tucked to his chest and his knees drawn up to his abdomen. Make sure his spine is curved and his back is at the edge of the bed (as shown below). This position widens the spaces between the vertebrae, easing insertion.

To help the patient maintain this position, place one of your hands behind his neck and the other hand behind his knees and pull gently. Hold the patient firmly in this position throughout the procedure to prevent accidental needle displacement.

NEEDLE INSERTION

Typically, the physician inserts the needle between the third and fourth lumbar vertebrae (as shown below).

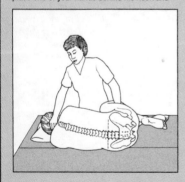

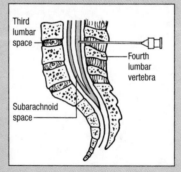

Third lumbar space

Fourth lumbar vertebra

Subarachnoid space

An anesthetic is given. If not included on the equipment tray, clean the injection port of a multidose vial of anesthetic with an alcohol pad. Invert the vial 45 degrees so the physician can insert a 25G needle and syringe and withdraw anesthetic.

Instruct the patient to remain still and breathe normally as the physician inserts the spinal needle.

Hold the patient firmly in position to prevent sudden movement.

The physician injects dye or anesthetic if contrast media or spinal anesthetic is needed.

The physician attaches a manometer when the needle is in place, to read CSF pressure.

Help the patient extend his legs to provide an accurate reading.

The physician detaches the manometer and allows CSF to drain from the needle hub into the collection tubes.

Mark the tubes in sequence (#1, #2, #3), insert a stopper, and label them.

If the physician suspects an obstruction in the spinal subarachnoid space, he may check for Queckenstedt's sign. After an initial CSF pressure reading, compress the patient's jugular vein for 10 seconds, as ordered. This increases ICP and, if no subarachnoid block exists, causes CSF pressure to rise. The physician takes pressure readings every 10 seconds until pressure stabilizes.

Put on sterile gloves.

After the spinal needle is removed, clean the puncture site with povidone-iodine and apply a small adhesive bandage.

Remove and discard gloves.

Send the CSF specimens to the laboratory immediately, with completed laboratory request forms.

SPECIAL CONSIDERATIONS

Watch closely for signs of adverse reaction: elevated pulse rate, pallor, and clammy skin. Alert the physician immediately of significant changes.

WARNING *The patient may be told to lie flat for 8 to 12 hours after the procedure. If necessary, place a patient-care reminder on his bed.*

Collected CSF specimens must be sent to the laboratory immediately.

COMPLICATIONS

- Headache (common)
- Anesthetic reaction
- Meningitis
- Epidural or subdural abscess
- Bleeding into the spinal canal
- CSF leakage through the dural defect remaining after needle withdrawal
- Local pain caused by nerve root irritation
- Edema or hematoma at the puncture site
- Transient difficulty voiding
- Fever

WARNING *The most serious complications of lumbar puncture, although rare, are tonsillar herniation and medullary compression.*

PATIENT TEACHING

Inform the patient he may experience headache after lumbar puncture, but reassure him that his cooperation during the procedure minimizes such an effect.

Emphasize the importance of remaining as still as possible to minimize discomfort and trauma.

DOCUMENTATION

- Record start and end times of the procedure.
- Note the patient's response.
- Document administration of drugs.
- Record the number of specimen tubes collected, time of transport to the laboratory, color, consistency, and other characteristics of collected specimens.

SELECTED REFERENCES

Abe, K.K., et al. "Lumbar Puncture Needle Length Determination," *American Journal of Emergency Medicine* 23(6):742-46, October 2005.

Clark, T., et al. "Lumbar Puncture in the Management of Adults with Suspected Bacterial Meningitis — A Survey of Practice," *Journal of Infection* 52(5):315-19, May 2006.

Hillemacher, T., et al. "Should Aspirin be Discontinued for Diagnostic Lumbar Puncture?" *Journal of the American Geriatrics Society* 54(1):181-82, January 2006.

Lawrence, R.H. "The Role of Lumbar Puncture as a Diagnostic Tool in 2005," *Critical Care and Resuscitation* 7(3):213-20, September 2005.

Seupaul, R.A. et al. "Prevalence of Postdural Puncture Headache after ED Performed Lumbar Puncture," *American Journal of Emergency Medicine* 23(7):913-15, November 2005.

Male incontinence device

DESCRIPTION

- The device reduces the risk of urinary tract infection from catheterization and promotes bladder retraining.
- It helps prevent skin breakdown and improves the patient's self-image.
- It consists of a condom catheter secured to the shaft of the penis and connects to a leg bag or drainage bag.

CONTRAINDICATIONS

- None known

 WARNING *Can cause skin irritation and edema.*

Condom catheter ◆ drainage bag ◆ extension tubing ◆ hypoallergenic tape or incontinence sheath holder ◆ commercial adhesive strip or skin-bond cement ◆ elastic adhesive or Velcro, if needed ◆ gloves ◆ clippers, if needed ◆ basin ◆ soap ◆ washcloth ◆ towel

PREPARATION

- Fill the basin with lukewarm water.
- Bring the basin and the remaining equipment to the patient's bedside.

- Confirm the patient's identity using two patient identifiers according to facility policy.
- Explain the procedure to the patient.

APPLYING THE DEVICE

- Provide privacy for the patient.
- Wash your hands and put on gloves.
- If the patient is circumcised, wash the penis with soap and water, rinse well, and pat dry with a towel.
- If the patient is uncircumcised, gently retract the foreskin and clean beneath it. Rinse well but don't dry because moisture provides lubrication and prevents friction during foreskin replacement. Replace the foreskin to avoid penile constriction.
- If necessary, clip hair from the base and shaft of the penis to prevent the adhesive strip or skin-bond cement from pulling pubic hair.
- If using a precut commercial adhesive strip, insert the glans penis through its opening, and position the strip 1″ (2.5 cm) from the scrotal area.
- If using uncut adhesive, cut a strip to fit around the shaft of the penis.
- Remove the protective covering from one side of the adhesive strip and press this side firmly to the penis to enhance adhesion. Remove the covering from the other side of the strip.
- If a commercial adhesive strip isn't available, apply skin-bond cement and let it dry for a few minutes.
- Position the rolled condom catheter at the tip of the penis, leaving a ½″ (1.3 cm) between the condom end and the tip of the penis, with the drainage opening at the urinary meatus.
- Unroll the catheter upward, past the adhesive strip on the shaft of the penis.
- Press the sheath against the strip until it adheres.
- After the condom catheter is in place, secure it with hypoallergenic tape or an incontinence sheath holder. (See *How to apply a condom catheter.*)

- Connect the condom catheter to the leg bag or drainage bag with extension tubing.
- Remove and discard your gloves.

REMOVING THE DEVICE
- Put on gloves.
- Simultaneously roll the condom catheter and adhesive strip off the penis and discard them.
- If you've used skin-bond cement rather than an adhesive strip, remove it with solvent.
- Remove and discard the hypoallergenic tape or incontinence sheath holder.
- Clean the penis with lukewarm water, rinse thoroughly, and dry.
- Check for swelling or signs of skin breakdown.

How to apply a condom catheter

Apply an adhesive strip to the shaft of the penis about 1″ (2.5 cm) from the scrotal area.

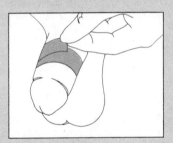

Roll the condom catheter onto the penis past the adhesive strip, leaving about ½″ (1.3 cm) clearance at the end. Press the sheath gently against the strip until it adheres.

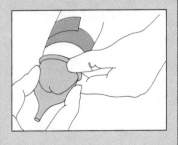

- Remove the leg bag by closing the drain clamp, unlatching the leg straps, and disconnecting the extension tubing at the top of the bag.
- Discard your gloves.

SPECIAL CONSIDERATIONS

- If hypoallergenic tape or an incontinence sheath holder isn't available, secure the condom with a strip of elastic adhesive or Velcro.
- Apply the strip snugly, but not too tightly, to prevent circulatory constriction.
- Inspect the condom catheter for twists and the extension tubing for kinks to prevent obstruction of urine flow, which could cause the condom to balloon, eventually dislodging it.

COMPLICATIONS
- Circulatory constriction
- Obstruction of urine flow
- Skin irritation and edema

PATIENT TEACHING

- Teach the patient how to apply the catheter.
- Instruct the patient about the signs and symptoms of infection.
- Teach the patient to check his penis for signs of irritation.

DOCUMENTATION

- Note the date and time of application and removal of incontinence device.
- Record skin condition.
- Note the patient's response to the device, including voiding pattern, to assist with bladder retraining.

SELECTED REFERENCES
Brodie, A. "A Guide to the Management of One-Piece Urinary Sheaths," *Nursing Times* 102(9):49, 51, February-March 2006.

Evans, D. "Lifestyle Solution for Men with Continence Problems," *Nursing Times* 101(2):61-62, 64, January 2005.

Milne, J.L., and Moore, K.N. "Factors Impacting Self-Care for Urinary Incontinence," *Urologic Nursing* 26(1):41-51, February 2006.

Newman, D.K. "Incontinence Products and Devices for the Elderly," *Urologic Nursing* 24(4):316-33, August 2004.

Manual ventilation

OVERVIEW

DESCRIPTION

◆ Manual ventilation delivers oxygen through a handheld resuscitation bag attached to a face mask, or an endotracheal (ET) or tracheostomy tube.

◆ It allows delivery of oxygen or room air to the lungs of a patient who can't breathe by himself.

◆ Used in an emergency, it maintains ventilation while patient is disconnected temporarily from a mechanical ventilator, during transport, or before suctioning.

◆ Oxygen administration with a resuscitation bag can help improve a compromised cardiopulmonary system.

CONTRAINDICATIONS

◆ None known

Using a positive end-expiratory pressure valve

Add positive end-expiratory pressure (PEEP) to manual ventilation by attaching a PEEP valve to the resuscitation bag. This may improve oxygenation if the patient hasn't responded to an increased fraction of inspired oxygen levels. Always use a PEEP valve to manually ventilate a patient who has been receiving PEEP on the ventilator.

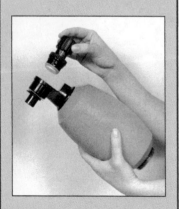

EQUIPMENT

Handheld resuscitation bag ◆ mask ◆ oxygen source (wall unit or tank) ◆ oxygen tubing ◆ nipple adapter attached to oxygen flowmeter ◆ gloves ◆ goggles ◆ oxygen accumulator, positive end-expiratory pressure valve (optional) (see *Using a positive end-expiratory pressure valve*)

PREPARATION

◆ Unless the patient is intubated or has a tracheostomy, select a mask that fits snugly over the mouth and nose.

◆ Attach the mask to the resuscitation bag.

◆ If oxygen is readily available, connect the handheld resuscitation bag to the oxygen.

◆ Attach one end of the tubing to the bottom of the bag and the other end to the nipple adapter on the flowmeter of the oxygen source.

◆ Turn on the oxygen, and adjust the flow rate according to the patient's condition. For example, if he has a low partial pressure of arterial oxygen, he'll need a higher fraction of inspired oxygen (FIO_2).

◆ To increase the concentration of inspired oxygen, you can add an oxygen accumulator (also called an *oxygen reservoir*). This device, which attaches to an adapter on the bottom of the bag, permits an FIO_2 of up to 100%.

◆ If time allows, set up suction equipment.

KEY STEPS

◆ Put on gloves and other personal protective equipment.

◆ Before using the handheld resuscitation bag, check the patient's upper airway for foreign objects.

◆ If present, remove them. This alone may restore spontaneous respirations. Also, foreign matter or secretions can obstruct the airway and impede resuscitation efforts.

◆ Suction the patient to remove any secretions that may obstruct the airway.

◆ If necessary, insert an oropharyngeal or nasopharyngeal airway to maintain airway patency.

◆ If the patient has a tracheostomy or ET tube in place, suction the tube.

◆ If appropriate, remove the bed's headboard and stand at the head of the bed so you can help keep the patient's neck extended and free up space at the side of the bed for other activities such as cardiopulmonary resuscitation.

◆ Tilt the patient's head backward, if not contraindicated, and pull his jaw forward to move the tongue away from the base of the pharynx and prevent obstruction of the airway. (See *How to use a bag-mask device.*)

◆ Using your nondominant hand, apply downward pressure to seal the mask against the patient's face.

◆ For the adult patient, use your dominant hand to compress the bag every 6 to 7 seconds to deliver approximately 1 L of air.

◆ Deliver breaths with the patient's inhalations, if any are present.

◆ Don't attempt to deliver a breath as he exhales.

◆ Observe his chest to make sure that it rises and falls with each compression.

◆ If ventilation fails to occur, check the fit of the mask and the patency of his airway; if necessary, reposition his head and ensure patency with an oral airway.

SPECIAL CONSIDERATIONS

◆ Avoid neck hyperextension if the patient has a possible cervical injury; instead, use the jaw-thrust technique to open the airway.
◆ If you need both hands to keep the mask in place and maintain hyperextension, use the lower part of your arm to compress the bag against your side.
◆ Observe for vomiting through the clear part of the mask.
◆ If vomiting occurs, stop immediately, lift the mask, wipe and suction vomitus, and resume resuscitation.
◆ The volume of air delivered to the patient varies with the type of bag used and the hand size of the person compressing the bag.
◆ An adult with a small or medium-sized hand may not consistently deliver 1 L of air.
◆ Have someone assist with the procedure, if possible, to lessen complications.

COMPLICATIONS

◆ Pneumonia due to aspiration of vomitus
◆ Gastric distention from air forced into the patient's stomach
◆ Underventilation commonly occurring because the handheld resuscitation bag is difficult to keep positioned tightly on the patient's face while ensuring an open airway

PATIENT TEACHING

◆ Tell the patient why manual ventilation is being done, as necessary.
◆ Explain the procedure, as needed, to lessen anxiety.

How to use a bag-mask device

Place the mask over the patient's face so the apex of the triangle covers the bridge of his nose and the base lies between his lower lip and chin.

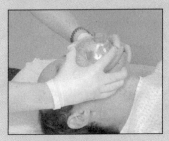

Make sure his mouth remains open underneath the mask. Attach the bag to the mask and the tubing leading to the oxygen source.

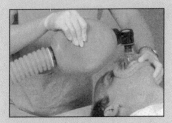

If the patient has a tracheostomy or endotracheal tube in place, remove the mask from the bag and attach the handheld resuscitation bag directly to the tube.

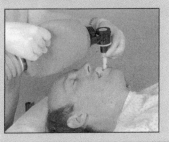

DOCUMENTATION

EMERGENCY DOCUMENTATION

◆ Note the date and time of procedure.
◆ Record manual ventilation efforts.
◆ Document complications and nursing action taken.
◆ Note the patient's response to treatment, according to facility protocol for respiratory arrest.

NONEMERGENCY DOCUMENTATION

◆ Note the date and time of procedure.
◆ Record the reason and length of time the patient was disconnected from mechanical ventilation and received manual ventilation.
◆ Document complications and nursing action taken.
◆ Note the patient's tolerance of the procedure.

SELECTED REFERENCES

Bennett, S., et al. "A Comparison of Three Neonatal Resuscitation Devices," *Resuscitation* 67(1):113-18, October 2005.

O'Donnell, C.P., et al. "Neonatal Resuscitation 2: An Evaluation of Manual Ventilation Devices and Face Masks," *Archives of Disease in Childhood: Fetal and Neonatal Edition* 90(5):F392-96, September 2005.

Pruitt, W.C. "Manual Ventilation by One or Two Rescuers," *Nursing* 34(11):43-45, November 2004.

Turki, M., et al. "Peak Pressures During Manual Ventilation," *Respiratory Care* 50(3):340-44, March 2005.

Mechanical debridement

DESCRIPTION

- Mechanical debridement removes necrotic tissue by mechanical, chemical, or surgical means.
- It's performed to remove eschar (hardened, dead tissue), control infection, promote healing, and prepare the wound surface to receive a graft.
- The procedure includes wet-to-dry dressings, irrigation, hydrotherapy, and excision of dead tissue with forceps and scissors.
- The procedure can be performed at bedside or a specially prepared area such as a hydrotherapy tub.
- A combination of debridement techniques may be used.
- Wet-to-dry dressings, used for wounds with extensive necrotic tissue and minimal drainage, require appropriate technique and dressing materials.
- Irrigation of a wound with a pressurized antiseptic solution cleans tissue and removes wound debris and excess tissue.
- Hydrotherapy involves immersing the patient in a tank of warm water, with intermittent agitation of the water.
- Local or general anesthesia is commonly used for surgical debridement.
- Other debridement techniques include chemical debridement (with wound-cleaning beads, or topical agents that remove exudate and debris) or surgical excision and skin grafting (usually reserved for deep burns or ulcers).
- Daily debridement prevents hemorrhage and the need for surgical intervention.

CONTRAINDICATIONS

- Closed blisters over partial-thickness burns

Ordered pain drug ◆ two pairs of sterile gloves ◆ two gowns or aprons ◆ mask ◆ cap ◆ sterile scissors ◆ sterile forceps ◆ 4″×4″ sterile gauze pads ◆ sterile solutions and drugs, as ordered ◆ hemostatic drug, as ordered

WET-TO-DRY DRESSINGS

Sterile saline solution ◆ waterproof trash bag ◆ 4″×4″ sterile gauze pads ◆ clean gloves ◆ tape or adhesive bandage

IRRIGATION

Prescribed irrigating solution ◆ irrigation syringe or catheter ◆ clean gloves

HYDROTHERAPY

Hydrotherapy tub ◆ sterile dressings ◆ waterproof trash bag ◆ clean gloves

TO CONTROL HEMORRHAGE

Needle holder ◆ gut suture with needle ◆ silver nitrate sticks

- Confirm he patient's identity using two patient identifiers according to facility policy.
- Explain the procedure to the patient to lessen anxiety and promote cooperation.
- Teach the patient distraction and relaxation techniques, if possible, to minimize discomfort.
- Provide privacy.
- Give an analgesic 20 minutes before debridement begins, or give an I.V. analgesic immediately before the procedure.

CONSERVATIVE SHARP DEBRIDEMENT

- Keep the patient warm.
- Expose only the area to be debrided to prevent chilling and fluid and electrolyte loss.
- Wash your hands and put on a cap, mask, gown or apron, and sterile gloves.
- Remove the burn dressings and clean the wound.
- Replace your gown or apron and gloves.
- Lift loosened edges of eschar with forceps.
- Use the blunt edge of scissors or forceps to probe the eschar.
- Cut the dead tissue from the wound with scissors.
- Leave a ¼″ (0.6 cm) edge on remaining eschar to avoid cutting into viable tissue.
- Because debridement removes only dead tissue, bleeding should be minimal. If bleeding occurs, apply gentle pressure on the wound with sterile 4″×4″ gauze pads and apply the hemostatic drug.
- If bleeding persists, notify the practitioner; maintain pressure on the wound until he arrives.
- Excessive bleeding or spurting vessels may require ligation.
- Perform additional procedures, such as application of topical drugs and dressing replacements, as ordered.

WET-TO-DRY DRESSING
◆ Put on clean gloves.
◆ Slowly remove the old dressing, using saline solution to moisten parts of the dressing that don't easily pull away. Discard old dressing and gloves in a waterproof trash bag.
◆ Put on clean gloves.
◆ Using sterile technique, moisten a gauze pad with saline solution and loosely pack it into the wound. Make sure the entire wound surface is lightly covered.
◆ Apply an outer dressing and secure it with tape or an adhesive bandage.
◆ Remove the dressing after it completely dries and becomes adherent to the necrotic tissue (4 to 6 hours).

IRRIGATION
◆ Using sterile technique, instill a slow, steady stream of solution into the wound with an irrigating syringe or catheter.

HYDROTHERAPY
◆ Prepare the tub and check the patient's vital signs.
◆ Assist the patient into the tub.
◆ After the affected area has been in the water for the prescribed time, put on clean gloves, remove old dressings, and discard items in a waterproof trash bag.
◆ Spray rinse and pat dry the patient before reapplying sterile dressings.

SPECIAL CONSIDERATIONS

◆ Work quickly, with an assistant if possible, to complete this painful procedure as soon as possible.
◆ Limit the procedure time to 20 minutes, if possible.
◆ Acknowledge the patient's discomfort and provide emotional support.
◆ Debride no more than a 4″ (10 cm) square area at one time.

COMPLICATIONS
◆ Infection
◆ Blood loss
◆ Fluid and electrolyte imbalances

PATIENT TEACHING

◆ Explain the procedure and why it's necessary.
◆ Tell the patient that the procedure is painful but that he'll be given pain medication.
◆ Teach the patient distraction and relaxation techniques to ease pain.

DOCUMENTATION

◆ Note the date and time of wound debridement.
◆ Record the area debrided.
◆ Document solutions and drugs used.
◆ Note wound condition, including signs of infection or skin breakdown.
◆ Record the patient's tolerance and reaction to the procedure.
◆ Document indications for additional therapy.

SELECTED REFERENCES
Anderson, I. "Debridement Methods in Wound Care," *Nursing Standard* 20(24):65-66, 68, 70, February 2006.
Beitz, J.M. "Wound Debridement: Therapeutic Options and Care Considerations," *Nursing Clinics of North America* 40(2):233-49, June 2005.
Davies, C.E., et al. "Exploring Debridement Options for Chronic Venous Leg Ulcers," *British Journal of Nursing* 14(7):393-97, April 2005.
Davies, P. "Current Thinking on the Management of Necrotic and Sloughy Wounds," *Professional Nurse* 19(10):34-36, June 2004.
Mosti, G., et al. "The Debridement of Hard to Heal Leg Ulcers by Means of a New Device Based on Fluidjet Technology," *International Wound Journal* 2(4):307-14, December 2005.

Mechanical traction

DESCRIPTION

- Mechanical traction exerts a pulling force on the spine, pelvis, or long bones of the arms and legs.
- It's used to reduce fractures, treat dislocations, correct or prevent deformities, improve or correct contractures, or decrease muscle spasms.
- There are two types:
- Skin traction is a light, temporary, intermittent force that provides immobilization over time by a pulling force on skin
- Skeletal traction involves a pin or wire inserted through the bone; it's used for longitudinal pulling force (tibia, femur, humerus fractures); weight applied is determined by body size and extent of injury.

CONTRAINDICATIONS

Skin traction
- Severe injury with open wounds
- Allergy to tape or other skin traction equipment
- Circulatory disturbances
- Dermatitis
- Varicose veins

Skeletal traction
- Infections such as osteomyelitis

CLAW-TYPE BASIC FRAME
102″ (259-cm) plain bar ◆ two 66″ (167.6-cm) swivel-clamp bars ◆ two upper-panel clamps ◆ two lower-panel clamps

I.V.-TYPE BASIC FRAME
102″ plain bar ◆ 27″ (68.6-cm) double-clamp bar ◆ 48″ (121.9-cm) swivel-clamp bar ◆ two 36″ (91.4-cm) plain bars ◆ four 4″ (10-cm) I.V. posts with clamps ◆ cross clamp

I.V.-TYPE BALKAN FRAME
Two 102″ plain bars ◆ two 27″ double-clamp bars ◆ two 48″ swivel-clamp bars ◆ five 36″ plain bars ◆ four 4″ I.V. posts with clamps ◆ eight cross clamps

ALL FRAME TYPES
Trapeze with clamp ◆ wall bumper or roller

SKELETAL TRACTION CARE
Sterile cotton-tipped applicators ◆ prescribed antiseptic solution ◆ sterile gauze pads ◆ povidone-iodine solution ◆ antimicrobial ointment (optional)

PREPARATION
- Have central supply transport traction equipment to patient's room on a traction cart.
- If appropriate, gather equipment for pin-site care at patient's bedside. Pin-site care protocols may vary with each facility or practitioner.

- Confirm the patient's identity using two patient identifiers according to facility policy.
- Explain the purpose of traction to the patient. Emphasize importance of maintaining proper body alignment after traction equipment is set up.

CLAW-TYPE BASIC FRAME SETUP
- Attach one lower-panel and one upper-panel clamp to each 66″ swivel-clamp bar.
- Fasten one bar to the footboard and one to the headboard by turning the clamp knobs clockwise until they're tight, then pulling back on the upper clamp's rubberized bar until it's tight.
- Secure the 102″ horizontal plain bar atop the two vertical bars, making sure the clamp knobs point up.
- Using the appropriate clamp, attach the trapeze to the horizontal bar about 24″ (61 cm) from the head of the bed.

I.V.-TYPE BASIC FRAME SETUP
- Attach one 4″ I.V. post with clamp to each end of both 36″ horizontal plain bars.
- Secure an I.V. post in each I.V. holder at the bed corners.
- Using a cross clamp, fasten the 48″ vertical swivel-clamp bar to the middle of the horizontal plain bar at the foot of the bed.
- Fasten the 27″ vertical double-clamp bar to the middle of the horizontal plain bar at the head of the bed.
- Attach the 102″ horizontal plain bar to the tops of the two vertical bars, making sure the clamp knobs point up.
- Using the appropriate clamp, attach the trapeze to the horizontal bar about 24″ from the head of the bed.

I.V.-TYPE BALKAN FRAME SETUP
- Attach one 4″ I.V. post with clamp to each end of two 36″ horizontal plain bars.
- Secure an I.V. post in each I.V. holder at the bed corners.

- Attach a 48″ vertical swivel-clamp bar, using a cross clamp, to each I.V. post clamp on the horizontal plain bar at the foot of the bed.
- Fasten one 36″ horizontal plain bar across the midpoints of the two 48″ swivel-clamp bars, using two cross clamps.
- Attach a 27″ vertical double-clamp bar to each I.V. post clamp on the horizontal bar at the head of the bed.
- Using two cross clamps, fasten a 36″ horizontal plain bar across the midpoints of two 27″ double-clamp bars.
- Clamp a 102″ horizontal plain bar onto the vertical bars on each side of the bed, making sure the clamp knobs point up.
- Use two cross clamps to attach a 36″ horizontal plain bar across the two overhead bars, about 24″ from the head of the bed.
- Attach the trapeze to this 36″ horizontal bar.

AFTER SETTING UP ANY FRAME
- Attach a wall bumper or roller to the vertical bar or bars at the head of the bed to protect walls from damage.

PROVIDING PATIENT CARE
- Show the patient how much movement he's allowed and instruct him not to adjust equipment.
- Tell the patient to report any pain or pressure from traction equipment.
- At least once per shift, make sure traction equipment connections are tight.
- Check for impingements, such as ropes getting caught between pulleys.
- Inspect equipment to ensure correct alignment.
- Inspect the ropes for fraying.
- Make sure ropes are positioned properly in the pulley track.
- Make sure all rope ends are taped above the knot.
- Inspect traction weights regularly to make sure they hang freely. Weights that touch the floor, bed, or each other reduce traction.
- About every 2 hours, check the patient for proper body alignment and reposition as needed.

- Assess neurovascular integrity based on the patient's condition, hospital routine, and practitioner's orders.
- Provide skin care, encourage coughing and deep-breathing exercises, and assist with ordered range-of-motion exercises for unaffected extremities.
- Apply elastic support stockings, if ordered.
- Check elimination patterns and provide laxatives, as ordered.
- For a skeletal traction patient, make sure protruding pin or wire ends are covered with cork.
- Check pin sites and surrounding skin regularly for signs of infection.

CLEANING THE PIN SITE
- Using sterile technique, put on gloves.
- Clean pin site and surrounding skin with cotton-tipped applicator dipped in ordered antiseptic.
- Apply antimicrobial ointment to pin sites, if ordered.

SPECIAL CONSIDERATIONS

- When using skin traction, apply ordered weights slowly and carefully to avoid jerking the affected extremity.
- To avoid injury if the ropes break, arrange weights so they don't hang over the patient.
- When applying Buck's traction, make sure the line of pull is always parallel to the bed and not angled downward to prevent pressure on the heel.
- Placing a flat pillow under the extremity may help as long as it doesn't alter the line of pull.

COMPLICATIONS
- Pressure ulcers
- Muscle atrophy
- Weakness or contractures
- Osteoporosis
- Constipation
- Urinary stasis and calculi
- Stasis of respiratory secretions, hypostatic pneumonia
- Circulatory stasis and thrombophlebitis

- Depression or other emotional disturbances
- Osteomyelitis caused by skeletal traction

PATIENT TEACHING

- Explain the procedure and why it's needed.
- Teach the patient diversional activities within the limits of the traction.
- Reinforce the need for bed exercises to prevent muscle deterioration in unaffected extremities.

DOCUMENTATION

- Record the amount of traction weight used daily.
- Note the application of additional weights and the patient's tolerance.
- Document equipment inspections.
- Record routine checks of neurovascular integrity.
- Note skin condition.
- Document respiratory status.
- Record elimination patterns.
- Note condition of the pin site and care given.

SELECTED REFERENCES
Garcia Crespo, R., et al. "Retrograde Nailing of Femur: Surgical Technique with Tibial Traction," *Journal of Orthopaedic Trauma* 18(5):310-11, May-June 2004.
Nigam, V., et al. "Local Antibiotics: Panacea for Long-term Skeletal Traction," *Injury* 36(1):199-202, January 2005.
Resch, S., et al. "Preoperative Skin Traction or Pillow Nursing in Hip Fractures: A Prospective, Randomized Study in 123 Patients," *Disability and Rehabilitation* 27(18-19):1191-95, September-October 2005.

Mechanical ventilation

DESCRIPTION

- Mechanical ventilation moves air in and out of lungs.
- Positive or negative pressure may be used.
- Conditions that may require mechanical ventilation include:
  - central nervous system disorders, such as cerebral hemorrhage and spinal cord transsection
  - acute respiratory distress syndrome
  - pulmonary edema
  - chronic obstructive pulmonary disease
  - flail chest
  - acute hypoventilation.
- The procedure doesn't ensure adequate gas exchange.

Positive-pressure ventilator

- Ventilator causes inspiration while increasing tidal volume.
- Inspiratory cycles vary in volume, pressure, or time.
- Types of ventilators include pressure-cycled, high-frequency, and time-cycled.

Negative-pressure ventilator

- Ventilator pulls the thorax outward, allowing air to flow into lungs.
- It's used to treat neuromuscular disorders, such as Guillain-Barré syndrome, myasthenia gravis, and poliomyelitis.

CONTRAINDICATIONS

- None known

Positive-pressure ventilator ◆ negative-pressure ventilator

PREPARATION

- In most facilities, respiratory therapists set up the ventilator.
- In most cases, add sterile distilled water to the humidifier and connect the ventilator to the appropriate gas source.

- Put on gloves and personal protective equipment.
- Connect the endotracheal tube to the ventilator.
- Observe for chest expansion and auscultate for bilateral breath sounds.
- Monitor the patient's arterial blood gas (ABG) values after initial ventilator setup (usually 20 to 30 minutes), after any changes in ventilator settings, and as the patient's clinical condition warrants.
- Adjust ventilator settings depending on ABG analysis.
- Check the ventilator tubing for condensation.
- Drain the condensate into a collection trap and empty.
- Don't drain the condensate into the humidifier.
- Monitor the in-line thermometer to ensure air is close to body temperature.
- When monitoring vital signs, count spontaneous and ventilator-delivered breaths.
- Change, clean, or dispose of ventilator tubing and equipment every 48 to 72 hours to reduce risk of bacterial contamination.
- When ordered, begin to wean the patient from the ventilator.

- Make sure ventilator alarms are on at all times. (See *Responding to ventilator alarms.*)
- If the problem can't be identified, disconnect patient from the ventilator and use a handheld resuscitation bag to ventilate him.
- Provide emotional support to reduce anxiety, even if the patient is unresponsive.
- Unless contraindicated, turn the patient from side to side every 1 to 2 hours.
- Perform active or passive range-of-motion exercises.
- If permitted, position the patient upright at regular intervals.
- Prevent condensation in the tubing from flowing into the lungs.
- Provide care for the patient's artificial airway as needed.
- Assess peripheral circulation and monitor urine output.
- Watch for fluid volume excess or dehydration.
- Place the call button within reach.
- Establish a method of communication, such as a communication board.
- Give a sedative or neuromuscular-blocking drug as ordered to relax patient and prevent spontaneous breathing efforts that interfere with the ventilator's action.
- Closely observe the patient with inability to breathe or talk.
- Reassure the patient and his family that the paralysis is temporary.
- Make sure that emergency equipment is readily available.
- Explain all procedures and ensure patient safety.
- Make sure that the patient gets adequate rest and sleep.
- Provide subdued lighting, low noise, and restricted staff.
- Observe for signs of hypoxia when weaning the patient.
- With the patient's input, schedule weaning around his daily regimen.
- As weaning progresses, encourage the patient to get out of bed.
- Suggest diversionary activities to take his mind off breathing.

COMPLICATIONS

- Tension pneumothorax
- Decreased cardiac output
- Oxygen toxicity
- Fluid volume excess

PATIENT TEACHING

- For home use, provide a teaching plan that covers ventilator care and settings, artificial airway care, suctioning, respiratory therapy, communication, nutrition, therapeutic exercise, signs and symptoms of infection, and troubleshooting minor equipment malfunctions.

- Have the caregiver demonstrate the ability to use the equipment.
- Refer the patient to a home health agency and durable medical equipment vendor.
- Refer the patient to community resources.

DOCUMENTATION

- Record the date and time of initiation of mechanical ventilation.
- Note the name, type, and settings of ventilator.
- Document responses to mechanical ventilation, including vital signs, breath sounds, use of accessory muscles, intake and output, and weight.
- Record complications and nursing actions taken.
- Note pertinent laboratory data.
- Document the weaning date, time, method, vital signs, oxygen saturation levels, and ABG values.
- Note level of consciousness, respiratory effort, arrhythmias, skin color, and need for suctioning.
- Document duration of spontaneous breathing if the patient received pressure support ventilation (PSV) or used a T-piece or tracheostomy collar.
- Record the time of each breath reduction and rate of spontaneous respirations if using intermittent mandatory ventilation, with or without PSV.

Responding to ventilator alarms

SIGNAL	POSSIBLE CAUSE	NURSING INTERVENTIONS
Low-pressure alarm	◆ Tube disconnected from ventilator ◆ Endotracheal (ET) tube displaced above vocal cords or tracheostomy tube extubated	◆ Reconnect tube to ventilator. ◆ Check tube placement and reposition if needed. If extubation or displacement has occurred, ventilate patient manually and call physician immediately.
	◆ Leaking tidal volume from low cuff pressure (from an underinflated or ruptured cuff or a leak in the cuff or one-way valve)	◆ Listen for a whooshing sound around tube, indicating an air leak. If you hear one, check cuff pressure. If you can't maintain pressure, call the physician; he may need to insert a new tube.
	◆ Ventilator malfunction	◆ Disconnect the patient from the ventilator and ventilate him manually if necessary. Obtain another ventilator.
	◆ Leak in ventilator circuitry (from loose connection or hole in tubing, loss of temperature-sensitive device, or cracked humidification jar)	◆ Make sure all connections are intact. Check for holes or leaks in tubing and replace if necessary. Check the humidification jar and replace if cracked.
High-pressure alarm	◆ Increased airway pressure or decreased lung compliance caused by worsening disease ◆ Patient biting on oral ET tube	◆ Auscultate the lungs for evidence of increasing lung consolidation, barotrauma, or wheezing. Call physician if indicated. ◆ Insert a bite block if needed. ◆ Consider an analgesic or sedation, if appropriate.
	◆ Secretions in airway	◆ Look for secretions in the airway. To remove them, suction the patient or have him cough.
	◆ Condensate in large-bore tubing	◆ Check tubing for condensate and remove any fluid.
	◆ Intubation of right mainstem bronchus	◆ Auscultate the lungs for evidence of diminished or absent breath sounds in the left lung fields. ◆ Check tube position. If it has slipped, call the physician; he may need to reposition it.
	◆ Patient coughing, gagging, or attempting to talk	◆ If the patient fights the ventilator, the physician may order a sedative or neuromuscular-blocking agent.
	◆ Chest wall resistance	◆ Reposition the patient to improve chest expansion. If repositioning doesn't help, administer the prescribed analgesic.
	◆ Failure of high-pressure relief valve	◆ Have faulty equipment replaced.
	◆ Bronchospasm	◆ Assess the patient for the cause. Report to the physician, and treat as ordered.

SELECTED REFERENCES

Christine, N. "Caring for the Mechanically Ventilated Patient: Part One," *Nursing Standard* 20(17):55-64, January 2006.

Goodman, S. "Implementing a Protocol for Weaning Patients Off Mechanical Ventilation," *Nursing in Critical Care* 11(1):23-32, January-February 2006.

Hampton, D.C., et al. "Evidence-Based Clinical Improvement for Mechanically Ventilated Patients," *Rehabilitation Nursing* 30(4):160-65, July-August 2005.

Manno, M.S. "Managing Mechanical Ventilation," *Nursing* 35(12):36-41, December 2005.

Rose, L., and Nelson, S. "Issues in Weaning from Mechanical Ventilation: Literature Review," *Journal of Advanced Nursing* 54(1):73-85, April 2006.

Mist tent therapy

DESCRIPTION

- A mist tent houses a nebulizer that transforms distilled water into mist.
- Mist tent therapy benefits the patient by providing a cool, moist environment. This atmosphere eases breathing and helps to decrease respiratory tract edema, liquefy secretions, and reduce fever.
- Oxygen may also be administered along with the mist.
- Mist tents are commonly used to treat croup and such infections or inflammations as bronchiolitis and pneumonia.
- It's also known as a *croupette* for infants or a *cool-humidity tent* for children.

CONTRAINDICATIONS

- None known

Mist tent frame and plastic tenting ◆ bed sheets ◆ plastic sheet or linen-saver pad ◆ two bath blankets ◆ nebulizer with water reservoir and filter ◆ oxygen flowmeter and oxygen analyzer, if ordered ◆ sterile distilled water ◆ optional: stockinette cap or booties, infant seat

PREPARATION

- Review facility policy to determine who sets up a mist tent. In some facilities the nurse sets up the tent; in others a respiratory therapist may do so.
- Whoever sets up the tent will first confirm the patient's identity using two patient identifiers according to facility policy, wash her hands and then place the tent frame and the plastic tenting at the head of the crib or bed.
- Then she'll cover the mattress with a bed sheet, cover the bed sheet with a plastic sheet or linen-saver pad (tucked under the mattress), and cover these layers with a bath blanket.
- Next, she'll fill the reservoir of the nebulizer with sterile distilled water and make sure that the inlet for air contains a clean filter.
- If the patient will have oxygen in the tent, make sure that the oxygen flowmeter connects to the tent. Then turn the flowmeter to the desired setting.
- Be sure to analyze the percentage of oxygen being delivered. Wait 2 minutes after mist begins filling the tent before placing the patient in it.

- Carefully explain the mist tent's purpose to the patient and his parents to alleviate anxiety and promote cooperation. Use terms that both generations can understand. When talking with the parents, you might compare the mist tent with a vaporizer. When talking with the patient, however, you might compare the tent with a teepee or a spaceship cabin.
- Elevate the head of the bed to a position that enhances patient comfort. If the patient is an infant, consider placing him in an infant seat. The more upright position will help him to mobilize secretions. If the patient will be in the room alone, position him on his side to prevent him from aspirating mucus from liquefied secretions and productive coughing.
- Use a stockinette cap, booties, and the other bath blanket, as needed, to keep the patient from becoming chilled as the mist condenses inside the tent.
- Change the patient's bed sheets and clothing as they dampen, and check his temperature frequently to detect impending hypothermia.
- Monitor the patient frequently for a change in condition, keeping in mind that the mist may make observation difficult.
- Encourage parents to stay with the patient. If he grows irritable and uncooperative while in the tent, the parents may enter the tent to comfort him because excessive irritability causes labored breathing and increases oxygen consumption.
- If secretions coat the inside of the tent, wipe the tent down with a hospital-approved cleaner such as soap and water. Also clean the reservoir with sterile water to prevent bacterial growth.

WARNING *Because the tent alone won't stop an infant or small child from falling out of bed, raise the side rails all the way. Check on the patient frequently; if possible, place him near the nurses' station.*

SPECIAL CONSIDERATIONS

◆ Allow the patient to have toys in the mist tent to provide distraction.
◆ To amuse infants, string plastic toys across the top bar of the tent. However, discourage playing with cloth or stuffed toys in the tent because these objects absorb moisture and supply a medium for bacterial growth.
◆ To prevent a fire, forbid toys or games that may spark or trigger an electric shock, such as battery-operated toys.
◆ Also, remove the electric call light, and give older children a hand bell instead.
◆ If the patient is receiving oxygen, analyze the percentage at least every 4 hours.
◆ For bathing, remove the patient from the tent to prevent hypothermia.

COMPLICATIONS
◆ None known

PATIENT TEACHING

◆ If the mist tent will be used at home, show the parents how to set up, use, and clean the tent properly.

DOCUMENTATION

◆ Record the date and time the patient was placed in the tent.
◆ Describe the patient's respiratory status, including breath sounds, sputum production, and perfusion.
◆ Record the patient's vital signs.
◆ Also note the date and time that the patient was removed from the tent.
◆ Record the percentage of oxygen being delivered, the date and time of all analyses, and the oxygen saturation.

SELECTED REFERENCES
Bjornson, C.L., and Johnson, D.W. "Croup — Treatment Update," *Pediatric Emergency Care* 21(12):863-70, December 2005.
Dykes, J. "Managing Children with Croup in Emergency Departments," *Emergency Nurse* 13(6):14-19, October 2005.
Scolnik, D., et al. "Controlled Delivery of High vs. Low Humidity vs. Mist Therapy for Croup in Emergency Departments: A Randomized Controlled Trial," *JAMA* 295(11):1274-80, March 2006.

Mixed venous oxygen saturation

OVERVIEW

DESCRIPTION
◆ The procedure uses a fiber-optic thermodilution pulmonary artery (PA) catheter to continuously monitor oxygen delivery to tissues and oxygen consumption by tissues.
◆ The process allows rapid detection of impaired oxygen delivery.
◆ It's used to evaluate the patient's response to drug therapy, endotracheal tube suctioning, ventilator setting changes, positive end-expiratory pressure, and fraction of inspired oxygen.
◆ Mixed venous oxygen saturation ($S\bar{v}o_2$) usually ranges from 60% to 80%; normal value is 75%.

CONTRAINDICATIONS
◆ None known

EQUIPMENT

Fiber-optic PA catheter ◆ co-oximeter (monitor) ◆ optical module and cable ◆ gloves

PREPARATION
◆ Review manufacturer's instructions for assembly and use of the fiber-optic PA catheter.
◆ Connect the optical module and cable to the monitor.
◆ Peel back catheter wrapping just enough to uncover the fiber-optic connector.
◆ Attach the fiber-optic connector to the optical module; don't remove the rest of the catheter.
◆ Calibrate the fiber-optic catheter.
◆ Assist with pulmonary catheter insertion.

KEY STEPS

◆ Confirm the patient's identity using two patient identifiers according to facility policy.
◆ Wash your hands and put on gloves.
◆ Explain the procedure to the patient.
◆ Assist with insertion of the fiber-optic catheter.
◆ After insertion, ensure correct positioning and function.
◆ Observe digital readout and record the $S\bar{v}o_2$ on graph paper. (See *$S\bar{v}o_2$ waveforms.*)
◆ Repeat readings at least hourly to monitor and document trends.
◆ Set alarms 10% above and 10% below patient's current $S\bar{v}o_2$ reading.

RECALIBRATING THE MONITOR
◆ Draw a blood sample from the distal port of the PA catheter and send it for laboratory analysis.
◆ Compare the laboratory's $S\bar{v}o_2$ reading with that of the fiber-optic catheter.
◆ If the catheter values and monitor values differ by more than 4%, follow the manufacturer's instructions to enter the $S\bar{v}o_2$ value obtained by the laboratory into the oximeter.
◆ Recalibrate the monitor every 24 hours or whenever the catheter has been disconnected from the optical module.

- If the patient's $S\bar{v}o_2$ drops below 60% or varies by more than 10% for 3 minutes or longer, reassess the patient.
- If the $S\bar{v}o_2$ doesn't return to the baseline value after nursing interventions, notify the physician. This could indicate hemorrhage, hypoxia, shock, or arrhythmias.
- $S\bar{v}o_2$ may also decrease as a result of increased oxygen demand from hyperthermia, shivering, or seizures.
- If the intensity of the tracing is low, make sure that all connections are secure and the catheter is patent and not kinked.
- If the tracing is damped or erratic, aspirate blood from the catheter to check for patency.
- If aspiration is unsuccessful, anticipate catheter replacement and notify the physician.
- Determine if the catheter is wedged by checking the PA waveform.
- If the catheter has wedged, turn the patient from side to side and instruct him to cough.
- If the catheter remains wedged, notify the physician immediately.
- Monitor for signs and symptoms of infection, such as redness or drainage at the catheter site.

COMPLICATIONS

- Thrombosis
- Thromboembolism
- Infection

- Explain the procedure to the patient, as necessary.

- Record the $S\bar{v}o_2$ value on a flowchart and attach a tracing.
- Note significant changes in the patient's status.
- For comparison, note the $S\bar{v}o_2$ as measured by the fiber-optic catheter whenever a blood sample is obtained for laboratory analysis of $S\bar{v}o_2$.

SELECTED REFERENCES

Kamijo, Y., et al. "Mixed Venous Oxygen Saturation Monitoring in Calcium Channel Blocker Poisoning: Tissue Hypoxia Avoidance Despite Hypotension," *American Journal of Emergency Medicine* 24(3):357-60, May 2006.

Rivers, E. "Mixed vs. Central Venous Oxygen Saturation May Not be Numerically Equal, but Both are Still Clinically Useful," *Chest* 129(3):507-508, March 2006.

Smartt, S. "The Pulmonary Artery Catheter: Gold Standard or Redundant Relic," *Journal of Perianesthesia Nursing* 20(6):373-79, December 2005.

Wang, X.R., et al. "A Preliminary Study on the Monitoring of Mixed Venous Oxygen Saturation through the Left Main Bronchus," *Critical Care* 10(1):R7, December 2005.

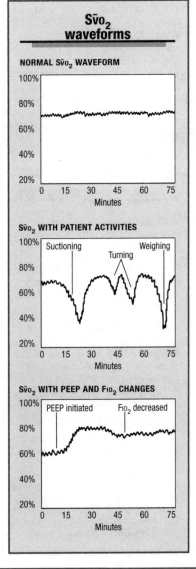

$S\bar{v}o_2$ waveforms

NORMAL $S\bar{v}o_2$ WAVEFORM

$S\bar{v}o_2$ WITH PATIENT ACTIVITIES

$S\bar{v}o_2$ WITH PEEP AND F_{IO_2} CHANGES

Mouth care

DESCRIPTION

◆ Mouth care involves brushing, flossing, and inspecting the patient's mouth.
◆ It's done to remove soft plaque deposits and calculus, clean and massage gums, reduce mouth odor, help prevent infection, and enhance food taste, aiding appetite and nutrition.
◆ Bedridden patients may need partial or full assistance.
◆ Comatose patients require suction to prevent aspiration.
◆ It should be given in morning, at bedtime, or after meals.

CONTRAINDICATIONS

◆ None known

EQUIPMENT

Towel or facial tissues ◆ emesis basin ◆ trash bag ◆ mouthwash ◆ toothbrush and toothpaste ◆ pitcher and glass ◆ drinking straw ◆ dental floss ◆ gloves ◆ dental floss holder ◆ small mirror ◆ oral irrigating device (optional)

COMATOSE OR DEBILITATED PATIENT

Linen-saver pad ◆ bite-block ◆ petroleum jelly ◆ cotton-tipped mouth swab ◆ oral suction equipment or gauze pads ◆ mouth-care kit ◆ tongue blade (optional)

PREPARATION

◆ Bring water and other equipment to the patient's bedside.
◆ If suctioning, connect the tubing to the suction bottle and suction catheter, insert plug, and check for correct operation.
◆ Devise a bite-block using a gauze pad and tongue blade, if needed.

KEY STEPS

◆ Confirm the patient's identity using two patient identifiers according to facility policy
◆ Wash your hands and put on gloves.
◆ Explain the procedure, as needed, and provide privacy.
◆ If allowed, place the patient in Fowler's position.

PERFORMING MOUTH CARE

◆ Adjust procedures as needed for a comatose patient or conscious patient.
◆ If the patient wears dentures, clean them thoroughly.
◆ Use an oral irrigating device if needed. (See *Using an oral irrigating device.*)
◆ Arrange the equipment on the overbed table or bedside stand.
◆ Raise the bed to a comfortable height to prevent back strain.

◆ Have the patient put his face over the edge of the pillow to facilitate drainage and prevent fluid aspiration.
◆ If a suction machine isn't available, use a sponge-tipped swab frequently.
◆ Use a linen-saver pad under his chin and an emesis basin near his cheek for drainage.
◆ Lubricate his lips with petroleum jelly.
◆ If needed, insert the bite-block to hold his mouth open.
◆ Use a dental floss holder and floss each tooth.
◆ Rinse with mouthwash and water in a glass. Have the patient use a straw.
◆ Wet the toothbrush with warm water. Apply toothpaste.
◆ Place the brush at a 45-degree angle to the gum line.
◆ Brush the lower teeth from the gum line up.
◆ Brush the upper teeth from the gum line down.

Using an oral irrigating device

Oral irrigating devices are useful for:
◆ massaging gums and removing debris and food particles
◆ cleaning areas missed by brushing
◆ providing mouthcare for patients undergoing head and neck irradiation and those with a fractured jaw or with mouth injuries that limit standard mouth care.

EQUIPMENT AND PREPARATION

◆ Assemble equipment: oral irrigating device, towel, emesis basin, pharyngeal suction apparatus, salt solution or mouthwash, and soap (optional).
◆ Wash your hands and put on gloves.
◆ Turn the patient to his side to prevent aspiration of water.
◆ Place a towel under the patient's chin and an emesis basin next to his cheek to absorb or catch drainage.
◆ Insert the oral irrigating device's plug.
◆ Remove the device's cover, turn it upside down, and fill it with lukewarm water or with a mouthwash or salt solution, as ordered.
◆ When using a salt solution, dissolve the salt beforehand in a separate container.
◆ Secure the cover to the base of the device.

◆ Remove the water hose handle from the base, and snap the jet tip into place.
◆ Adjust the pressure dial to the patient's comfort. Choose a low setting if the gums are sensitive or bleed.
◆ Adjust the water jet, place the jet tip in the patient's mouth, and turn on the device.
◆ Instruct the alert patient to keep his lips partially closed to avoid spraying water.
◆ Direct the water at a right angle to the gum line of each tooth and between teeth.
◆ Avoid directing water under the patient's tongue.
◆ After irrigating each tooth, instruct the patient to expectorate the water or solution into the emesis basin.
◆ If the patient is unable to do so, suction it.
◆ After irrigating all teeth, turn off the device, and remove the jet tip from the patient's mouth.
◆ Empty the remaining water or solution from the cover, remove the jet tip from the handle, and return the handle to the base.
◆ Clean the jet tip with soap and water, rinse the cover, and dry them both and return to storage.

- Brush the facial surfaces (toward the cheek) and lingual surfaces (toward the tongue) of the bottom and top teeth.
- Brush the biting surfaces of the top and bottom teeth, using a back-and-forth motion.
- Rinse frequently, if needed.
- After brushing, use a moist sponge-tipped mouth swab to gently stroke the gums, buccal surfaces, palate, and tongue.

AFTER MOUTH CARE

- Assess the patient's mouth for cleanliness and tooth and tissue condition.
- Rinse the toothbrush, and clean the emesis basin and glass.
- Empty and clean the suction bottle, if used. Then remove your gloves.
- Place a clean suction catheter on the tubing.
- Return reusable equipment to the appropriate storage location, and properly discard disposable equipment.

SPECIAL CONSIDERATIONS

- Use sponge-tipped mouth swabs for patients with sensitive gums.
- Clean the mouth of the toothless comatose patient by wrapping a gauze pad around your index finger, moistening it with mouthwash or hydrogen peroxide and water, and then swab the oral tissues.
- Moisten his mouth and lips regularly with moistened sponge-tipped swabs or water.
- If you use water as the lubricant, put a straw in a glass of water with your finger over the end. Take the straw out with your finger in place, put it in the patient's mouth, and release your finger to let the water flow out gradually.

COMPLICATIONS
- Aspiration

WARNING *If the patient is comatose, suction excess water to prevent aspiration.*

PATIENT TEACHING

- Encourage the bedridden, self-care patient to perform his own mouth care.
- Instruct the patient to floss his teeth while looking into the mirror.
- Observe and correct flossing technique if needed.
- Provide mouthwash, water, straw, and emesis basin for rinsing.
- Encourage frequent rinsing. Provide facial tissues as needed.

DOCUMENTATION

- Record the date and time of mouth care.
- Note unusual conditions, such as bleeding, edema, mouth odor, excessive secretions, or plaque on the tongue.

SELECTED REFERENCES

Bailey, R., et al. "The Oral Health of Older Adults: An Interdisciplinary Mandate," *Journal of Gerontological Nursing* 31(7):11-17, July 2005.

Chalmers, J., and Pearson, A. "Oral Hygiene Care for Residents with Dementia: A Literature Review," *Journal of Advanced Nursing* 52(4):410-19, November 2005.

Gillam, J.L., and Gillam, D.G. "The Assessment and Implementation of Mouth Care in Palliative Care: A Review," *Journal of the Royal Society of Health* 126(1):33-37, January 2006.

Gil-Montoya, J.A., et al. "Oral Health Protocol for the Dependent Institutionalized Elderly," *Geriatric Nursing* 27(2):95-101, March-April 2006.

Mucus clearance device

DESCRIPTION

- The mucus clearance device is used for patients who need mucus secretions removed from their lungs and those with chronic respiratory disorders.
- A handheld mucus clearance device (known as the *flutter*) helps patients cough up secretions more easily. (See *Flutter valve device*.)
- Vibrations propagate throughout airway during expiration, loosening the mucus.
- Mucus progressively moves up airways until it can be coughed out easily.
- A licensed practitioner determines the frequency and duration of device use.

CONTRAINDICATIONS

- None known

Mucus clearance device ◆ emesis basin ◆ tissues

- Confirm the patient's identity using two patient identifiers according to facility policy.
- Explain the procedure to the patient.
- Tell the patient this device will move mucus through his airway so he can eventually expectorate it.
- Position the patient sitting with his back straight and his head tilted backward slightly to open his throat and trachea.
- If the patient places his elbows on a table the height should prevent slouching.
- Tell the patient to hold the device so that the stem is horizontal.
- Have the patient draw a deep breath and hold it for 2 to 3 seconds.
- Have the patient place the device in his mouth and exhale at a steady rate for as long as possible.
- Quick or forceful exhalations prevent vibration and flutter.
- Tell the patient to keep his cheeks as flat and hard as possible while exhaling.
- To teach the patient the technique, have him hold his cheeks lightly with his other hand.
- After the patient exhales completely, instruct him to remove the device from his mouth, take in another full breath, and cough. Repeat several times.
- Alternatively, after completely exhaling:
  - the patient can leave the device in his mouth
  - draw another big breath through his nose
  - hold it for 2 to 3 seconds
  - repeat the exhalation maneuver.
- He can breathe through the device up to five times before taking the final breath and cough.
- Provide an emesis basin and tissues.

Flutter valve device

When the patient exhales through the flutter valve device, both positive end-expiratory pressure and high-frequency oscillations help move mucus.

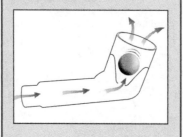

SPECIAL CONSIDERATIONS

◆ To help the patient achieve the best fluttering effect, place one hand on his back and the other on his chest as he exhales through the device.
◆ If the patient is achieving the maximum effect, you'll feel vibrations in his lungs as he exhales.
◆ If results are unsatisfactory at first, tell the patient to adjust the angle at which he's holding the device until optimal fluttering occurs.
◆ If the patient's final cough doesn't seem to work, he can try repeated, controlled, short, rapid exhalations to aid mucus removal.
◆ After the procedure, thoroughly clean the device. All parts should be rinsed under a stream of hot tap water, wiped with a clean towel, and reassembled and stored in a clean, dry place.
◆ Auscultate the patient for breath sounds.

COMPLICATIONS
◆ None known

PATIENT TEACHING

◆ Explain the procedure and why it's needed.
◆ Teach the patient how to use the device.
◆ Teach the patient how to clean the device after each use.
◆ Instruct the patient to clean it more thoroughly every 2 days in a solution of mild soap or detergent.
◆ Tell the patient not to use bleach or other chlorine-containing products.
◆ Teach the patient how to use controlled, short, rapid exhalations to help remove loosened mucus.

DOCUMENTATION

◆ Note patient teaching.
◆ Record the patient's tolerance of the procedure.
◆ Document the amount, color, and odor of secretions.
◆ Note the patient's breath sounds before and after treatment.
◆ Record the number of repetitions and success of coughing efforts.

SELECTED REFERENCES
Pruitt, B., and Jacobs, M. "Clearing Away Pulmonary Secretions," *Nursing* 35(7):36-41, July 2005.
Vuorisalo, S., et al. "Comparison between Flutter Valve Drainage Bag and Underwater Seal Device for Pleural Drainage after Lung Surgery," *Scandinavian Journal of Surgery* 94(1):56-58, 2005.
Wolkove, N., et al. "A Randomized Trial to Evaluate the Sustained Efficacy of a Mucus Clearance Device in Ambulatory Patients with Chronic Obstructive Pulmonary Disease," *Canadian Respiratory Journal* 11(8):567-72, November-December 2004.

Nasal drug instillation

OVERVIEW

DESCRIPTION
- Nasal drugs are instilled by drops, spray, or aerosol; they produce local (not systemic) effects.
- Drops can be directed at a specific area; sprays and aerosols diffuse drug throughout nasal passages.
- Most nasal drugs are vasoconstrictors, which relieve nasal congestion.
- Vasoconstrictors may be absorbed systemically; they're usually contraindicated in hypersensitive patients.
- Other types of nasal drugs include antiseptics, anesthetics, and corticosteroids.
- Local anesthetics may be given during rhinolaryngologic examination, laryngoscopy, bronchoscopy, and endotracheal intubation.
- Corticosteroids reduce inflammation in allergic or inflammatory conditions and nasal polyps.

CONTRAINDICATIONS
- Patient sensitivity

EQUIPMENT

Prescribed drug ◆ patient's drug record and chart ◆ emesis basin (with nose drops only) ◆ facial tissues ◆ pillow, small piece of soft rubber or plastic tubing ◆ gloves (optional)

KEY STEPS
- Verify the drug order.
- Note the concentration of the drug.
- Verify the expiration date.
- Confirm the patient's identity using two patient identifiers according to facility policy.
- If your facility uses a bar-code scanning system, be sure to scan your ID badge, the patient's ID bracelet, and the medication's bar code.
- Explain the procedure and provide privacy.
- Wash your hands and put on gloves, if necessary.

INSTILLING NOSE DROPS
- Position the patient so the drops flow back into the nostrils toward the affected area. (See *Positioning the patient for nose drop instillation.*)
- Draw up some drug into the dropper.
- Push the tip of the patient's nose up slightly.
- Position the dropper just above the nostril, and direct its tip toward the midline of the nose.
- Insert the dropper about ⅜" (1 cm) into the nostril, not letting the dropper touch the sides of the nostril.
- Instill the prescribed number of drops.
- Observe the patient carefully for signs of discomfort.
- To prevent the drops from leaking out of the nostrils, ask her to keep her head tilted back for at least 5 minutes and to breathe through her mouth.
- Keep an emesis basin handy.
- Use a facial tissue to wipe any excess drug from the patient's nostrils and face.
- Clean the dropper by separating the plunger and pipette and flushing them with warm water. Allow them to air-dry.

USING A NASAL SPRAY
- Have the patient sit upright with her head tilted back slightly or lying on her back with her shoulders elevated, neck hyperextended, and head tilted back over the edge of the bed.

Positioning the patient for nose drop instillation

To reach the ethmoid and sphenoid sinuses, have the patient lie on her back with her neck hyperextended and head tilted back over the edge of the bed. Support her head with one hand to prevent neck strain.

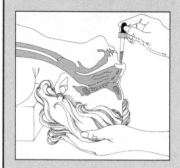

To reach the maxillary and frontal sinuses, have the patient lie on her back with her head toward the affected side and hanging slightly over the edge of the bed. Ask her to rotate her head laterally after hyperextension. Support her head with one hand to prevent neck strain.

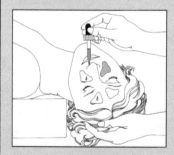

To administer drops to relieve ordinary nasal congestion, help the patient to a reclining or supine position with her head tilted slightly toward the affected side. Aim the dropper upward toward her eye, rather than downward toward her ear.

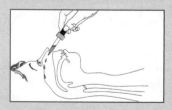

- Support her head with one hand to prevent neck strain.
- Remove the protective cap from the atomizer.
- Occlude one of her nostrils with your finger. Insert the atomizer tip into the open nostril.
- Instruct her to inhale.
- Squeeze the atomizer once, quickly and firmly.
- Tell the patient to exhale through her mouth.
- If ordered, spray the nostril again. Then repeat the procedure in the other nostril.
- Instruct the patient to keep her head tilted back for several minutes and to breathe slowly through her nose.
- Tell her not to blow her nose for several minutes.

USING A NASAL AEROSOL

- Instruct the patient to blow her nose to clear her nostrils.
- Insert the drug cartridge according to the manufacturer's directions.
- Shake the aerosol well before each use and remove the protective cap.
- Hold the aerosol between your thumb and index finger, with your index finger positioned on top of the drug cartridge.
- Tilt the patient's head back, and carefully insert the adapter tip in one nostril while sealing the other nostril with your finger.
- Press the adapter and cartridge together firmly to release one measured dose of drug.
- Shake the aerosol and repeat the procedure in the other nostril.
- Remove the drug cartridge and wash the nasal adapter in lukewarm water daily.
- Allow the adapter to dry before reinserting the cartridge.

SPECIAL CONSIDERATIONS

AGE FACTOR Before instilling nose drops in a young child, attach a small piece of tubing to the end of the dropper. Do the same for an uncooperative patient.

- If using a metered-dose pump spray system, prime the delivery system with four sprays or until a fine mist appears.
- Reprime the system with two sprays or until a fine mist appears if 3 or more days have lapsed since the last use.
- When using an aerosol, be careful not to puncture or incinerate the pressurized cartridge.
- Store at temperatures below 120° F (48.9° C).
- To prevent spread of infection, label the drug bottle so it will be used only for that patient.

COMPLICATIONS

- Rebound effect (causing drug to lose its effectiveness) by using nasal drugs longer than prescribed
- Restlessness, palpitations, nervousness, and other systemic effects

PATIENT TEACHING

- Teach the patient how to instill nasal drugs correctly so she can continue treatment after discharge, if necessary.
- Teach the patient good oral and nasal hygiene.
- Inform the patient of therapeutic effects and possible adverse reactions.

DOCUMENTATION

- Record the drug name, concentration, dosage, and in which nostril drug was given.
- Note the time and date of instillations.
- Document adverse events.

SELECTED REFERENCES

Djupesland, P.G., et al. "Breath Actuated Device Improves Delivery to Target Sites beyond the Nasal Valve," *Laryngoscope* 116(3):466-72, March 2006.

Loder, E. "Post-Marketing Experience with an Opioid Nasal Spray for Migraine: Lessons for the Future," *Cephalalgia* 26(2):89-97, February 2006.

Stjarne, P., et al. "A Randomized Controlled Trial of Mometasone Furoate Nasal Spray for the Treatment of Nasal Polyposis," *Archives of Otolaryngology — Head & Neck Surgery* 132(2):179-85, February 2006.

Wolfe, T.R., and Bernstone, T. "Intranasal Drug Delivery: An Alternative to Intravenous Administration in Selected Emergency Cases," *Journal of Emergency Nursing* 30(2):141-47, April 2004.

Nasal irrigation

DESCRIPTION

- Nasal irrigation soothes irritated mucous membranes and washes away crusted mucus, secretions, and foreign matter (deposits impede sinus drainage and nasal airflow and cause headaches, infections, and unpleasant odors).
- It's performed with a bulb syringe or electronic oral irrigating device.
- It benefits the patient with acute or chronic nasal conditions, including sinusitis, rhinitis, Wegener's granulomatosis, and Sjögren's syndrome.
- It may help those who regularly inhale allergens or toxins (such as paint fumes, sawdust, pesticides, or coal dust).
- It's recommended after some nasal surgeries to enhance healing by removing postoperative eschar and to aid remucosolization of the sinus cavities and ostia.

CONTRAINDICATIONS

- Advanced destruction of sinuses
- Frequent nosebleeds
- Foreign bodies in nasal passages

Bulb syringe or an oral irrigating device (such as a Waterpik) ◆ rigid or flexible disposable irrigation tips (for one-patient use) ◆ hypertonic saline solution ◆ plastic sheet ◆ apron or towels ◆ facial tissues ◆ bath basin ◆ gloves

PREPARATION

- Warm the saline solution to about 105° F (40.6° C).
- If using a bulb syringe, draw some irrigant into the bulb, then expel it to remove residual solution.
- If using an oral irrigating device, plug the instrument into an electrical outlet near the patient.
- Run about 8 oz (236.6 ml) of saline solution through the tubing to remove residual solution.
- Fill the reservoir of the device with warm saline solution.

- Confirm the patient's identity using two patient identifiers according to facility policy.
- Wash your hands and put on gloves.
- Explain the procedure to the patient.
- Place an apron or towel on his upper body to protect his clothing.
- Place a plastic sheet on the bed, if indicated.
- Position the patient to allow the bulb or catheter tip to enter his nose and the returning irrigant to flow into the bath basin or sink. (See *Positioning the patient for nasal irrigation.*)
- Remind the patient to keep his mouth open and breathe rhythmically during irrigation.
- Instruct the patient not to speak or swallow during irrigation.
- Remove the irrigating tip from the patient's nostril if he needs to sneeze or cough.

USING A BULB SYRINGE

- Fill the bulb syringe with saline solution and insert the tip about ½" (1.3 cm) into the patient's nostril.
- Squeeze the bulb until a gentle stream of warm irrigant washes through the nose.
- Avoid forceful squeezing, which may drive debris into the sinuses or eustachian tubes and introduce infection.
- Alternate nostrils until the return irrigant runs clear.

USING AN ORAL IRRIGATING DEVICE

- Insert the irrigation tip into the nostril ½" to 1" (1.3 to 2.5 cm) and turn on the irrigating device.
- Begin with a low pressure setting (increase as needed) to obtain a gentle stream.
- Irrigate both nostrils.
- Note the color, viscosity, or volume of irrigant and report changes.
- Report blood or necrotic material.

CONCLUDING THE PROCEDURE

◆ A few minutes after irrigation, have the patient blow excess fluid from both nostrils.
◆ Clean the bulb syringe or irrigating device with soap, water, and disinfectant.
◆ Rinse and dry the device.
◆ Remove your gloves.

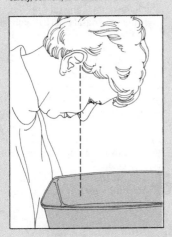

Positioning the patient for nasal irrigation

When performing nasal irrigation, teach the patient how to hold her head for optimal safety, comfort, and effectiveness.

Help the patient sit upright with her head bent forward over the basin or sink and flexed on her chest. Her nose and ear should be on the same vertical plane.

Explain that she's less likely to breathe in the irrigant when holding her head in this position, which should also keep the irrigant from entering the eustachian tubes because they lie above the level of the irrigation stream.

SPECIAL CONSIDERATIONS

◆ Fluid will drain from the patient's nose for a brief time after irrigation.
◆ Insert the irrigation tip far enough to make sure that the irrigant cleans the nasal membranes before draining out. A typical amount of irrigant ranges from 500 to 1,000 ml.

COMPLICATIONS

◆ Infection caused by nasal material traveling to the sinuses or eustachian tube

PATIENT TEACHING

◆ For home irrigations, teach the patient how to prepare saline solution.
◆ Tell the patient to fill a clean 1-L plastic bottle with bottled or distilled water (4 cups + 1 oz = 1 L), add 1 tsp of salt, and shake the solution until the salt dissolves.
◆ Teach the patient how to disinfect used irrigation devices.

DOCUMENTATION

◆ Note the time and duration of the procedure.
◆ Record the amount of irrigant used.
◆ Document the appearance of returned solution.
◆ Record the patient's comfort level and breathing ease before and after the procedure.
◆ Document patient-teaching content.

SELECTED REFERENCES

Elliott, K.A., and Stringer, S.P. "Evidence-Based Recommendations for Antimicrobial Nasal Washes in Chronic Rhinosinusitis," *American Journal of Rhinology* 20(1):1-6, January-February 2006.

Plaut, M., and Valentine, M.D. "Clinical Practice: Allergic Rhinitis," *New England Journal of Medicine* 353(18):1934-44, November 2005.

Rabago, D., et al. "The Efficacy of Hypertonic Saline Nasal Irrigation for Chronic Sinonasal Symptoms," *Otolaryngology — Head and Neck Surgery* 133(1):3-8, July 2005.

Rabago, D., et al. "Nasal Irrigation to Treat Acute Bacterial Rhinosinusitis," *American Family Physician* 72(9):1661-62, November 2005.

Schlegel-Wagner, C., et al. "Non-Invasive Treatment of Intractable Posterior Epistaxis with Hot-Water Irrigation," *Rhinology* 44(1):90-93, March 2006.

Nasal packing

DESCRIPTION
- Nasal packing is performed when routine therapeutic measures fail to control epistaxis.
- There are two main types of epistaxis: anterior bleeding and posterior bleeding.
- The procedure is typically performed with a nurse assisting the physician.

CONTRAINDICATIONS
- Nasal trauma that might involve internal structure injury
- Coagulopathy
- Potential cerebrospinal fluid leak

EQUIPMENT

ANTERIOR AND POSTERIOR PACKING
Gowns ◆ goggles ◆ masks ◆ sterile gloves ◆ emesis basin ◆ facial tissue ◆ patient drape ◆ nasal speculum and tongue depressors ◆ directed illumination source, or fiber-optic nasal endoscope ◆ suction apparatus with sterile suction-connecting tubing and sterile nasal aspirator tip ◆ sterile bowl and sterile normal saline solution for flushing ◆ sterile towels ◆ sterile cotton-tipped applicators ◆ local anesthetic spray or solution (such as 2% lidocaine or 1% to 2% lidocaine with epinephrine 1:100,000) ◆ sedative or analgesic ◆ sterile cotton balls or cotton pledgets ◆ 10-ml syringe with 22G 1½″ needle ◆ silver nitrate sticks ◆ electrocautery device ◆ topical vasoconstrictor ◆ absorbable hemostatic ◆ sterile normal saline solution (1-g container and 60-ml syringe with luer-lock tip) ◆ hypoallergenic tape ◆ antibiotic ointment ◆ petroleum jelly

ANTERIOR PACKING
Two packages of 1½″ (4-cm) petroleum strips ◆ gauze (36″ to 48″ [0.9 to 1.2 m]) ◆ two nasal tampons

POSTERIOR PACKING
Two #14 or #16 French catheters with 30-cc balloon or two single- or double-chamber nasal balloon catheters ◆ bayonet forceps ◆ marking pen

ASSESSMENT AND BEDSIDE USE
Tongue blades ◆ flashlight ◆ long hemostats or sponge forceps ◆ 60-ml syringe for deflating balloons (if applicable)

PREPARATION
- Wash your hands.
- Assemble all equipment at the patient's bedside.
- Plug in and test the suction apparatus, and connect the tubing from the collection bottle to the suction source.
- Create a sterile field at the bedside and, using aseptic technique, place all sterile equipment on the sterile field.
- If the practitioner will inject a local anesthetic rather than spray, place the 22G 1½″ needle attached to the 10-ml syringe on the sterile field.
- When the practitioner readies the syringe, clean the stopper and hold the vial so he can withdraw the anesthetic.
- Open the packages containing the sterile suction-connecting tubing and aspirating tip, and place them on the sterile field.
- Fill the sterile bowl with normal saline solution to flush the suction tubing.
- Thoroughly lubricate the anterior or posterior packing with antibiotic ointment.
- Test a balloon for leaks by inflating the catheter with normal saline solution.
- Remove the solution before insertion.

- Confirm patient's identity using two patient identifiers according to facility policy.
- Wear a gown, gloves, and goggles during insertion of packing to prevent contamination.
- Check vital signs, and observe for hypotension with postural changes.

⚡ **WARNING** *Hypotension in the patient with a nosebleed suggests significant blood loss.*

- Monitor airway patency.

⚡ **WARNING** *The patient with an uncontrolled nosebleed is at risk for aspirating or vomiting swallowed blood.*

- Explain the procedure to the patient and offer reassurance.
- If ordered, give a sedative or analgesic to reduce anxiety and pain and decrease sympathetic stimulation, which can exacerbate a nosebleed.
- Help the patient sit with his head tilted forward.
- Turn on the suction apparatus and attach the connecting tubing.
- To inspect the nasal cavity, the physician will use a nasal speculum and an external light source or a fiber-optic nasal endoscope.
- To remove collected blood and help visualize the bleeding vessel, the physician will use suction or cotton-tipped applicators.
- The nose may be treated early with a topical vasoconstrictor such as phenylephrine to slow bleeding and aid visualization.

❂ **AGE FACTOR** *Heavy posterior bleeding that's difficult to treat is most common in elderly patients.*

ANTERIOR NASAL PACKING
- Help the practitioner apply a topical vasoconstrictor or use chemical cautery to control bleeding.
- To enhance the vasoconstrictor's action, apply manual pressure to the nose for about 10 minutes.
- If bleeding persists, you may help insert an absorbable hemostatic nasal pack directly on the bleeding site.

- If these methods fail, prepare to assist with electrocautery or insertion of petroleum strip gauze.
- While the anterior pack is in place, apply petroleum jelly to the patient's lips and nostrils to prevent drying and cracking.

POSTERIOR NASAL PACKING
- Wash your hands and put on sterile gloves.
- Lubricate the soft catheters to ease insertion.
- Instruct the patient to open his mouth and breathe normally.
- Help the physician insert the packing as directed.
- Help the patient assume a position with his head elevated 45 to 90 degrees.
- Assess the patient for airway obstruction or any respiratory changes.
- Monitor vital signs regularly.

SPECIAL CONSIDERATIONS

⚡ **WARNING** *Nasal packing is very uncomfortable and promotes hypoxia and hypoventilation, which can be fatal if patient isn't properly monitored.*
- If mucosal oozing persists, apply a moustache dressing.
- Change the pad when soiled.
- Test the patient's call bell to make sure he can summon help.

⚡ **WARNING** *Keep emergency equipment at patient's bedside to speed packing removal if it becomes displaced and occludes the airway.*
- Obtain a patient history to determine the underlying cause of nosebleed.
- Laboratory work may include complete blood count and coagulation profile.
- A blood transfusion may be necessary.
- Arterial blood gas analysis may be ordered.
- Supplemental humidified oxygen with a face mask may be needed.
- Provide thorough mouth care often.
- The patient should be on modified bed rest.

- Give nonaspirin analgesics, decongestants, sedatives, and antibiotics.
- Nasal packing is usually removed in 2 to 5 days.

COMPLICATIONS
- Blood loss
- Infection (such as otitis media and sinusitis)
- Hypoxemia
- Airway obstruction
- Mucosal pressure necrosis
- Hypotension
- Septal hematoma-perforation
- Vasovagal episode
- Migration of packing

PATIENT TEACHING

- After an anterior pack is removed, tell the patient to avoid picking, inserting any object, or blowing his nose forcefully for 48 hours or as ordered.
- Tell the patient to expect reduced smell and taste ability.
- Make sure the patient has a working smoke detector at home.
- Advise the patient to eat soft foods because of eating and swallowing impairment.
- Instruct the patient to drink fluids or use artificial saliva to cope with dry mouth.
- Teach the patient how to prevent nosebleeds and have him seek medical help if he can't stop bleeding.

DOCUMENTATION

- Note the type of pack used to ensure its removal at the appropriate time.
- Record estimated blood loss and all fluids given.
- Document vital signs.
- Note response to sedation or position changes.
- Record laboratory results.
- Document drugs given, including topical agents.
- Note any complications.
- Document discharge instructions and clinical follow-up plans.

SELECTED REFERENCES
Badran, K. "Blood Clots Should Be Evacuated Before Nasal Packing: The Problem of the Yankauer Sucker," *Clinical Otolaryngology* 31(1):74-75, February 2006.

Bugten, V., et al. "Effects of Nonabsorbable Packing in Middle Meatus after Sinus Surgery," *Laryngoscope* 116(1):83-88, January 2006.

Eliashar, R., et al. "Packing in Endoscopic Sinus Surgery: Is It Really Required?" *Otolaryngology — Head and Neck Surgery* 134(2):276-79, February 2006.

Sariguney, Y., et al. "Vertically Split Merocel Tampon has Advantages in Nasal Packing," *Plastic and Reconstructive Surgery* 117(5):1646-47, April 2006.

Skilbeck, C.J., and Oakley, R. "The Fist Model for Nasal Packing," *European Journal of Emergency Medicine* 13(2):97-98, April 2006.

Nasoenteric-decompression tube care

DESCRIPTION

- Care is performed after the nasoenteric-decompression tube is inserted nasally and advanced beyond the stomach into the intestinal tract; the patient requires encouragement and support while the tube is in place.
- Care involves continuous monitoring to ensure tube patency, maintain suction and bowel decompression, and detect complications, such as skin breakdown and fluid-electrolyte imbalances.

CONTRAINDICATIONS

- Nasal polyps, deviated septum, or other obstruction that prevents insertion

EQUIPMENT

Suction apparatus with intermittent suction capability (stationary or portable unit) ◆ container of water ◆ intake and output record sheets ◆ mouthwash and water mixture ◆ petroleum jelly or water-soluble lubricant ◆ cotton-tipped applicators ◆ safety pin ◆ tape or rubber band ◆ disposable irrigation set ◆ irrigant ◆ labels for tube lumens ◆ throat comfort measures such as gargle, viscous lidocaine, throat lozenges, ice collar, sour hard candy, or gum (optional)

PREPARATION

- Assemble the suction apparatus and set up the suction unit.
- Test the unit.

KEY STEPS

- Confirm the patient's identity using two patient identifiers according to facility policy
- Explain the procedure to the patient and family and answer questions.
- After tube insertion, have the patient lie quietly on his right side for about 2 hours to promote the tube's passage.
- After the tube advances past the pylorus, it can be advanced 2″ (5 cm) per hour.
- After the tube advances to desired position, coil excess external tubing and secure to the patient's gown or bed linens; secure the tube's position by taping to the patient's face.
- Maintain slack in the tubing so the patient can move safely in bed.
- Show the patient how far he can move without dislodging the tube.
- After securing the tube, connect it to the tubing on the suction machine to begin decompression.
- Check the suction machine every 2 hours to confirm proper function, tube patency, and bowel decompression.
- Excessive negative pressure may draw the mucosa into the tube openings, impair the suction's effectiveness, and injure the mucosa. Intermittent suction may prevent these problems.
- To check functioning in an intermittent suction unit, look for drainage in the connecting tube and dripping into the collecting container.
- Empty the container every 8 hours and measure the contents.
- After decompression and before extubation, as ordered, provide a clear-to-full liquid diet to assess bowel function.
- Record intake and output to monitor fluid balance.
- If you irrigate the tube, its length may prohibit aspiration of the irrigant, so record the amount of instilled irrigant as "intake."

- Normal saline solution is preferred over water as irrigant.
- Watch for signs and symptoms of pneumonia related to the patient's inability to clear his pharynx or cough effectively with a tube in place.
- Be alert for fever, chest pain, tachypnea or labored breathing, and diminished breath sounds over the affected area.
- Observe drainage characteristics: color, amount, consistency, odor, and unusual changes.
- Provide mouth care frequently, and encourage the patient to brush his teeth or rinse his mouth with the mouthwash and water mixture.
- Lubricate his lips with petroleum jelly applied with a cotton-tipped applicator.
- At least every 4 hours, clean and lubricate his external nostrils with either petroleum jelly or water-soluble lubricant on a cotton-tipped applicator to prevent skin breakdown.
- Watch for peristalsis to resume, signaled by bowel sounds, passage of flatus, decreased abdominal distention and, possibly, a spontaneous bowel movement.

SPECIAL CONSIDERATIONS

- Label the other lumen "Suction." Marking the tube may prevent accidentally instilling irrigant into the wrong lumen.
- If the suction machine doesn't work, replace it immediately.
- If the machine works properly but no drainage accumulates in the collection container, there may be an obstruction in the tube.
- As ordered, irrigate the tube with the irrigation set to clear the obstruction. (See *Clearing a nasoenteric-decompression tube obstruction*.)
- If the tube connects to a portable suction unit, the patient may move short distances while connected to the unit.
- If ordered, the tube can be disconnected briefly and clamped while he moves about.
- For throat irritation, offer mouthwash, gargles, viscous lidocaine, throat lozenges, an ice collar, sour hard candy, or gum, as appropriate.
- If the tip of the balloon falls below the ileocecal valve (confirmed by X-ray), the tube can't be removed nasally. It must be advanced and removed through the anus.
- If the balloon at the end of the tube protrudes from the anus, notify the practitioner.

COMPLICATIONS

- Fluid and electrolyte imbalance
- Pneumonia
- Intussusception of the bowel

PATIENT TEACHING

- Explain the purpose of the procedure and advise the patient what to expect during and after insertion.
- Explain signs and symptoms to report.
- Tell the patient when the tube will be removed.

Clearing a nasoenteric-decompression tube obstruction

If the tube appears to be obstructed, notify the practitioner right away. He may order the following measures to restore patency:
- Disconnect the tube from the suction source and irrigate with normal saline solution. Use gravity flow to help clear the obstruction unless ordered otherwise.
- If irrigation doesn't reestablish patency, the tube may be obstructed by its position against the gastric mucosa. Tug slightly on the tube to move it away from the mucosa.
- If gentle tugging doesn't restore patency, the tube may be kinked and may need additional manipulation. Before proceeding, assess these precautions:
  – If the patient has had GI surgery, don't reposition or irrigate a nasoenteric-decompression tube without a practitioner's order.
  – Avoid manipulating a tube that was inserted during surgery to avoid disturbing new sutures.
  – Don't try to reposition a tube in the patient who was difficult to intubate.

DOCUMENTATION

- Record the frequency and type of mouth and nose care given.
- Note therapeutic effect.
- Document the amount, color, consistency, and odor of drainage.
- Record the amount of drainage on intake and output sheet.
- Note the amount of any irrigant or other fluid introduced through the tube or taken orally by the patient.
- Document length of time of any suction machine malfunctions and nursing actions.
- Note the amount and character of vomitus.
- Record the patient's tolerance of the tube's insertion and removal.

SELECTED REFERENCES

Gallagher, J.J. "How to Recognize and Manage Abdominal Compartment Syndrome," *Nursing Management* (Suppl):36-42, 2004.

Gowen, G.F. "Long Tube Decompression is Successful in 90% of Patients with Adhesive Small Bowel Obstruction," *American Journal of Surgery* 185(6): 512-15, June 2003.

McClave, S.A., and Ritchie, C.S. "The Role of Endoscopically Placed Feeding or Decompression Tubes," *Gastroenterology Clinics of North America* 35(1):83-100, March 2006.

Shayani, V., and Sarker, S. "Diagnosis and Management of Acute Gastric Distention Following Laparoscopic Adjustable Gastric Banding," *Obesity Surgery* 14(5):702-704, May 2004.

Nasoenteric-decompression tube use

OVERVIEW

DESCRIPTION
◆ A nasoenteric-decompression tube is inserted nasally and advanced beyond the stomach into the intestinal tract.
◆ Many tubes are weighted at the end to stimulate peristalsis and facilitate the tube's passage through the pylorus and into the intestinal tract. (See *Common types of nasoenteric-decompression tubes*.)
◆ It's used to aspirate intestinal contents for analysis and treat intestinal obstruction.
◆ Its use may prevent abdominal distention after GI surgery.
◆ The tube is usually inserted and removed by the physician; a trained nurse may remove the tube.

CONTRAINDICATIONS
◆ None known

EQUIPMENT

Sterile 10-ml syringe ◆ 21G needle ◆ nasoenteric-decompression tube ◆ container of water ◆ 5 to 10 ml of water ◆ suction-decompression equipment ◆ gloves ◆ towel or linen-saver pad ◆ water-soluble lubricant ◆ 4″ × 4″ gauze pad ◆ ½″ hypoallergenic tape ◆ bulb syringe or 60-ml catheter-tip syringe ◆ rubber band ◆ safety pin ◆ clamp ◆ specimen container ◆ basin of ice or warm water ◆ penlight ◆ waterproof marking pen ◆ glass of water with straw ◆ local anesthetic ◆ ice chips (optional)

PREPARATION
◆ Stiffen a flaccid tube by chilling it in a basin of ice to facilitate insertion.
◆ To make a stiff tube flexible, dip it in warm water.
◆ Check the tube's balloon for leaks.
◆ If using a Cantor or Harris tube, inject 10 cc of air into the balloon with a 10-ml syringe and 21G needle.
◆ If using an Anderson Miller-Abbott or Dennis tube, attach a 10-ml syringe to the distal balloon port.
◆ Immerse the balloon in a container of water and watch for air bubbles.
◆ Air or water is added to the balloon either before or after insertion of the tube, depending on the type of tube used.
◆ Set up and test suction-decompression equipment.

KEY STEPS

◆ Confirm the patient's identity using two patient identifiers according to facility policy.
◆ Explain the procedure to the patient.
◆ Provide privacy and adequate lighting.
◆ Wash your hands and put on gloves.
◆ Put the patient in semi-Fowler's or high Fowler's position.
◆ Protect his chest with a linen-saver pad or towel.
◆ Devise a signal the patient can use to stop insertion briefly, if necessary.

ASSISTING WITH INSERTION
◆ The physician assesses patency of the patient's nostrils.
◆ To decide how far the tube must be inserted, the physician places the tube's distal end at the tip of the patient's nose, then extends the tube to the earlobe and down to the xiphoid process and marks the tube.
◆ Apply water-soluble lubricant to the first few inches of the tube to reduce friction and tissue trauma and facilitate insertion.
◆ If the balloon already contains water, the physician holds it so the fluid runs to the bottom. He then pinches the balloon closed to retain the fluid as insertion begins.
◆ Tell the patient to breathe or pant through his mouth as the balloon enters his nostril.
◆ After the balloon begins its descent, the physician releases his grip on it, allowing the weight of the fluid to pull the tube into the nasopharynx.
◆ When the tube reaches the nasopharynx, the physician has the patient lower his chin and swallow. The patient may sip water through a straw to facilitate swallowing.
◆ The tube is advanced slowly to prevent it from curling or kinking in the stomach.
◆ To confirm the tube's passage into the stomach, the physician aspirates stomach contents with a bulb syringe.

Common types of nasoenteric-decompression tubes

The tube chosen will depend on the size of the patient and his nostrils, the estimated duration of intubation, and the reason for the procedure.

Most tubes are impregnated with a radiopaque mark so X-ray or other imaging technique can confirm placement.

Tubes such as the preweighted Andersen Miller-Abbott type intestinal tube (shown at right), have a tungsten-weighted inflatable latex balloon tip designed for temporary management of mechanical obstruction in the small or large intestine.

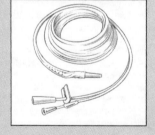

- To keep the tube out of the patient's eyes and avoid skin irritation, fold a 4″ × 4″ gauze pad in half and tape it to his forehead with the fold directed toward his nose.
- Position the patient as directed to help advance the tube. He'll typically lie on his right side until the tube clears the pylorus (about 2 hours).
- The physician confirms passage by X-ray.
- After the tube clears the pylorus, you may advance it 2″ to 3″ (5 to 7.5 cm) every hour and reposition the patient until the premeasured mark reaches his nostril.
- Keep the remaining premeasured length of tube lubricated to ease passage and prevent irritation.
- When the mark reaches the nostril, confirm tube positioning with X-ray.
- After the tube is in place, secure the external tubing with tape.
- Loop a rubber band around the tube and pin the rubber band to the patient's gown with a safety pin.
- If ordered, attach the tube to intermittent suction.

REMOVING THE TUBE
- Put the patient in semi-Fowler's or high Fowler's position.
- Drape a linen-saver pad or towel across his chest.
- Wash your hands and put on gloves.
- Clamp the tube and disconnect it from the suction.
- Slowly withdraw 6″ to 8″ (15 to 20.5 cm) of tube at a time, then wait 10 minutes. Continue until the tube reaches the patient's esophagus (about 18″ [45.7 cm] of tube remaining inside patient). Then withdraw the tube completely.

SPECIAL CONSIDERATIONS

- For a double- or triple-lumen tube, note which lumen accommodates balloon inflation and which accommodates drainage.
- An alternative method for removing a single-lumen tube is to withdraw it into the pharynx. Ask the patient to open his mouth. Grasp the tube and pull it out of the patient's mouth.
- Never forcibly remove a tube if you meet resistance; notify the physician.
- If the patient has pain, apply a local anesthetic to the nostril or back of the throat or let the patient gargle with a liquid anesthetic, or have him suck on ice chips to sooth his throat.

COMPLICATIONS
- Reflux esophagitis, nasal or oral inflammation, and nasal, laryngeal, or esophageal ulceration

PATIENT TEACHING

- Explain the procedure, as needed, to lessen anxiety.
- Teach the patient relaxation techniques, such as breathing and guided imagery, to use during insertion of the tube.

DOCUMENTATION

- Record the dates and times of procedures.
- Note who inserted and removed the tube.
- Note the patient's tolerance of procedures.
- Document the type of tube used.
- Record the amount, color, and consistency of drainage.

SELECTED REFERENCES
Gallagher, J.J. "How to Recognize and Manage Abdominal Compartment Syndrome," *Nursing Management* (Suppl):36-42, 2004.
McClave, S.A., and Ritchie, C.S. "The Role of Endoscopically Placed Feeding or Decompression Tubes," *Gastroenterology Clinics of North America* 35(1):83-100, March 2006.
Shayani, V., and Sarker, S. "Diagnosis and Management of Acute Gastric Distention Following Laparoscopic Adjustable Gastric Banding," *Obesity Surgery* 14(5):702-704, May 2004.

Nasogastric tube care

OVERVIEW

DESCRIPTION
- After a nasogastric (NG) tube is inserted, careful monitoring of the patient and equipment is required.
- Specific care varies only slightly for the most commonly used NG tubes (the single-lumen Levin tube and the double-lumen Salem sump tube).

CONTRAINDICATIONS
- None known

EQUIPMENT

Irrigant (usually normal saline solution) ◆ irrigant container ◆ 60-ml catheter-tip syringe ◆ bulb syringe ◆ suction equipment ◆ toothbrush and toothpaste ◆ petroleum jelly ◆ ½" or 1" hypoallergenic tape ◆ water-soluble lubricant ◆ gloves ◆ pH test strip ◆ linen-saver pad ◆ emesis basin (optional)

PREPARATION
- Make sure the suction equipment works properly. (See *Common gastric suction devices*.)
- When using a Salem sump tube with suction, connect the larger, primary lumen (for drainage and suction) to the suction equipment and select the appropriate setting, as ordered (usually low constant suction).
- If the practitioner doesn't specify the setting, follow the manufacturer's directions.
- A Levin tube usually calls for intermittent low suction.

KEY STEPS

- Confirm the patient's identity using two patient identifiers according to facility policy.
- Explain the procedure to the patient and provide privacy.
- Wash your hands and put on gloves.

IRRIGATING AN NG TUBE
- Review the irrigation schedule (usually every 4 hours), if the practitioner orders this procedure.
- Aspirate stomach contents to check correct positioning in the stomach and prevent the patient from aspirating the irrigant.
- Examine the aspirate and place a small amount on the pH test strip. Correct gastric placement is likely if the aspirate has a gastric fluid appearance (grassy-green, clear and colorless with mucus shreds, or brown) and the pH is 5.0 or less.
- Measure the amount of irrigant (usually 10 to 20 ml) in the syringe (bulb or 60-ml catheter-tip) for accurate input and output monitoring.
- When using suction with a Salem sump tube or a Levin tube, unclamp and disconnect the tube from the suction equipment while holding it over a linen-saver pad or an emesis basin.
- Slowly instill the irrigant into the NG tube.
- Aspirate the solution with the bulb syringe or 60-ml catheter-tip syringe or connect the tube to the suction equipment, as ordered.
- Report any bleeding.

Common gastric suction devices

Various wall-mounted suction devices are available for applying negative pressure to nasogastric (NG) and other drainage tubes. Two common types are shown here.

PORTABLE SUCTION MACHINE
In the portable suction machine, a vacuum created intermittently by an electric pump draws gastric contents up the NG tube and into the collecting bottle.

STATIONARY SUCTION MACHINE
A stationary wall-unit apparatus can provide intermittent or continuous suction. On-off switches and variable power settings let you set and adjust the suction force on either machine.

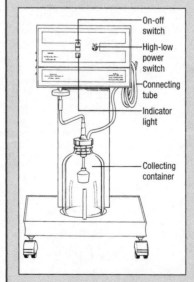

On-off switch
High-low power switch
Connecting tube
Indicator light
Collecting container

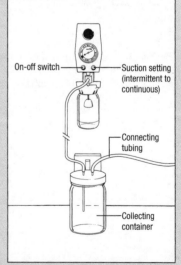

On-off switch
Suction setting (intermittent to continuous)
Connecting tubing
Collecting container

◆ Reconnect the tube to suction after completing irrigation.

INSTILLING A SOLUTION THROUGH AN NG TUBE

◆ If the practitioner orders instillation, inject the solution, and don't aspirate it.
◆ Note the amount of instilled solution on the intake and output record.
◆ Reattach the tube to suction, as ordered.
◆ After attaching the Salem sump tube's primary lumen to suction, instill 10 to 20 cc of air into the vent lumen to verify patency.
◆ Listen for a soft hiss in the vent. If you don't hear this sound, suspect a clogged tube.
◆ Recheck patency by instilling 10 ml of normal saline solution and 10 to 20 cc of air in the vent.

MONITORING THE PATIENT'S COMFORT AND CONDITION

◆ Provide mouth care once per shift or as needed.
◆ Depending on the patient's condition, use sponge-tipped swabs to clean his teeth or assist him with brushing.
◆ Coat the patient's lips with petroleum jelly.
◆ Change the tape securing the tube as needed or at least daily. Clean the skin, apply fresh tape, and dab water-soluble lubricant on the nostrils, as needed.
◆ Regularly check the tape securing the tube.
◆ Assess bowel sounds regularly.
◆ Measure drainage and update intake and output record every 8 hours.
◆ Be alert for electrolyte imbalances with excessive gastric output.
◆ Inspect gastric drainage and note its color, consistency, odor, and amount.
◆ Immediately report any drainage with a coffee-bean color.
◆ If you suspect the drainage contains blood, perform an occult blood screening.

SPECIAL CONSIDERATIONS

◆ Irrigate the NG tube with 30 ml of irrigant before and after instilling the drug.
◆ Wait about 30 minutes, or as ordered, after instillation before reconnecting suction equipment to allow sufficient time for the drug to be absorbed.
◆ When no drainage appears, check the suction equipment for proper function.
◆ Holding the NG tube over a linen-saver pad or emesis basin, separate the tube and the suction source.
◆ Check suction by placing the suction tubing in an irrigant container. If the apparatus draws water, check the NG tube for proper function.
◆ Note the amount of water drawn into the suction container on the intake and output record.
◆ A dysfunctional NG tube may be clogged or incorrectly positioned. Attempt to irrigate the tube, reposition the patient, or rotate and reposition the tube. If the tube was inserted during surgery, avoid this maneuver to avoid interfering with gastric or esophageal sutures; notify the physician.
◆ If you can move the patient and interrupt suction, disconnect the NG tube from the suction equipment.
◆ Clamp the tube to prevent stomach contents from draining out of the tube.
◆ If the patient has a Salem sump tube, watch for gastric reflux in the vent lumen when pressure in the stomach exceeds atmospheric pressure.
◆ Assess the suction equipment for proper functioning.
◆ Irrigate the NG tube and instill 30 cc of air into the vent tube to maintain patency. Don't attempt to stop reflux by clamping the vent tube.
◆ Unless contraindicated, elevate the patient's torso more than 30 degrees, and keep the vent tube above his midline to prevent a siphoning effect.

COMPLICATIONS

◆ Epigastric pain and vomiting
◆ Perforation
◆ Dehydration and electrolyte imbalances
◆ Nasal skin breakdown and discomfort
◆ Increased mucous secretions
◆ Aspiration pneumonia
◆ Damage of the gastric mucosa from suctioning
◆ Aggravation of esophagitis, ulcers, or esophageal varices, causing hemorrhage
◆ Pain, swelling, and salivary dysfunction may signal parotitis, which occurs in dehydrated, debilitated patients

PATIENT TEACHING

◆ Instruct the patient about the procedure and why it's being performed, as needed.

DOCUMENTATION

◆ Note tube placement confirmation.
◆ Record fluid intake and output, including the instilled irrigant.
◆ Document the irrigation schedule and actual time of each irrigation.
◆ Note drainage color, consistency, odor, and amount.
◆ Record tape change times and condition of the nostrils.
◆ Record the pH of the aspirate.

SELECTED REFERENCES

Best, C. "Caring for the Patient with a Nasogastric Tube," *Nursing Standard* 20(3):59-65, September-October 2005.

Ellett, M.L. "What is Known about Methods of Correctly Placing Gastric Tubes in Adults and Children," *Gastroenterology Nursing* 27(6):253-59, November-December 2004.

McKay, L. "Nasogastric Intubation," *Nursing Standard* 20(24):63, February 2006.

Nasogastric tube drug instillation

OVERVIEW

DESCRIPTION

- It provides an alternate means of nourishment.
- It allows direct instillation of drugs into the GI system of patients who can't ingest drugs orally.

CONTRAINDICATIONS

- Tube obstruction
- Improper tube position
- Absent bowel sounds
- Oily drugs
- Enteric-coated or sustained-release tablets or capsules
- Vomiting around tube

EQUIPMENT

Patient's drug record and chart ◆ prescribed drug ◆ towel or linen-saver pad ◆ 50- or 60-ml piston-type catheter-tip syringe ◆ feeding tubing ◆ two 4″×4″ gauze pads ◆ pH test strip ◆ gloves ◆ diluent ◆ cup for mixing drug and fluid ◆ spoon ◆ 50 ml of water ◆ rubber band ◆ gastrostomy tube and funnel ◆ juice, water, or nutritional supplement for diluting the drug ◆ mortar and pestle, clamp (optional)

PREPARATION

- Gather the equipment for use at bedside.
- Liquids should be at room temperature.
- Giving cold liquids through a nasogastric (NG) tube can cause abdominal cramping.
- Make sure the cup, syringe, spoon, and gauze are clean.

KEY STEPS

- Verify the order.
- Wash your hands and put on gloves.
- Check the label on the drug three times before preparing it for administration.
- Request liquid forms of drugs, if available. If the prescribed drug is in tablet form, crush the tablets.
- Bring the drug and equipment to the patient's bedside.
- Confirm the patient's identity using two patient identifiers according to facility policy.
- If your facility uses a bar code scanning system, be sure to scan your ID badge, the patient's ID bracelet, and the medication's bar code.
- Explain the procedure and provide privacy.
- Unpin the tube from the patient's gown.
- To avoid soiling the sheets, drape her chest with a towel or linen-saver pad.
- Elevate the head of the bed so the patient is in Fowler's position.
- After unclamping the tube, attach a syringe to the end of the tube and check tube placement by attempting to aspirate gastric secretions.
- If no gastric contents appear when you draw back on the syringe, the tube may have risen into the esophagus, and you'll have to advance it before proceeding.
- If you meet resistance when aspirating, stop the procedure. Resistance may indicate a nonpatent tube or improper tube placement.
- Examine the aspirate and place a small amount on the pH test strip. Correct gastric placement is likely if the aspirate has a typical gastric fluid appearance (grassy-green, clear and colorless with mucus shreds, or brown) and the pH is 5.0 or less.
- If you confirm that the tube is in the stomach, resistance probably means the tube is lying against the stomach wall. To relieve resistance, withdraw the tube slightly or turn the patient.
- After you have established that the tube is patent and in the correct position, clamp the tube, detach the sy-

ringe, and lay the end of the tube on the 4″×4″ gauze pad.
- Mix the crushed tablets or liquid drug with the diluent.
- If the drug is in capsule form, open the capsules and empty their contents into the liquid.
- Pour liquid drugs directly into the diluting liquid. Stir well with the spoon. (If the drug was in tablet form, make sure particles are small enough to pass through the eyes at the distal end of the tube.)
- Reattach the syringe, without the piston, to the end of the tube and open the clamp.
- Deliver the drug slowly and steadily. (See *Giving drugs through an NG tube*.)
- If the drug flows smoothly, slowly administer until the entire dose has been given; if the drug doesn't flow properly, don't force it.
- If it's too thick, dilute it with water. If you suspect that tube placement is inhibiting flow, stop the procedure and check tube placement.
- Watch the patient's reaction throughout instillation. If there's any discomfort, stop the procedure immediately.
- As the last of the drug flows out of the syringe, irrigate the tube by adding 30 to 50 ml of water.

  ◆ **AGE FACTOR** *For a child, irrigate the tube using only 15 to 30 ml of water.*
- When the water stops flowing, quickly clamp the tube. Detach the syringe and discard properly.
- Fasten the NG tube to the patient's gown.
- Remove the towel or linen-saver pad and replace bed linens.
- Leave the patient in Fowler's position, or have her lie on her right side with the head of the bed partially elevated for 30 minutes.
- You may be asked to deliver drugs through a gastrostomy tube.
- If drug is prescribed for a patient with a gastrostomy feeding button, ask the prescriber to order the liquid form of the drug, if possible. If not, you may give a tablet or capsule if dissolved in 30 to 50 ml of warm water (15 to 30 ml for children).

- To give drug this way, use the same procedure as for feeding the patient through the button.
- Draw up the dissolved drug into a syringe and inject it into the feeding tube.
- Withdraw the drug syringe, and flush the tube with 50 ml of warm water.

🏶 **AGE FACTOR** *For a child, flush the tube with 30 ml of water.*

- Then replace the safety plug, and keep the patient upright at a 30-degree angle for 30 minutes after giving the drug.

Giving drugs through an NG tube

Holding the nasogastric (NG) tube above the patient's nose, pour up to 30 ml of diluted drug into the syringe barrel. To prevent air from entering the patient's stomach, hold the tube at a slight angle and add more drug before the syringe empties. If necessary, raise the tube slightly higher to increase flow rate.

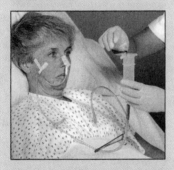

After you've delivered the whole dose, position the patient on her right side, head slightly elevated, to minimize esophageal reflux.

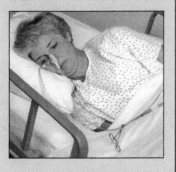

SPECIAL CONSIDERATIONS

- Before instillation, patency and positioning of the tube must be carefully checked for obstruction or improper positioning.
- Crushing enteric-coated or sustained-released tablets to facilitate transport through the tube destroys intended properties.
- To prevent instillation of too much fluid (more than 400 ml of liquid at one time for an adult), avoid scheduling drug instillation with the patient's regular tube feeding. If you must schedule a tube feed and drug instillation simultaneously, give the drug first.
- Remember to avoid giving foods that interact adversely with the drug. Tube feedings of Osmolite or Isocal must be held 2 hours before and 2 hours after phenytoin administration.
- If the patient receives continuous tube feedings, stop the feeding and check the quantity of residual stomach contents. If it's more than 50% of the previous hour's intake, withhold the drug and feeding and notify the physician. An excessive amount of residual contents may indicate intestinal obstruction or paralytic ileus.
- If the NG tube is attached to suction, be sure to turn off the suction for 20 to 30 minutes after giving drug.

COMPLICATIONS
- None known

PATIENT TEACHING

- If necessary, teach the patient who requires long-term treatment how to instill the drug himself through the NG tube.
- Remain with the patient when he performs the procedure for the first few times.
- Encourage the patient and correct any errors, as necessary.

DOCUMENTATION

- Record the date and time of instillation.
- Document the dose.
- Note the patient's tolerance of procedure.
- Record the amount of fluid instilled on the intake and output sheet.

SELECTED REFERENCES

Goorhuis, J.F., et al. "Buccal vs. Nasogastric Tube Administration of Tacrolimus after Pediatric Liver Transplantation," *Pediatric Transplantation* 10(1):74-77, February 2006.

Messaouik, D., et al. "Comparative Study and Optimisation of the Administration Mode of Three Proton Pump Inhibitors by Nasogastric Tube," *International Journal of Pharmaceutics* 299(1-2), 65-72, August 2005.

Mohammedi, I., et al. "Plasma Levels of Voriconazole Administered via a Nasogastric Tube to Critically Ill Patients," *European Journal of Clinical Microbiology & Infectious Diseases* 24(5):358-60, May 2005.

Nasogastric tube insertion and removal

OVERVIEW

DESCRIPTION

◆ A nasogastric (NG) tube is usually inserted to decompress the stomach.
◆ The tube can prevent vomiting after major surgery.
◆ It's used to assess and treat upper GI bleeding, collect gastric contents for analysis, perform gastric lavage, aspirate gastric secretions, and give drugs and nutrients.
◆ It requires close observation of the patient and verification of proper placement.
◆ The tube must be inserted with care in pregnant patients and those with increased risk of complications.
◆ The most common tubes are the Levin tube (one lumen) and Salem sump tube (two lumens [air flows through the vent lumen to protect the gastric mucosa should the tube adhere to the stomach lining]).

CONTRAINDICATIONS

◆ Coma
◆ Facial or basilar skull fracture with cribriform plate injury
◆ Hypothermia (insertion can cause myocardial irritability leading to ventricular fibrillation)

EQUIPMENT

NG TUBE INSERTION

Tube (usually #12, #14, #16, or #18 French for a normal adult) ◆ towel or linen-saver pad ◆ facial tissues ◆ emesis basin ◆ penlight ◆ 1″ or 2″ hypoallergenic tape ◆ gloves ◆ water-soluble lubricant ◆ cup or glass of water with straw (if appropriate) ◆ pH test strip ◆ tongue blade ◆ catheter-tip or bulb syringe or irrigation set ◆ safety pin ◆ ordered suction equipment

NG TUBE REMOVAL

Stethoscope ◆ gloves ◆ catheter-tip syringe ◆ normal saline solution ◆ towel or linen-saver pad ◆ adhesive remover ◆ clamp (optional)

PREPARATION

◆ Inspect the NG tube for defects.
◆ Check the tube's patency by flushing it with water.

KEY STEPS

◆ Provide privacy.
◆ Wash your hands and put on gloves.
◆ Identify the proper tube.

INSERTING AN NG TUBE

◆ Confirm the patient's identity using two patient identifiers according to facility policy.
◆ Explain the procedure to the patient.
◆ Emphasize that swallowing will ease the tube's advancement.
◆ Agree on a signal the patient can use if he wants you to stop briefly during the procedure.
◆ Put the patient in high Fowler's position, unless contraindicated.
◆ Drape the towel or linen-saver pad over his chest.
◆ Have the patient blow his nose to clear his nostrils.
◆ Place the facial tissues and emesis basin within reach.
◆ Help the patient face forward with his neck in a neutral position.
◆ To determine how long the NG tube must be to reach the stomach, hold the end of the tube at the tip of his nose, then extend the tube to his earlobe and down to the xiphoid process.
◆ Mark this distance on the tubing with tape. It may be necessary to add 2″ (5 cm) for tall individuals to ensure entry into the stomach.
◆ To determine which nostril will allow easier access, use a penlight and inspect for a deviated septum or other abnormalities, ask if he ever had nasal surgery or a nasal injury, and assess airflow in both nostrils.
◆ Lubricate the first 3″ (7.6 cm) of the tube with a water-soluble gel.
◆ Instruct the patient to hold his head straight and upright.
◆ Grasp the tube with the end pointing downward, curve it if necessary, and carefully insert it into the more patent nostril.

◆ Aim the tube downward and toward the ear closer to the chosen nostril.
◆ Advance it slowly to avoid pressure on the turbinates and resultant pain and bleeding. When the tube reaches the nasopharynx, you'll feel resistance.
◆ Instruct the patient to lower his head slightly to close the trachea and open the esophagus.
◆ Rotate the tube 180 degrees toward the opposite nostril.
◆ Unless contraindicated, offer the patient a cup or glass of water with a straw.
◆ Direct the patient to sip and swallow as you slowly advance the tube.
◆ Watch for respiratory distress as you advance the tube.
◆ Stop advancing the tube when the tape mark reaches the patient's nostril.

ENSURING PROPER NG TUBE PLACEMENT

◆ Use a tongue blade and penlight to examine the patient's mouth and throat for signs of a coiled section of tubing.
◆ Attach a catheter-tip or bulb syringe and try to aspirate stomach contents.
◆ Examine the aspirate and place a small amount on the pH test strip.
◆ Correct gastric placement is likely if the aspirate has a typical gastric fluid appearance (grassy-green, clear and colorless with mucus shreds, or brown) and the pH is 5.0 or less.

⚡ *WARNING When confirming tube placement, never place the tube's end in a container of water. If the tube is in the trachea, the patient may aspirate water. Bubbles don't confirm proper placement as the tube may be coiled in the trachea or the esophagus.*
◆ If you still can't aspirate stomach contents, advance the tube 1″ to 2″ (2.5 to 5 cm). Then inject 10 cc of air into the tube.
◆ If tests don't confirm proper tube placement, you'll need X-ray verification.
◆ Secure the NG tube to the patient's nose with hypoallergenic tape.

- Alternatively, stabilize the tube with a prepackaged product that secures and cushions it at the nose.
- Tie a slipknot around the tube with a rubber band, then secure the rubber band to the patient's gown with a safety pin.
- Fasten the tape tab to the patient's gown.
- Attach the tube to suction equipment, if ordered, and set the designated suction pressure.
- Provide frequent nose and mouth care while the tube is in place.

REMOVING AN NG TUBE

- Explain the procedure to the patient.
- Assess bowel function by auscultating for peristalsis or flatus.
- Help the patient into semi-Fowler's position.
- Wash your hands and put on gloves.
- Drape a towel or linen-saver pad across his chest.
- Using a catheter-tip syringe, flush the tube with 10 ml of normal saline solution to make sure that the tube doesn't contain stomach contents.
- Untape the tube from the patient's nose and unpin it from his gown.
- Clamp the tube by folding it in your hand.
- Ask the patient to hold his breath to close the epiglottis.
- Slowly withdraw the tube.
- Immediately cover and discard the tube.
- Assist the patient with thorough mouth and skin care.
- For the next 48 hours, monitor for signs of GI dysfunction.
- GI dysfunction may necessitate reinsertion of the tube.

SPECIAL CONSIDERATIONS

- If the tube position can't be confirmed, the practitioner may order fluoroscopy to verify placement.
- If the patient has a deviated septum or other nasal condition that prevents nasal insertion, pass the tube orally. Sliding the tube over the tongue, proceed as you would for nasal insertion.
- When using the oral route, coil the end of the tube around your hand.
- If your patient is unconscious, tilt the chin toward his chest to close the trachea.
- Advance the tube between respirations.
- While advancing the tube, watch for signs that it entered the trachea, such as choking or breathing difficulties in a conscious patient and cyanosis in an unconscious patient or a patient without a cough reflex. If these signs occur, remove the tube immediately.
- Allow the patient time to rest, then try to reinsert the tube.
- After tube placement, vomiting suggests tubal obstruction or incorrect position. Assess immediately to determine the cause.

COMPLICATIONS

- Skin erosion at the nostril
- Sinusitis
- Esophagitis
- Esophagotracheal fistula
- Gastric ulceration
- Pulmonary and oral infection
- Electrolyte imbalances and dehydration

PATIENT TEACHING

- Tell the patient what to expect during insertion.
- Explain signs and symptoms to report, as needed.
- Tell the patient to avoid food and drink for several hours after tube removal.

DOCUMENTATION

- Record the type and size of the NG tube.
- Note the date, time, and route of insertion and removal.
- Note the patient's tolerance of the procedure.
- Document the type, color, odor, consistency, and amount of gastric drainage.
- Record the patient's tolerance of the procedure.
- Record the signs and symptoms of complications.
- Note subsequent irrigation procedures and continuing problems after irrigation.
- Note any unusual events following NG removal, such as nausea, vomiting, abdominal distention, and food intolerance.

SELECTED REFERENCES

Crisp, C.L. "Nasogastric Tube Insertion in a Child with Neurodevelopmental Disabilities: Size Does Matter: A Case Study," *Gastroenterology Nursing* 29(2):108-110, March-April 2006.

Higgins, D. "Nasogastric Tube Insertion," *Nursing Times* 101(37):28-29, September 2005.

Jones, A.P., et al. "Insertion of a Nasogastric Tube Under Direct Vision," *Anaesthesia* 61(3):305, March 2006.

Puttaswamy, R.K., et al. "A Novel Method for Replacement of a Blocked Fine-Bore Nasogastric Tube," *Journal of Laryngology and Otology* 118(8):659-60, August 2004.

Rushing, J. "Inserting a Nasogastric Tube," *Nursing* 35(5):22, May 2005.

Nasopharyngeal airway insertion and care

DESCRIPTION

- Insertion of this soft rubber or latex uncuffed catheter establishes or maintains a patent airway.
- It's used after oral surgery or facial trauma and for patients with loose, cracked, or avulsed teeth.
- It protects the nasal mucosa from injury when the patient needs frequent nasotracheal suctioning.
- The airway follows the curvature of the nasopharynx, passes through the nose, and extends from the nostril to the posterior pharynx.
- The bevel-shaped pharyngeal end allows easier insertion; the funnel-shaped nasal end prevents slippage.
- This method is preferred when an oropharyngeal airway is contraindicated or fails to maintain a patent airway.

CONTRAINDICATIONS

- Anticoagulant therapy
- Hemorrhagic disorder
- Sepsis
- Pathologic nasopharyngeal deformity

AIRWAY INSERTION

Nasopharyngeal airway of proper size ◆ tongue blade ◆ water-soluble lubricant ◆ gloves ◆ suction equipment (optional)

AIRWAY CARE

Hydrogen peroxide ◆ water ◆ basin ◆ pipe cleaner (optional)

PREPARATION

- Measure the diameter of the patient's nostril and the distance from the tip of his nose to his earlobe.
- Select an airway slightly smaller than the nostril's diameter and slightly longer (1″ [2.5 cm]) than measured length.
- Recommended sizes are: large adult, 8 to 9 mm; medium adult, 7 to 8 mm; small adult, 6 to 7 mm.
- Lubricate the distal half of the airway's surface with a water-soluble lubricant to prevent traumatic injury during insertion.

- Wash your hands and put on gloves.
- In nonemergency situations, confirm the patient's identity using two patient identifiers according to facility policy and explain the procedure to the patient.
- Lubricate the airway and insert it properly. (See *Inserting a nasopharyngeal airway*.)
- After the airway is inserted, check it regularly to detect dislodgment or obstruction.
- When the patient's natural airway is patent, remove the airway in one smooth motion.
- If the airway sticks, apply lubricant around the nasal end of the tube and around the nostril; then rotate the airway until it's free.

Inserting a nasopharyngeal airway

Hold the airway beside the patient's face to make sure it's the proper size (shown at right). It should be slightly smaller than the patient's nostril diameter and slightly longer than the distance from the tip of his nose to his earlobe.

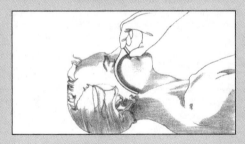

To insert the airway, hyperextend the patient's neck (unless contraindicated). Then push the tip of his nose up and pass the airway into his nostril (shown at right). Avoid pushing against any resistance to prevent tissue trauma and airway kinking.

To check for correct airway placement, close the patient's mouth and then place your finger over the tube's opening to detect air exchange. Also, depress his tongue with a tongue blade and look for the airway tip behind the uvula.

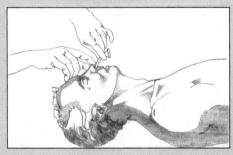

SPECIAL CONSIDERATIONS

◆ Use a chin-lift or jaw-thrust technique when inserting the airway.
◆ Assess the patient's respirations immediately after inserting.
◆ If absent or inadequate, initiate artificial positive-pressure ventilation with a mouth-to-mask technique, a handheld resuscitation bag, or an oxygen-powered breathing device.
◆ If the patient coughs or gags, the tube may be too long. Replace it with a shorter one.
◆ Remove the airway at least every 8 hours to check nasal mucous membranes for irritation or ulceration.
◆ Clean the airway by rinsing with hydrogen peroxide followed by water.
◆ If secretions remain, use a pipe cleaner to remove them.
◆ Reinsert the clean airway into the other nostril.

COMPLICATIONS

◆ Sinus infection
◆ Gastric distention and hypoventilation during artificial ventilation
◆ Laryngospasm and vomiting
◆ Bleeding and possibly aspiration of blood into the trachea caused by nasal mucosa injury

PATIENT TEACHING

◆ Explain the procedure and answer questions, as needed.

DOCUMENTATION

◆ Record the dates and times of the airway insertion and removal.
◆ Note the size of the airway.
◆ Record shifts from one nostril to the other.
◆ Note the condition of the mucous membranes.
◆ Document suctioning.
◆ Record complications and nursing action taken.
◆ Note the patient's reaction to the procedure.

SELECTED REFERENCES

Holm-Knudsen, R., et al. "Using a Nasopharyngeal Airway during Fiber-optic Intubation in Small Children with a Difficult Airway," *Pediatric Anesthesia* 15(10):839-45, October 2005.

Isono, S. "Developmental Changes of Pharyngeal Airway Patency: Implications for Pediatric Anesthesia," *Pediatric Anesthesia* 16(2):109-22, February 2006.

Martin, J.E., et al. "Intracranial Insertion of a Nasopharyngeal Airway in a Patient with Craniofacial Trauma," *Military Medicine* 169(6):496-97, June 2004.

Roberts, K., et al. "The Nasopharyngeal Airway: Dispelling Myths and Establishing the Facts," *Emergency Medical Journal* 22(6):394-96, June 2005.

Nebulizer therapy

OVERVIEW

DESCRIPTION
- Nebulizer therapy aids bronchial hygiene by restoring and maintaining mucous blanket continuity, hydrating dried secretions, promoting secretion expectoration, humidifying inspired oxygen, and delivering drugs.
- It may be given through nebulizers that have large or small volume, are ultrasonic, or are placed inside ventilator tubing:
- Large-volume nebulizers provide humidity for an artificial airway.
- Small-volume nebulizers are used to deliver drugs such as bronchodilators.
- Ultrasonic nebulizers are electrically driven and use high-frequency vibrations to break up surface water into particles; resultant dense mist can penetrate smaller airways, hydrate secretions, and induce coughing.
- In-line nebulizers are used to deliver drugs to patients being mechanically ventilated.

CONTRAINDICATIONS
- None known

EQUIPMENT

LARGE-VOLUME NEBULIZER (SUCH AS VENTURI JET)
Pressurized gas source ◆ flowmeter ◆ large-bore oxygen tubing ◆ nebulizer bottle ◆ sterile distilled water ◆ heater (if ordered) ◆ in-line thermometer (if using heater)

SMALL-VOLUME NEBULIZER (SUCH AS A MINI-NEBULIZER)
Pressurized gas source ◆ flowmeter ◆ oxygen tubing ◆ nebulizer cup ◆ mouthpiece or mask ◆ normal saline solution ◆ prescribed drug

ULTRASONIC NEBULIZER
Ultrasonic gas-delivery device ◆ large-bore oxygen tubing ◆ nebulizer couplet compartment

IN-LINE NEBULIZER
Pressurized gas source ◆ flowmeter ◆ nebulizer cup ◆ normal saline solution ◆ prescribed drug

PREPARATION
Large-volume nebulizer
- Fill with distilled water to indicated level.
- Avoid using normal saline solution to prevent corrosion.
- Add a heating device, if ordered.
- Ensure delivery of prescribed oxygen percentage.

Small-volume nebulizer
- Draw up drug, inject it into the nebulizer cup, and add the prescribed amount of normal saline solution or water.
- Attach the mouthpiece, mask, or other gas-delivery device.

Ultrasonic nebulizer
- Fill the couplet compartment to level indicated.

In-line nebulizer
- Draw up the drug and diluent, remove the nebulizer cup, quickly inject the drug, then replace the cup.
- If using an intermittent positive-pressure breathing machine, attach the mouthpiece and mask to the machine.

KEY STEPS

- Confirm the patient's identity using two patient identifiers according to facility policy.
- Explain the procedure to the patient.
- Wash your hands.
- Take the patient's vital signs, and auscultate his lungs.
- Place the patient in a sitting or high Fowler's position.

LARGE-VOLUME NEBULIZER
- Attach the delivery device to the patient.
- Encourage the patient to cough and expectorate, or suction as needed.
- Check the water level in the nebulizer and refill as indicated.
- When refilling a reusable container, discard the old water.
- Change the nebulizer unit and tubing according to facility policy.
- If the nebulizer is heated, tell the patient to report discomfort.
- Use the in-line thermometer to monitor the temperature of the gas the patient is inhaling.
- If you turn off the flow for more than 5 minutes, unplug the heater.

SMALL-VOLUME NEBULIZER
- Attach the flowmeter to the gas source. Attach the nebulizer to the flowmeter. Adjust the flow to at least 10 L.
- Check the outflow port to ensure adequate misting.
- Remain with the patient during the treatment.
- Take vital signs and monitor for adverse reactions.
- Encourage the patient to cough and expectorate, or suction as necessary.
- Change the nebulizer cup and tubing according to facility policy.

ULTRASONIC NEBULIZER

◆ Administer an inhaled bronchodilator to prevent bronchospasm.
◆ Turn the machine on and check the outflow port for proper misting.
◆ Monitor the patient for adverse reactions.
◆ Watch for labored respirations.
◆ Take the patient's vital signs, and auscultate his lung fields.
◆ Encourage the patient to cough and expectorate, or suction as needed.

IN-LINE NEBULIZER

◆ Turn on the machine and check for proper misting.
◆ Remain with the patient during the treatment.
◆ Take vital signs and monitor for adverse reactions.
◆ Encourage the patient to cough, and suction excess secretions as necessary.
◆ Auscultate the patient's lungs to evaluate effectiveness of therapy.

SPECIAL CONSIDERATIONS

◆ Efficacy of aerosol therapy, what type of fluids to use, types of drugs that can be delivered, and effectiveness of therapy haven't been established.
◆ Be alert for overhydration, especially in pediatric patients or those with a delicate fluid balance.
◆ Carefully monitor for adequate flow if oxygen is being delivered at the same time.

COMPLICATIONS

◆ Mucosa irritation
◆ Bronchospasm
◆ Dyspnea
◆ Airway burns
◆ Infection
◆ Adverse drug reactions

PATIENT TEACHING

◆ Encourage the patient to take slow, even breaths to derive maximum benefit.

DOCUMENTATION

◆ Record the date, time, and duration of therapy.
◆ Note the type and amount of drug.
◆ Document the fraction of inspired oxygen or oxygen flow.
◆ Record baseline and subsequent vital signs and breath sounds.
◆ Note the patient's response to treatment.

SELECTED REFERENCES

Dubus, J.C., and Anhoj, J. "Inhaled Steroid Delivery from Small-Volume Holding Chambers Depends on Age, Holding Chamber, and Interface in Children," *Journal of Aerosol Medicine* 17(3):225-30, Fall 2004.

Lentz, Y.K., et al. "DNA Acts as a Nucleation Site for Transient Cavitation in the Ultrasonic Nebulizer," *Journal of Pharmaceutical Sciences* 95(3):607-19, March 2006.

Mathews, P.J., et al. "The Latest in Respiratory Care," *Nursing Management* Suppl:18, 20-21, 2005.

Wan, G.H., et al. "A Large-Volume Nebulizer Would Not Be an Infectious Source for Severe Acute Respiratory Syndrome," *Infection Control and Hospital Epidemiology* 25(12):1113-115, December 2004.

Nephrostomy and cystostomy tube care

OVERVIEW

DESCRIPTION

- Urinary diversion techniques ensure adequate drainage from kidneys or bladder and help prevent urinary tract infection or kidney failure. (See *Urinary diversion techniques.*)
- A nephrostomy tube drains urine directly from a kidney when a disorder (such as calculi in the ureter or ureteropelvic junction or an obstructing tumor) inhibits normal urine flow.
- The tubes are usually placed percutaneously; sometimes they're surgically inserted.
- Draining urine with a nephrostomy tube allows kidney tissue damaged by obstructive disease to heal.
- A cystostomy tube drains urine from the bladder, diverting it from the urethra.
- The tubes are used after certain gynecologic procedures, bladder surgery, prostatectomy, and for severe urethral strictures or traumatic injury.
- They're inserted about 2″ (5 cm) above the symphysis pubis; a cystostomy tube may be used alone or with an indwelling urethral catheter.

CONTRAINDICATIONS

- None known

EQUIPMENT

DRESSING CHANGES

4″ × 4″ gauze pads ◆ povidone-iodine solution or povidone-iodine pads ◆ sterile cup or emesis basin ◆ paper bag ◆ linen-saver pad ◆ clean gloves (for dressing removal) ◆ sterile gloves (for new dressing) ◆ precut 4″ × 4″ drain dressings or transparent semipermeable dressings ◆ adhesive tape (preferably hypoallergenic)

NEPHROSTOMY-TUBE IRRIGATION

3-ml syringe ◆ alcohol pad or povidone-iodine pad ◆ normal saline solution ◆ hemostat (optional)

PREPARATION

- Wash your hands.
- Assemble equipment at the patient's bedside.
- Open several packages of gauze pads, place them in the sterile cup or emesis basin, and pour the povidone-iodine solution over them.
- Open a commercially packaged kit (if available), using aseptic technique.
- Fill the cup with antiseptic solution.
- Open the paper bag and place it away from the other equipment to avoid contaminating the sterile field.

KEY STEPS

- Confirm the patient's identity using two patient identifiers according to facility policy.
- Wash your hands and provide privacy.
- Explain the procedure to the patient.

CHANGING A DRESSING

- Put the patient on his back (for a cystostomy tube) or the side opposite the tube (for a nephrostomy tube).
- Place the linen-saver pad under the patient to absorb drainage.
- Put on clean gloves.
- Carefully remove the tape around the tube.
- Remove wet or soiled dressings.
- Discard the tape and dressing in the paper bag.
- Remove the gloves and discard them in the bag.
- Put on sterile gloves.
- Pick up a saturated pad or dip a dry one into the cup of antiseptic solution.
- To clean the wound, wipe only once with each pad or sponge, moving from the insertion site outward.
- Discard the used pad or sponge in the paper bag.
- To avoid contaminating your gloves, don't touch the bag.

Urinary diversion techniques

A cystostomy or a nephrostomy can be used to create a permanent urinary diversion, to relieve obstruction from an inoperable tumor, or provide an outlet for urine after cystectomy.

A temporary diversion can relieve obstruction from a calculus or ureteral edema.

In a cystostomy, a catheter is inserted percutaneously through the suprapubic area into the bladder. In a nephrostomy, a catheter is inserted percutaneously through the flank into the renal pelvis.

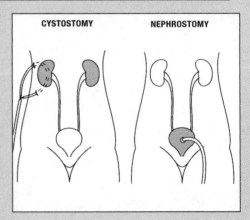

- Pick up a sterile 4" × 4" drain dressing and place it around the tube.
- If necessary, overlap two drain dressings to provide maximum absorption. Alternatively, depending on your facility's policy, apply a transparent semipermeable dressing over the site and tubing to allow observation of the site.
- Secure the dressing with hypoallergenic tape.
- Tape the tube to the patient's lateral abdomen to prevent tension.
- Dispose of all equipment appropriately.
- Clean the patient as necessary.

IRRIGATING A NEPHROSTOMY TUBE

- Fill the 3-ml syringe with the normal saline solution.
- Clean the junction of the nephrostomy tube and drainage tube with the alcohol pad or povidone-iodine pad, and disconnect the tubes.
- Insert the syringe into the nephrostomy tube opening, and instill 2 to 3 ml of normal saline solution into the tube.
- Slowly aspirate the solution back into the syringe.
- Never pull back on the plunger.

TROUBLESHOOTER *If the solution doesn't return, remove the syringe from the tube and reattach it to the drainage tubing to allow the solution to drain by gravity.*

- Dispose of all equipment appropriately.

SPECIAL CONSIDERATIONS

- Change dressings once per day or more often as needed.

WARNING *Never irrigate a nephrostomy tube with more than 5 ml of solution because the capacity of the renal pelvis is usually between 4 and 8 ml. (The purpose of irrigation is to keep the tube patent, not to lavage the renal pelvis.)*

- Irrigate a cystostomy tube as you would an indwelling urinary catheter.
- Perform irrigation to avoid damaging any suture lines.
- Curve a cystostomy tube to prevent kinks; kinks are likely if the patient lies on the insertion site.
- Check a nephrostomy tube frequently for kinks or obstructions.
- Suspect an obstruction when the amount of urine in the drainage bag decreases or the amount of urine around the insertion site increases.

TROUBLESHOOTER *If a blood clot or mucus plug obstructs a nephrostomy or cystostomy tube, try milking the tube to restore its patency.*

- Check cystostomy hourly for postoperative urologic patients.
- To check tube patency, note the amount of urine in the drainage bag and check the patient's bladder for distention.
- Keep the drainage bag below the level of the kidney at all times.
- Notify the practitioner immediately if the tube becomes dislodged.
- Cover the site with a sterile dressing.
- While clamping the nephrostomy tube, assess the patient for flank pain and fever, and monitor urine output.

COMPLICATIONS

- Infection

PATIENT TEACHING

- Explain how to clean the insertion site with soap and water, check for skin breakdown, and change dressing daily.
- Teach the patient how to change the leg bag or drainage bag.
- Explain how and when to wash the drainage bag.
- Encourage the patient to increase fluid intake to 3 qt (3 L) daily, if no contraindications.
- Explain signs of infection and have the patient report them to his physician.

DOCUMENTATION

- Record the color and amount of drainage.
- Note the amount and type of irrigant used.
- Document whether you obtained a complete return.

SELECTED REFERENCES

Jou, Y.C., et al. "Nephrostomy Tube-Free Percutaneous Nephrolithotomy for Patients with Large Stones and Staghorn Stones," *Urology* 67(1):30-34, January 2006.

Kim, S.C., et al. "Using and Choosing a Nephrostomy Tube after Percutaneous Nephrolithotomy for Large or Complex Stone Disease: A Treatment Strategy," *Journal of Endourology* 19(3):348-52, April 2005.

Modi, P., et al. "Laparoscopic Ureteroneocystostomy for Distal Ureteral Injuries," *Urology* 66(4):751-53, October 2005.

Neurologic vital sign assessment

DESCRIPTION

- This procedure supplements measurement of temperature, pulse rate, and respirations by evaluating level of consciousness (LOC), pupillary activity, and orientation to place, time, date, and person.
- LOC (measure of environmental- and self-awareness) reflects cortical function and provides early sign of central nervous system deterioration.
- Pupillary activity changes may signal increased intracranial pressure (ICP) associated with a space-occupying lesion.
- Evaluating muscle strength and tone, reflexes, and posture helps identify nervous system damage.
- Vital sign changes alone don't indicate neurologic compromise; changes should be evaluated in light of complete neurologic assessment.

CONTRAINDICATIONS

- None known

EQUIPMENT

Penlight ◆ thermometer ◆ sterile cotton ball or cotton-tipped applicator ◆ stethoscope ◆ sphygmomanometer ◆ pupil size chart ◆ pencil or pen

KEY STEPS

- Confirm the patient's identity using two patient identifiers according to facility policy.
- Explain the procedure to the patient, even if he's unresponsive.
- Wash your hands and provide privacy.

ASSESSING LEVEL OF CONSCIOUSNESS AND ORIENTATION

- Use the Glasgow Coma Scale. (See *Using the Glasgow Coma Scale.*)
- Measure the patient's response to verbal, tactile (touch), or painful (nail bed pressure) stimuli.
- Ask the patient his full name.
- Assess his orientation to time, date, place, and person.
- Assess the quality of responses.
- Assess his ability to understand and follow one-step commands that require a motor response.
- Note whether the patient can maintain his LOC.
- If the patient doesn't respond to commands or touch, apply a painful stimulus.
- Check motor responses bilaterally to rule out monoplegia and hemiplegia.

EXAMINING PUPILS AND EYE MOVEMENT

- Ask the patient to open his eyes.
- If he doesn't respond, lift his upper eyelids.
- Inspect each pupil's size and shape, and compare for equality.
- Pupil size varies; some patients have normally unequal pupils (anisocoria).
- Note if the pupils are positioned in, or deviate from, the midline.

TESTING DIRECT LIGHT RESPONSE

- Darken the room before testing.
- Hold each eyelid open in turn, keeping the other eye covered.
- Swing a penlight from the patient's ear toward the midline of the face.
- Shine the light directly into the eye. Normally, the pupil constricts immediately.
- When you remove the penlight, the pupil should dilate immediately.
- Wait about 20 seconds before testing the other pupil.

TESTING CONSENSUAL LIGHT RESPONSE

- Hold both eyelids open, but shine light into one eye only.

Using the Glasgow Coma Scale

The Glasgow Coma Scale provides a standard reference for assessing or monitoring level of consciousness in a patient with a suspected or confirmed brain injury. The scale measures three responses to stimuli — eye opening, motor response, and verbal response — and assigns a number to each possible response within these categories.

A score of 3 is lowest and 15 is highest. A score of 7 or less indicates coma.

CHARACTERISTICS	RESPONSE	SCORE
Eye opening response	◆ Spontaneous	4
	◆ To verbal command	3
	◆ To pain	2
	◆ No response	1
Best motor response	◆ Obeys commands	6
	◆ To painful stimuli	
	– Localizes pain; pushes stimulus away	5
	– Flexes and withdraws	4
	– Abnormal flexion	3
	– Extension	2
	– No response	1
Best verbal response (Arouse patient with painful stimuli, if necessary.)	◆ Oriented and converses	5
	◆ Disoriented and converses	4
	◆ Uses inappropriate words	3
	◆ Makes incomprehensible sounds	2
	◆ No response	1
		Total: 3 to 15

- Watch for constriction in the other pupil, which indicates proper nerve function of the optic chiasm.
- Brighten the room and have the conscious patient open his eyes.
- Observe the eyelids for ptosis or drooping.
- Check extraocular movements.
- Watch for involuntary jerking or oscillating eye movements (nystagmus).

CHECKING ACCOMMODATION

- Hold up one finger midline to the patient's face and several feet away.
- Have the patient focus on your finger.
- Gradually move your finger toward his nose while he focuses on your finger. This should cause his eyes to converge and both pupils to constrict equally.
- Test the corneal reflex by touching a wisp of cotton ball to the cornea. This normally causes an immediate blink reflex.
- Repeat for the other eye.
- If patient is unconscious, test the oculocephalic (doll's eye) reflex.

WARNING *Never test the doll's eye reflex if you know or suspect the patient has a cervical spine injury. Permanent spinal cord damage may result.*

- Hold the patient's eyelids open.
- Quickly turn patient's head to one side, then the other. If his eyes move in the opposite direction from the side to which you turn the head, the reflex is intact.

EVALUATING MOTOR FUNCTION

- If the patient is conscious, test his grip strength in both hands at the same time.
- Test arm strength.
- Test leg strength.

WARNING *If decorticate or decerebrate posturing develops in response to stimuli, notify the practitioner immediately. (See* Identifying warning postures.*)*

- Flex and extend the extremities on both sides to evaluate muscle tone.
- Test the plantar reflex in all patients.
- Watch for a positive Babinski's sign (dorsiflexion of the great toe with fanning of the other toes), indicating an upper motor neuron lesion.

- Take patient's temperature, pulse rate, respiratory rate, and blood pressure.
- Pulse pressure is especially important because widening pulse pressure can indicate increasing ICP.

SPECIAL CONSIDERATIONS

WARNING *If a previously stable patient suddenly develops a change in neurologic or routine vital signs, further assess his condition, and notify the practitioner immediately.*

COMPLICATIONS
- None known

PATIENT TEACHING

- Explain the procedures as you are performing them in an effort to elicit a response.

DOCUMENTATION

- Baseline data require detailed documentation. Subsequent notes can be brief unless patient's condition changes.
- Record the patient's LOC and orientation, pupillary activity, motor function, and routine vital signs.
- Note the patient's behavior.

SELECTED REFERENCES
Fairley, D., and Pearce, A. "Assessment of Consciousness: Part One," *Nursing Times* 102(4):26-27, January-February 2006.

Iacono, L.A., and Lyones, K.A. "Making GCS as Easy as 1, 2, 3, 4, 5, 6," *Journal of Trauma Nursing* 12(3):77-81, July-September 2005.

Morgan, A. "Neurological Assessment," *Nursing Standard* 20(14-16):67, December 2005-January 2006.

Schollenberger, J., et al. "Brain Monitors," *RN* 69(1):44-49, January 2006.

Identifying warning postures

Decorticate and decerebrate postures are ominous signs of central nervous system deterioration.

DECORTICATE (ABNORMAL FLEXION)
The arms are adducted and flexed, with wrists and fingers flexed on the chest. The legs may be stiffly extended and internally rotated, with plantar flexion of the feet.

The decorticate posture may indicate a lesion of the frontal lobe, internal capsule, or cerebral peduncles.

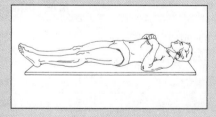

DECEREBRATE (EXTENSION)
The patient's arms are adducted and extended with wrists pronated and fingers flexed. One or both legs may be stiffly extended, with plantar flexion of the feet.

The decerebrate posture may indicate lesions of the upper brain stem.

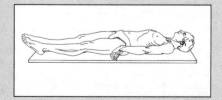

Neutropenic precautions

DESCRIPTION

- There are two types of neutropenic precautions: protective precautions and reverse isolation.
- They protect a patient at increased risk for infection.
- They're used primarily for patients with extensive noninfected burns, leukopenia or a depressed immune system, and those receiving immunosuppressive treatments. (See *Conditions and treatments requiring neutropenic precautions*.)
- They require a private room equipped with positive air pressure.
- They may require thorough hand-washing technique; limitation of traffic into the room; the use of gowns, gloves, and masks by staff members and visitors; a patient isolator unit; and sterile linens, gowns, gloves, and head and shoe coverings.
- All items taken into the room should be sterilized or disinfected.
- The patient's diet may be modified to eliminate raw fruits and vegetables and allow only cooked foods and possibly only sterile beverages.

CONTRAINDICATIONS

- None known

Gloves ◆ gowns ◆ masks ◆ shoe covers, if required ◆ NEUTROPENIC PRECAUTIONS door card ◆ thermometer ◆ stethoscope ◆ blood pressure cuff

PREPARATION

- Assemble all equipment in advance so you don't have to leave the isolation room unnecessarily.
- Keep supplies in a clean, enclosed cart or in an anteroom outside the room.

- Confirm the patient's identity using two patient identifiers according to facility policy.
- Put the patient in a private room.
- Explain isolation precautions to patient and family to ease anxiety and promote compliance.
- Place the NEUTROPENIC PRECAUTIONS card on the door to caution those entering the room.
- Wash your hands with an antiseptic agent before putting on gloves, after removing gloves, and as indicated during patient care.
- Wear gloves and gown according to standard precautions, unless the patient's condition warrants sterile gown, gloves, and mask.
- Avoid transporting the patient out of the room.
- If the patient must be moved, make sure he wears a gown and mask.
- Notify the receiving department or area so that the precautions will be maintained and the patient will be returned to the room promptly.
- Don't allow visits by anyone known to be ill or infected.

Conditions and treatments requiring neutropenic precautions

CONDITION OR TREATMENT	PRECAUTIONARY PERIOD
Acquired immunodeficiency syndrome	Until white blood cell count reaches 1,000/µl or more or according to facility guidelines
Agranulocytosis	Until remission
Burns (extensive noninfected)	Until skin surface heals substantially
Dermatitis, noninfected vesicular, bullous, or eczematous disease (when severe and extensive)	Until skin surface heals substantially
Immunosuppressive therapy	Until patient's immunity is adequate
Lymphomas and leukemia, especially late stages of Hodgkin's disease or acute leukemia	Until clinical improvement is substantial

SPECIAL CONSIDERATIONS

◆ Don't perform invasive procedures such as urethral catheterization unless absolutely necessary because these procedures risk serious infection in the patient with impaired resistance.
◆ Instruct housekeeping staff to put on gowns, gloves, and masks before entering the room.
◆ No ill or infected person should enter the room.
◆ Make sure that the room is cleaned with new or scrupulously clean equipment.
◆ Because the patient doesn't have a contagious disease, materials leaving the room need no special precautions beyond standard precautions.

COMPLICATIONS
◆ None known

PATIENT TEACHING

◆ Explain why precautions are being instituted.
◆ Explain how precautions protect the patient from infection.

DOCUMENTATION

◆ Note the need for neutropenic precautions on the nursing care plan.
◆ Record other documentation as required by facility policy.

SELECTED REFERENCES
Chalmers, C., and Straub, M. "Standard Principles for Preventing and Controlling Infection," *Nursing Standard* 20(23):57-65, February 2006.
Larson, E., and Nirenberg, A. "Evidence-Based Nursing Practice to Prevent Infection in Hospitalized Neutropenic Patients with Cancer," *Oncology Nursing Forum* 31(4):717-25, July 2004.
Padilla, G., and Ropka, M.E. "Quality of Life and Chemotherapy-Induced Neutropenia," *Cancer Nursing* 28(3):167-71, May-June 2005.
Weber, J., et al. "Infection Control in Burn Patients," *Burns* 30(8):A16-24, December 2004.

Obstructed airway management (foreign body)

OVERVIEW

DESCRIPTION
- Obstructed airway can occur when a foreign body lodges in the throat or bronchus; when the patient aspirates blood, mucus, or vomitus; when the tongue blocks the pharynx; or when the patient experiences traumatic injury, bronchoconstriction, or bronchospasm.
- The patient will display such symptoms as grabbing his throat with his hand, inability to speak, weak and ineffective coughing, or high-pitched sounds while inhaling.
- Airway obstruction causes anoxia, which leads to brain damage and death in 4 to 6 minutes.
- If the patient is unconscious, an abdominal thrust should be used.
- For pregnant patients, markedly obese patients, and patients who have recently undergone abdominal surgery, a chest thrust should be used.

CONTRAINDICATIONS
- Incomplete or partial airway obstruction
- Patients who can maintain adequate ventilation to dislodge the foreign body by effective coughing

EQUIPMENT

No specific equipment needed

KEY STEPS

- Determine the patient's level of consciousness by shouting, "Are you choking? Can you speak?"
- Assess for airway obstruction.
- Don't intervene if the person is coughing forcefully and able to speak; a strong cough can dislodge the object.
- Give each individual thrust with the intent of relieving the obstructing object. It may be necessary to repeat thrusts to dislodge the obstruction and clear the airway.

AGE FACTOR *Don't use abdominal thrusts to relieve choking in infants.*

CONSCIOUS ADULT AND CHILDREN OVER AGE 1
- Tell the patient that you'll try to dislodge the foreign body.
- Stand behind him, and wrap your arms around his waist.
- Make a fist with one hand, and place the thumb side of your fist against his abdomen, in the midline, slightly above the umbilicus and well below the xiphoid process.
- Grasp your fist with the other hand.
- Press your fist into the victim's abdomen with quick inward and upward thrusts.
- Each thrust should be a separate and distinct movement; each should be forceful enough to create an artificial cough that will dislodge the object.
- Repeat thrusts until the object is expelled from the airway or the victim becomes unresponsive.
- Make sure you have a firm grasp on the patient because he may lose consciousness and need to be lowered to the floor.
- If the patient loses consciousness, lower him to the floor, support his head and neck to prevent injury and place him supine.
- Call for help, activate the emergency response system, and begin cardiopulmonary resuscitation (CPR).

- Open the airway with the tongue-jaw lift, perform a finger-sweep only if you can see the object, and attempt to ventilate.
- If the chest doesn't rise, reposition the airway and attempt to ventilate again.
- If ventilation is unsuccessful, begin CPR.

UNCONSCIOUS ADULT
- Establish unresponsiveness. Call for help, activate the emergency response system.
- Open the airway (head tilt-chin lift or jaw-thrust) and check for breathing; if not breathing, attempt to ventilate.

WARNING *Each time you open the airway to give breaths, open the victim's mouth wide and look for the object. If you see the object, remove it with your fingers. If you do not see the object, continue CPR.*
- If you're unable to ventilate him, reposition his head and try again.
- Lift the jaw to draw the tongue away from the back of the throat and away from any foreign body.
- If you can see the object, remove it by inserting your index finger and perform a sweeping motion to remove the obstruction.
- You can assess if you have successfully removed the object in the unresponsive victim if you feel air movement and see the chest rise when you give breaths or if you see and remove the foreign body from the victim's pharynx.
- After the object is removed, try to ventilate the patient.
- Assess for spontaneous respirations, and check for a pulse.
- Proceed with CPR if necessary.

OBESE OR PREGNANT ADULT
- If the patient is conscious, stand behind the patient, and place your arms under the armpits and around the chest.
- Place the thumb side of your clenched fist against the middle of the sternum, avoiding the margins of the ribs and the xiphoid process.
- Grasp your fist with your other hand, and perform a chest thrust with enough force to expel the foreign body.
- Continue until the patient expels the obstruction or loses consciousness.
- If the patient loses consciousness, lower him to the floor, support his head and neck to prevent injury and place him supine.
- Call for help, activate the emergency response system, and begin cardiopulmonary resuscitation (CPR).
- Open the airway with the tongue-jaw lift, perform a finger-sweep only if you can see the object, and attempt to ventilate.
- If the chest doesn't rise, reposition the airway and attempt to ventilate again.
- If ventilation is unsuccessful, begin CPR.

UNCONSCIOUS, OBESE, OR PREGNANT ADULT
- Establish unresponsiveness.
- Call for help and activate the emergency response system.
- Open the airway with the tongue-jaw lift, perform a finger-sweep, and attempt to ventilate.
- If the chest doesn't rise, reposition the airway and attempt to ventilate again.
- If ventilation is unsuccessful, begin CPR.

SPECIAL CONSIDERATIONS

- If the patient vomits, wipe out his mouth to prevent additional obstruction.
- Even if efforts to clear the airway don't seem to be effective, keep trying.

COMPLICATIONS
- Nausea
- Regurgitation
- Injuries caused by chest thrusts

PATIENT TEACHING

- Explain what you're doing to gain the patient's cooperation, as needed.

DOCUMENTATION

- Record the date and time of the procedure.
- Note the patient's actions before the obstruction.
- Document the approximate length of time it took to clear the airway.
- Record the type and size of object removed.
- Note vital signs after the procedure.
- Document complications and nursing actions taken.

SELECTED REFERENCES
Lankster, M.A., and Brasfield, M.S., 3rd. "Update on Pediatric Advanced Life Support Guidelines," *Critical Care Nursing Clinics of North America* 17(1):59-64, March 2005.
Rodenberg, H. "The Heimlich in Near-Drownings," *Journal of Emergency Medical Services* 29(7):26, July 2004.
St. John, R.E. "Airway Management," *Critical Care Nurse* 24(2):93-96, April 2004.
Wick, R., et al. "Café Coronary Syndrome-Fatal Choking on Food: An Autopsy Approach," *Journal of Clinical Forensic Medicine* 13(3):135-38, April 2006.
Wrenn, K. "The Perils of Vinegar and the Heimlich Maneuver," *Annals of Emergency Medicine* 47(2):207-208, February 2006.

Ommaya reservoir drug infusion

OVERVIEW

DESCRIPTION

- The Ommaya reservoir is also known as a *subcutaneous cerebrospinal fluid (CSF) reservoir*.
- It allows delivery of long-term drug therapy to the CSF via the brain's ventricles.
- It spares the patient repeated lumbar punctures to administer chemotherapeutic drugs, analgesics, antibiotics, and antifungals.
- It permits consistent and predictable drug distribution throughout the subarachnoid space and central nervous system (CNS) and allows for measurement of intracranial pressure (ICP). (See *How the Ommaya reservoir works.*)
- It's most commonly used for chemotherapy and pain management, treating CNS leukemia, malignant CNS disease, and meningeal carcinomatosis.
- The device is a mushroom-shaped silicone apparatus with an attached catheter.
- It's surgically implanted beneath the patient's scalp in the nondominant lobe; the catheter is threaded into the ventricle through a burr hole in the skull.
- The patient may receive a local or general anesthetic.
- After an X-ray confirms placement, a pressure dressing is applied for 24 hours, followed by gauze dressing for 1 or 2 days.
- Sutures are removed in about 10 days; the reservoir can be used within 48 hours to deliver drugs, obtain CSF pressure measurements, drain CSF, and withdraw CSF specimens.
- The practitioner usually injects drugs into the Ommaya reservoir, but a specially trained nurse may perform this procedure if facility policy allows.

CONTRAINDICATIONS

- None known

EQUIPMENT

Equipment varies, may include: preservative-free prescribed drug ◆ gloves ◆ povidone-iodine solution ◆ sterile towel ◆ two 3-ml syringes ◆ 25G needle or 22G Huber needle ◆ sterile gauze pad ◆ collection tubes for CSF (if ordered) ◆ vial of bacteriostatic normal saline solution ◆ sterile label ◆ sterile marker

PREPARATION

- Using the sterile towel, establish a sterile field near the patient.
- Prepare a syringe with the preservative-free drug to be instilled and place it, the CSF collection tubes, and the normal saline solution on the sterile field.
- Label all medications, medication containers, and solution containers on and off the sterile field.

KEY STEPS

- Confirm the patient's identity using two patient identifiers according to facility policy.
- Explain the procedure before reservoir insertion.
- Reassure the patient that hair shaved for the implant will grow back.

INSTILLING THE DRUG

- Obtain baseline vital signs.
- Position the patient so he's either sitting or reclining.
- Put on gloves and prepare his scalp with the povidone-iodine solution, working in a circular motion from the center outward.
- Placing the 25G needle at a 45-degree angle, insert it into the reservoir and aspirate 3 ml of clear CSF into a syringe. (If aspirate isn't clear, check with the practitioner before continuing.)
- Continue aspirating as many milliliters of CSF as you'll instill of the drug.
- Detach the syringe from the needle hub, attach the drug syringe, and instill the drug slowly, monitoring for headache, nausea, and dizziness. (Some facilities use the CSF instead of a preservative-free diluent to deliver the drug.)
- Tell the patient to lie quietly for about 15 to 30 minutes after the procedure to prevent meningeal irritation leading to nausea and vomiting.
- Cover the site with a sterile gauze pad, and apply gentle pressure until superficial bleeding stops.
- Monitor the patient for adverse drug reactions and signs of increased ICP, such as nausea, vomiting, pain, and dizziness.
- Assess for adverse reactions every 30 minutes for 2 hours, then every hour for 2 hours, and finally every 4 hours.

SPECIAL CONSIDERATIONS

◆ An antiemetic may be ordered and administered 30 minutes before the procedure to control nausea and vomiting.
◆ The patient may resume normal activities after the reservoir is implanted.

COMPLICATIONS
◆ Infection
◆ Increased ICP symptoms: headache and nausea
◆ Slow filling, suggesting catheter migration or blockage and need for surgical correction

PATIENT TEACHING

◆ Discuss potential complications and answer any questions.
◆ Instruct the patient to protect the site from bumps and traumatic injury.
◆ Inform the patient that the reservoir may function for years, unless there are complications.
◆ Instruct the patient about signs and symptoms of infection and when to notify the practitioner.

DOCUMENTATION

◆ Note the appearance of the reservoir insertion site before and after access.
◆ Document the patient's tolerance of the procedure.
◆ Record the amount of CSF withdrawn and its appearance.
◆ Note the name and dose of the drug instilled.

SELECTED REFERENCES
Dickerman, R.D., and Eisenberg, M.B. "Preassembled Method for Insertion of Ommaya Reservoir," *Journal of Surgical Oncology* 89(1):36-38, January 2005.
Ishii, K., et al. "Intracranial Ectopic Recurrence of Craniopharyngioma After Ommaya Reservoir Implantation," *Pediatric Neurosurgery* 40(5): 230-33, September-October 2004.
Yoshida, S., and Morii, K. "Intrathecal Chemotherapy for Patients With Meningeal Carcinomatosis," *Surgical Neurology* 63(1):52-55, January 2005.

How the Ommaya reservoir works

To insert an Ommaya reservoir, the physician drills a burr hole and inserts the catheter's device through the patient's nondominant frontal lobe into the lateral ventricle. The reservoir, which has a self-sealing silicone injection dome, rests over the burr hole under a scalp flap. This creates a slight, soft bulge on the scalp about the size of a quarter. Usually, drugs are injected into the dome with a syringe.

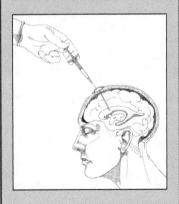

Oral drug administration

DESCRIPTION
- Oral drug administration is usually the safest, most convenient, and least expensive administration method; most drugs are given orally.
- Oral drugs are available as tablets, enteric-coated tablets, capsules, syrups, elixirs, oils, liquids, suspensions, powders, and granules.
- They may require special preparation before administration, such as mixing with juice to make more palatable; oils, powders, and granules usually require preparation.
- They're sometimes prescribed in higher dosages than parenteral equivalents because after absorption through the GI system, the liver immediately breaks them down before they reach systemic circulation.

CONTRAINDICATIONS
- Unconscious patients
- Nausea and vomiting
- Inability to swallow

   AGE FACTOR *Oral dosages normally prescribed for adults may be dangerous for elderly or young patients.*

Patient's drug record and chart ◆ prescribed drug ◆ drug cup ◆ drinking straw ◆ pill crushing device ◆ appropriate vehicle, such as jelly or applesauce, for crushed pills (commonly used with children or elderly patients) and juice, water, or milk for swallowing drugs

PREPARATION
- Prepare drugs as indicated.
- Determine if special preparation is needed, such as crushing drug and mixing with food or drink, as appropriate.

- Verify the order.
- Wash your hands.
- Check the label on the drug three times before administering.
- Confirm the patient's identity using two patient identifiers according to facility policy.
- Assess the patient's condition, including level of consciousness, swallowing ability, and vital signs.
- Give the patient his drugs and an appropriate vehicle or liquid to aid swallowing, minimize adverse effects, and promote absorption.
- Stay with the patient until he has swallowed the drug.
- If he seems confused or disoriented, check his mouth to make sure he has swallowed it.

Measuring liquid drugs

To measure liquids, hold the drug cup at eye level. Use your thumb to mark the correct level on the cup. Set the cup down, and read the bottom of the meniscus at eye level to ensure accuracy. If you've poured too much medication into the cup, discard the excess. Don't return it to the bottle.

Here are a few additional tips:
- Hold the container so the drug flows from the side opposite the label to keep it from running down the container and staining or obscuring the label.
- Remove drips from the lip of the bottle first, then from the sides, using a clean, damp paper towel.
- For a liquid measured in drops, use only the dropper supplied with the medication.

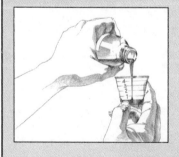

SPECIAL CONSIDERATIONS

- ◆ Make sure you have a written order for every drug given.
- ◆ Verbal orders should be signed by the practitioner within a specified time.
- ◆ Notify the practitioner about drugs withheld.
- ◆ If the patient questions you about his drug or the dosage, check his drug record again. If the drug is correct, reassure him. Make sure you tell him about changes in his drug or dosage.
- ◆ Accurately measure the prescribed dose of any liquid oral drug. (See *Measuring liquid drugs*.)
- ◆ Don't give a drug from a poorly labeled or unlabeled container.
- ◆ Don't attempt to label or reinforce drug labels yourself.
- ◆ Don't give a drug prepared by someone else.
- ◆ Never allow your drug cart or tray out of your sight.
- ◆ Don't return unwrapped or prepared drugs to stock containers. Dispose of them and notify the pharmacy.
- ◆ Disposal of an opioid drug must be cosigned by another nurse, as mandated by law.
- ◆ Administer iron preparations through a straw to avoid damaging or staining the patient's teeth.
- ◆ For those who can't swallow whole pills, use liquids if available, crush if possible, or administer by another route.
- ◆ Enteric-coated or time-release drugs and gelatin capsules shouldn't be crushed.
- ◆ Obtain an order to change the route of administration if necessary.

AGE FACTOR *Oral drugs are relatively easy to give to infants because of their natural sucking instinct and, in infants younger than age 4 months, their undeveloped sense of taste.*

COMPLICATIONS

- ◆ Aspiration (if swallowing ability is impaired)

PATIENT TEACHING

- ◆ Instruct the patient about possible adverse effects, as appropriate.
- ◆ Advise the patient that drugs must be taken as prescribed and review prescribed administration times.
- ◆ For home administration, teach the patient any necessary preparation.

DOCUMENTATION

- ◆ Record the drug given, dose, and date and time.
- ◆ Note the patient's response.
- ◆ Document the patient's refusal and actions taken regarding refusal.
- ◆ Record drug omission or withholding, and give the reason.
- ◆ Document opioids given on the appropriate record.

SELECTED REFERENCES

Ferguson, A. "Administration of Oral Medication," *Nursing Times* 101(45): 24-25, November 2005.

Hohenhaus, S.M. "Giving Liquid Medications to Pediatric Patients," *Journal of Emergency Nursing* 32(1):69-70, February 2006.

Morris, H. "Administering Drugs to Patients with Swallowing Difficulties," *Nursing Times* 101(39):28-30, September-October 2005.

Riordan, S.W., et al. "Introducing Patient-Controlled Oral Analgesia," *Nursing* 34(9):20, September 2004.

Turnbull, G.B. "The Issue of Oral Medications and a Fecal Ostomy," *Ostomy/ Wound Management* 51(3):14, 16, March 2005.

Oronasopharyngeal suction

DESCRIPTION

◆ Oronasopharyngeal suction removes secretions from the pharynx by a suction catheter inserted through the mouth or nostril.
◆ The procedure is used to maintain a patent airway; it helps the patient who can't clear his airway effectively with coughing and expectoration.
◆ The procedure is aseptic and requires sterile equipment; however, clean technique may be used for a tonsil tip suction device.
◆ An alert patient can use a tonsil tip suction device himself to remove secretions.

CONTRAINDICATIONS

◆ Deviated septum
◆ Nasal polyps
◆ Nasal obstruction
◆ Traumatic injury
◆ Epistaxis
◆ Mucosal swelling

EQUIPMENT

Wall suction or portable suction apparatus ◆ collection bottle ◆ connecting tubing ◆ water-soluble lubricant ◆ normal saline solution ◆ disposable sterile container ◆ sterile suction catheter (a #12 or #14 French for an adult, #8 or #10 French for a child, or pediatric feeding tube for an infant) ◆ sterile gloves ◆ clean gloves ◆ goggles ◆ overbed table ◆ waterproof trash bag ◆ soap ◆ water ◆ 70% alcohol for cleaning catheters ◆ nasopharyngeal or oropharyngeal airway (optional for frequent suctioning) ◆ tongue blade, tonsil tip suction device (optional)

PREPARATION

◆ Check for a history of deviated septum, nasal polyps, nasal obstruction, traumatic injury, epistaxis, or mucosal swelling.
◆ Some facilities use a commercially prepared kit that contains a sterile catheter, disposable container, and sterile gloves.

◆ Determine if a practitioner's order is required.
◆ Review the patient's blood gas or oxygen saturation values.
◆ Check the patient's vital signs.
◆ Evaluate the patient's ability to cough and deep breathe.
◆ Gather the suction equipment, and place it on the patient's overbed table or bedside stand.
◆ Position the table to facilitate suctioning.
◆ Attach the collection bottle to the suctioning unit, and attach the connecting tubing to it.
◆ Date and open the bottle of normal saline solution.
◆ Open the waterproof trash bag.

KEY STEPS

◆ Confirm the patient's identity using two patient identifiers according to facility policy.
◆ Explain the procedure to the patient, even if he's unresponsive.
◆ Reassure him throughout the procedure.
◆ Ask which nostril is more patent.
◆ Wash your hands, and put on appropriate personal protective equipment.
◆ Place the patient in semi-Fowler's or high Fowler's position.
◆ Turn on the suction from the wall or portable unit, and set the pressure according to facility policy (usually between 80 and 120 mm Hg).

⚡ WARNING *Suctioning with excessively higher pressure causes trauma to the mucosa.*

◆ Occlude the end of the connecting tubing to check suction pressure.
◆ Using strict sterile technique, open the suction catheter kit or the packages containing the sterile catheter, container, and gloves.
◆ Put on the gloves; consider your dominant hand sterile and your nondominant hand nonsterile.
◆ Using your nondominant hand, pour the normal saline solution into the sterile container.

◆ With your nondominant hand, place a small amount of water-soluble lubricant on the sterile area.
◆ Pick up the catheter with your dominant hand, and attach it to the connecting tubing.
◆ Use your nondominant hand to control the suction valve while your dominant hand manipulates the catheter.
◆ Instruct the patient to cough and breathe slowly and deeply several times before beginning suction. (See *Tips on airway clearance.*)

NASAL INSERTION

◆ Raise the tip of the patient's nose with your nondominant hand to straighten the passageway and facilitate insertion of the catheter.
◆ Without applying suction, gently insert the suction catheter.
◆ Roll the catheter between your fingers to help it advance through the turbinates.
◆ Continue to advance the catheter 5″ to 6″ (12.5 to 15 cm) until you reach the pool of secretions or the patient begins to cough.

ORAL INSERTION

◆ Without applying suction, gently insert the catheter into the patient's mouth.
◆ Advance it 3″ to 4″ (7.5 to 10 cm) along the side of the patient's mouth until you reach the pool of secretions or the patient begins to cough.
◆ Suction both sides of the patient's mouth and pharyngeal area.

REMOVING SECRETIONS

◆ Withdraw the catheter with a continuous rotating motion to minimize invagination of the mucosa into the catheter's tip and side ports.
◆ Apply suction for only 10 to 15 seconds at a time to minimize tissue trauma.
◆ Between passes, wrap the catheter around your dominant hand to prevent contamination.
◆ Clear the lumen of the catheter by dipping it in normal saline solution and applying suction.

- Repeat the procedure until respirations are quiet or secretions are minimal.
- After completing suctioning, pull your sterile glove off over the coiled catheter and discard it and the nonsterile glove along with the container of water.
- Flush the connecting tubing with normal saline solution, replace the used items so they're ready for the next suctioning, and wash your hands.

Tips on airway clearance

Deep breathing and coughing are vital for removing secretions from the lungs. Other techniques used to help clear the airways include diaphragmatic breathing and forced expiration.

DIAPHRAGMATIC BREATHING

Place patient in supine position with his head elevated 15 to 20 degrees on a pillow.

Tell him to place one hand on his abdomen and then inhale so that he can feel his abdomen rise. Explain that this is known as "breathing with the diaphragm."

Tell him to exhale slowly, preferably through pursed lips, while letting his abdomen collapse. Explain that this action decreases his respiratory rate and increases his tidal volume. Suggest that he perform this exercise for 30 minutes several times a day. To enhance the effectiveness of exercise, he may manually compress the lower costal margins, perform straight-leg lifts, and coordinate the breathing technique with a physical activity such as walking.

FORCED EXPIRATION

Explain to the patient that forced expiration helps clear secretions while causing less traumatic injury than coughing.

Tell the patient to forcefully expire without closing his glottis, starting with a middle to low lung volume. Tell him to follow this expiration with a period of diaphragmatic breathing and relaxation. Inform him that if his secretions are in the central airways, he may have to use a more forceful expiration or a cough to clear them.

SPECIAL CONSIDERATIONS

- Be sure to observe pulse oximetry during suctioning, if available.
- If the patient has no history of nasal problems, alternate suctioning between nostrils to minimize injury.
- If repeated oronasopharyngeal suctioning is required, the use of a nasopharyngeal or oropharyngeal airway will help with catheter insertion, reduce traumatic injury, and promote a patent airway.
- To facilitate catheter insertion for oropharyngeal suctioning, depress the patient's tongue with a tongue blade.
- If the patient has excessive oral secretions, consider using a tonsil tip catheter.
- Let the patient rest after suctioning while you continue to observe him.

COMPLICATIONS

- Increased dyspnea
- Hypoxia
- Bloody aspirate
- Nasal trauma

PATIENT TEACHING

- For suctioning at home, instruct the patient to use clean technique rather than sterile technique.
- Instruct the patient that properly cleaned catheters can be reused.
- Instruct the patient to wash catheters in soapy water, then boil them for 10 minutes or soak them in 70% alcohol for 3 to 5 minutes.
- Tell the patient to rinse with normal saline solution or tap water.

DOCUMENTATION

- Record the date, time, reason for suctioning, and technique used.
- Note the amount, color, consistency, and odor of the secretions.
- Document the patient's respiratory status before and after the procedure.
- Record complications and nursing actions taken.
- Note the patient's tolerance of the procedure.

SELECTED REFERENCES

Castledine, G. "Nurse Negligence in Oral/Nasal Suctioning Caused Patients Distress and Put Them at Risk," *British Journal of Nursing* 15(2):67, January-February 2006.

Gungor, S., et al. "Oronasopharyngeal Suction Versus No Suction in Normal, Term and Vaginally Born Infants: A Prospective Randomised Controlled Trial," *Australian and New Zealand Journal of Obstetrics and Gynaecology* 45(5):453-56, October 2005.

Vain, N.E., et al. "Oropharyngeal and Nasopharyngeal Suctioning of Meconium-Stained Neonates before Delivery of their Shoulders: Multicentre, Randomised Controlled Trial," *Lancet* 364(9434):597-602, August 2004.

Oropharyngeal airway insertion and care

OVERVIEW

DESCRIPTION
- Intended for short-term use, an oropharyngeal airway is used to maintain a patient's airway.
- It conforms to the curvature of the palate, removing obstruction, allowing air to pass around and through the tube, and facilitating oropharyngeal suctioning.
- It may be left in place longer as an airway adjunct to prevent an orally intubated patient from biting the endotracheal tube.

CONTRAINDICATIONS
- Conscious patient

EQUIPMENT

INSERTING
Oral airway of appropriate size ◆ tongue blade ◆ padded tongue blade ◆ gloves ◆ suction equipment, handheld resuscitation bag or oxygen-powered breathing device (optional)

CLEANING
Hydrogen peroxide ◆ water basin ◆ pipe cleaner (optional)

REFLEX TESTING
Cotton-tipped applicator

PREPARATION
- Select an appropriate sized airway: small (size 1 or 2) for an infant or child, medium (size 4 or 5) for an average adult, and large (size 6) for a large adult.
- Confirm the correct size. The airway curve should reach to the angle of the jaw.

KEY STEPS

- Confirm the patient's identity using two patient identifiers according to facility policy.
- Explain the procedure to the patient even if he appears not to be alert.
- Provide privacy.
- Put on gloves.
- Remove dentures if any.
- Suction the patient if necessary.
- Place the patient in a supine position with his neck hyperextended, unless contraindicated.
- Insert the airway using either the cross-finger or the tongue-blade technique. (See *Inserting an oral airway.*)
- Auscultate the patient's lungs to ensure adequate ventilation.
- After insertion, position the patient on his side to prevent aspiration.
- Perform mouth care every 2 to 4 hours and as needed.
- To remove, hold the patient's jaws open with a padded tongue blade, and remove the airway.
- Place the airway in a basin, and rinse it with hydrogen peroxide and then water. If secretions remain, use a pipe cleaner to remove them.
- While the airway is removed, examine the patient's mouth for tissue irritation or ulceration.
- Complete standard mouth care and reinsert the airway.
- Frequently check the airway's position.
- Remove the airway when the patient regains consciousness, pulling it outward and downward.
- Test the patient's cough and gag reflexes: for gag reflex, use a cotton-tipped applicator to touch both sides of the posterior pharynx.
- For cough reflex, gently touch the posterior oropharynx with the cotton-tipped applicator.

SPECIAL CONSIDERATIONS

◆ To prevent injury, make sure that the patient's lips and tongue aren't between his teeth and the airway.
◆ If respirations are absent or inadequate, initiate artificial positive-pressure ventilation by using a mouth-to-mask technique, a handheld resuscitation bag, or an oxygen-powered breathing device.
◆ In an unconscious patient, the tongue usually obstructs the posterior pharynx.
◆ Clear breath sounds on auscultation indicate that the airway is the proper size and in the correct position.
◆ Avoid taping the airway in place to reduce the risk of aspiration.
◆ When the patient begins to gag or cough, remove the airway.

COMPLICATIONS

◆ Tooth damage or loss, tissue damage, or bleeding resulting from insertion
◆ Complete airway obstruction if the airway is too long
◆ Upper airway obstruction due to improper insertion

PATIENT TEACHING

◆ Explain to the patient's family members the need for oropharyngeal airway insertion.

Inserting an oral airway

As shown below, hyperextend the patient's head (unless contraindicated); then use either the cross-finger or tongue-blade insertion method.

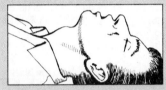

To insert an oral airway using the cross-finger method, place your thumb on the patient's lower teeth and your index finger on his upper teeth. Open his mouth by pushing his teeth apart (as shown below).

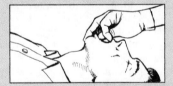

Insert the airway upside down to avoid pushing the tongue toward the pharynx. Slide it over the tongue toward the back of the mouth. Rotate the airway as it approaches the posterior wall of the pharynx so that it points downward (as shown below).

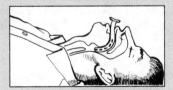

To use the tongue-blade technique, open the patient's mouth, and depress his tongue with the blade. Guide the airway over the back of the tongue as you did for the cross-finger technique.

DOCUMENTATION

◆ Record the date and time of airway insertion.
◆ Note the size of the airway.
◆ Document removal and cleaning of the airway.
◆ Record the condition of mucous membranes and when oral care is performed.
◆ Note suctioning.
◆ Document adverse reactions and nursing actions taken.
◆ Record the patient's tolerance of procedure.

SELECTED REFERENCES

Hagberg, C., et al. "An Evaluation of the Insertion and Function of a New Supraglottic Airway Device, the King LT, During Spontaneous Ventilation," *Anesthesia and Analgesia* 102(2):621-25, February 2006.
Matioc, A.A., and Olson, J. "Use of the Laryngeal Tube in Two Unexpected Difficult Airway Situations: Lingual Tonsillar Hyperplasia and Morbid Obesity," *Canadian Journal of Anaesthesia* 51(10):1018-21, December 2004.
Tong, J.L., and Smith, J.E. "Cardiovascular Changes Following Insertion of Oropharyngeal and Nasopharyngeal Airways," *British Journal of Anaesthesia* 93(3):339-42, September 2004.

Oropharyngeal handheld inhalers

DESCRIPTION

- These devices include the metered-dose inhaler or nebulizer, the turbo-inhaler, and the nasal inhaler.
- Inhalers use pressurized air to produce a mist containing tiny droplets of the drug.
- The device delivers topical drugs to the respiratory tract, traveling deep into the lungs and producing local and systemic effects.
- The mucosal lining of the respiratory tract absorbs the inhalant almost immediately.

CONTRAINDICATIONS

- Inability to form an airtight seal around the device
- Lack of coordination or clear vision needed to assemble the turbo-inhaler
- Use of specific inhalant drugs
- Use of bronchodilators, if patient has tachycardia or a history of cardiac arrhythmias associated with tachycardia

EQUIPMENT

Patient's drug record and chart ◆ metered-dose inhaler ◆ turbo-inhaler or nasal inhaler ◆ prescribed drug ◆ normal saline solution (or other appropriate solution) for gargling ◆ emesis basin (optional)

KEY STEPS

- Verify the practitioner's order.
- Confirm the patient's identity using two patient identifiers according to facility policy.
- Wash your hands.
- Check the label on the inhaler against the drug record.
- Verify the expiration date.
- Explain the procedure to the patient.

USING A METERED-DOSE INHALER

- Shake the inhaler bottle to mix the drug and aerosol propellant.
- Remove the mouthpiece and cap.
- Some metered-dose inhalers have a spacer built into the inhaler. Pull the spacer away from the section holding the drug canister until it clicks into place.
- Insert the metal stem on the bottle into the small hole on the flattened portion of the mouthpiece, and turn the bottle upside down.
- Have the patient exhale, place the mouthpiece in his mouth, and close his lips around it.
- As you firmly push the bottle down against the mouthpiece, ask the patient to inhale slowly until his lungs feel full. This draws the drug into his lungs.
- Compress the bottle against the mouthpiece once.
- Remove the mouthpiece from the patient's mouth.
- Tell the patient to hold his breath for several seconds.
- Have the patient exhale slowly through pursed lips.
- Offer normal saline solution (or other appropriate solution) to gargle for removing drug from the mouth and the back of the throat.
- Provide an emesis basin if the patient needs one.
- Rinse the mouthpiece thoroughly with warm water.

USING A TURBO-INHALER

- Hold the mouthpiece in one hand. With the other hand, slide the sleeve away from the mouthpiece as far as possible.
- Unscrew the tip of the mouthpiece by turning it counterclockwise.
- Firmly press the colored portion of the drug capsule into the propeller stem of the mouthpiece.
- Screw the inhaler together again securely.
- Holding the inhaler with the mouthpiece at the bottom, slide the sleeve all the way down, then up again to puncture the capsule and release the drug. Do this only once.
- Have the patient exhale and tilt his head back.
- Tell the patient to place the mouthpiece in his mouth, close his lips around it, and quickly inhale.
- Tell the patient to hold his breath for several seconds.
- Instruct the patient not to exhale through the mouthpiece.
- Remove the inhaler from his mouth, and tell him to exhale as much air as possible.
- Repeat the procedure until all of the drug is inhaled.
- Offer normal saline solution (or other solution) to gargle.
- Provide an emesis basin if patient needs one.
- Discard the empty drug capsule.
- Place the inhaler in its can, and secure the lid.
- Rinse the inhaler with warm water at least once a week.

USING A NASAL INHALER

- Have the patient blow his nose to clear his nostrils.
- Shake the drug cartridge; then insert it in the adapter.
- Before inserting a refill cartridge, remove the protective cap from the adapter tip.
- Hold the inhaler with your index finger on top of the cartridge and your thumb under the nasal adapter. The adapter tip should point toward the patient.
- Have the patient tilt his head back.

- Tell the patient to place the adapter tip into one nostril while closing the other with his finger.
- Tell the patient to inhale gently as he presses the adapter and the cartridge together firmly to release a measured dose of drug.
- Follow the manufacturer's instructions; some drugs shouldn't be inhaled during administration.
- Tell the patient to remove the inhaler and exhale through his mouth.
- Shake the inhaler.
- Have the patient repeat the procedure in the other nostril.
- Offer normal saline solution (or other solution) to gargle.
- Remove the drug cartridge from the nasal inhaler.
- Wash the nasal adapter in lukewarm water.
- Let the adapter dry thoroughly before reinserting the cartridge.

SPECIAL CONSIDERATIONS

- The lungs retain about 10% of the inhalant; most of the remainder is exhaled.
- When using a turbo-inhaler or a nasal inhaler, make sure the pressurized cartridge isn't punctured or incinerated.
- Store the drug cartridge below 120° F (48.9° C).
- When using a turbo-inhaler, keep the drug capsules wrapped until needed to prevent deterioration.
- Spacer inhalers may be recommended for children and those having difficulty with coordination.
- A spacer attachment is an extension to the inhaler's mouthpiece.
- It provides more dead-air space for mixing the drug.
- Some inhalers have built-in spacers.

COMPLICATIONS
- Adverse reaction to medication

PATIENT TEACHING

- Teach the patient how to use the inhaler so treatments can continue after discharge.
- Explain that overdosage (which is common) can cause drug to lose its effectiveness.
- Tell the patient to record the date and time of each inhalation and his response to treatment.
- Inform the patient of possible adverse reactions.
- If more than one inhalation is ordered, advise the patient to wait at least 2 minutes before repeating the procedure.
- If the patient is also using a steroid inhaler, instruct him to use the bronchodilator first, then wait 5 minutes before using the steroid. This allows the bronchodilator to open the air passages for maximum effectiveness.

DOCUMENTATION

- Record the name of the inhalant and dose given.
- Record the date and time given.
- Note significant change in heart rate.
- Document patient's response to treatment.

SELECTED REFERENCES
Bower, L.M. "Is Your Patient's Metered-Dose Inhaler Technique Up to Snuff?" *Nursing* 35(8):50-51, August 2005.

Capriotti, T. "Changes in Inhaler Devices for Asthma and COPD," *Medsurg Nursing* 14(3):185-94, June 2005.

Flower, J., and Saewyc, E.M. "Assessing the Capability of School-Age Children With Asthma to Safely Self-Carry an Inhaler," *Journal of School Nursing* 21(5):283-92, October 2005.

Joyce, M., et al. "The Use of Nebulized Opioids in the Management of Dyspnea: Evidence Synthesis," *Oncology Nursing Forum* 31(3):551-61, May 2004.

Meadows-Oliver, M., and Banasiak, N.C. "Asthma Medication Delivery Devices," *Journal of Pediatric Health Care* 19(2): 121-23, March-April 2005.

Oxygen administration

DESCRIPTION

- Oxygen administration is used for hypoxemia resulting from respiratory or cardiac emergency or increase in metabolic function.
- In a respiratory emergency, the procedure enables reduction of ventilatory effort by boosting alveolar oxygen levels.
- In a cardiac emergency, it helps meet increased myocardial workload as the heart tries to compensate for hypoxemia.
- When metabolic demand is high, oxygen administration supplies the body with enough oxygen to meet cellular needs.
- It's useful in the patient with reduced blood oxygen-carrying capacity (such as with carbon monoxide poisoning or sickle cell crisis).
- The procedure's effectiveness is determined by arterial blood gas (ABG) analysis, oximetry monitoring, and clinical examinations.
- Disease, physical condition, and age help determine the most appropriate means of administration.
- Typically, a practitioner's order is needed for oxygen administration except in emergency situations. Check facility policy.

CONTRAINDICATIONS

- Decreased respiratory drive in patients with chronic obstructive pulmonary disease.

Oxygen source (wall unit, cylinder, liquid tank, or concentrator) ◆ flowmeter ◆ adapter, if using a wall unit; pressure-reduction gauge, if using a cylinder ◆ sterile humidity bottle and adapters ◆ sterile distilled water ◆ OXYGEN PRECAUTION sign ◆ appropriate oxygen delivery system (nasal cannula, simple mask, partial rebreather mask or non-rebreather mask — for low-flow and variable oxygen concentrations, Venturi mask, aerosol mask, endotracheal tube, tracheostomy collar, tent or oxygen hood for high-flow and specific oxygen concentrations) ◆ small-diameter and large-diameter connection tubing ◆ flashlight (for nasal cannula) ◆ water-soluble lubricant ◆ gauze pads ◆ tape (for oxygen masks) ◆ jet adapter for Venturi mask (if adding humidity) ◆ oxygen analyzer (optional)

PREPARATION

- A respiratory therapist usually sets up, maintains, and manages equipment, but you should have a working knowledge of the oxygen system being used.
- Check the oxygen outlet port to verify flow.
- Pinch the tubing near the prongs to ensure that an audible alarm will sound if the oxygen flow stops.

- Verify the order.
- Confirm the patient's identity using two patient identifiers according to facility policy.
- Assess the patient's condition; verify an open airway.
- Explain the procedure to the patient.
- Perform a safety check of the patient's room to make sure it's safe for oxygen use.

AGE FACTOR *For a child in an oxygen tent, remove all toys that may produce a spark. Oxygen supports combustion, and the smallest spark can cause a fire.*

- Place an OXYGEN PRECAUTION sign over the patient's bed and on the door to his room.
- Fit the oxygen delivery device to the patient.
- Monitor his response to oxygen therapy.
- Check his ABG values to make adjustments to oxygen concentrations.
- When stable, use pulse oximetry instead.
- Check the patient frequently for signs of hypoxia.
- Observe the patient's skin integrity to prevent skin breakdown.
- Wipe moisture from the patient's face and mask.
- Watch for signs of oxygen toxicity.
- Remind the patient to cough and deep breathe frequently.

SPECIAL CONSIDERATIONS

⚡ **WARNING** *Don't administer oxygen by nasal cannula at more than 2 L/minute to a patient with chronic lung disease, unless ordered. Long-term oxygen therapy (12 to 17 hours daily) may help patients with chronic lung disease sleep better, survive longer, and have reduced incidence of pulmonary hypertension.*

◆ Monitor or measure ABG and pulse oximetry values 20 to 30 minutes after adjusting the oxygen flow.
◆ Monitor the patient for adverse response to a change in oxygen flow.

COMPLICATIONS

◆ Disrupted skin integrity from ill-fitting oxygen delivery device

PATIENT TEACHING

◆ Explain different types of oxygen and available services. (See *Types of home oxygen therapy*.)
◆ If the patient is receiving transtracheal oxygen therapy, teach him how to clean and care for the catheter.
◆ Advise the patient to keep the skin surrounding the insertion site clean and dry to prevent infection.
◆ Evaluate the patient and family's ability and motivation to administer oxygen therapy at home.
◆ Review rationale and safety issues with the patient and family.
◆ Teach the patient and his family proper use and care of equipment and supplies.
◆ Check to see if home oxygen is covered by patient's insurance. If it isn't, identify criteria for coverage.

DOCUMENTATION

◆ Record the date and time of oxygen administration.
◆ Record ABG results and pulse oximetry readings.
◆ Note the type of delivery device.
◆ Document oxygen flow rate.
◆ Note vital signs, skin color, respiratory effort, and lung sounds.
◆ Record subjective patient response before and after initiation of therapy.
◆ Document patient or family teaching.

SELECTED REFERENCES

Considine, J. "The Reliability of Clinical Indicators of Oxygenation: A Literature Review," *Contemporary Nurse* 18(3): 258-67, April-June 2005.

Demir, F., and Dramali, A. "Requirement for 100% Oxygen Before and After Closed Suction," *Journal of Advanced Nursing* 51(3):245-51, August 2005.

Edwards, M. "Caring for Patients With COPD on Long-Term Oxygen Therapy," *British Journal of Community Nursing* 10(9):404, 406, 408-410, September 2005.

Higgins, D. "Oxygen Therapy," *Nursing Times* 101(4):30-31, January 2005.

Kbar, F.A., and Campbell, I.A. "Oxygen Therapy in Hospitalized Patients: The Impact of Local Guidelines," *Journal of Evaluation in Clinical Practice* 12(1): 31-36, February 2006.

Mathews, P.J., et al. "The Latest in Respiratory Care," *Nursing Management* (suppl):18, 20-21, 2005.

Types of home oxygen therapy

Oxygen therapy can be administered at home using an oxygen tank, an oxygen concentrator, or liquid oxygen.

OXYGEN TANK

An oxygen tank is commonly used for patients who need oxygen on a standby basis or who need a ventilator at home. Disadvantages include its cumbersome design and the need for frequent refills. Because oxygen is stored under high pressure, the oxygen tank also poses a potential explosion hazard.

OXYGEN CONCENTRATOR

The oxygen concentrator, which extracts oxygen molecules from room air, can be used for low oxygen flow (less than 4 L/minute) and doesn't need to be refilled. Its main disadvantage is that it runs on electricity and won't function during a power failure.

LIQUID OXYGEN

Liquid oxygen is commonly used by patients who are oxygen-dependent but still mobile. The liquid oxygen system includes a large liquid reservoir for home use. When the patient wants to leave the house, he fills a portable unit worn over the shoulder; this supplies oxygen for up to 3 hours, depending on the liter flow.

Pacemaker (permanent) insertion and care

DESCRIPTION

- A pacemaker is a self-contained heart pacing device implanted in a pocket beneath the patient's skin, designed to operate 3 to 8 years, depending on usage.
- The device is inserted in an operating room, cardiac catheterization laboratory, or electrophysiology laboratory.
- Nursing responsibilities involve monitoring cardiac rhythm and the insertion site.
- It's used in patients with myocardial infarction, persistent bradyarrhythmia, complete heart block or slow ventricular rates, Stokes-Adams syndrome, Wolff-Parkinson-White syndrome, and sick sinus syndrome.
- A biventricular pacemaker may benefit the patient with heart failure.
- Pacemaker functions in the demand mode, which allows the patient's heart to beat on its own but prevents it from falling below a preset level.
- Pacing electrodes can be placed in the atria, ventricles, or in both chambers; most common pacing codes are VVI for single-chamber pacing and DDD for dual-chamber pacing. (See *Understanding pacemaker codes.*)

CONTRAINDICATIONS

- None known

EQUIPMENT

Sphygmomanometer ◆ stethoscope ◆ electrocardiogram (ECG) monitor and strip-chart recorder ◆ sterile dressing tray ◆ povidone-iodine ointment ◆ hair clippers ◆ sterile gauze dressing ◆ hypoallergenic tape ◆ sedatives ◆ alcohol pads ◆ emergency resuscitation equipment ◆ sterile gown and mask ◆ I.V. line for emergency medications (optional)

KEY STEPS

- Confirm the patient's identity using two patient identifiers according to facility policy.
- Explain the procedure to the patient.
- Provide and review literature from the manufacturer or the American Heart Association.
- Emphasize to the patient that the pacemaker augments his natural heart rate.
- Obtain informed consent.
- Ask the patient if he's allergic to anesthetics or iodine.

PREOPERATIVE CARE
Pacemaker insertion

- Clip hair on the patient's chest from the axilla to the midline and from the clavicle to the nipple line on the side selected by the practitioner.
- Establish an I.V. line and infuse fluids at a keep-vein-open rate.
- Obtain baseline vital signs and a baseline ECG.
- Provide sedation as ordered.

In operating room

- Put on a gown and mask.
- Place the patient on a cardiac monitor; run a baseline rhythm strip. Check for adequate paper.
- In transvenous placement, the pacing leads are guided by a fluoroscope and passed through the cephalic or external jugular vein until they reach the right ventricle.
- The leads are attached to the pulse generator, inserted into the chest wall, and sutured closed.

POSTOPERATIVE CARE

- Monitor the patient's cardiac rhythm.
- Monitor the I.V. fluid flow rate; the I.V. line is usually kept in place for 24 to 48 hours postoperatively to allow for possible emergency treatment of arrhythmias.

Understanding pacemaker codes

A permanent pacemaker uses a three or five-letter programming code. The first letter represents the chamber that's paced. The second represents the chamber that's sensed. The third represents how the pulse generator responds. The fourth denotes the pacemaker's programmability. The fifth denotes the pacemaker's response to a tachyarrhythmia.

FIRST LETTER	SECOND LETTER	THIRD LETTER	FOURTH LETTER	FIFTH LETTER
A = atrium V = ventricle D = dual (both chambers) O = not applicable	A = atrium V = ventricle D = dual (both chambers) O = not applicable	I = inhibited T = triggered D = dual (inhibited and triggered) O = not applicable	P = basic functions programmable M = multiprogrammable parameters C = communicating functions such as telemetry R = rate responsiveness O = none	P = pacing ability S = shock D = dual ability to shock and pace O = none

EXAMPLES OF TWO COMMON PROGRAMMING CODES

DDD

Pace: Atrium and ventricle
Sense: Atrium and ventricle
Response: Inhibited and triggered
This is the most common dual-chamber pacemaker setting, allowing the heart's intrinsic pacemaker cells to function whenever possible.

VVI

Pace: Ventricle
Sense: Ventricle
Response: Inhibited
This is a single-chamber pacemaker which will pace the ventricle only when an intrinsic contraction doesn't occur.

- Check the dressing for signs of bleeding and infection.
- Explain movement restrictions for the first 24 to 48 hours.
- Prophylactic antibiotics may be ordered for up to 7 days after implantation.
- Change the dressing and apply povidone-iodine ointment at least once every 24 to 48 hours.
- If the dressing becomes soiled or the site is exposed to air, change the dressing immediately.
- Check vital signs and level of consciousness (LOC) every 15 minutes for the first hour, every hour for the next 4 hours, every 4 hours for the next 48 hours, and then once every shift.

AGE FACTOR *Confused, elderly patients with second-degree heart block won't show immediate improvement in LOC.*

WARNING *Report to the practitioner signs and symptoms of a perforated ventricle, with resultant cardiac tamponade: persistent hiccups, distant heart sounds, pulsus paradoxus, hypotension with narrow pulse pressure, increased venous pressure, cyanosis, jugular vein distention, decreased urine output, restlessness, or complaints of fullness in the chest.*

SPECIAL CONSIDERATIONS

- A biventricular pacemaker has three leads instead of one or two; one lead is placed in the right atrium and the other two are placed in each of the ventricles, improving pumping efficiency by allowing both ventricles to beat in synchrony.
- Provide the patient with an identification card that lists the pacemaker type and manufacturer, serial number, pacemaker rate setting, date implanted, and practitioner's name.
- Watch for signs of pacemaker malfunction such as loss of capture.

COMPLICATIONS
- Infection
- Lead displacement
- Perforated ventricle
- Cardiac tamponade
- Lead fracture and disconnection
- Pacemaker malfunction

PATIENT TEACHING

- Tell the patient to inform his practitioners, dentist, and other health care personnel that he has a pacemaker.
- Advise the patient to use a cellular phone on the side opposite the pacemaker.
- Caution the patient to move away from electrical equipment if he experiences light-headedness or dizziness. Moving away should restore normal pacemaker function.
- Teach the patient to clean the pacemaker site gently with soap and water when taking a shower or a bath. Tell him to leave the incision exposed to the air.
- Instruct the patient to inspect the skin around the incision. Advise him that a slight bulge is normal, but to call the practitioner if he feels discomfort or notices swelling, redness, discharge, or other problems.
- Teach the patient how to check his pulse for 1 minute on the side of his neck, inside his elbow, or on the thumb side of his wrist. The pulse rate should be the same as his pacemaker rate or faster. Instruct him to contact the practitioner if he thinks his heart is beating too fast or too slow.
- Advise the patient to take medications, including those for pain, as prescribed.
- Advise the patient to notify the practitioner if he experiences signs of pacemaker failure, such as palpitations, a fast heart rate, a slow heart rate (5 to 10 beats less than the pacemaker's setting), dizziness, fainting, shortness of breath, swollen ankles or feet, anxiety, forgetfulness, or confusion.
- Explain to the patient that the pacemaker will need to be checked on a regular basis by the cardiologist and that can usually be accomplished using a telephone device.

DOCUMENTATION

- Record the type, serial number, and manufacturer of the pacemaker.
- Document the pacing rate.
- Record the date of implantation.
- Note the practitioner's name.
- Document whether the pacemaker successfully treated the arrhythmias.
- Note the condition of the incision site.
- Document the cardiac rhythm.

SELECTED REFERENCES
Arslan, S., et al. "Images in Cardiology. Permanent Pacemaker Lead Thrombosis Leading to Recurrent Pulmonary Embolism," *Heart* 92(5):597, May 2006.

Erdogan, H.B., et al. "Risk Factors for Requirement of Permanent Pacemaker Implantation after Aortic Valve Replacement," *Journal of Cardiac Surgery* 21(3):211-15, May-June 2006.

Hsieh, M.J., et al. "Permanent Pacing Using a Coronary Sinus Lead in a Patient with Univentricular Physiology: An Extended Application of Biventricular Pacing Technology," *Europace* 8(2): 147-50, February 2006.

Taylor, B.A. "Cutting Surgical-Site Infection Rates for Pacemakers and ICDs," *Nursing* 36(3):18-19, March 2006.

Thompson, C., et al. "Can Pacemakers Cause Life-Threatening Arrhythmias?" *Progress in Cardiovascular Nursing* 20(4):184-85, Fall 2005.

Pacemaker (temporary) insertion and care

OVERVIEW

DESCRIPTION

- The device is usually inserted in an emergency to correct conduction disturbances; it may help diagnose conduction abnormalities.
- It has an external, battery-powered pulse generator and lead or electrode system.
- There are four types of temporary pacemakers: transcutaneous, transvenous, transthoracic (rare), and epicardial.
- In a life-threatening situation, a transcutaneous pacemaker is the best choice; it's quick and effective, but used only until transvenous pacing can be done.
- It works by sending an electrical impulse from the pulse generator to the patient's heart by way of two electrodes, placed on the front and back of the patient's chest.
- A transvenous pacemaker is more comfortable and reliable than a transcutaneous pacemaker.
- Transvenous pacing involves threading an electrode catheter through a vein into the patient's right ventricle. The electrode then attaches to an external pulse generator, providing a direct electrical stimulus to the endocardium.
- A transthoracic pacemaker is used as an elective surgical procedure or as an emergency measure during cardiopulmonary resuscitation (CPR).
- Epicardial pacing involves insertion of electrodes through epicardium of the right ventricle and atrium during cardiac surgery; electrodes remain externally available for temporary pacing.

CONTRAINDICATIONS

- Pulseless electrical activity
- Severe hypothermia
- Ventricular fibrillation

EQUIPMENT

TRANSCUTANEOUS PACING

Transcutaneous pacing generator ◆ transcutaneous pacing electrodes ◆ cardiac monitor

OTHER TYPES OF TEMPORARY PACING

Temporary pacemaker ◆ generator with new battery ◆ guide wire or introducer ◆ electrode catheter ◆ sterile gloves ◆ sterile dressings ◆ adhesive tape ◆ povidone-iodine solution ◆ nonconducting tape or rubber surgical glove ◆ emergency cardiac drugs ◆ intubation equipment ◆ defibrillator ◆ monitor with strip-chart recorder ◆ equipment to start a peripheral I.V. line ◆ if appropriate, I.V. fluids ◆ sedative ◆ restraints ◆ elastic bandage or gauze strips (optional)

TRANSVENOUS PACING

All equipment listed for temporary pacing ◆ bridging cable ◆ introducer tray or venous cutdown tray ◆ sterile gowns ◆ linen-saver pad ◆ soap ◆ pads ◆ vial of 1% lidocaine ◆ 5-ml syringe ◆ fenestrated drape ◆ sutures ◆ receptacle for infectious waste

TRANSTHORACIC PACING

All equipment listed for temporary pacemaker ◆ transthoracic or cardiac needle

EPICARDIAL PACING

All equipment listed for temporary pacemakers ◆ atrial epicardial wires ◆ ventricular epicardial wires ◆ sterile rubber finger cot ◆ sterile dressing materials (if wires won't be connected to pulse generator)

KEY STEPS

TRANSCUTANEOUS PACING

- Clip rather than shave the hair over areas of electrode placement.
- Attach monitoring electrodes to the patient in lead I, II, or III position, even if the patient is already on telemetry monitoring.
- If you select the lead II position, adjust the LL electrode placement to accommodate the anterior pacing electrode and the patient's anatomy.
- Plug the patient cable into the electrocardiogram (ECG) input connection on the front of the pacing generator.
- Set the selector switch to the MONITOR ON position. You should see the ECG waveform on the monitor.
- Adjust the R-wave beeper volume and press the ALARM ON button.
- Set the alarm for 10 to 20 beats lower and 20 to 30 beats higher than the intrinsic rate.
- Press the START/STOP button for a printout of the waveform.
- Make sure the patient's skin is clean and dry.
- Remove the protective strip from the posterior electrode (marked "Back"); apply the electrode on the left side of the back below the scapula and left of the spine.
- The anterior pacing electrode (marked "Front") has two protective strips — one covering the jellied area and one covering the outer rim. Expose the jellied area and apply it to the skin in the anterior position — to the left side of the precordium in the usual V_2 to V_5 position. (See *Proper electrode placement*.)
- Adjust the electrode to get the best waveform, expose the electrode's outer rim, and firmly press it to the skin.
- After making sure the energy output in milliamperes (mA) is on 0, connect the electrode cable to the monitor output cable.
- Check the waveform, looking for a tall QRS complex in lead II.
- Turn the selector switch to PACER ON.

- Tell the patient that he may feel a thumping or twitching sensation.
- Offer medication if he can't tolerate the discomfort.
- Set the rate dial to 10 to 20 beats higher than the patient's intrinsic rhythm.
- Look for pacer artifact or spikes, which will appear as you increase the rate.
- If the patient doesn't have an intrinsic rhythm, set the rate at 60.
- Slowly increase the amount of energy delivered to the heart by adjusting the "Output mA" dial. Do this until capture is achieved — you'll see a pacer spike followed by a widened QRS complex that resembles a premature ventricular contraction. This is the pacing threshold.
- To ensure consistent capture, increase output by 10%.
- With full capture, the patient's heart rate should be approximately the same as the pacemaker rate set on the machine. The usual pacing threshold is between 40 and 80 mA.

TRANSVENOUS PACING
- Check the patient's history for hypersensitivity to local anesthetics.

- Attach the cardiac monitor to the patient, and obtain baseline assessment of vital signs, skin color, level of consciousness (LOC), heart rate and rhythm, and emotional state.
- Insert a peripheral I.V. catheter if one isn't present.
- Infuse normal saline at a keep-vein-open rate.
- Put a new battery into the external pacemaker generator and test it.
- Connect the bridging cable to the generator, and align the positive and negative poles.
- Place the patient in the supine position.
- Clip the hair around the insertion site.
- Open the supply tray while maintaining a sterile field.
- Using sterile technique, clean the insertion site with antimicrobial soap; wipe the area with povidone-iodine solution.
- Cover the insertion site with a fenestrated drape.
- Wear a protective apron if fluoroscopy is used during placement of leadwires.
- Provide the practitioner with the local anesthetic.

- An electrode catheter will be inserted and advanced with a guide wire or an introducer through the brachial, femoral, subclavian, or jugular vein.
- Watch for large P waves and small QRS complexes when the electrode catheter reaches the right atrium.
- Watch for P waves becoming smaller while QRS complexes enlarge as the catheter reaches the right ventricle.
- Watch for elevated ST segments and premature ventricular contractions when the catheter touches the right ventricular endocardium.
- When in the right ventricle, the electrode catheter sends an impulse to the myocardium, causing depolarization.
- Continuously monitor the patient's cardiac status and treat arrhythmias.
- Assess the patient for jaw pain and earache, which indicate the electrode catheter has moved into the neck instead of the superior vena cava.
- After the electrode catheter is in place, attach the catheter leads to the bridging cable, lining up the positive and negative poles.
- Set the pacemaker as ordered.
- The catheter will be sutured to the insertion site.
- Put on sterile gloves, and apply a sterile dressing to the site.
- Label the dressing with the date and time of application.

TRANSTHORACIC PACING
- Clean the skin to the left of the xiphoid process with povidone-iodine solution. Work quickly because CPR must be interrupted for the procedure.
- A transthoracic needle is inserted through the patient's chest wall to the left of the xiphoid process into the right ventricle.
- The needle is followed with the electrode catheter.
- Connect the electrode catheter to the generator, lining up the positive and negative poles.
- Watch the cardiac monitor for signs of ventricular pacing and capture.
- Apply a sterile $4'' \times 4''$ gauze dressing to the site, and tape it securely.

(continued)

Proper electrode placement

Place the two pacing electrodes for a noninvasive temporary pacemaker at heart level on the patient's chest and back (as shown at right). This placement ensures that the electrical stimulus must travel only a short distance to the heart.

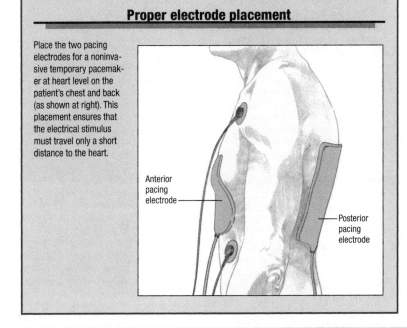

Anterior pacing electrode

Posterior pacing electrode

- Label the dressing with the date and time of application.
- Check the patient's peripheral pulses and vital signs to assess cardiac output. Continue CPR if pulses are absent.
- If the patient has a palpable pulse, assess the patient's vital signs, ECG, and LOC.

EPICARDIAL PACING
- Inform the patient that epicardial pacemaker wires may be placed during cardiac surgery.
- During cardiac surgery, atrial, ventricular, or both types of wires are hooked into the epicardium before the end of surgery.
- If indicated, connect the electrode catheter to the generator, lining up the positive and negative poles.
- Set the pacemaker as ordered.
- If the wires won't be connected to an external pulse generator, place them in a sterile rubber finger cot.
- Cover both the wires and the insertion site with a sterile, occlusive dressing. This will help protect the patient from microshock as well as infection.

SPECIAL CONSIDERATIONS
- Take care to prevent microshock. This includes warning the patient not to use any electrical equipment that isn't grounded.
- Place a plastic cover supplied by the manufacturer over the pacemaker controls to avoid accidental setting changes.
- Insulate the pacemaker by covering all exposed metal parts with nonconducting tape, or place the pacing unit in a dry, rubber surgical glove.
- If the patient is disoriented or uncooperative, provide measures to prevent accidental removal of pacemaker wires.
- If the patient needs emergency defibrillation, place the paddles away from the pacemaker generator and insertion site.
- When using a transcutaneous pacemaker, don't place the electrodes over a bony area because bone conducts current poorly.
- With female patients, place the anterior electrode of a transcutaneous pacemaker under the patient's breast but not over her diaphragm.
- Immobilize the patient's arm or leg if the practitioner inserts the electrode of a transvenous pacemaker through the brachial or femoral vein.
- Assess the patient's vital signs, skin color, LOC, and peripheral pulses to determine the effectiveness of the paced rhythm.
- Perform a 12-lead ECG to serve as a baseline. Perform additional ECGs daily or with clinical changes, monitoring them and noting capture, sensing, rate, intrinsic beats, and competition of paced and intrinsic rhythms.
- Obtain a rhythm strip before, during, and after pacemaker placement, when settings are changed, and when complications arise; continuously monitor cardiac rhythm.
- If the pacemaker is sensing correctly, the sense indicator on the pulse generator should flash with each beat. (See *When a temporary pacemaker malfunctions.*)

- If the patient has epicardial pacing wires in place, clean the insertion site with povidone-iodine solution, and change the dressing daily.
- Monitor the site for signs of infection.
- Keep the pulse generator nearby in case pacing becomes necessary.

COMPLICATIONS
- Microshock
- Competitive or fatal arrhythmias
- Transcutaneous pacemakers: skin breakdown, muscle pain and twitching
- Transvenous pacemakers: pneumothorax or hemothorax, cardiac perforation and tamponade, diaphragmatic stimulation, pulmonary embolism, thrombophlebitis, infection; threading electrode through antecubital or femoral vein may cause venous spasm, thrombophlebitis, and lead displacement
- Transthoracic pacemakers: pneumothorax, cardiac tamponade, emboli, sepsis, lacerations of myocardium or coronary artery, perforation of a cardiac chamber
- Epicardial pacemakers: infection, cardiac arrest, and diaphragmatic stimulation

When a temporary pacemaker malfunctions

Occasionally, a temporary pacemaker may fail to function appropriately. When this occurs, you'll need to take immediate action to correct the problem. Take the steps described below when your patient's pacemaker fails to pace, capture, or sense intrinsic beats.

FAILURE TO PACE

This happens when the pacemaker either doesn't fire or fires too often. The pulse generator may not be working properly, or it may not be conducting the impulse to the patient.

Nursing interventions

◆ If the pacing or sensing indicator flashes, check the connections to the cable and the position of the pacing electrode in the patient (by X-ray). The cable may have come loose, or the electrode may have been dislodged, pulled out, or broken.

◆ If the pulse generator is turned on but the indicators still aren't flashing, change the bat-

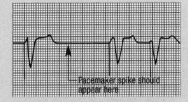

Pacemaker spike should appear here

tery. If that doesn't help, use a different pulse generator.

◆ Check the settings if the pacemaker is firing too rapidly. If they're correct, or if altering them (according to facility policy or practitioner's order) doesn't help, change the pulse generator.

FAILURE TO CAPTURE

Here, you see the pacemaker spikes, but the heart isn't responding. This may be caused by changes in the pacing threshold from ischemia, an electrolyte imbalance (high or low potassium or magnesium levels), acidosis, an adverse reaction to a medication, a perforated ventricle, fibrosis, or the position of the electrode.

Nursing interventions

◆ If the patient's condition has changed, notify the practitioner, and ask him for new settings.

◆ If the pacemaker settings have been altered by the patient (or his family members), return them to their correct positions. Then make sure the face of the pacemaker is covered with a plastic shield. Tell the patient and his family members not to touch the dials.

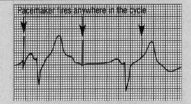

Pacemaker spikes, but no response from heart

◆ If the heart isn't responding, try these suggestions: Carefully check all connections, making sure they're placed properly and securely; increase the milliamperes slowly (according to facility policy or practitioner's order); turn the patient on his left side, then on his right (if turning him to the left didn't help); schedule an anteroposterior or lateral chest X-ray to determine the position of the electrode.

FAILURE TO SENSE INTRINSIC BEATS

This could cause ventricular tachycardia or ventricular fibrillation if the pacemaker fires on the vulnerable T wave. This could be caused by the pacemaker sensing an external stimulus as a QRS complex, which could lead to asystole, or by the pacemaker not being sensitive enough, which means it could fire anywhere within the cardiac cycle.

Nursing interventions

◆ If the pacing is undersensing, turn the sensitivity control completely to the right. If it's oversensing, turn it slightly to the left.

◆ If the pacemaker isn't functioning correctly, change the battery or the pulse generator.

◆ Remove items in the room that may be causing electromechanical interference (such as electrical razors, radios, and cautery devices). Check the ground wires on the bed and

Pacemaker fires anywhere in the cycle

other equipment for obvious damage. Unplug each piece, and see if the interference stops. When you locate the cause, notify the staff engineer, and ask him to check it.

◆ If the pacemaker is still firing on the T wave and all else has failed, turn off the pacemaker. Make sure atropine is available in case the patient's heart rate drops. Be prepared to call a code and institute cardiopulmonary resuscitation if necessary.

PATIENT TEACHING

◆ Tell the patient why a pacemaker is needed and how it's inserted.
◆ Explain the importance of not changing pacemaker settings or touching the pulse generator or wires.
◆ Explain how to prevent microshock.
◆ Caution the patient about possible sensations or discomforts felt with transcutaneous pacing.
◆ Explain signs and symptoms of complications and when to report them to the nurse.

DOCUMENTATION

◆ Record the reason for pacing.
◆ Document cardiac rhythms with an ECG or rhythm strip.
◆ Note the date and time the pacing started.
◆ Document electrode locations.
◆ Note what type of pacing was done.
◆ Record pacemaker settings.
◆ Document the patient's response to the procedure.
◆ Note complications and nursing actions taken.

SELECTED REFERENCES

Craig, K. "How to Provide Transcutaneous Pacing," *Nursing* 36(Suppl Cardiac):22-23, Spring 2006.

Hidaka, N., et al. "Is Intrapartum Temporary Pacing Required for Women With Complete Atrioventricular Block? An Analysis of Seven Cases," *BJOG* 113(5):605-607, May 2006.

James, M., et al. "An Unusual Complication of Transvenous Temporary Pacing," *Heart* 89(4):448, April 2003.

Yeh, K., et al. "Two-Dimensional Echocardiography for the Diagnosis of Interventricular Septum Perforation by a Temporary Pacing Catheter," *American Journal of the Medical Sciences* 331(2):95-96, February 2006.

Pain management

DESCRIPTION

- Procedures are used to assess and manage pain; the nurse depends on patient's subjective description in addition to objective tools.
- Pain management includes use of analgesics (opioid analgesics if pain is severe), emotional support, comfort measures, or complementary and alternative therapies (such as cognitive techniques) that distract the patient.
- Pain management may also require invasive measures, such as epidural analgesia or patient-controlled analgesia (PCA).

CONTRAINDICATIONS

- Inability to utilize certain management techniques

EQUIPMENT

Pain assessment tool or scale ◆ oral hygiene supplies ◆ non-opioid analgesic (such as aspirin or acetaminophen) ◆ PCA device ◆ opioid (such as oxy-codone or codeine) ◆ strong opioid (such as morphine or hydromorphone)

KEY STEPS

- Explain how pain drugs and pain management therapies work together.
- Explain that pain management aims to keep pain at a low level.
- Use pain assessment tools or scale, or ask key questions such as duration, severity, and location of pain. (See *How to assess pain.*)
- Note the patient's reaction to pain.
- Look for physiologic or behavioral clues to the pain's severity.
- Develop a nursing care plan with the patient, including prescribed drugs, emotional support, comfort measures, complementary and alternative therapies, and pain management education.
- Emphasize the importance of maintaining good bowel habits, respiratory functions, and mobility.
- Implement your care plan.

GIVING MEDICATIONS

- Verify the order.
- Confirm the patient's identity using two patient identifiers according to facility policy.
- Give a nonopioid analgesic if the patient is allowed oral intake.
- Give a mild opioid if relief isn't achieved with a nonopioid as ordered.
- Administer a strong opioid if the patient needs more relief as ordered.
- Administer oral drugs if possible.
- Check the appropriate drug information for each drug given.
- If ordered, teach the patient how to use a PCA device.

PROVIDING EMOTIONAL SUPPORT

- Spend time talking with the patient.
- Provide reassurance that measures are being taken to relieve pain.

PERFORMING COMFORT MEASURES

- Reposition the patient every 2 hours.
- Increase the angle of the bed to reduce pull on an abdominal incision.
- Elevate a limb to reduce swelling, inflammation, and pain.
- Splint or support abdominal and chest incisions with a pillow when coughing or changing position.
- Give a back massage, and provide hygiene as needed.
- Perform passive range-of-motion exercises.

PERFORMING COMPLEMENTARY AND ALTERNATIVE THERAPIES

- If he feels persistent pain, begin teaching distraction techniques through short, simple relaxation exercises.
- Dim the lights, remove restrictive clothing, and eliminate noise.
- Have him recall a pleasant experience or focus his attention on an enjoyable activity.
- Have him close his eyes and concentrate on listening to music, raising or lowering the volume as his pain increases or subsides.
- As needed, use guided imagery, deep breathing, and relaxation techniques.

How to assess pain

To assess pain, consider the patient's description and your observations of physical and behavioral responses. Start by asking the following questions (consider that the patient's responses will be shaped by his prior experiences, self-image, and beliefs about his condition):

- Where is the pain located?
- How long does it last?
- How often does it occur?
- Can you describe the pain?
- What triggers the pain?
- What relieves the pain or makes it worse?

Ask the patient to rank his pain on a scale of 0 to 10, with 0 denoting no pain and 10 denoting the worst pain. This helps the patient verbally evaluate pain therapies.

Observe the patient's behavioral and physiologic responses to pain. Physiologic responses may be sympathetic or parasympathetic.

BEHAVIORAL RESPONSES

Behavioral responses include altered body position, moaning, sighing, grimacing, withdrawal, crying, restlessness, muscle twitching, irritability, and immobility.

SYMPATHETIC RESPONSES

Sympathetic responses are commonly associated with mild to moderate pain and include pallor, elevated blood pressure, dilated pupils, skeletal muscle tension, dyspnea, tachycardia, and diaphoresis.

PARASYMPATHETIC RESPONSES

Parasympathetic responses are commonly associated with severe, deep pain and include pallor, decreased blood pressure, bradycardia, nausea and vomiting, weakness, dizziness, and loss of consciousness.

- For guided imagery:
  - guide the patient to concentrate on a peaceful, pleasant image
  - ask about its sight, sound, smell, taste, and touch
  - have the patient visualize the goal and picture himself taking action to achieve it.
- For deep breathing:
  - have the patient stare at an object
  - have him slowly inhale and exhale as he counts aloud
  - ask him to concentrate on the rise and fall of his abdomen
  - encourage him to feel increasingly weightless with each breath.
- For muscle relaxation:
  - have the patient focus on a particular muscle group
  - ask him to tense the muscles and note the sensation
  - after 5 to 7 seconds, tell him to relax his muscles and concentrate on the relaxed state
  - have him describe the difference between the tense and relaxed states
  - after he tenses and relaxes one muscle group, have him proceed to another and another until he has covered his entire body.

SPECIAL CONSIDERATIONS

- Evaluate your patient's response to pain management.
- Reassess and alter your care plan as appropriate.
- During intense pain, know that the patient's ability to concentrate diminishes.
- If your patient is in severe pain, help him select a cognitive technique that's easy to use and encourage him to use it consistently.
- Remind the patient that cognitive therapy results improve with practice.
- Cultural beliefs affect behavioral responses to pain and treatment, so consider patient expectations when developing the care plan.

AGE FACTOR *Provide pain relief for the elderly patient using pharmacologic and nonpharmacologic approaches. Identify age-related factors that affect assessment and pain management in the elderly patient. Avoid such drugs as meperidine and propoxyphene due to adverse effects.*

AGE FACTOR *Developmental factors make pain assessment in children more difficult. Look for behavioral cues in infants and young children, such as crying, facial grimacing, or eye closing, and use pain tools such as the Wong and Baker Faces Pain Rating Scale.*

- Opioid analgesics may lead to tolerance, dependence, or addiction; however, addiction resulting from acute pain treatment is less than 1%.
- If a preexisting drug addiction problem exists, make appropriate referrals to experts to develop an effective pain management plan.

COMPLICATIONS

- Respiratory depression (most serious)
- Sedation
- Constipation
- Nausea
- Vomiting
- Tolerance
- Dependence
- Addiction

PATIENT TEACHING

- Teach the patient distraction, guided imagery, deep breathing, and relaxation techniques, as appropriate.
- Teach about prescribed medications, including dosage, administration, and possible adverse effects.

DOCUMENTATION

- Record subjective information from the patient, including exact words.
- Note the location, quality, and duration of pain.
- Document precipitating and relieving factors.
- Note the pain-relief method selected.
- Note alternative treatments to consider if pain isn't relieved.
- Record nursing interventions and patient response.
- Document complications of drug therapy.
- Document the patient's rating of pain before and after interventions.

SELECTED REFERENCES

D'Arcy, Y. "How to Care for a Surgical Patient With Chronic Pain," *Nursing* 36(3):17, March 2006.

Doughty, D.B. "Strategies for Minimizing Chronic Wound Pain," *Advances in Skin & Wound Care* 19(2):82-85, March 2006.

Morrison, R.S., et al. "Improving the Management of Pain in Hospitalized Adults," *Archives of Internal Medicine* 166(9):1033-39, May 2006.

Savory, J., and Bennett, M. "Managing Children's Pain," *Nursing Times* 102(9): 57-59, February-March 2006.

Sofer, D. "PCA Pumps: An Illusion of Safety?" *American Journal of Nursing* 105(2):22, February 2005.

Williams, H. "Assessing, Diagnosing and Managing Neuropathic Pain," *Nursing Times* 102(16):22-24, April 2006.

Wilson, B., and McSherry, W. "A Study of Nurses' Inferences of Patients' Physical Pain," *Journal of Clinical Nursing* 15(4):459-68, April 2006.

Papanicolaou test

DESCRIPTION

- Also known as a *Pap test* or *Pap smear*; this cytologic test allows early detection of cervical cancer.
- The test involves scraping cells from the cervix, spreading them on a slide, and coating the slide with fixative spray or solution to preserve specimen cells for nuclear staining.
- Cytologic evaluation outlines cell maturity, morphology, and metabolic activity.
- The ThinPrep Pap test is a relatively new tool for early detection of cervical cancer. (See *ThinPrep Pap test.*)

CONTRAINDICATIONS

- Menses

ThinPrep Pap test

Since 1996, the ThinPrep Pap test has been used as a replacement for the conventional papanicolaou (Pap) test for cervical cancer screening.

Most laboratories in the United States can process this test, which is significantly more effective than traditional tests for detecting cervical abnormalities for many patient populations.

The ThinPrep Pap test can also be used to test for human papillomavirus, a sexually transmitted disease causally linked to cervical cancer and to diagnose *Chlamydia trachomatis* and *Neisseria gonorrhoeae*.

Bivalve vaginal speculum ◆ gloves ◆ Pap stick (wooden spatula) ◆ long cotton-tipped applicator ◆ three glass microscope slides ◆ fixative (a commercial spray or 95% ethyl alcohol solution) ◆ adjustable lamp ◆ drape ◆ laboratory request forms

PREPARATION

- Select a speculum of appropriate size.
- Gather the equipment in the examining room.
- Label the glass slides with the patient's name and "E," "C," and "V" to differentiate endocervical, cervical, and vaginal specimens.

- Confirm the patient's identity using two patient identifiers according to facility policy.
- Explain the procedure to the patient.
- Wash your hands.
- Instruct the patient to void before the examination.
- Provide privacy.
- Instruct the patient to undress below the waist.
- Instruct the patient to sit on the examination table and drape her genital region.
- Place the patient in the lithotomy position, with her feet in the stirrups and her buttocks extended slightly beyond the edge of the table.
- Adjust the drape.
- Adjust the lamp so that it fully illuminates the genital area.
- Fold back the corner of the drape to expose the perineum.
- Put on gloves.
- Take the speculum in your dominant hand, and moisten it with warm water to ease insertion.
- Avoid using water-soluble lubricants, which interfere with accurate laboratory testing.
- Warn the patient that you're about to touch her to avoid startling her.
- Gently separate the labia with the thumb and forefinger of your nondominant hand.
- Instruct the patient to take several deep breaths.
- Insert the speculum into the vagina.
- When it's in place, slowly open the blades to expose the cervix.
- Lock the blades in place.
- Insert a cotton-tipped applicator through the speculum ⅕″ (5 mm) into the cervical os.
- Rotate the applicator 360 degrees to obtain an endocervical specimen.
- Remove the applicator, and gently roll it in a circle across the slide marked "E."
- To prevent cell destruction, don't rub the applicator on the slide.
- Immediately place the slide in a fixative solution, or spray it with a fixative, to prevent drying of cells.

- Insert the small curved end of the Pap stick through the speculum, and place it directly over the cervical os.
- Rotate the stick gently but firmly to scrape cells loose.
- Remove the stick, spread the specimen across the slide marked "C," and fix it immediately, as before.
- Insert the opposite end of the Pap stick or a cotton-tipped applicator through the speculum, and scrape the posterior fornix or vaginal pool, an area that collects cells from the endometrium, vagina, and cervix.
- Remove the stick or applicator, spread the specimen across the slide marked "V," and fix it immediately.
- Unlock the speculum to ease removal and avoid accidentally pinching the vaginal wall. Then withdraw the speculum.
- Remove your gloves and discard.
- Remove the patient's feet from the stirrups, and help her to a sitting position.
- Provide privacy for the patient to dress.
- Fill out the appropriate laboratory request forms, including the date of the patient's last menses.

SPECIAL CONSIDERATIONS

- Many preventable factors can interfere with the Pap test's accuracy.
- Instruct the patient to avoid sexual intercourse, vaginal douching, or administering vaginal medications 48 hours before specimen collection.
- Schedule the test 5 to 6 days before menses or 1 week after.
- Application of topical antibiotics promotes rapid, heavy shedding of cells and requires postponement of the Pap test for at least 1 month.
- If the patient has had a complete hysterectomy, collect test specimens from the vaginal pool and cuff.

COMPLICATIONS

- Pinching of vaginal tissue due to failure to unlock speculum blades before removal
- Severe cramping from rough handling of speculum
- Slight bleeding due to scraping an inflamed cervix with the Pap stick

PATIENT TEACHING

- Explain the procedure, and answer any questions to lessen the patient's anxiety.
- Tell the patient that she will be notifed with the results of the test.

DOCUMENTATION

- Record the date and time of specimen collection.

SELECTED REFERENCES

Bond, S., American College of Obstetrics and Gynecology, American Cancer Society, United States Preventive Services Task Force, "New Guidelines for Pap Screening and Management of Results," *Journal of Midwifery & Women's Health* 49(1):57-59, January-February 2004.

Christie, L., et al. "Women's Views of Registered Nurses as Papanicolaou Smear Providers: A Pilot Study," *Contemporary Nurse* 20(2):159-68, December 2005.

Kubovchik, M. "Abnormal Pap Anxiety," *Nurse Practitioner* 29(1):10, January 2004.

Wright, D., et al. "Speculum 'Self-Insertion': A Pilot Study," *Journal of Clinical Nursing* 14(9):1098-111, October 2005.

Paracentesis, abdominal

DESCRIPTION

◆ A bedside procedure, abdominal paracentesis involves aspiration of fluid from the peritoneal space through a needle, trocar, or cannula inserted in the abdominal wall.

◆ It's used to diagnose and treat massive ascites resistant to other therapy; it helps determine cause of ascites while relieving pressure created by ascites.

◆ It's used to detect intra-abdominal bleeding after traumatic injury and obtain a peritoneal fluid specimen for laboratory analysis.

◆ It may precede other procedures, including radiography, peritoneal dialysis, and surgery.

◆ Nursing responsibilities include preparing the patient, monitoring his condition, providing emotional support during the procedure, assisting the practitioner, and obtaining specimens for laboratory analysis.

CONTRAINDICATIONS

◆ Abnormal bleeding
◆ Suspected abdominal adhesions
◆ Severely distended bowel
◆ Cellulitis of abdominal wall
◆ Uncooperative or agitated patient

Tape measure ◆ sterile gloves ◆ clean gloves ◆ gown ◆ goggles ◆ linen-saver pads ◆ Vacutainer laboratory tubes ◆ large glass ◆ Vacutainer bottles (1,000 ml or larger) ◆ dry, sterile pressure dressing ◆ laboratory request forms ◆ povidone-iodine solution ◆ local anesthetic (multidose vial of 1% or 2% lidocaine with epinephrine) ◆ 4″ × 4″ sterile gauze pads ◆ paracentesis tray (containing needle, trocar, cannula, three-way stopcock), usually disposable ◆ sterile drapes ◆ marking pen ◆ 5-ml syringe with 22G or 25G needle ◆ alcohol pad ◆ 50-ml syringe ◆ sterile label ◆ sterile marker ◆ suture materials ◆ salt-poor albumin ◆ povidone-iodine ointment (optional)

◆ Verify order.

◆ Confirm the patient's identity using two patient identifiers according to facility policy.

◆ Explain the procedure to the patient.

◆ Reassure the patient that he shouldn't feel pain, but explain he may feel a stinging sensation and pressure.

◆ Make sure a signed consent has been obtained.

◆ Have the patient void before the procedure.

◆ If the patient is unable to void, insert an indwelling urinary catheter if ordered.

◆ Identify and record baseline values, including vital signs, weight, and abdominal girth. Indicate the abdominal area measured with a felt-tipped marking pen. Baseline data will be used to monitor the patient's status.

◆ Help the patient sit up in bed, on the side of the bed, or in a chair so fluid accumulates in the lower abdomen.

◆ Expose the patient's abdomen from diaphragm to pubis.

◆ Place a linen-saver pad under the patient.

◆ Remind the patient to stay as still as possible during the procedure.

◆ Wash your hands.

◆ Open the paracentesis tray using aseptic technique.

◆ Put on clean gloves.

◆ The practitioner will prepare the patient's abdomen with povidone-iodine solution, drape the operative site with sterile drapes, and administer the local anesthetic.

◆ If the paracentesis tray doesn't contain a sterile ampule of anesthetic, wipe the top of a multidose vial of anesthetic solution with an alcohol pad, and invert the vial at a 45-degree angle to allow the practitioner to insert the sterile 5-ml syringe with the 22G or 25G needle and withdraw the anesthetic without touching the nonsterile vial.

◆ Label all medications, medication containers, and solution containers on and off the sterile field.

- A small incision may be made before inserting the needle or trocar and cannula (usually 1″ to 2″ [2.5 to 5 cm] below the umbilicus).
- Listen for a popping sound. This signifies that the needle or trocar has pierced the peritoneum.
- Assist the practitioner in collecting specimens in proper containers.
- If the practitioner orders substantial drainage, connect the three-way stopcock and tubing to the cannula.
- Run the other end of the tubing to a large sterile Vacutainer, or aspirate the fluid with a three-way stopcock and 50-ml syringe.
- Gently turn the patient from side to side to enhance drainage.
- As the fluid drains, monitor the patient's vital signs every 15 minutes.
- Watch closely for vertigo, faintness, diaphoresis, pallor, heightened anxiety, tachycardia, dyspnea, and hypotension — especially if more than 1,500 ml of peritoneal fluid was aspirated at one time, which may induce a fluid shift and hypovolemic shock. Immediately report signs of shock to the practitioner.
- Salt-poor albumin may be ordered I.V. to prevent hypovolemia and a decline in renal function.
- The incision may be sutured after the needle or trocar and cannula are removed.
- Wearing sterile gloves, apply the dry, sterile pressure dressing and povidone-iodine ointment to the site.
- Help the patient assume a comfortable position.
- Monitor the patient's vital signs and check the dressing for drainage every 15 minutes for 1 hour, every 30 minutes for 2 hours, every hour for 4 hours, and then every 4 hours for 24 hours to detect delayed reactions to the procedure.
- Note color, amount, and character of drainage.
- Label the Vacutainer specimen tubes, and send them to the laboratory for testing.
- If the patient is receiving antibiotics, note this on the request form.
- Remove and dispose of equipment properly.

SPECIAL CONSIDERATIONS

- Help the patient remain still throughout the procedure.
- If the patient shows signs of hypovolemic shock, reduce the vertical distance between the needle or the trocar and cannula and the drainage collection container to slow the drainage rate. If necessary, stop the drainage.
- To prevent fluid shifts and hypovolemia, limit aspirated fluid to between 1,500 and 2,000 ml.
- If peritoneal fluid doesn't flow easily, reposition the patient.
- Verify suction in the Vacutainer collection bottle when you connect it to the drainage tubing.
- Use macrodrip tubing without a backflow device.
- After the procedure, observe for peritoneal fluid leakage, and notify the practitioner if this develops.
- Maintain daily patient weight and abdominal girth records, and compare these values with the baseline figures.

COMPLICATIONS

- Hypotension
- Oliguria
- Hyponatremia
- Perforation of abdominal organs
- Wound infection
- Peritonitis
- If excessive fluid (more than 2 L) is removed, ascitic fluid tending to form again

PATIENT TEACHING

- Explain the procedure to the patient.
- Instruct the patient that he need not restrict food and fluids.
- Provide support to decrease the patient's anxiety during the procedure.

DOCUMENTATION

- Record the date and time of the procedure.
- Note the puncture site location and appearance.
- Document whether the wound was sutured.
- Record the amount, color, viscosity, and odor of aspirated fluid in your notes and in fluid intake and output record.
- Note vital signs, weight, and abdominal girth measurements before and after procedure.
- Document the patient's tolerance of the procedure.
- Record signs and symptoms of complications from the procedure.
- Note the number of specimens sent to the laboratory.

SELECTED REFERENCES

Becker, G., et al. "Malignant Ascites: Systematic Review and Guideline for Treatment," *European Journal of Cancer* 42(5):589-97, March 2006.

Blaivas, M. "Emergency Diagnostic Paracentesis to Determine Intraperitoneal Fluid Identity Discovered on Bedside Ultrasound of Unstable Patients," *Journal of Emergency Medicine* 29(4):461-65, November 2005.

Lin, C.H., et al. "Should Bleeding Tendency Deter Abdominal Paracentesis?" *Digestive and Liver Disease* 37(12):946-51, December 2005.

Parra, M.W., et al. "Paracentesis for Resuscitation-Induced Abdominal Compartment Syndrome: An Alternative to Decompressive Laparotomy in the Burn Patient," *Journal of Trauma* 60(5): 1119-21, May 2006.

Passive range-of-motion exercises

OVERVIEW

DESCRIPTION
◆ Exercises performed to move patient's joints through as full a range of motion (ROM) as possible.
◆ Passive ROM exercises improve or maintain joint mobility and help prevent contractures; they require recognition of the patient's limits of motion and support of all joints during movement.
◆ Performed by the nurse, physical therapist, or caregiver, exercises are indicated for the patient with temporary or permanent loss of mobility, sensation, or consciousness.

CONTRAINDICATIONS
◆ Septic joints
◆ Acute thrombophlebitis
◆ Severe arthritic joint inflammation
◆ Recent trauma with possible hidden fractures or internal injuries
◆ Severe pain
◆ Hemodynamic instability

EQUIPMENT

No specific equipment needed

KEY STEPS

◆ Confirm the patient's identity using two patient identifiers according to facility policy.
◆ Before you begin, raise the bed to a comfortable working height.
◆ Determine the joints that need ROM exercises.
◆ Consult the practitioner or physical therapist about limitations or precautions.
◆ Specific exercises should be done for all joints. (See *Glossary of joint movements.*)
◆ Exercises don't need to be performed in given order or all at once.
◆ Perform exercises slowly, gently, and to the end of the normal ROM or to the point of pain, but no further.

EXERCISING THE NECK
◆ Support the patient's head with your hands and extend the neck, flex the chin to the chest, and tilt the head laterally toward each shoulder.
◆ Rotate the patient's head from right to left.

EXERCISING THE SHOULDERS
◆ Support the patient's arm in an extended, neutral position.
◆ Extend the forearm and flex it back.
◆ Abduct the arm outward from the side of the body.
◆ Adduct it back to the side.
◆ Rotate the shoulder so the arm crosses the midline; bend the elbow so the hand touches the opposite shoulder, then touches the bed for complete internal rotation.
◆ Return the shoulder to a neutral position; with the elbow bent, push the arm backward so the back of the hand touches the mattress for complete external rotation.

EXERCISING THE ELBOW
◆ Place the patient's arm at his side with his palm facing up.
◆ Flex and extend the arm at the elbow.

EXERCISING THE FOREARM
◆ Stabilize the patient's elbow; then twist the hand to bring the palm up (supination).
◆ Twist it back again to bring the palm down (pronation).

EXERCISING THE WRIST
◆ Stabilize the forearm, and flex and extend the wrist.
◆ Rock the hand sideways for lateral flexion, and rotate the hand in a circular motion.

EXERCISING THE FINGERS AND THUMB
◆ Extend the patient's fingers, and flex the hand into a fist.
◆ Repeat extension and flexion of each joint of each finger and thumb separately.
◆ Spread two adjoining fingers apart (abduction) and then bring them together (adduction).
◆ Oppose each fingertip to the thumb, and rotate the thumb and each finger in a circle.

EXERCISING THE HIP AND KNEE
◆ Fully extend the patient's leg, and then bend the hip and knee toward the chest, allowing full joint flexion.
◆ Move the straight leg sideways, out and away from the other leg and then back, over, and across it.
◆ Rotate the straight leg internally toward the midline, and then rotate it externally away from the midline.

EXERCISING THE ANKLE
◆ Bend the patient's foot so the toes push upward, and then bend the foot so the toes push downward.
◆ Rotate the ankle in a circular motion.
◆ Invert the ankle so that the sole of the foot faces the midline, and evert the ankle so that the sole faces away from the midline.

EXERCISING THE TOES
◆ Flex the patient's toes toward the sole, and then extend them back toward the top of the foot.
◆ Spread two adjoining toes apart and bring them together.

♦ Joints begin to stiffen within 24 hours of disuse.
♦ Start passive ROM exercises as soon as possible.
♦ Perform them at least once per shift.
♦ Use proper body mechanics, and repeat each exercise at least three times, if the patient can tolerate it.

COMPLICATIONS

♦ Pain

♦ Patients undergoing prolonged bed rest or limited activity without profound weakness can be taught to perform active ROM exercises, or isometric exercises, as needed.
♦ If the patient requires long-term rehabilitation after discharge, consult with a physical therapist, and teach a family member or caregiver to perform passive ROM exercises.

♦ Record the joints exercised.
♦ Note edema or pressure areas.
♦ Record pain resulting from the exercises.
♦ Note limitation of ROM.
♦ Record the patient's tolerance of the exercises.

SELECTED REFERENCES

Corio, F., et al. "The Effect of Oral and Intrathecal Baclofen Treatment on Passive Range of Motion of the Knee in Children Diagnosed with Cerebral Palsy," *Pediatric Physical Therapy* 17(1):71-72, Spring 2005.

Huang, R.C., et al. "Correlation Between Range of Motion and Outcome After Lumbar Total Disc Replacement: 8.6 Year Follow-up," *Spine* 30(12):1407-11, June 2005.

"Performing Passive Range-of-Motion Exercises," *Nursing* 36(3):50-51, March 2006.

Tully, E. "The Practical Guide to Range of Motion Assessment," *British Journal of Sports Medicine* 39(4):245, April 2005.

Glossary of joint movements

Joints should be exercised to the point of discomfort, but not pain. They should be moved in the intended direction of function, holding the position a few seconds, then returning to the rest position.

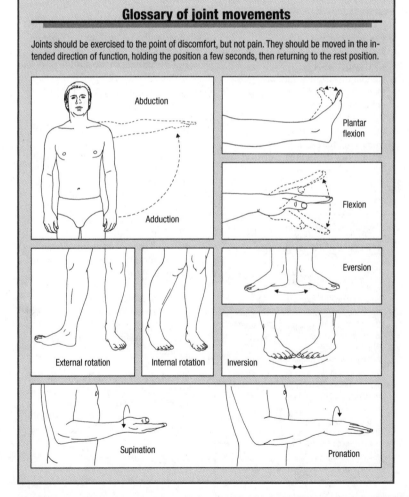

Pericardiocentesis

DESCRIPTION

- Pericardiocentesis involves a needle aspiration of pericardial fluid for analysis.
- This diagnostic procedure is therapeutic and is most useful as an emergency measure to relieve cardiac tamponade — a potentially lethal syndrome marked by increased intrapericardial pressure that prevents complete ventricular filling and reduces cardiac output.
- The fluid sample is used to confirm and identify the cause of pericardial effusion (excess pericardial fluid) and determine appropriate therapy.
- Excess pericardial fluid may accumulate after inflammation, cardiac surgery, rupture, or penetrating trauma (gunshot or stab wounds) of the pericardium.
- Rapidly forming effusions may induce cardiac tamponade.
- Slowly forming effusions pose less immediate danger and allow the pericardium more time to adapt to accumulating fluid.
- The pericardium normally contains 10 to 50 ml of sterile fluid.
- Pericardial fluid is clear and straw colored, without evidence of pathogens, blood, or malignant cells.
- The white blood cell count in the fluid is usually less than $1,000/\mu l$.
- Its glucose concentration should approximate the glucose levels in the blood.
- Pericardial effusions are typically classified as transudates or exudates. (See *Pericardial effusions: Transudates and exudates*.)

CONTRAINDICATIONS

- None known

Povidone-iodine solution ◆ 1% procaine or 1% lidocaine for local anesthetic ◆ sterile needles (25G for anesthetic and 14G, 16G, and 18G 4″ or 5″ cardiac needles) ◆ 50-ml syringe with Luer-lock tip ◆ 7-ml sterile test tubes (one red-top with clot activator, one green-top with heparin, and one lavender-top with EDTA) ◆ sterile specimen container for culture ◆ 4″ × 4″ gauze pads ◆ sterile bandage ◆ sterile marker ◆ sterile labels ◆ vial of heparin 1,000 units/ml ◆ three-way stopcock ◆ electrocardiograph (ECG) or bedside monitor ◆ pulse oximeter ◆ Kelly clamp ◆ alligator clips ◆ defibrillator and emergency drugs ◆ gloves ◆ protective eyewear

PREPARATION

- Use a prepackaged pericardiocentesis tray if available.
- Needle insertion is generally guided by electrocardiogram (ECG) or echocardiogram.
- Connect the patient to the bedside monitor, set to read lead V_1.
- Make sure that a defibrillator and emergency drugs are nearby.

Pericardial effusions: Transudates and exudates

Transudates are protein-poor effusions that usually arise from mechanical factors altering fluid formation or resorption, such as increased hydrostatic pressure, decreased plasma oncotic pressure, or obstruction of the pericardial lymphatic drainage system by a tumor.

Exudates result from inflammation and contain large amounts of protein. Inflammation damages the capillary membrane, allowing protein molecules to leak into the pericardial fluid.

Both effusion types occur in pericarditis, neoplasms, acute myocardial infarction, tuberculosis, rheumatoid disease, and systemic lupus erythematosus.

- Confirm the patient's identity using two patient identifiers according to facility policy.
- Explain the procedure and answer questions.
- A consent form should be signed unless the procedure is done emergently.
- Inform the patient that he may feel pressure when the needle is inserted into the pericardial sac.
- Provide privacy.
- Wash your hands.
- Open the equipment tray on an overbed table, being careful not to contaminate the sterile field.
- Provide adequate lighting at the puncture site.
- Adjust the height of the patient's bed to allow the practitioner to perform the procedure comfortably.
- Put the patient in the supine position with his thorax elevated 60 degrees.
- Wash your hands again, and put on gloves and protective eyewear.
- The skin is cleaned by the practitioner with sterile gauze pads soaked in povidone-iodine solution.
- If no ampule of anesthetic is included on the equipment tray, clean the injection port of a multidose vial of anesthetic with an alcohol pad. Invert the vial 45 degrees so the practitioner can insert a needle and syringe and withdraw the anesthetic.
- Label all medications, medication containers, and solution containers on and off the sterile field.
- Tell the patient the anesthetic may cause brief burning and local pain.
- The practitioner attaches a 50-ml syringe to one end of a three-way stopcock and the cardiac needle to the other.
- The V_1 lead (precordial leadwire) of the ECG may be attached to the hub of the aspirating needle using the alligator clips to help determine if the needle has come in contact with the epicardium during the procedure.

- The practitioner will insert the needle through the chest wall into the pericardial sac, maintaining aspiration until fluid appears in the syringe.
- The needle should be angled 35 to 45 degrees toward the tip of the right scapula between the left costal margin and the xiphoid process. This minimizes risk of lacerating the coronary vessels or the pleura.
- After the needle is positioned, the practitioner attaches a Kelly clamp to the skin surface so it won't advance further.
- Assist the practitioner by labeling all specimen containers on and off the sterile field, numbering the specimen tubes, and cleaning the top of the tube used for culture and sensitivity with povidone-iodine solution.
- If bacterial culture and sensitivity tests are ordered, record on the laboratory request any antimicrobial drugs the patient is receiving.
- If anaerobic organisms are suspected, consult the laboratory about proper collection technique to avoid exposing the aspirate to air.
- Send specimens to the laboratory immediately.
- When the needle is withdrawn, immediately apply pressure to the site with sterile gauze pads for 3 to 5 minutes.
- Apply a sterile bandage and assess for complications.
- Check blood pressure, pulse, respirations, oxygen saturation, and heart sounds every 15 minutes until stable, then every half hour for 2 hours, every hour for 4 hours, and every 4 hours thereafter. Your facility may require more frequent monitoring.
- Monitor continually for cardiac arrhythmias.
- Document rhythm strips according to facility policy.
- Return equipment to the proper location.
- Dispose of equipment according to facility policy.

SPECIAL CONSIDERATIONS

- Observe the ECG tracing when the cardiac needle is being inserted.
- ST-segment elevation indicates that the needle has reached the epicardial surface and should be retracted slightly.
- An abnormally shaped QRS complex may indicate perforation of the myocardium.
- Premature ventricular contractions usually indicate that the needle has touched the ventricular wall.
- Watch for grossly bloody fluid aspirate, which may indicate inadvertent puncture of a cardiac chamber.
- After the procedure, be alert for respiratory and cardiac distress.
- Watch especially for signs of cardiac tamponade: muffled and distant heartbeat, jugular vein distention, paradoxical pulse, tachycardia, hypotension, and shock.

COMPLICATIONS

WARNING *To minimize risk of complications, echocardiography should precede pericardiocentesis to determine the effusion site.*

- Laceration of a coronary artery or the myocardium (potentially fatal)
- Ventricular fibrillation
- Vasovagal arrest
- Pleural infection
- Accidental puncture of lung, liver, or stomach

PATIENT TEACHING

- Explain the procedure to the patient and answer questions.
- Inform the patient that he'll be monitored closely during and after the procedure.

DOCUMENTATION

- Note the initiation and completion time of the procedure.
- Record the patient's response, vital signs, and cardiac rhythm.
- Document drugs administered.
- Note the amount, color, and consistency of fluid.
- Record the number of specimen tubes collected.
- Document the time of transport to the laboratory.
- Note patient and family education, complications, and interventions.

SELECTED REFERENCES

Ben-Horin, S., et al. "Large Symptomatic Pericardial Effusion as the Presentation of Unrecognized Cancer: A Study in 173 Consecutive Patients Undergoing Pericardiocentesis," *Medicine (Baltimore)* 85(1):49-53, January 2006.

Cubero, G.I., et al. "Pericardial Effusion: Clinical and Analytical Parameters Clues," *International Journal of Cardiology* 108(3):404-405, April 2006.

Humphreys, M. "Pericardial Conditions: Signs, Symptoms and Electrocardiogram Changes," *Emergency Nurse* 14(1):30-36, April 2006.

Little, W.C., and Freeman, G.L. "Pericardial Disease," *Circulation* 113(12): 1622-32, March 2006.

Perineal care

DESCRIPTION

◆ Care of the perineal area to promote cleanliness and prevent infection.
◆ Care removes irritating and odorous secretions, such as smegma, that collect under the foreskin of the penis and on the inner surface of the labia.
◆ Care of the external genitalia and anal area should be performed during daily bath and, if necessary, at bedtime and after urination and bowel movements.
◆ For the patient with perineal skin breakdown, frequent bathing followed by application of ointment or cream aids healing.
◆ Standard precautions must be followed when providing perineal care.

CONTRAINDICATIONS

◆ None known

Gloves ◆ washcloths ◆ clean basin ◆ mild soap ◆ bath towel or bath blanket ◆ toilet tissue ◆ linen-saver pad ◆ trash bag ◆ peri bottle ◆ antiseptic soap ◆ petroleum jelly ◆ zinc oxide cream ◆ vitamin A and D ointment ◆ ABD pad ◆ bedpan (optional)

PREPARATION

◆ Following genital or rectal surgery, you may need to use sterile supplies, including sterile gloves, gauze, and cotton balls.
◆ Obtain ointment or cream as needed.
◆ Fill the basin two-thirds full with warm water.
◆ Fill the peri bottle with warm water if needed.

◆ Assemble equipment at the patient's bedside and provide privacy.
◆ Wash your hands and put on gloves.
◆ Explain the procedure to the patient.
◆ Adjust the bed to a comfortable working height to prevent back strain; lower the head of the bed if allowed.
◆ Provide privacy, and help the patient to a supine position.
◆ Place a linen-saver pad under the patient's buttocks to protect the bed from stains and moisture.

PERINEAL CARE FOR THE FEMALE PATIENT

◆ To minimize the patient's exposure, place the bath blanket over her with corners head to foot and side to side.
◆ Wrap each leg with a side corner, tucking it under the hip.
◆ Fold back the corner between the legs to expose the perineum.
◆ Ask the patient to bend her knees slightly and spread her legs.
◆ Separate the patient's labia with one hand and wash with the other, using downward strokes from the front to the back of the perineum to prevent intestinal organisms from contaminating the urethra or vagina.
◆ Avoid the area around the anus, and use a clean section of washcloth for each stroke by folding each used section inward. This prevents the spread of contaminated secretions or discharge.
◆ Using a clean washcloth, rinse thoroughly from front to back; soap residue can cause skin irritation.
◆ Pat the area dry with a bath towel because moisture can also cause skin irritation and discomfort.
◆ Apply ordered ointments or creams.
◆ Turn the patient on her side to Sims' position, if possible, to expose the anal area.
◆ Clean, rinse, and dry the anal area, starting at the posterior vaginal opening and wiping from front to back.

PERINEAL CARE FOR THE MALE PATIENT

◆ Drape the patient's legs to minimize exposure of the genital area.
◆ Hold the shaft of the penis with one hand and wash with the other, beginning at the tip and working in a circular motion from the center to the periphery to avoid introducing microorganisms into the urethra.
◆ Use a clean section of washcloth for each stroke to prevent spread of contaminated secretions or discharge.
◆ Rinse thoroughly, using the same circular motion.
◆ For the uncircumcised patient, gently retract the foreskin and clean beneath it. Rinse well but don't dry because moisture provides lubrication and prevents friction when replacing the foreskin. Replace the foreskin to avoid constriction of the penis, which causes edema and tissue damage.
◆ Wash the rest of the penis, using downward strokes toward the scrotum.
◆ Rinse well, and pat dry with a bath towel.
◆ Handle the scrotum gently to avoid causing discomfort.
◆ Turn the patient on his side. Clean the bottom of the scrotum and the anal area.
◆ Rinse well and pat dry.

SPECIAL CONSIDERATIONS

◆ Give perineal care in a matter-of-fact way to minimize embarrassment.
◆ If the patient is incontinent, first remove excess feces.
◆ Position him on a bedpan, and add a small amount of antiseptic soap to a peri bottle to eliminate odor.
◆ Irrigate the perineal area to remove any remaining fecal matter.
◆ After cleaning the perineum, apply ointment or cream (petroleum jelly, zinc oxide cream, or vitamin A and D ointment) to prevent skin breakdown.

COMPLICATIONS
◆ None known

PATIENT TEACHING

◆ Explain the procedure to the patient.
◆ Assure the patient that you'll protect his privacy.

DOCUMENTATION

◆ Record perineal care and special treatments.
◆ Note need for continued treatment, if necessary, in your care plan.
◆ Describe perineal skin condition and odor or discharge.

SELECTED REFERENCES

Grant, B.M., et al. "Vulnerable Bodies: Competing Discourses of Intimate Bodily Care," *Journal of Nursing Education* 44(11):498-504, November 2005.
Holloway, S., and Jones, V. "The Importance of Skin Care and Assessment," *British Journal of Nursing* 14(22):1172-76, December 2005-January 2006.
Nix, D., and Ermer-Seltun, J. "A Review of Perineal Skin Care Protocols and Skin Barrier Product Use," *Ostomy/Wound Management* 50(12):59-67, December 2004.
Rader, J., et al. "The Bathing of Older Adults with Dementia,"*AJN* 106(4): 40-48, April 2006.

Peripheral I.V. catheter insertion

DESCRIPTION

◆ Peripheral I.V. catheter insertion allows administration of fluids, medication, blood, and blood components.

◆ Device and site selection depend on the type of solution used; frequency and duration of infusion; patency and location of accessible veins; patient's age, size, and condition; and, if possible, patient's preference.

◆ If possible, a vein in the nondominant arm or hand should be chosen.

◆ Preferred venipuncture sites are the cephalic and basilic veins in the lower arm and veins in the dorsum of the hand.

◆ Antecubital veins can be used if no other venous access is available.

CONTRAINDICATIONS

◆ Sclerotic vein
◆ Edematous or impaired arm or hand
◆ Postmastectomy arm
◆ Burns
◆ Arteriovenous fistula

EQUIPMENT

Alcohol pads or an approved antimicrobial solution such as chlorhexidine ◆ gloves ◆ tourniquet ◆ I.V. access device with safety device ◆ I.V. solution with attached and primed administration set ◆ I.V. pole ◆ a transparent semipermeable dressing ◆ sterile tape or catheter stabilization device

PREPARATION

◆ Make sure that I.V. solution container label includes the patient's name and room number, type of solution, time and date of preparation, preparer's name, and ordered infusion rate.

◆ Select an appropriate-gauge device.

◆ If using a winged infusion set, connect the adapter to the administration set, and unclamp the line until fluid flows from the open end of the needle cover.

◆ Close the clamp, and place the needle on a sterile surface.

◆ If using a catheter device, open its package to allow easy access.

KEY STEPS

◆ Hang the I.V. solution with primed administration set on the I.V. pole.

◆ Confirm the patient's identity using two patient identifiers according to facility policy.

◆ Wash your hands.

◆ Explain the procedure to the patient.

SELECTING THE SITE

◆ If long-term therapy is anticipated, start with a vein at the most distal site so you can move proximally as needed for subsequent sites.

◆ For infusion of an irritating medication, choose a large vein distal to any nearby joint.

◆ Make sure the intended vein can accommodate the cannula.

◆ Place the patient in a comfortable, reclining position, leaving the arm in a dependent position to increase venous fill of the lower arms and hands.

◆ If the patient's skin is cold, warm it by rubbing his arm or covering it with warm packs or submerging it in warm water for 5 to 10 minutes.

APPLYING THE TOURNIQUET

◆ Apply a tourniquet 4″ to 6″ (10 to 15 cm) above the puncture site.

◆ Leave the tourniquet in place no longer than 3 minutes.

◆ Check for a radial pulse. If it isn't present, release the tourniquet, and reapply it with less tension to prevent arterial occlusion.

◆ Lightly palpate the vein with the index and middle fingers of your nondominant hand.

◆ Stretch the skin to anchor the vein. If the vein feels hard or ropelike, select another.

◆ If you've selected a vein in the arm or hand that's palpable but not sufficiently dilated, tell the patient to open and close his fist several times.

PREPARING THE SITE

◆ Put on gloves, and if necessary, clip the hair around the insertion site.

◆ Clean the site with a facility-approved antimicrobial solution. Use a vigorous side-to-side motion. Allow the solution to dry.

◆ If ordered, and if the patient isn't sensitive to lidocaine, administer a local anesthetic.

◆ Lightly press the skin with the thumb of your nondominant hand about 1½″ (4 cm) from the intended insertion site.

◆ If using a winged infusion device, hold the short edges of the wings (with the needle's bevel facing upward) between the thumb and forefinger of your dominant hand, and squeeze the wings together.

◆ If you're using an over-the-needle cannula, grasp the plastic hub with your dominant hand, remove the cover, and examine the cannula tip. If the edge isn't smooth, discard it and replace the device.

◆ Using the thumb of your nondominant hand, pull the skin taut below the puncture site to stabilize the vein.

◆ Tell the patient you're about to insert the device.

◆ Hold the needle bevel up, and enter the skin directly over the vein at a 0- to 15-degree angle.

◆ Push the needle through the skin and into the vein in one motion.

◆ Check the flashback chamber behind the hub for a blood return.

◆ Level the insertion device slightly by lifting the tip of the device up to prevent puncturing the back wall of the vessel.

◆ If using a winged infusion device, advance the needle fully and hold it in place.

◆ Release the tourniquet, open the administration set, clamp slightly, and check for a free flow or an infiltration.

◆ If using an over-the-needle cannula, advance the device to at least half of its length to ensure that the cannula itself, not just the introducer needle, has entered the vein. Remove the tourniquet.

◆ Grasp the cannula hub to hold it in the vein, and withdraw the needle. As you withdraw it, press slightly on the catheter tip to prevent bleeding.

◆ Advance the cannula up to the hub or until you meet resistance.

- Using sterile technique, attach the I.V. tubing and begin the infusion.
- While stabilizing the vein with one hand, use the other to advance the catheter into the vein.
- Decrease the I.V. flow rate when the catheter is advanced.
- To advance the cannula before starting the infusion, release the tourniquet, stabilize the vein and needle, and advance the catheter off the needle and further into the vein up to the hub.
- Remove the inner needle quickly using sterile technique; attach the I.V. tubing.

DRESSING THE SITE
- Clean the skin completely.
- Use tape or a catheter stabilization device to secure the device.
- Cover with a transparent semipermeable dressing.
- Loop the I.V. tubing on the patient's limb, and secure the tubing with tape.
- Label the dressing with the type and length of the cannula, the gauge of needle, the date and time of insertion, and your initials.

REMOVING THE I.V. LINE
- Clamp the I.V. tubing to stop the flow of solution.
- Gently remove the transparent dressing and tape from the skin.
- Using aseptic technique, open the gauze pad and adhesive bandage, and place it within reach.
- Put on gloves.
- Hold the sterile gauze pad over the puncture site with one hand; use the other to withdraw the cannula slowly, keeping it parallel to the skin.
- Inspect the cannula tip; if it isn't smooth, assess the patient immediately and notify the practitioner.

- Using the gauze pad, apply firm pressure over the puncture site for 1 to 2 minutes after removal or until bleeding stops.
- Clean the site and apply the adhesive bandage or, if blood oozes, apply a pressure bandage.
- If drainage appears at the puncture site, swab the tip of the device across an agar plate.
- Clean the area and apply a sterile dressing.
- Obtain an order from the practitioner and send the specimen to the laboratory.
- Tell the patient to restrict activity for about 10 minutes and to leave the dressing in place for at least 1 hour.
- If tenderness persists at the site, apply warm packs and notify the practitioner.

SPECIAL CONSIDERATIONS

- If you fail to see flashback after the needle enters the vein, pull back slightly and rotate the device. If that doesn't work, remove the cannula and try again, or proceed according to your facility's policy.
- Change a gauze or transparent dressing whenever you change the administration set (every 48 to 72 hours or according to facility policy).
- Rotate the I.V. site, usually every 72 hours or according to facility policy.

COMPLICATIONS
- Infection
- Phlebitis
- Embolism
- Circulatory overload
- Infiltration
- Sepsis
- Allergic reaction

PATIENT TEACHING

- Instruct the patient on movement restrictions.
- Tell the patient to call the nurse if the I.V. fluid stops, an alarm goes off, or he has pain at the site.

DOCUMENTATION

- Record the date and time of venipuncture.
- Note the type, gauge, and length of the cannula or needle.
- Document the anatomic location of the insertion site.
- Note the reason for site changes.
- Document the number of attempts at venipuncture.
- Record the type and flow rate of the I.V. solution, including additives.
- Document adverse reactions and actions taken.
- Record patient teaching.

SELECTED REFERENCES
Blaivas, M. "Ultrasound-Guided Peripheral I.V. Insertion in the ED," *American Journal of Nursing* 105(10):54-57, October 2005.

Fein, J.A., and Gorelick, M.H. "The Decision to Use Topical Anesthetic for Intravenous Insertion in the Pediatric Emergency Department," *Academic Emergency Medicine* 13(3):264-68, March 2006.

Marders, J. "Sounding the Alarm for I.V. Infiltration," *Nursing* 35(4):18, 20, April 2005.

Moureau, N.L. "Tips for Inserting an I.V. in an Older Patient," *Nursing* 34(7):18, July 2004.

Rosenthal, K. "Selecting the Best I.V. Site for an Obese Patient," *Nursing* 34(11):14, November 2004.

Rosenthal, K. "Tailor Your I.V. Insertion Techniques Special Populations," *Nursing* 35(5):36-41, May 2005.

Peripheral I.V. catheter maintenance

OVERVIEW

DESCRIPTION
- Peripheral I.V. catheter maintenance includes regular assessment and rotation of site and periodic changes of dressing, tubing, and solution.
- Maintenance helps prevent complications, such as thrombophlebitis and infection.
- Gauze I.V. dressings are changed every 48 hours or when a dressing becomes wet, soiled, or nonocclusive.
- Transparent semipermeable dressings are changed when I.V. tubing is changed (every 48 to 72 hours or according to policy). I.V. solution is changed every 24 hours or as needed.
- The I.V. site should be assessed every 24 hours if a transparent semipermeable dressing is used or with every dressing change and should be rotated every 48 to 72 hours.

CONTRAINDICATIONS
- None known

EQUIPMENT

DRESSING CHANGES
Sterile gloves ◆ povidone-iodine or alcohol pads ◆ adhesive bandage ◆ sterile 2″ × 2″ gauze pad or transparent semipermeable dressing ◆ 1″ adhesive tape

SOLUTION CHANGES
Solution ◆ container ◆ alcohol pad

TUBING CHANGES
I.V. administration set ◆ sterile gloves ◆ sterile 2″ × 2″ gauze pad ◆ adhesive tape for labeling ◆ hemostat

I.V. SITE CHANGE
Alcohol pads or an approved antimicrobial solution such as chlorhexidine ◆ gloves ◆ tourniquet ◆ I.V. access device ◆ transparent semipermeable dressing ◆ 1″ hypoallergenic tape

PREPARATION
- Use a commercial dressing change kit if available.
- Keep I.V. equipment and dressings nearby.
- If you're changing the solution and the tubing, attach and prime the I.V. administration set before entering the patient's room.

KEY STEPS
- Confirm the patient's identity using two patient identifiers according to facility policy.
- Explain the procedure to the patient.
- Wash your hands.

CHANGING THE DRESSING
- Remove old dressing, open supply packages, and put on sterile gloves.
- Hold the cannula in place with your nondominant hand.
- Assess the venipuncture site for signs of infection (redness and pain at the puncture site), infiltration (coolness, blanching, and edema at the site), and thrombophlebitis (redness, firmness, pain along the path of the vein, and edema).
- If any signs are present, cover the area with a sterile 2″ × 2″ gauze pad, and remove the catheter or needle.
- Apply pressure to the area until bleeding stops, then apply an adhesive bandage.
- Using fresh equipment and solution, insert an I.V. catheter in another appropriate site, preferably on the opposite extremity.
- If the venipuncture site is intact, stabilize the cannula, and carefully clean around the puncture site with a povidone-iodine or alcohol pad.
- Work in a circular motion outward from the site to avoid introducing bacteria into the clean area.
- Allow the area to dry completely.
- Cover the site with a transparent semipermeable dressing.
- Place it over the insertion site to halfway up the hub of the cannula.

CHANGING THE SOLUTION
- Wash your hands.
- Inspect the new solution container for damage.
- Check the solution for discoloration, turbidity, and particulates.
- Note the date and time the solution was mixed and its expiration date.
- Clamp the tubing when inverting it to prevent air from entering the tubing.
- Keep the drip chamber one-half full.

- If replacing a bag, remove the seal or tab from the new bag, and remove the old bag from the pole.
- Remove the spike, insert it into the new bag, and adjust the flow rate.
- If you're replacing a bottle, remove the cap and seal from the new bottle, and wipe the rubber port with an alcohol pad.
- Clamp the line, remove the spike from the old bottle, and insert the spike into the new bottle.
- Hang the new bottle and adjust the flow rate.

CHANGING THE TUBING
- Prime the new system using new I.V. solution.
- Hang the new I.V. container and primed set on the pole, and grasp the new adapter in one hand.
- Stop the flow rate in the old tubing.
- Put on sterile gloves.
- Place a sterile gauze pad under the needle or cannula hub to create a sterile field.
- Press one of your fingers over the cannula to prevent bleeding.
- Gently disconnect the old tubing, being careful not to dislodge or move the I.V. device.
- Use a hemostat if needed to hold the hub securely while twisting the tubing to remove it, or use one hemostat on the venipuncture device and another on the hard plastic end of the tubing.
- Pull the hemostats in opposite directions. Don't clamp the hemostats shut; this may crack the tubing adapter or the venipuncture device.
- Remove the protective cap from the new tubing, and connect the new adapter to the cannula tip.
- Hold the hub securely to prevent dislodging the needle or cannula tip.
- Observe for blood backflow into the new tubing to verify that the needle or cannula is still in place.
- Adjust the clamp to maintain the appropriate flow rate.
- Retape the cannula hub and I.V. tubing. Recheck the I.V. flow rate because taping may alter it.
- Label the new tubing and container with the date and time.

- Label the solution container with a time strip.

SPECIAL CONSIDERATIONS
- Check the prescribed I.V. flow rate before each solution change to prevent errors.
- If you crack the adapter or hub (or if you accidentally dislodge the cannula from the vein), remove the cannula.
- Apply pressure and an adhesive bandage to stop bleeding.
- Perform a venipuncture at another site, and restart the I.V. solution.

COMPLICATIONS
- Accidental dislodgement of I.V. catheter

PATIENT TEACHING
- Explain the procedure to the patient and enlist his cooperation with movement restriction.

DOCUMENTATION
- Note the time, date, rate, and type of solution (and additives) on the I.V. flowchart.
- Record dressing and tubing changes.
- Document the appearance of the site in your notes.

SELECTED REFERENCES
Higgins, D. "Priming an I.V. Infusion Set," *Nursing Times* 100(47):32-33, November 2004.
Rosenthal, K. "Documenting Peripheral I.V. Therapy," *Nursing* 35(7):28, July 2005.
Wotton, K., et al. "Flushing an I.V. Line: A Simple but Potentially Costly Procedure for Both Patient and Health Unit," *Contemporary Nurse* 17(3):264-73, October 2004.
Zahourek, R. "Nursing the I.V. Tubing," *AJN* 105(10):15, October 2005.

Peripherally inserted central catheter insertion and

DESCRIPTION

- A single-, double-, or triple-lumen central catheter that's inserted via a peripheral vein is the best option for the patient who needs prolonged central venous therapy or requires repeated venous access.
- It helps avoid complications that may occur with a central venous line.
- Made of silicone or polyurethane, the peripherally inserted central catheter (PICC) is soft and flexible with increased biocompatibility.
- Catheters range from 16G to 23G in diameter and 16″ to 24″ (40.5 to 61 cm) in length.
- Common infusions include total parenteral nutrition, chemotherapy, antibiotics, opioids, and analgesics.
- A PICC works best when introduced early in treatment.
- If state law permits, a specially trained nurse may perform the procedure.

CONTRAINDICATIONS

- History of deep vein thrombosis (DVT)
- Mastectomy arm shouldn't be used

EQUIPMENT

Prepackaged catheter insertion kit (if available) ◆ three alcohol swabs or other approved antimicrobial solution, such as 10% povidone-iodine or tincture of iodine ◆ 2% povidone-iodine ointment ◆ 3-ml vial of heparin (100 units/ml) ◆ injection port with short extension tubing ◆ sterile and clean measuring tape ◆ vial of normal saline solution ◆ sterile gauze pads ◆ tape ◆ linen-saver pad ◆ sterile drapes ◆ tourniquet ◆ sterile transparent semipermeable dressing ◆ two pairs of sterile gloves ◆ sterile gown ◆ mask ◆ goggles ◆ clean gloves ◆ sterile labels ◆ sterile markers

KEY STEPS

- Describe the procedure to the patient.
- Wash your hands before procedures.
- Assemble equipment for each procedure as needed.

INSERTING THE CATHETER

- Confirm the patient's identity using two patient identifiers according to facility policy.
- Select an insertion site, and place the tourniquet on the patient's arm.
- Determine the catheter tip placement or spot at which the catheter tip will rest after insertion.
- For placement in the superior vena cava, measure the distance from the insertion site to the shoulder and from his shoulder to the sternal notch. Then add 3″ (7.6 cm) to the measurement.
- Have the patient lie in a supine position with his arm at a 90-degree angle to his body.
- Place a linen-saver pad under his arm.
- Open the PICC tray and place the rest of the sterile items onto the sterile field.
- Label all medications, medication containers, and solution containers on and off the sterile field.
- Put on a sterile gown, mask, goggles, and gloves.
- Using the sterile measuring tape, cut the distal end of the catheter according to the specific manufacturer's recommendations and guidelines.
- Withdraw 5 ml of normal saline solution, and remove the needle from the syringe.
- Attach the syringe to the hub of the catheter and flush.
- Prepare the insertion site by rubbing it with three alcohol swabs or other approved antimicrobial solution. Use a back-and-forth motion, working outward from the site to about 6″ (15 cm) away from the site.
- Allow the area to dry.

- Take off your gloves and apply the tourniquet about 4″ (10 cm) above the antecubital fossa.
- Put on new sterile gloves and put a sterile drape under the patient's arm and another on top of his arm.
- Put a sterile 4″ × 4″ gauze pad on the tourniquet.
- Stabilize the patient's vein and insert the catheter introducer at a 10-degree angle directly into the vein.
- After successful vein entry, you'll see a blood return in the flashback chamber.
- Gently advance the plastic introducer sheath until you're sure the tip is well within the vein.
- Remove the tourniquet using the sterile 4″×4″ gauze pad.
- Carefully withdraw the needle while holding the introducer still.
- Using sterile forceps, insert the catheter into the introducer sheath, and advance it into the vein 2″ to 4″ (5 to 10 cm).
- Advance the catheter to the shoulder, then ask the patient to turn his head toward the affected arm and place his chin on his chest.
- Advance the catheter until about 4″ remain.
- Pull the introducer sheath out of the vein and away from the venipuncture site.
- Grab the tabs of the introducer sheath, and flex them toward its distal end to split the sheath completely.
- Discard the sheath.
- Advance the catheter until it's completely inserted.
- Flush with normal saline solution followed by heparin according to facility policy.
- With the patient's arm below heart level, remove the syringe, and connect the capped extension set to the hub of the catheter.
- Apply a sterile transparent semipermeable dressing over the site. Leave this dressing on for 24 hours.
- After the initial 24 hours, apply a new sterile transparent semipermeable dressing, and flush with heparin.

removal

ADMINISTERING DRUGS

◆ Check for blood return, and flush with 3 ml of normal saline solution in a 10 ml syringe before and after administering a drug.
◆ Flush with normal saline solution between infusions of incompatible drugs or fluids.

CHANGING THE DRESSING

◆ Change the dressing every 3 to 7 days, or more frequently if needed.
◆ Use aseptic technique.
◆ To prevent embolism, position the patient with his arm extended away from his body at a 45- to 90-degree angle so the insertion site is below heart level.
◆ Put on a sterile mask.
◆ Open a package of sterile gloves, and use the inside of the package as a sterile field.
◆ Open the transparent semipermeable dressing, and drop it onto the field.
◆ Put on clean gloves and remove the old dressing.
◆ Remove the clean gloves and put on sterile gloves.
◆ Clean the area thoroughly with three alcohol swabs or other approved antimicrobial solution, starting at the insertion site and working back and forth.
◆ Repeat the step three times with antimicrobial solution and let dry.
◆ Apply the dressing.
◆ Secure the tubing to the edge of the dressing over the tape with ¼" adhesive tape.

REMOVING THE CATHETER

◆ Remove the tape holding the extension tubing.
◆ Open two sterile gauze pads on a clean, flat surface.
◆ Put on clean gloves.
◆ Stabilize the catheter at the hub with one hand.
◆ Without dislodging the catheter, use your other hand to gently remove the dressing by pulling it toward the insertion site.
◆ Withdraw the catheter in small, slow increments. If you feel resistance, stop.

◆ Apply slight tension to the line by taping it down.
◆ Try to remove it again after a few minutes. If you still feel resistance, notify the practitioner for further instructions.
◆ Once you remove the catheter, apply manual pressure to the site with a sterile gauze pad for 1 minute.
◆ Inspect the catheters. If any part has broken off during removal, notify the practitioner immediately, and monitor the patient for signs of distress.

⚡ **WARNING** *If a portion of the catheter breaks during removal, immediately apply a tourniquet to the upper arm, close to the axilla, to prevent the catheter piece from advancing into the right atrium. Check the patient's radial pulse. If you don't detect the radial pulse, the tourniquet is too tight. Keep the tourniquet in place until an X-ray can be obtained, the practitioner is notified, and surgical retrieval is attempted.*

◆ Cover the site with povidone-iodine ointment, and tape a new folded gauze pad in place.

SPECIAL CONSIDERATIONS

◆ The practitioner or nurse inserts a PICC by way of the basilic, median cubital, or cephalic vein. It's then threaded to the superior vena cava or subclavian vein.
◆ Flush the catheter per facility policy.
◆ Use a declotting agent to clear a clotted PICC per manufacturer's recommendations and facility policy.
◆ Assess the catheter insertion site through the transparent semipermeable dressing every 12 hours.
◆ Assess for bleeding, redness, drainage, swelling, and pain.
◆ Although oozing is common for the first 24 hours after insertion, excessive bleeding after that should be evaluated.

COMPLICATIONS

◆ Air embolism
◆ Catheter tip migration or breakage on removal
◆ Catheter occlusion
◆ DVT

PATIENT TEACHING

◆ Explain the procedure, as needed, to lessen the patient's anxiety.

DOCUMENTATION

◆ Record the entire procedure and any problems.
◆ Note the size, length, and type of catheter.
◆ Document the insertion site.

SELECTED REFERENCES

DeLegge, M.H., et al. "Central Venous Access in the Home Parenteral Nutrition Population-You PICC," *Journal of Parenteral and Enteral Nutrition* 29(6): 425-28, November-December 2005.

Falkowski, A. "Improving the PICC Insertion Process," *Nursing* 36(2):26-27, February 2006.

Knue, M., et al. "Peripherally Inserted Central Catheters in Children: A Survey of Practice Patterns," *Journal of Infusion Nursing* 29(1):28-33, January-February 2006.

Moureau, N. "Vascular Safety: It's All About PICCs," *Nursing Management* 37(5):22-27, May 2006.

Todd, J., and Hammond, P. "Choice and Use of Peripherally Inserted Central Catheters by Nurses," *Professional Nurse* 19(9):493-97, May 2004.

Peritoneal dialysis

DESCRIPTION

- Dialysate, solution instilled into the peritoneal cavity by a catheter to draw waste products, excess fluid, and electrolytes from the blood across the semipermeable peritoneal membrane. (See *How peritoneal dialysis works.*)
- After a prescribed period, dialysate is drained from the peritoneal cavity, removing impurities with it.
- Indicated for chronic renal failure with cardiovascular instability, vascular access problems that prevent hemodialysis, fluid overload, or electrolyte imbalances.
- The catheter is inserted in the operating room or, in acute situations, at the patient's bedside with nursing assistance.
- Specially trained nurses may perform dialysis, either manually or using an automatic or semiautomatic cycle machine.

CONTRAINDICATIONS

- Extensive abdominal or bowel surgery
- Extensive abdominal trauma
- Severe vascular disease
- Obesity
- Respiratory distress
- Abdominal infection

All equipment must be sterile. Commercially packaged dialysis kits or trays are available.

CATHETER PLACEMENT AND DIALYSIS

Prescribed dialysate ◆ warmer ◆ heating pad or water bath ◆ three face masks ◆ medication such as heparin ◆ ordered dialysis administration set with drainage bag ◆ two pairs of sterile gloves ◆ I.V. pole ◆ fenestrated sterile drape ◆ vial of 1% or 2% lidocaine ◆ iodine pads ◆ 3-ml syringe with 25G 1″ needle ◆ scalpel (with #11 blade) ◆ ordered type of multi-eyed nylon peritoneal catheter ◆ peritoneal stylet ◆ sutures or hypoallergenic tape ◆ povidone-iodine solution (to prepare abdomen) ◆ sterile marker ◆ sterile labels ◆ precut drain dressings ◆ cap for catheter ◆ small, sterile plastic clamp ◆ 4″ × 4″ gauze pads ◆ protein or potassium supplement ◆ specimen container ◆ 10-ml syringe with 22G 1½″ needle (optional)

DRESSING CHANGES

One pair of sterile gloves ◆ 10 sterile cotton-tipped applicators or sterile 2″ × 2″ gauze pads ◆ povidone-iodine ointment ◆ two precut drain dressings ◆ adhesive tape ◆ povidone-iodine solution or normal saline solution ◆ two sterile 4″ × 4″ gauze pads

PREPARATION

- Bring all equipment to the patient's bedside.
- Warm the dialysate to body temperature with a heating pad or commercial warmer.

- Confirm the patient's identity using two patient identifiers according to facility policy.

How peritoneal dialysis works

Peritoneal dialysis works through a combination of diffusion and osmosis.

DIFFUSION

In diffusion, particles move through a semipermeable membrane from an area of high-solute concentration to an area of low-solute concentration.

In peritoneal dialysis, the water-based dialysate being infused contains glucose, sodium chloride, calcium, magnesium, acetate or lactate, and no waste products. Waste products and excess electrolytes in the blood cross through the semipermeable peritoneal membrane into the dialysate. Removing waste-filled dialysate and replacing it with fresh solution keeps waste concentration low and encourages further diffusion.

OSMOSIS

In osmosis, fluids move through a semipermeable membrane from an area of low-solute concentration to an area of high-solute concentration. In peritoneal dialysis, dextrose is added to the dialysate to give it a higher solute concentration than the blood, creating a high osmotic gradient. Water migrates from the blood through the membrane at the beginning of each infusion, when the osmotic gradient is highest.

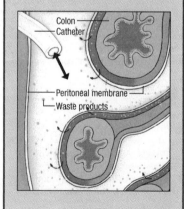

Colon — Catheter — Peritoneal membrane — Waste products

- Explain the procedure to the patient.
- Assess and record vital signs, weight, and abdominal girth to establish baseline levels.
- Review recent laboratory values, including blood urea nitrogen, creatinine, sodium, potassium, and complete blood count.
- Assess the patient's hepatitis B and human immunodeficiency virus status if known.

CATHETER PLACEMENT AND DIALYSIS

- Have the patient try to urinate.
- If he can't urinate and you suspect his bladder isn't empty, obtain an order for straight catheterization to empty his bladder.
- Put the patient in the supine position, and have him put on a sterile face mask.
- Wash your hands.
- Inspect the warmed dialysate, which should appear clear and colorless.
- Put on a sterile face mask.
- Prepare to add prescribed drug to the dialysate, using strict aseptic technique to avoid contaminating the solution.
- Label all medications, medication containers, and solution containers on and off the sterile field.
- Prepare the dialysis administration set. (See *Setup for peritoneal dialysis.*)
- Close the clamps on all lines.
- Place the drainage bag below the patient to facilitate gravity drainage, and connect the drainage line to it.
- Connect the dialysate infusion lines to the bottles or bags of dialysate using aseptic technique.
- Hang the bottles or bags on the I.V. pole at the patient's bedside.
- Prime the tubing and close all clamps.
- The practitioner cleans the patient's abdomen with povidone-iodine solution and drapes it with a sterile drape.

- Wipe the stopper of the lidocaine vial with povidone-iodine, and allow it to dry.
- Invert the vial, so the practitioner can withdraw lidocaine using the 3-ml syringe with the 25G 1″ needle.
- The practitioner anesthetizes a small area of the patient's abdomen below the umbilicus.
- The practitioner makes a small incision with the scalpel, inserts the catheter into the peritoneal cavity — using the stylet to guide the catheter — and sutures or tapes the catheter in place.
- If the catheter is already in place, clean the site with povidone-iodine solution in a circular outward motion before each dialysis treatment.
- Connect the catheter to the administration set using strict aseptic technique to prevent contamination of

the catheter and solution, which may cause peritonitis.
- Open the drain dressing and the 4″×4″ gauze pad packages, and put on the other pair of sterile gloves.
- Apply the precut drain dressings around the catheter, cover them with the gauze pads, and tape them securely.
- Unclamp the lines to the patient.
- Rapidly instill 500 ml of dialysate into the peritoneal cavity to test the catheter's patency.
- Clamp the lines to the patient.
- Immediately unclamp the lines to the drainage bag to allow fluid to drain into the bag. Outflow should be brisk.
- Having established the catheter's patency, clamp the lines to the drainage bag, and unclamp the lines to the patient to infuse the prescribed volume

(continued)

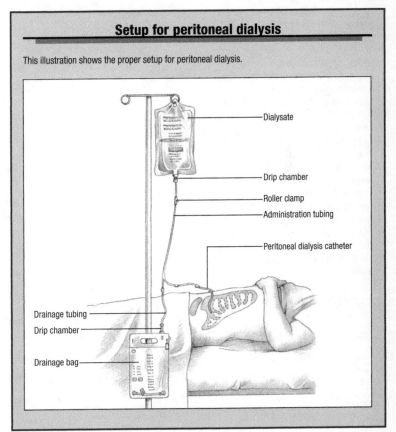

Setup for peritoneal dialysis

This illustration shows the proper setup for peritoneal dialysis.

- Dialysate
- Drip chamber
- Roller clamp
- Administration tubing
- Peritoneal dialysis catheter
- Drainage tubing
- Drip chamber
- Drainage bag

of solution over a period of 5 to 10 minutes.

- As soon as the dialysate container empties, clamp the lines to the patient to prevent air from entering the tubing.
- Allow the solution to dwell in the peritoneal cavity for the prescribed time (10 minutes to 4 hours).
- Warm the solution for the next infusion.
- At the end of the prescribed dwell time, unclamp the line to the drainage bag, and allow the solution to drain from the peritoneal cavity into the drainage bag (normally 20 to 30 minutes).
- Repeat the infusion-dwell-drain cycle until the prescribed number of fluid exchanges have been completed.
- If the practitioner or facility policy requires a dialysate specimen, collect one after every 10 infusion-dwell-drain cycles (always during the drain phase), after every 24-hour period, or as ordered.
- To do this, attach the 10-ml syringe to the 22G 1½" needle, insert it into the injection port on the drainage line using strict aseptic technique, and aspirate the drainage sample.
- Transfer the sample to the specimen container.
- Label it, and send it to the laboratory with a request form.
- After completing the prescribed number of exchanges, clamp the catheter and put on sterile gloves.
- Disconnect the administration set from the peritoneal catheter.
- Place the sterile protective cap over the catheter's distal end.
- Dispose of used equipment appropriately.

DRESSING CHANGES

- Explain the procedure to the patient.
- Wash your hands.
- Carefully remove the old dressings.
- Put on the sterile gloves.
- Saturate the sterile applicators or the 2"×2" gauze pads with povidone-iodine.
- Clean the skin around the catheter, moving in concentric circles from the catheter site outward.
- Remove crusted material.
- Inspect the catheter site for drainage.
- Inspect the tissue around the site for redness and swelling.
- Apply povidone-iodine ointment to the catheter site with a sterile gauze pad.
- Place two precut drain dressings around the catheter site.
- Tape the 4"×4" gauze pads over them to secure the dressing.

SPECIAL CONSIDERATIONS

- Monitor the patient during and after dialysis.
- Monitor the patient's vital signs every 10 to 15 minutes for the first 1 to 2 hours of exchanges, then every 2 to 4 hours, or more frequently if necessary.
- Notify the practitioner of abrupt changes in the patient's condition.
- To reduce the risk of peritonitis, use strict aseptic technique during catheter insertion, dialysis, and dressing changes.
- Masks should be worn by all personnel in the room whenever the dialysis system is opened or entered.
- Change the dressing at least every 24 hours or whenever it becomes wet or soiled.
- To prevent respiratory distress, position the patient for maximal lung expansion.
- Promote lung expansion through turning and deep-breathing exercises.

WARNING If the patient suffers severe respiratory distress during the dwell phase of dialysis, drain the peritoneal cavity and notify the practitioner.

- To prevent protein depletion, the practitioner may order a high-protein diet or a protein supplement. He'll also monitor albumin levels.
- Dialysate is available in three concentrations — 4.25% dextrose, 2.5% dextrose, and 1.5% dextrose. The 4.25% solution removes the largest amount of fluid from the blood.
- If your patient receives this concentrated solution, monitor him carefully to prevent excess fluid loss.
- Some of the glucose in the 4.25% solution may enter the patient's bloodstream, causing hyperglycemia severe enough to require an insulin injection or an insulin addition to the dialysate.
- Patients with low potassium levels may require the addition of potassium to the dialysate solution to prevent further losses.

- Monitor fluid volume balance, blood pressure, and pulse.
- Assess fluid balance at the end of each infusion-dwell-drain cycle.
- Notify the practitioner if the patient retains 500 ml or more of fluid for three consecutive cycles or loses at least 1 L of fluid for three consecutive cycles.
- Weigh the patient daily to help determine fluid loss.
- If inflow and outflow are slow or absent, check the tubing for kinks, raise the I.V. pole, or reposition the patient to increase the inflow rate.
- Repositioning the patient or applying manual pressure to the lateral aspects of his abdomen may help increase drainage.
- If these maneuvers fail, notify the practitioner.
- Improper positioning of the catheter or an accumulation of fibrin may obstruct the catheter.
- Always examine outflow fluid (effluent) for color and clarity.
- If the effluent remains pink-tinged or is grossly bloody, suspect bleeding into the peritoneal cavity, and notify the practitioner.
- Notify the practitioner if the outflow contains feces, which suggests bowel perforation, or if it's cloudy, which suggests peritonitis.
- Patient discomfort at the start of the procedure is normal.
- If the patient experiences pain during the procedure, determine when it occurs, its quality and duration, and whether it radiates to other body parts. Notify the practitioner as necessary.
- Pain during infusion usually results from a dialysate that's too cool or acidic or from rapid inflow.
- Severe, diffuse pain with rebound tenderness and cloudy effluent may indicate peritoneal infection.
- Pain that radiates to the shoulder commonly results from air accumulation under the diaphragm.
- Severe perineal or rectal pain can result from improper catheter placement.

- The patient undergoing peritoneal dialysis requires assistance in his daily care.
- To minimize discomfort, perform daily care during a drain phase in the cycle, when his abdomen is less distended.

COMPLICATIONS
- Peritonitis
- Protein depletion
- Respiratory distress
- Constipation
- Hypovolemia
- Hypotension
- Shock
- Blood volume expansion
- Hypertension
- Peripheral edema
- Pulmonary edema
- Heart failure
- Electrolyte imbalance
- Hyperglycemia
- Catheter occlusion or dislodgement

PATIENT TEACHING
- Explain the procedure to the patient to lessen anxiety.
- Teach the patient signs and symptoms of infection and when to report them.
- Explain the need for follow-up home care if peritoneal dialysis will continue after discharge.

DOCUMENTATION
- Record the amount of dialysate infused and drained.
- Note drugs added to the solution.
- Document the color and character of effluent.
- Record daily weight and fluid balance.
- Record vital signs and tolerance of the treatment.
- Document abrupt changes in the patient's condition.
- Record each time you notify the practitioner of an abnormality.
- Complete a peritoneal dialysis flowchart every 24 hours.
- Note the condition of the patient's skin at the dialysis catheter site.
- Document the patient's reports of unusual discomfort or pain.
- Record your interventions and outcomes.

SELECTED REFERENCES
Bernardini, J. "Peritoneal Dialysis: Myths, Barriers, and Achieving Optimum Outcomes," *Nephrology Nursing Journal* 31(5):494-98, September-October 2004.

Kelley, K.T. "How Peritoneal Dialysis Works," *Nephrology Nursing Journal* 31(5):481-82, 488-89, September-October 2004.

Redmond, A., and Doherty, E. "Peritoneal Dialysis," *Nursing Standard* 19(40): 55-65, June 2005.

Zorzanello, M.M. "Peritoneal Dialysis and Hemodialysis: Similarities and Differences," *Nephrology Nursing Journal* 31(5):588-89, September-October 2004.

Peritoneal dialysis, continuous ambulatory

DESCRIPTION
- Use of a permanent peritoneal catheter (such as a Tenckhoff catheter), which serves as a port to circulate dialysate continuously in the peritoneal cavity.
- The catheter is inserted under local anesthetic; the catheter is sutured in place, and the distal portion is tunneled subcutaneously to the skin surface.
- It's commonly used for patients with end-stage renal disease.
- It can be a helpful alternative to hemodialysis; it also gives the patient more independence and requires less travel for treatments.
- It provides more stable fluid and electrolyte levels than conventional hemodialysis.

CONTRAINDICATIONS
- Recent abdominal surgery
- Abdominal adhesions
- Infected abdominal wall
- Diaphragmatic tears
- Ileus
- Respiratory insufficiency

EQUIPMENT

All equipment for infusing dialysate and discontinuing procedure must be sterile. Commercially prepared sterile continuous ambulatory peritoneal dialysis kits are available.

INFUSING DIALYSATE
Prescribed amount of dialysate (usually in 2-L bags) ◆ heating pad or commercial warmer ◆ three face masks ◆ 42" (106.7 cm) connective tubing with drain clamp ◆ six to eight packages of sterile 4" × 4" gauze pads ◆ povidone-iodine pads ◆ hypoallergenic tape ◆ plastic snap-top container ◆ povidone-iodine solution ◆ sterile basin ◆ container of alcohol ◆ sterile gloves ◆ belt or fabric pouch ◆ two sterile waterproof paper drapes (one fenestrated) ◆ educational materials (if ordered) ◆

syringes and labeled specimen container (optional)

DISCONTINUING DIALYSIS TEMPORARILY
Three sterile waterproof paper barriers (two fenestrated) ◆ 4" × 4" gauze pads (for cleaning and dressing the catheter) ◆ two face masks ◆ sterile basin ◆ hypoallergenic tape ◆ povidone-iodine solution ◆ sterile gloves ◆ sterile rubber catheter cap

PREPARATION
- Check the concentration of the dialysate against the practitioner's order.
- Check the expiration date.
- Ensure the solution is clear, not cloudy.
- Warm the solution to body temperature with a heating pad or commercial warmer, not a microwave oven.
- Wash your hands, and put on a surgical mask.
- Remove the dialysate container from the warming setup, and remove its protective wrapper.
- Squeeze the bag firmly to check for leaks.
- If ordered, use a syringe to add prescribed medication to the dialysate, using sterile technique.
- Insert the connective tubing into the dialysate container.
- Open the drain clamp to prime the tube, and then close the clamp.
- Place a povidone-iodine pad on the dialysate container's port.
- Cover the port with a dry gauze pad, and secure the pad with tape.
- Remove and discard the surgical mask.
- Commercial devices with povidone-iodine pads are available for covering the dialysate container and tubing connection.

KEY STEPS

- Weigh the patient to establish a baseline level. Weigh him at the same time every day.
- Explain all procedures before performing them.

INFUSING DIALYSATE
- Confirm the patient's identity using two patient identifiers according to facility policy.
- Prepare the sterile field by placing a waterproof, sterile paper drape on a dry surface near the patient.
- Fill the snap-top container with povidone-iodine solution, and place it on the sterile field.
- Place the basin on the sterile field.
- Place four pairs of sterile gauze pads in the sterile basin, and saturate them with the povidone-iodine solution.
- Drop the remaining gauze pads on the sterile field.
- Loosen the cap on the alcohol container, and place it next to the sterile field.
- Put on a clean surgical mask, and provide one for the patient.
- Carefully remove and discard the dressing covering the peritoneal catheter.
- Be careful not to touch the catheter or skin.
- Check skin integrity at the catheter site, and look for signs of infection.
- If drainage is present, obtain a swab specimen, put it in a labeled specimen container, and notify the practitioner.
- Put on the sterile gloves, and palpate the insertion site and subcutaneous tunnel route for tenderness or pain. If these symptoms occur, notify the practitioner.

⚡ **WARNING** *If the patient has drainage, tenderness, or pain, don't proceed with the infusion without specific orders.*

- Wrap one gauze pad saturated with povidone-iodine solution around the distal end of the catheter, and leave it in place for 5 minutes.
- Clean the catheter and insertion site with the rest of the gauze pads, moving in concentric circles away from the insertion site.
- Use straight strokes to clean the catheter, beginning at the insertion site and moving outward.
- Use a clean area of the pad for each stroke.

- Loosen the catheter cap one notch, and clean the exposed area.
- After using the third pair of pads, place the fenestrated paper drape around the base of the catheter.
- Continue cleaning the catheter for another minute with one of the remaining pads soaked with povidone-iodine.
- Remove the povidone-iodine pad on the catheter cap, remove the cap, and use the remaining povidone-iodine pad to clean the end of the catheter hub.
- Attach the connective tubing from the dialysate container to the catheter and secure tightly.
- Open the drain clamp on the dialysate container to allow the solution to enter the peritoneal cavity by gravity over a period of 5 to 10 minutes.
- Close the drain clamp.
- Fold the bag and secure it with a belt, or tuck it in the patient's clothing or a small fabric pouch.
- After the prescribed dwell time (usually 4 to 6 hours), unfold the bag, open the clamp, and allow peritoneal fluid to drain back into the bag by gravity.
- When drainage is complete, attach a new bag of dialysate, and repeat the infusion.
- Discard used supplies appropriately.

DISCONTINUING DIALYSIS TEMPORARILY
- Wash your hands, and put on a surgical mask.
- Provide a surgical mask for the patient.
- Using sterile gloves, remove the dressing over the peritoneal catheter.
- Set up a sterile field next to the patient. Maintain the drape's sterility.
- Put equipment on the sterile field; place the 4″ × 4″ gauze pads in the basin.
- Saturate them with the povidone-iodine solution.
- Open the 4″ × 4″ gauze pads to be used as the dressing, and drop them onto the sterile field.
- Tape the dialysate tubing to the bedside rail to keep the catheter and tubing off the patient's abdomen.

- Change to another pair of sterile gloves.
- Place one of the fenestrated drapes around the base of the catheter.
- Use a pair of povidone-iodine pads to clean about 6″ (15 cm) of the dialysis tubing.
- Clean for 1 minute, moving away from the catheter.
- Clean the catheter, moving from the insertion site to the junction of the catheter and dialysis tubing.
- Use two more pairs of pads to clean the junction for a total of 3 minutes.
- Place the second fenestrated paper drape over the first at the base of the catheter.
- With the fourth pair of pads, clean the junction of the catheter and 6″ of the dialysate tubing for another minute.
- Disconnect the dialysate tubing from the catheter.
- Pick up the catheter cap, and fasten it to the catheter, making sure it fits securely over both notches of the hard plastic catheter tip.
- Clean the insertion site and a 2″ (5-cm) radius around it with povidone-iodine pads, working from the insertion site outward.
- Let the skin air-dry before applying the dressing.
- Discard used supplies appropriately.

SPECIAL CONSIDERATIONS
- If inflow or outflow are slow or absent, check the tubing for kinks, or try raising the solution or repositioning the patient to increase the flow.
- Repositioning the patient or applying manual pressure to the lateral aspects of the patient's abdomen may also help increase drainage.

COMPLICATIONS
- Peritonitis with possible septicemia and death
- Excessive fluid loss
- Excessive fluid retention
- Catheter obstruction or dislodgement

PATIENT TEACHING
- Explain the procedure to the patient to reduce anxiety.

DOCUMENTATION
- Record the type and amount of fluid instilled and returned for each exchange.
- Note the time and duration of exchange.
- Document drugs added to the dialysate.
- Record the color and clarity of the returned exchange fluid.
- Note the presence of mucus, pus, or blood.
- Note the patient's weight, blood pressure, and pulse rate after his last fluid exchange for the day.

SELECTED REFERENCES
Borazan, A., et al. "The Comparison in Terms of Early Complications of a New Technique and Percutaneous Method for the Placement of CAPD Catheters," *Renal Failure* 28(1):37-42, 2006.

Chow, K.M., et al. "Continuous Ambulatory Peritoneal Dialysis in Patients with Hepatitis B Liver Disease," *Peritoneal Dialysis International* 26(2):213-17, March-April 2006.

Garcia-Urena, M.A., et al. "Prevalence and Management of Hernias in Peritoneal Dialysis Patients," *Peritoneal Dialysis International* 26(2):198-202, March-April 2006.

Schuetz, C.E. "Training a Continuous Ambulatory Peritoneal Dialysis Patient with One Functional Arm," *Advances in Peritoneal Dialysis* 21:146-47, 2005.

Wright, L.S. "Training a Patient With Visual Impairment on Continuous Ambulatory Peritoneal Dialysis," *Nephrology Nursing Journal* 32(6): 675, 677, November-December 2005.

Peritoneal lavage

DESCRIPTION

◆ Procedure used to detect bleeding in the peritoneal cavity in a patient who's experienced blunt abdominal trauma.

◆ The practitioner inserts the catheter through the abdominal wall into the peritoneal cavity and aspirates peritoneal fluid with a syringe.

◆ The medical team maintains strict aseptic technique to avoid introducing microorganisms into the peritoneum, which may cause peritonitis.

CONTRAINDICATIONS

◆ Presence of multiple abdominal operations or adhesions

◆ Abdominal wall hematoma

◆ Unstable patient in need of immediate surgery

◆ Patient who can't be catheterized before the procedure

EQUIPMENT

Indwelling urinary catheter ◆ catheter insertion kit ◆ drainage bag ◆ nasogastric (NG) tube ◆ gastric suction machine ◆ shaving kit ◆ I.V. pole ◆ macrodrip I.V. tubing ◆ I.V. solutions (1 L of warmed, balanced saline solution, usually lactated Ringer's solution or normal saline solution) ◆ sterile specimen labels ◆ sterile marker ◆ three containers for specimen collection including one sterile tube for a culture and sensitivity ◆ antiseptic ointment ◆ 4″ × 4″ gauze pads ◆ alcohol pads ◆ 1″ hypoallergenic tape ◆ 2-0 and 3-0 sutures ◆ peritoneal dialysis tray with: sterile gloves, gown, goggles, antiseptic solution (such as povidone-iodine), 3-ml syringe with 25G 1″ needle, bottle of 1% lidocaine with epinephrine, 8″ (20.3 cm) #14 intracatheter, extension tubing, small sterile hemostat (to clamp tubing), 30-ml syringe, one 20G 1½″ needle, and sterile towels

PREPARATION

◆ If using a commercially prepared peritoneal dialysis kit (containing a #15 peritoneal dialysis catheter, trocar, and extension tubing with roller clamp), make sure the macrodrip I.V. tubing doesn't have a reverse flow (or back-check) valve that prevents infused fluid from draining out of the peritoneal cavity.

KEY STEPS

◆ Confirm the patient's identity using two patient identifiers according to facility policy.

◆ Provide privacy and wash your hands.

◆ Reinforce the practitioner's explanation of the procedure.

◆ Put on the gown and goggles.

◆ Advise the patient to expect a sensation of abdominal fullness.

◆ Inform him that he may experience a chill if the lavage solution isn't warmed or doesn't reach his body temperature.

◆ Catheterize the patient with the indwelling urinary catheter, and connect this catheter to a drainage bag.

◆ Insert an NG tube and attach to the gastric suction machine (set for low intermittent suction).

◆ Using the shaving kit, clip or shave the hair, as ordered, from the area between the patient's umbilicus and pubis.

◆ Place the lavage solution container on the I.V. pole.

◆ Attach the macrodrip tubing to the container, and clear air from the tubing.

◆ Using aseptic technique, open the peritoneal dialysis tray.

◆ Label all medications, medication containers, and solution containers on and off the sterile field.

◆ The practitioner will wipe the patient's abdomen from the costal margin to the pubic area and from flank to flank with the antiseptic solution.

◆ He'll drape the area with sterile towels to create a sterile field.

◆ Using aseptic technique, hand the practitioner the 3-ml syringe and the 25G 1″ needle.

◆ If the peritoneal dialysis tray doesn't contain a sterile ampule of anesthetic, wipe the top of a multidose vial of 1% lidocaine with epinephrine with an alcohol pad, and invert the vial at a 45-degree angle so the practitioner can insert the needle and withdraw the anesthetic without touching the nonsterile vial.

◆ The practitioner injects the anesthetic directly below the umbilicus.

◆ When the area is numb, he makes an incision, inserts the catheter or trocar, withdraws fluid, and checks the findings.

◆ If findings are positive, the procedure ends, and you'll prepare the patient for laparotomy and further measures.

◆ Even if retrieved fluid looks normal, lavage will continue.

◆ Wearing gloves, connect the catheter extension tubing to the I.V. tubing, if ordered, and instill 500 to 1,000 ml (10 ml/kg body weight) of the warmed I.V. solution into the peritoneal cavity over 5 to 10 minutes.

◆ Clamp the tubing with a hemostat.

◆ Unless contraindicated, turn the patient from side to side to distribute the fluid throughout the peritoneal cavity.

◆ If the patient's condition contraindicates turning, the practitioner may gently palpate the sides of the abdomen to distribute the fluid.

◆ After 5 to 10 minutes, place the I.V. container below the level of the patient's body, and open the clamp on the I.V. tubing to drain the fluid.

◆ Drain as much fluid as possible from the peritoneal cavity to the container.

◆ Be careful not to disconnect the tubing from the catheter.

◆ The peritoneal cavity may take 20 to 30 minutes to drain completely.

◆ Although you don't need to vent a plastic bag container, be sure to vent glass I.V. containers with a needle to promote flow.

- To obtain a fluid specimen, put on gloves and use a 30-ml syringe and 20G 1½" needle to withdraw between 25 and 30 ml of fluid from a port in the I.V. tubing.
- Clean the top of each specimen container with an alcohol pad.
- Deposit fluid specimens in containers, and send specimens to the laboratory for culture and sensitivity analysis, Gram stain, red and white blood cell counts, amylase and bile level determinations, and spun-down sediment evaluation.
- If you didn't obtain the culture and sensitivity specimen first, change the needle before drawing this fluid sample to avoid contaminating the specimen.
- Label the specimens, and send them to the laboratory immediately.
- With positive test results, the practitioner will usually perform a laparotomy. If test results are normal, the practitioner will close the incision with sutures.
- Wearing sterile gloves, apply antiseptic ointment to the site, and dress the incision with a 4" × 4" gauze pad secured with 1" hypoallergenic tape.
- Discard disposable equipment.
- Return reusable equipment to the appropriate department for cleaning and sterilization.

SPECIAL CONSIDERATIONS

- After lavage, monitor vital signs frequently.
- Report signs of shock, such as tachycardia, decreased blood pressure, diaphoresis, dyspnea or shortness of breath, and vertigo, immediately.
- Assess the incision site frequently for bleeding.
- If the practitioner orders abdominal X-rays, they'll should be done before peritoneal lavage. X-ray films made after lavage may be unreliable because of air introduced into the peritoneal cavity.

COMPLICATIONS

- Bleeding from lacerated blood vessels
- Peritonitis and subsequent laparotomy for repair
- Respiratory distress and respiratory arrest
- Bladder laceration or puncture
- Infection at the incision site

PATIENT TEACHING

- Explain the procedure as needed to lessen the patient's anxiety.

DOCUMENTATION

- Record the type and size of peritoneal dialysis catheter used.
- Note the type and amount of solution instilled.
- Document the amount and color of fluid returned.
- Note whether the fluid flowed freely into and out of the abdomen.
- Note which specimens were obtained and sent to the laboratory.
- Document complications and actions taken.

SELECTED REFERENCES

Klein, Y., et al. "Diagnostic Peritoneal Lavage Through an Abdominal Stab Wound," *American Journal of Emergency Medicine* 21(7):559-60, November 2003.

Platell, C. "The Role of Peritoneal Lavage," *ANZ Journal of Surgery* (Suppl 75):A45, May 2005.

Xu, Ping, et al. "Peritoneal Lavage for the Treatment of Severe Acute Pancreatitis," *Journal of Gastroenterology & Hepatology* 19(Suppl 5):A581, October 2004.

Pneumatic antishock garment application and removal

DESCRIPTION

- A pneumatic antishock garment (PASG), also known as a *medical antishock trousers (MAST) suit*, consists of inflatable bladders sandwiched between double layers of fabric.
- It's used to treat shock when systolic blood pressure falls below 80 mm Hg — or below 100 mm Hg when accompanied by signs of shock.
- When inflated, it places external pressure on lower extremities and abdomen, creating an autotransfusion effect that squeezes blood and increases blood volume to the heart, lungs, and brain by up to 30%.
- It controls abdominal and lower extremity hemorrhage and also helps stabilize and splint pelvic and femoral fractures.

CONTRAINDICATIONS

- Cardiogenic shock
- Heart failure
- Pulmonary edema
- Tension pneumothorax
- Increased intracranial pressure

PASG foot pump ◆ resuscitation equipment (optional)

AGE FACTOR *PASGs come in a pediatric size for patients 3½' to 5' [1 to 1.5 m] tall and an adult size for patients taller than 5'*

PREPARATION

- Spread the PASG open on a smooth surface or blanket to avoid puncturing.
- Make sure stopcock valves are open.
- Attach the foot pump.

- Explain the procedure to the patient and answer any questions.

APPLYING A PNEUMATIC ANTISHOCK GARMENT

- Take vital signs to establish baseline measurements.
- Assess for contraindications.
- Assess for injuries, and determine best method for placing the patient on the PASG. (See *Applying a pneumatic antishock garment.*)
- You can also set up the PASG on a stretcher and place the patient on it in a supine position.
- Double-check to ensure stopcocks are open.

Applying a pneumatic antishock garment

Open the garment with Velcro fasteners down.

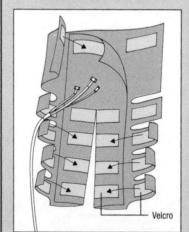

Velcro

Open all stopcock valves; then attach the foot pump tubing to the valve on the pressure control unit. If the patient can be turned, place the garment next to him, and roll him onto it. If he can't be turned, slide the garment under him.

Before closing the garment, remove sharp objects, such as pieces of glass, stones, keys, or a buckle that could injure the patient or tear the garment. As appropriate, pad pressure points and apply lanolin to protect the patient's skin from irritation.

Place the upper edge of the garment below the patient's lowest rib. Wrap the right leg compartment around his right leg. Secure the compartment by fastening all the Velcro straps from the ankle to the thigh.

Repeat the procedure for the left leg; then wrap the abdomen. Double-check that all valves are properly positioned.

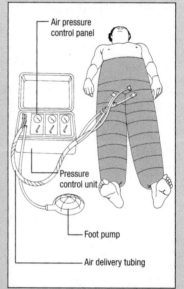

Air pressure control panel

Pressure control unit

Foot pump

Air delivery tubing

- Inflate the legs, then the abdominal segment, to about 20 to 30 mm Hg initially.
- Monitor the patient's blood pressure, pulse rate, and respirations every 5 minutes.
- Continue inflating until systolic blood pressure reaches the desired level, usually 100 mm Hg.
- Close all stopcocks to prevent accidental air loss.
- Check pedal pulses and temperature periodically.
- Notify the practitioner if circulation in the feet seems impaired.

REMOVING A PNEUMATIC ANTISHOCK GARMENT
- Before deflation, make sure that I.V. catheters are patent, a practitioner is attending, and emergency resuscitation equipment is available.
- Open the abdominal stopcock, and start releasing small amounts of air. If blood pressure drops 5 mm Hg, close the stopcock.

WARNING *Deflating the garment too quickly can allow circulating blood to rush to the abdomen or extremities and cause potentially irreversible shock.*

- If blood pressure drops, increase the flow rate of I.V. solutions.
- Deflate the abdominal section and the legs simultaneously.
- When the PASG is loose enough, gently pull it off.
- Clean the PASG as required, but don't autoclave it or use solvents.

SPECIAL CONSIDERATIONS
- A therapeutic response occurs at about 25 mm Hg.
- A morbidity effect occurs at about 50 mm Hg.
- Safety features include Velcro straps, pop-off valves, or gauges that prevent inflation beyond 104 mm Hg.
- The PASG shouldn't be left inflated for more than 2 hours.
- A range of 25 to 50 mm Hg can usually be maintained for up to 48 hours.
- For prolonged use, inflate at a lower pressure than normal.
- X-rays can be taken with a PASG on due to being radiolucent.

COMPLICATIONS
- Vomiting from compression of abdomen
- Metabolic acidosis caused by anaerobic metabolism
- Prolonged use may lead to skin breakdown, tissue sloughing, or amputation

PATIENT TEACHING
- Explain the procedure and the reason it's being performed.

DOCUMENTATION
- Record the application and removal time.
- Record pressures used for the garment.
- Note the patient's vital signs before, during, and after procedure.

SELECTED REFERENCES
Higgins, T.F., and Swanson, E.R. "Pelvic Antishock Sheeting," *Air Medical Journal* 25(2):88-90, March-April 2006.

Kemeny, A., and Geddes, L.A. "Retrospectroscope. Military Antishock Trousers," *IEEE Engineering in Medicine and Biology Magazine* 24(4):80, 91, July-August 2005.

Salomone, J.P., et al. "Opinions of Trauma Practitioners Regarding Prehospital Interventions for Critically Injured Patients," *Journal of Trauma* 58(3): 509-15, March 2005.

Postmortem care

DESCRIPTION

- Postmortem care involves preparation of a deceased patient for family viewing, arranging transportation to morgue or funeral home, and determining disposition of the patient's belongings.
- Care usually begins after the practitioner certifies the patient's death.
- Care also entails comforting and supporting the patient's family and friends and providing for their privacy.
- If the patient died violently or under suspicious circumstances, postmortem care may be postponed until the medical examiner completes an autopsy.

CONTRAINDICATIONS

- None known

Gauze or soft string ◆ ties ◆ gloves ◆ chin straps ◆ ABD pads ◆ cotton balls ◆ plastic shroud or body wrap ◆ three identification tags ◆ adhesive bandages to cover wounds or punctures ◆ plastic bag for patient's belongings ◆ water-filled basin ◆ soap ◆ towels ◆ washcloths ◆ stretcher ◆ protective equipment

- Put on gloves and protective equipment.
- Place the body in the supine position, with arms at sides and head on a pillow.
- Elevate the head of the bed 30 degrees.
- Insert dentures if your facility's policy permits, and close the mouth.
- Close the eyes with gentle pressure.
- If the eyes don't stay closed, place moist cotton balls on the eyelids for a few minutes, and then try again.
- Place a folded towel under the chin to keep the jaw closed.
- Remove all catheters, tubes, and tape.
- Apply adhesive bandages to puncture sites.
- Replace soiled dressings.
- Collect valuables. If you're unable to remove a ring, cover it with gauze, tape it in place, and tie the gauze to the wrist to prevent slippage and subsequent loss.
- Clean the body thoroughly.
- Place ABD pads between the buttocks to absorb rectal discharge or drainage.
- Cover the body up to the chin with a clean sheet.
- Offer emotional support to the family and friends.
- Provide them privacy while viewing the patient.
- Ask if jewelry should remain with the patient.
- After the family leaves, remove the towel.
- Pad the chin, apply chin straps, tie them loosely.
- Pad the wrists and ankles, and tie pads with gauze or soft string.
- Each identification tag should include the deceased patient's name, room and bed numbers, date and time of death, and practitioner's name.
- Tie one identification tag to the hand or foot.
- Don't remove hospital identification.
- Place the shroud or body wrap on the morgue stretcher.

- Transfer the body to the stretcher.
- Wrap the body, and tie the shroud with the string provided.
- Attach an identification tag to the front of the shroud or wrap.
- Cover with a clean sheet.
- If a shroud or wrap isn't available, use a clean gown and sheet.
- Attach the third identification to the bag of personal belongings.
- If the patient died of an infectious disease, label the body according to facility policy.
- Transport the body to the morgue.
- Close doors to nearby rooms.
- Use the service elevator.

SPECIAL CONSIDERATIONS

- Ask the family if they need the support of a clergy member.
- Ask the family if they need help contacting a funeral director.
- If the patient was a child, ask the parents or other family members if they would like to assist with the postmortem care. For some families, this helps to begin the grieving process.
- Give personal belongings to the family or bring them to the morgue.
- Ask a coworker to witness the transfer of valuables.
- Obtain a family member's signature to verify the receipt of valuables or to state their preference that jewelry remain on the patient.
- Express sympathy for the family, and don't remove the patient's body until the family is ready.
- Bathe and handle the patient's body according to the family's wishes. Some cultures have rules and rituals for treatment of the body.

COMPLICATIONS

- None known

PATIENT TEACHING

- None

DOCUMENTATION

- Record that postmortem care was provided.
- Note the disposition of the patient's possessions, including valuables.
- Document the date and time transport to the morgue took place.
- Document any assistance given in helping the family make funeral arrangements.
- Document special handling of the patient's body based on the family's requests.
- Note whether family members assisted with preparation of the patient's body.
- Document if the patient's body was transported to the medical examiner's office for an autopsy.

SELECTED REFERENCES

Blum, C.A. "'Til Death Do Us Part?' The Nurse's Role in the Care of the Dead: A Historical Perspective: 1850-2004," *Geriatric Nursing* 27(1):58-63, January-February 2006.

Bucaro, P.J., et al. "Bereavement Care: One Children's Hospital's Compassionate Plan for Parents and Families," *Journal of Emergency Nursing* 31(3):305-308, June 2005.

Flanagan, R.J., et al. "Analytical Toxicology: Guidelines for Sample Collection Postmortem," *Toxicology Reviews* 24(1):63-71, 2005.

Teasdale, K. "Care of the Bereaved When Postmortems are Required," *Nursing Times* 100(36):32-33, September 2004.

Postoperative care

DESCRIPTION

◆ Care of the patient after surgery begins when the patient arrives in the postanesthesia care unit (PACU) and continues as he moves on to the short procedure unit, medical-surgical unit, or critical care area.

◆ Techniques aim to minimize postoperative complications by early detection and prompt treatment.

◆ After anesthesia, the patient may experience pain, inadequate oxygenation, or adverse physiologic effects of sudden movement.

◆ Recovery from general anesthesia takes longer than induction because anesthetic is retained in fat and muscle.

◆ Recovery time varies with the patient's amount of body fat, overall condition, premedication regimen, and type, dosage, and duration of anesthesia.

CONTRAINDICATIONS

◆ None known

Thermometer ◆ watch with second hand ◆ stethoscope ◆ sphygmomanometer ◆ postoperative flowchart or documentation tool ◆ pulse oximetry ◆ cardiac monitor (if ordered)

PREPARATION

◆ Assemble the necessary equipment at the patient's bedside.

◆ Obtain the patient's record from the PACU nurse.

◆ Confirm the patient's identity using two patient identifiers according to facility policy.

◆ Transfer the patient from the stretcher to the bed, and position him properly.

◆ Use caution when transferring the patient who has had orthopedic surgery or skeletal traction.

◆ Provide comfort and ensure safety (raise the bed's side rails).

◆ Assess level of consciousness, skin color, and mucous membranes.

◆ Monitor breathing rate, depth, and breath sounds.

◆ Administer oxygen and initiate oximetry.

◆ Attach to cardiac monitor, if ordered.

◆ Monitor the patient's pulse rate and blood pressure.

◆ Make sure that preoperative and postoperative blood pressures are within 20% of each other.

◆ Make sure body temperature is at least 95° F (35° C). If it's lower, use blankets or the Bair Hugger patient-warming system.

◆ Assess infusion sites for redness, pain, swelling, or drainage. If infiltration occurs, discontinue the I.V. and restart.

◆ Assess wound dressings. If soiled, note characteristics of drainage and outline the soiled area. Note the date and time of assessment on the dressing.

◆ If the drainage area enlarges, reinforce the dressing and alert the practitioner.

◆ Note the presence and condition of drains and tubes.

◆ Note the color, type, odor, and amount of drainage and urine output.

◆ Make sure all drains are properly connected and free of obstructions.

◆ For a vascular or orthopedic surgery, assess all extremities.

- Perform neurovascular checks; assess color, temperature, sensation, movement, and presence and quality of pulses. Notify the practitioner of abnormalities.
- Be alert for signs of airway obstruction and hypoventilation.
- Assess for cardiovascular complications (arrhythmias or hypotension).
- Encourage coughing and deep-breathing exercises. (Exceptions: nasal, ophthalmic, or neurologic surgery.)
- Administer postoperative drugs.
- Obtain laboratory specimens as ordered.
- Assess the gag reflex before offering fluids.
- Monitor the patient's intake and output.
- Assess for bowel sounds and flatus before offering food.

SPECIAL CONSIDERATIONS

- Monitor fear, pain, anxiety, hypothermia, confusion, and immobility, which can affect patient safety and recovery.
- Offer emotional support, and refer for ongoing emotional support if indicated.
- Avoid talking about the patient in his presence because hearing returns first.
- Cough and gag reflexes reappear and, if the patient can lift his head, he's usually able to breathe on his own.
- After spinal anesthesia, the patient should remain supine with the bed adjusted between 0 and 20 degrees for at least 6 hours. Reassure him that sensation and mobility will return to his legs.
- Monitor respiratory status for those using epidural analgesia infusion for postoperative pain control.
- Monitor for nausea, vomiting, itching, or sensorimotor loss.

COMPLICATIONS

- Arrhythmias
- Bleeding
- Hypotension
- Hypovolemia
- Septicemia
- Septic shock
- Atelectasis
- Respiratory failure
- Pneumonia
- Thrombophlebitis
- Pulmonary embolism
- Urine retention
- Wound infection
- Wound dehiscence
- Evisceration
- Abdominal distention
- Paralytic ileus
- Constipation
- Altered body image
- Postoperative psychosis

PATIENT TEACHING

- Tell the patient what to expect postoperatively before he has surgery.
- Advise the patient that he may feel some discomfort from the surgery, but that analgesia will be available.
- Teach the patient how to use the patient-controlled analgesia if one has been ordered.

DOCUMENTATION

- Record vital signs.
- Note the condition of dressings, drains, and characteristics of drainage.
- Document interventions taken to alleviate pain and anxiety and the patient's responses to them.
- Record complications and interventions taken.

SELECTED REFERENCES

Beke, D.M., et al. "Management of the Pediatric Postoperative Cardiac Surgery Patient," *Critical Care Nursing Clinics of North America* 17(4):405-16, xi, December 2005.
Litwack, K. "Adjusting Postsurgical Care for Older Patients," *Nursing* 36(1): 66-67, January 2006.
Pirie, S. "New Procedures in the Recovery Unit," *British Journal of Perioperative Nursing* 15(10):414-16, 418-19, October 2005.
Stanhope, N. "Temperature Measurement in the Phase I PACU," *Journal of Perianesthesia Nursing* 21(1):27-33, February 2006.

Preoperative care

OVERVIEW

DESCRIPTION
- Care of the patient begins when surgery is planned and ends with administration of anesthesia.
- Preoperative care includes:
- preoperative interview and assessment to collect baseline subjective and objective data from patient and family
- diagnostic tests such as urinalysis, complete blood count, electrolyte studies, electrocardiogram, and chest radiography
- preoperative teaching
- signed informed consent from the patient
- physical preparation.

CONTRAINDICATIONS
- None known

EQUIPMENT

Thermometer ◆ sphygmomanometer ◆ stethoscope ◆ watch with second hand ◆ weight scale ◆ tape measure

PREPARATION
- Assemble needed equipment at the patient's bedside or admission area.

KEY STEPS

- For same-day surgery, instruct the patient not to eat or drink for 8 hours before surgery.
- Confirm arrival time, and instruct him to leave valuables at home.
- Verify arrangements for postsurgery transportation or admission.
- Obtain a health history, including previous medical or surgical procedures.
- Assess the patient's readiness: knowledge, perceptions, and expectations.
- Assess psychosocial needs: occupational, financial, support systems, mental status, and cultural.
- Obtain a drug history of prescriptions, over-the-counter drugs, supplements, and herbal preparations and when they were last taken.
- Assess for known allergies to foods, drugs, and latex.
- Obtain height, weight, and vital signs.
- Identify risk factors including age, general health, drug use, mobility, nutritional status, fluid and electrolyte disturbances, lifestyle considerations, disorder's duration, location, and nature of the procedure.
- Explain procedures to reduce postoperative anxiety and pain, increase compliance, hasten recovery, and decrease length of stay. Explain sequence of events, holding area, surgical dress, equipment, incision, dressings, and staples or sutures.
- Explain that minimal conversation will help the preoperative medication take effect.
- Discuss transfer procedures and techniques, and describe sensations the patient will experience.
- Discuss postoperative exercises such as deep breathing and coughing, (exceptions: ophthalmic or neurologic surgery), extremity exercises, and movement and ambulation to minimize respiratory and circulatory complications.

- Discuss procedures on the day of surgery (morning care, verifying a signed informed consent form, preoperative medications, preoperative checklist, and chart). (See *Obtaining informed consent.*)
- Discuss preoperative interventions such as restricting food and fluids for about 8 hours before surgery, enemas before abdominal or GI surgery, and antibiotics for 2 or 3 days preoperatively to prevent contamination of the peritoneal cavity by GI bacteria.
- Remove hairpins, nail polish, and jewelry. Note whether dentures, contact lenses, or prosthetic devices have been removed or left in place. Verify with the patient that the correct surgical site has been marked.
- Before transport to the surgical area, ensure the following are in place: hospital gown, identification band, vital signs recorded.

SPECIAL CONSIDERATIONS

- Administer preoperative medications on time.
- Make sure the patient has had no food or drink preoperatively.
- Raise the bed's side rails after giving preoperative medications.
- If present, direct family to the appropriate waiting area, and offer support as needed.
- The chart and the surgical checklist must accompany the patient to surgery.

COMPLICATIONS
- None known

PATIENT TEACHING

- Teach the patient coughing and deep-breathing exercises before surgery as appropriate.
- Inform the patient that he may have surgical dressings, surgical drains, an I.V. line, and a urinary catheter after the surgery.
- Advise the patient that he'll feel discomfort, but that pain medication will be available, and he should ask for it when he feels pain.
- Tell the patient that he'll be in a postsurgical recovery area for at least 1 hour after surgery to monitor his vital signs.

DOCUMENTATION

- Document using preoperative checklist used by your facility.
- Note nursing care measures.
- Document preoperative drugs.
- Record the results of diagnostic tests.
- Note time the patient is transferred to the surgical area.

SELECTED REFERENCES

Barnett, J.S. "An Emerging Role for Nurse Practitioners — Preoperative Assessment," *AORN Journal* 82(5):825-30, 833-34, November 2005.

Hurley, C., and McAleavy, J. "Preoperative Assessment and Intraoperative Care Planning," *Journal of Perioperative Practice* 16(4):187-90, 192-94, April 2006.

Justus, R., et al. "Preparing Children and Families for Surgery: Mount Sinai's Multidisciplinary Perspective," *Pediatric Nursing* 32(1):35-43, January-February 2006.

Saufl, N.M. "Preparing the Older Adult for Surgery and Anesthesia," *Journal of Perianesthesia Nursing* 19(6):372-78, December 2004.

Pressure ulcer care

DESCRIPTION

- Pressure ulcer care involves relieving skin pressure, restoring circulation, promoting adequate nutrition, and resolving or managing related disorders in order to decrease pressure ulcer incidence and promote healing of existing pressure ulcers.
- Care may require special pressure-reducing devices, such as beds, mattresses, mattress overlays, and chair cushions.
- Other measures include decreasing risk factors, use of topical treatments, wound cleansing, debridement, and use of dressings to support moist wound healing.
- Standard precaution guidelines of the Centers for Disease Control and Prevention should be used when giving care.
- Effectiveness and duration of treatment depends on the pressure ulcer's characteristics and patient's health status.

CONTRAINDICATIONS

- None known

EQUIPMENT

Hypoallergenic tape or elastic netting ◆ overbed table ◆ piston-type irrigating system ◆ two pairs of gloves ◆ normal saline solution as ordered ◆ sterile 4″ × 4″ gauze pads ◆ sterile cotton swabs ◆ selected topical dressing ◆ linen-saver pads ◆ impervious plastic trash bag ◆ disposable wound-measuring device

PREPARATION

- Assemble equipment at patient's bedside.
- Cut tape into strips.
- Loosen lids on cleaning solutions and drugs.
- Loosen existing dressing edges and tapes.
- Put on gloves.
- Attach an impervious plastic trash bag to the overbed table.

KEY STEPS

- Wash your hands.
- Review the principles of standard precautions.
- Provide privacy.

CLEANING THE PRESSURE ULCER

- Explain the procedure to allay fear and promote cooperation.
- Position patient for comfort and easy access to site.
- Cover bed linens with a linen-saver pad to prevent soiling.
- Open the normal saline solution container and the piston syringe.
- Pour the solution carefully into a clean or sterile irrigation container.
- Put the piston syringe into the opening of the irrigation container.
- Open the packages of supplies.
- Put on gloves before removing the old dressing and exposing the pressure ulcer.
- Discard the soiled dressing in the impervious plastic trash bag.
- Inspect the wound. Note the color, amount, and odor of any drainage or necrotic debris.
- Measure the wound perimeter with a disposable wound-measuring device.
- Apply full force of the piston syringe to irrigate the ulcer, remove necrotic debris, and decrease bacteria in the wound.
- For nonnecrotic wounds, use pressure to prevent damage.
- Remove and discard your soiled gloves, and put on a clean pair.
- Insert a gloved finger or sterile cotton swab into the wound to assess wound tunneling or undermining.
- Assess and note the condition of the clean wound and surrounding skin.
- Notify a wound care specialist if adherent necrotic material is present.
- Apply the appropriate topical dressing.

APPLYING A MOIST SALINE GAUZE DRESSING

- Irrigate the ulcer with normal saline solution. Blot the surrounding skin dry.

- Moisten the gauze dressing with normal saline solution.
- Gently place the dressing over the surface of the ulcer.
- To separate surfaces within the wound, gently place a dressing between opposing wound surfaces. Don't pack the gauze tightly.
- Change the dressing often enough to keep the wound moist.

APPLYING A HYDROCOLLOID DRESSING

- Irrigate the ulcer with normal saline solution. Blot the surrounding skin dry.
- Choose a clean, dry, presized dressing, or cut one to overlap the pressure ulcer by about 1″ (2.5 cm).
- Remove the dressing from its package, remove the release paper, and apply the dressing to the wound. Carefully smooth wrinkles as you apply the dressing.
- If using tape to secure the dressing, apply a skin sealant to the intact skin around the ulcer.
- When dry, tape the dressing to the skin. Avoid tension or pressure.
- Remove and discard your gloves and other refuse.
- Wash your hands.
- Change a hydrocolloid dressing every 2 to 7 days.
- Discontinue if signs of infection are present.

APPLYING A TRANSPARENT DRESSING

- Irrigate the ulcer with normal saline solution. Blot the surrounding skin dry.
- Clean and dry the wound as described above.
- Select a dressing to overlap the ulcer by 2″ (5 cm).
- Gently lay the dressing over the ulcer. Don't stretch it.
- Press firmly on the edges of the dressing to promote adherence.
- Tape the edges to prevent them from curling.
- If necessary, aspirate the accumulated fluid with a 21G needle and syringe.
- Clean the site with an alcohol pad

and cover it with a transparent dressing.
◆ Change the dressing every 3 to 7 days, depending on drainage.

APPLYING AN ALGINATE DRESSING
◆ Irrigate the ulcer with normal saline solution. Blot the surrounding skin dry.
◆ Apply alginate dressing to the ulcer surface. Cover with a second dressing (such as gauze pads). Secure with tape or elastic netting.
◆ If drainage is heavy, change the dressing once or twice daily for the first 3 to 5 days.
◆ As drainage decreases, change the dressing less frequently — every 2 to 4 days or as ordered.
◆ When drainage stops or the wound bed looks dry, stop using alginate dressing.

APPLYING A FOAM DRESSING
◆ Irrigate the ulcer with normal saline solution. Blot the surrounding skin dry.
◆ Lay the foam dressing over the ulcer.
◆ Use tape, elastic netting, or gauze to hold the dressing in place.
◆ Change the dressing when the foam no longer absorbs the exudate.

APPLYING A HYDROGEL DRESSING
◆ Irrigate the ulcer with normal saline solution. Blot surrounding skin dry.
◆ Apply gel to the wound bed.
◆ Cover the area with a second dressing.
◆ Change the dressing as needed to keep the wound bed moist.
◆ If you choose a sheet form dressing, cut it to match the wound base.
◆ Hydrogel dressings also come in a prepackaged, saturated gauze to fill "dead space." Follow the manufacturer's directions.

PREVENTING PRESSURE ULCERS
◆ Turn and reposition the patient every 1 to 2 hours unless contraindicated.
◆ Use an air or gel mattress for those who can't turn themselves or those who are turned on a schedule.

◆ Low- or high-air-loss therapy may be indicated.
◆ Implement active or passive range-of-motion exercises.
◆ To save time, combine exercises with bathing if applicable.
◆ Lift rather than slide the patient when turning.
◆ Use a turning sheet and get help from coworkers.
◆ Use pillows to position the patient and increase his comfort.
◆ Eliminate sheet wrinkles.
◆ Post a turning schedule at his bedside.
◆ Avoid the trochanter position. Instead, position at a 30-degree angle.
◆ Avoid raising the bed more than 30 degrees for long periods.
◆ Adjust or pad appliances, casts, or splints, to ensure proper fit.
◆ Gently apply lotion after bathing to keep skin moist.
◆ Clean and dry soiled skin. Apply a protective moisture barrier.

SPECIAL CONSIDERATIONS

◆ Prevention helps avoid extensive therapy; measures include ensuring adequate nourishment and mobility to relieve pressure and promote circulation.
◆ Direct the patient in a chair or wheelchair to shift his weight every 15 minutes.
◆ Instruct a paraplegic to shift his weight by doing push-ups.
◆ Tell the patient to avoid heat lamps and harsh soaps.
◆ Avoid using elbow and heel protectors with a single narrow strap.
◆ Avoid using artificial sheepskin. It doesn't reduce pressure.
◆ Repair of stages 3 and 4 ulcers may require surgical intervention.

COMPLICATIONS
◆ Infection that produces foul-smelling drainage, persistent pain, severe erythema, induration, and elevated skin and body temperatures
◆ Infection that may lead to cellulitis and septicemia

PATIENT TEACHING

◆ Teach the patient and family the importance of prevention, position changes, and treatment. Teach proper methods and encourage participation.
◆ Encourage the patient to follow a diet with adequate calories, protein, and vitamins.

DOCUMENTATION

◆ Record the date and time of initial and subsequent treatments.
◆ Detail preventive strategies performed.
◆ Note the location, size (length, width, depth), color, and appearance of ulcer.
◆ Record the amount, odor, color, and consistency of the drainage.
◆ Document the condition and temperature of surrounding skin.
◆ Record body temperature daily.
◆ Reassess pressure ulcers at least weekly, and update the care plan.
◆ Record practitioner notification.

SELECTED REFERENCES
Jones, J. "Evaluation of Pressure Ulcer Prevention Devices: A Critical Review of the Literature," *Journal of Wound Care* 14(9):422-25, October 2005.
Niezgoda, J.A., and Mendez-Eastman, S. "The Effective Management of Pressure Ulcers," *Advances in Skin & Wound Care* 19(suppl 1):3-15, January-February 2006.
Ohura, N., et al. "Evaluating Dressing Materials for the Prevention of Shear Force in the Treatment of Pressure Ulcers," *Journal of Wound Care* 14(9): 401-404, October 2005.
Stevens, J., and Gray, W. "New Guidelines on Preventing and Managing Pressure Ulcers," *Nursing Times* 101(46):40-42, November 2005.

Prone positioning

DESCRIPTION

◆ Prone positioning, also known as *proning,* involves physically turning the patient from supine position to a face-down position to improve oxygenation and pulmonary mechanics.
◆ Criteria for the procedure include acute onset of acute respiratory failure; hypoxemia, specifically a partial pressure of arterial oxygen (Pao_2)/fraction of inspired oxygen (Fio_2) ratio of 300 or less for acute lung injury or a Pao_2/Fio_2 ratio of 200 or less for acute respiratory distress syndrome (ARDS); and radiological evidence of diffuse bilateral pulmonary infiltrates.
◆ It's usually performed for 6 or more hours per day, for as long as 10 days, until requirement for high concentration of inspired oxygen resolves.
◆ It may improve oxygenation in patients by shifting blood flow to better ventilated regions of the lung.
◆ It facilitates better movement of the diaphragm by allowing the abdomen to expand more fully.
◆ It helps correct severe hypoxemia and maintain adequate oxygenation (Pao_2 greater than 60%) while avoiding ventilator-induced lung injury.
◆ It's indicated to support mechanically ventilated patients with ARDS, who require high concentrations of inspired oxygen.
◆ Patients with extrapulmonary ARDS (such as ARDS due to multiple trauma) appear to respond consistently to prone positioning.

CONTRAINDICATIONS

◆ Increased intracranial pressure
◆ Spinal instability
◆ Unstable bone fractures
◆ Multiple trauma
◆ Left-sided heart failure
◆ Shock
◆ Abdominal compartment syndrome
◆ Abdominal surgery
◆ Extreme obesity (greater than 300 lb [136 kg])
◆ Pregnancy
◆ Hemodynamic instability

◆ Inability to tolerate face-down position
◆ Patient whose head can't be supported in position

Vollman prone positioner (HillRom) or other prone-positioning device ◆ gloves

PREPARATION

◆ Clean the positioner device between turns and when discontinuing.

◆ Confirm the patient's identity using two patient identifiers according to facility policy.
◆ Assess the patient's hemodynamic and neurologic status.
◆ Explain the procedure to the patient and his family.
◆ Before turning the patient, wash your hands and put on gloves.
◆ Provide eye care (lubrication and taping of eyelid if indicated).
◆ Protect the tongue. Use a bite block if edematous or protruding.
◆ Secure the endotracheal (ET) tube or tracheotomy tube.
◆ Perform anterior body wound care and dressing changes.
◆ Empty ileostomy or colostomy drainage bags.
◆ Reposition anterior electrocardiogram leads to the patient's back after he's prone.
◆ Engage the bed brake.
◆ Attach the surface of the prone positioner to the bed frame.
◆ Position staff, one on either side of the bed and one at the head of the bed.
◆ Position upper torso lines over the right or left shoulder.
◆ Position chest tubes at the foot of the bed.
◆ Position lower torso lines at the foot of the bed.
◆ Turn the patient's face away from the ventilator, placing the ET tubing on

the side of the patient's face that's turned away from the ventilator.
◆ Loop the remaining tubing above the patient's head.
◆ Place the straps under the patient's head, chest, and pelvic area.
◆ Attach the prone positioner device by placing the frame on top of the patient.
◆ Position the chest piece to rest between clavicles and sixth ribs.

⚡ **WARNING** *If the patient has a short neck or limited neck range of motion, align the chest piece lower — at the third intercostal space. Move both head pieces up to the top of the frame so only the forehead is supported by the head cushion and the chin is suspended, to reduce risk of skin breakdown.*

◆ Adjust the pelvic piece so it rests ½" (1.3 cm) above the iliac crest.
◆ Evaluate the distance between the chest and pelvic pieces to ensure suspension of the abdomen, while preventing bowing of the patient's back.
◆ Adjust the chin and forehead pieces to provide facial support in either a face-down or side-lying position without interfering with the ET tube.
◆ Fasten all adjustable straps on one side before tightening them on the opposite side. When secured, lift the positioner to ensure a secure fit.
◆ To help ensure a secure fit, look for cushion compression. If the frame isn't tightly secured, shear and friction injuries to the chest and pelvic area may occur.
◆ Lower the side rails.
◆ Move the patient with a draw sheet to the edge of the bed farthest from the ventilator.
◆ Tuck the straps to the center of the bed underneath the patient.
◆ Tuck the arm and hand, resting in the center of the bed, under the buttocks.
◆ Cross the leg closest to the edge of the bed over the opposite leg at the ankle.
◆ If the patient's arm can't be straightened and tucked under his buttocks, tuck the arm into the open space between the chest and pelvic pads.
◆ Turn the patient toward the ventilator at a 45-degree angle. Always turn

the patient in the direction of the mechanical ventilator.

◆ The person on the side of the bed with the ventilator grasps the upper steel bar.

◆ The person on the other side grasps the lower steel bar or turning straps of the device.

◆ Lift the patient by the frame into the prone position.

◆ Move the patient's tucked arm and hand so they're comfortable.

⚡ **WARNING** *To prevent placing stress on the shoulder capsule, don't extend the arm to a 90-degree angle.*

◆ Loosen the straps if the patient is clinically stable.

⚡ **WARNING** *Keeping the straps securely fastened for an unstable patient allows rapid supine repositioning in an emergency.*

◆ Support the patient's feet with a pillow or towel roll.

◆ Pad his elbows to prevent ulnar nerve compression.

◆ Monitor vital signs, pulse oximetry, and mixed venous oxygen saturation.

◆ Obtain arterial blood gases within ½ hour of proning and within ½ hour before returning the patient to the supine position.

◆ Reposition the patient's head hourly.

◆ Provide range of motion to shoulders, arms, and legs every 2 hours.

RETURNING PATIENT TO SUPINE POSITION

◆ Fasten the positioning device straps securely.

◆ Position the patient on the edge of the bed closest to the ventilator.

◆ Adjust tubing and monitoring lines to prevent dislodgment.

◆ Straighten the patient's arms, and rest them on either side.

◆ Cross his leg closest to the edge of the bed over the opposite leg.

◆ Using the steel bars of the device, turn the patient to a 45-degree angle away from the ventilator, and then roll him to the supine position.

◆ Position the patient's arms parallel to his body.

◆ Unfasten the positioning device, and remove it from the patient.

SPECIAL CONSIDERATIONS

◆ A practitioner's order is usually required.

◆ Some patients may require increased sedation during the procedure.

◆ Use capnography to verify correct ET tube placement.

◆ Reposition the patient every 4 to 6 hours.

◆ Discontinue when the patient no longer demonstrates improved oxygenation with the position change.

COMPLICATIONS

◆ Inadvertent ET extubation

◆ Airway obstruction

◆ Decreased oxygen saturation

◆ Apical atelectasis

◆ Obstructed chest tube

◆ Pressure injuries on weight-bearing parts of body

◆ Hemodynamic instability

◆ Dislodgment of central venous access

◆ Transient arrhythmias

◆ Reversible dependent edema of the face and anterior chest wall

◆ Contractures

◆ Enteral feeding intolerance and aspiration after repositioning

◆ Corneal ulceration

PATIENT TEACHING

◆ Explain the procedure to the patient to lessen anxiety.

DOCUMENTATION

◆ Note the patient's response to therapy.

◆ Record the patient's ability to tolerate the turning procedure.

◆ Document length of time in the position.

◆ Note positioning schedule.

◆ Record monitoring, complications, and interventions.

SELECTED REFERENCES

Essat, Z. "Prone Positioning in Patients with Acute Respiratory Distress Syndrome," *Nursing Standard* 20(9):52-55, November 2005.

Griffiths, H., and Gallimore, D. "Positioning Critically Ill Patients in Hospital," *Nursing Standard* 19(42):56-64, June-July 2005.

Suter, P.M. "Reducing Ventilator-Induced Lung Injury and Other Organ Injury by the Prone Position," *Critical Care* 10(2): 139, April 2006.

Vollman, K.M. "Prone Positioning in the Patient Who Has Acute Respiratory Distress Syndrome: The Art and Science," *Critical Care Nursing Clinics of North America* 16(3):319-36, viii, September 2004.

Pulmonary artery pressure and wedge pressure

DESCRIPTION

- Monitoring of pulmonary artery pressure (PAP) and pulmonary artery wedge pressure (PAWP) measurements evaluates left ventricular function and preload.
- Procedures are useful for aiding diagnosis, refining assessment, guiding interventions, and projecting patient outcomes.
- PAP monitoring is especially useful for these conditions:
  – hemodynamic instability
  – fluid management
  – continuous cardiopulmonary assessment
  – shock
  – trauma
  – pulmonary or cardiac disease
  – multiorgan disease
  – use of multiple cardioactive drugs.
- The Swan-Ganz catheter, also called *a pulmonary artery (PA) catheter*, has up to six lumens, allowing more hemodynamic information to be gathered.
- The PA catheter has distal and proximal lumens used to measure pressures, a balloon inflation lumen that inflates the balloon for PAWP measurement, and a thermistor connector lumen that allows cardiac output measurement.
- Some catheters have a pacemaker wire lumen that provides a port for pacemaker electrodes and measures continuous mixed venous oxygen saturation.
- The pulmonary artery, right atrium, and right ventricle produce characteristic pressures and waveforms that can be observed on the monitor to help track catheter-tip location.
- The PA catheter is inserted into the heart's right side with the distal tip lying in the pulmonary artery.
- Left-sided pressures can be assessed indirectly.

CONTRAINDICATIONS

- Abnormal bleeding
- Right heart mass
- Tricuspid or pulmonary valve prosthesis or endocarditis

Balloon-tipped, flow-directed PA catheter ◆ prepared pressure transducer system ◆ I.V. solutions ◆ sterile gloves ◆ alcohol pads ◆ "medication-added" label ◆ monitor and monitor cable ◆ I.V. pole with transducer mount ◆ emergency resuscitation equipment ◆ electrocardiogram (ECG) monitor ◆ ECG electrodes ◆ armboard (for antecubital insertion) ◆ lead aprons (if fluoroscope is necessary) ◆ sutures ◆ sterile 4″ × 4″ gauze pads, or other dry, occlusive dressing material ◆ shaving materials (for femoral insertion site) ◆ small sterile basin ◆ sterile water ◆ prepackaged introducer kit ◆ dextrose 5% in water (optional)

If a prepackaged introducer kit is unavailable, obtain the following: introducer (one size larger than the catheter) ◆ sterile tray containing instruments for procedure ◆ masks ◆ sterile gowns ◆ sterile gloves ◆ sterile drapes ◆ iodine ointment and solution ◆ sutures ◆ two 10-ml syringes ◆ anesthetic (1% to 2% lidocaine) ◆ one 5-ml syringe, 25G ½″ needle ◆ 1″ and 3″ tape

PREPARATION

- The pressure monitoring system and bedside monitor must be properly calibrated and zeroed.
- Make sure the monitor has correct pressure modules.
- Calibrate according to manufacturer's instructions.
- Prepare the pressure monitoring system according to facility policy.
- Have emergency resuscitation equipment on hand (defibrillator, oxygen, and supplies for intubation and emergency drug administration).
- Prepare a sterile field for insertion of the introducer and catheter.

- Confirm the patient's identity using two patient identifiers according to facility policy.
- Check the patient's chart for heparin sensitivity, which contraindicates adding heparin to the flush solution.
- Explain that the catheter will monitor pressures from the pulmonary artery and heart.
- Reassure him that the catheter poses little danger and rarely causes pain.
- Tell him that if pain occurs at the introducer insertion site, an analgesic or sedative will be given.
- Position the patient at the proper height and angle.
- For superior approach: Place the patient in a flat, slight Trendelenburg position. Remove the pillow.
- Turn the patient's head to the side opposite the insertion site.
- For inferior approach: Place the patient in a supine position.

PREPARING THE CATHETER

- Maintain aseptic technique and use standard precautions.
- Clean the insertion site with a povidone-iodine solution, and drape it.
- Put on a mask.
- Help the practitioner put on a sterile mask, gown, and gloves.
- Open the outer packaging of catheter, revealing the inner sterile wrapping.
- The practitioner opens the inner wrapping and picks up the catheter.
- Take the catheter lumen hubs when he hands them to you.
- Flush the catheter with normal saline solution to remove air and verify patency.
- For multiple pressure lines, ensure the distal PA lumen hub is attached to the pressure line being monitored.
- Inadvertently attaching the distal PA line to the proximal lumen hub will prevent the proper waveform from appearing during insertion.
- Make sure the scale on the monitor is appropriate for lower pressures. A scale of 0 to 25 mm Hg or 0 to 50 mm Hg (more common) is preferred.

monitoring

- To verify the integrity of the balloon, the practitioner inflates it with air (usually 1.5 cc) before handing you the lumens to attach to the pressure monitoring system.
- The balloon is checked for symmetrical shape and for leaks by submerging it in a small, sterile basin filled with sterile water.

INSERTING THE CATHETER

- Assist the practitioner as he inserts the introducer to access the vessel.
- A percutaneous or, less commonly, a cutdown insertion is done.
- After the introducer is placed, the practitioner inserts the catheter through the introducer with the balloon deflated, directing the curl of the catheter toward the patient's midline.
- As insertion begins, observe the bedside monitor for waveform variations.
- When the catheter exits the end of the introducer sheath and reaches the junction of the superior vena cava and right atrium (at the 15- to 20-cm mark on the catheter shaft), the monitor shows oscillations that correspond to the patient's respirations.
- The balloon is then inflated with the recommended volume of air to allow normal blood flow to aid catheter insertion.
- The catheter is advanced through the heart chambers, moving rapidly to the pulmonary artery.
- When the mark on the catheter shaft reaches 15 to 20 cm, the catheter enters the right atrium.
- The waveform shows two small, upright waves; pressure is low (from 2 to 4 mm Hg).
- Read the pressure values in the mean mode because systolic and diastolic values are similar.
- The catheter is quickly advanced into the right ventricle to minimize irritation.
- Sharp systolic upstrokes and lower diastolic dips are seen on the waveform.

- Depending on the size of the patient's heart, the catheter should be at the 30- to 35-cm mark.
- Record systolic and diastolic pressures.
- As the catheter floats into the pulmonary artery, note that the upstroke from right ventricular systole is smoother, and systolic pressure is nearly the same as right ventricular systolic pressure.
- Record systolic, diastolic, and mean pressures.
- A dicrotic notch on the diastolic portion of the waveform indicates pulmonic valve closure.

WEDGING THE CATHETER

- To obtain a wedge tracing, the practitioner lets the inflated balloon float with the blood flow to a smaller, more distal branch of the pulmonary artery.
- When the catheter lodges, occlusion of right ventricular and pulmonary artery diastolic pressures occurs.
- The tracing resembles the right atrial tracing because the catheter tip is recording left atrial pressure. The waveform shows two small uprises.
- Record PAWP in the mean mode.
- A PAWP waveform, or wedge tracing, usually appears when the catheter has been inserted 45 to 50 cm.
- In a large heart, a longer catheter length — up to 55 cm — is typically required but shouldn't be inserted more than 60 cm.
- Allow 30 to 45 seconds to elapse from insertion time to the wedge tracing.
- The balloon is then deflated, and the catheter drifts out of the wedge position and back into the pulmonary artery— its normal resting place.
- To verify balloon deflation, observe the monitor for return of the pulmonary artery tracing.
- If the appropriate waveforms don't appear at the expected times during catheter insertion, the catheter may be coiled in the right atrium and ventricle.

- The practitioner will pull the catheter back and attempt advancement again until the correct position is achieved.
- A portable chest X-ray is ordered to confirm catheter position.
- Apply a sterile occlusive dressing to the insertion site.

OBTAINING INTERMITTENT PULMONARY ARTERY PRESSURE VALUES

- After inserting the catheter and recording initial pressure readings, record subsequent PAP values and monitor waveforms.
- To ensure accurate values, make sure the transducer is properly leveled and zeroed.
- If possible, obtain PAP values at end expiration (when the patient completely exhales). If you obtain a reading during other phases of the respiratory cycle, respiratory interference may occur.
- For patients with a rapid respiratory rate and subsequent variations, you may have trouble identifying end expiration.
- Obtain a printout of the digital readings over time and readings obtained during a full respiratory cycle.
- Use the averaged values obtained through the full respiratory cycle.
- To analyze trends accurately, record values at consistent times during the respiratory cycle.

(continued)

TAKING A PULMONARY ARTERY WEDGE PRESSURE READING

◆ PAWP is recorded by inflating the balloon and letting it float in a distal artery.

◆ Some facilities allow only practitioners or specially trained nurses to take a PAWP reading because of the risk of pulmonary artery rupture — a rare but life-threatening complication.

◆ If allowed to perform this procedure, do so with extreme caution, and make sure you're thoroughly familiar with intracardiac waveform interpretation.

◆ Verify that the transducer is properly leveled and zeroed.

◆ Detach the syringe from the balloon inflation hub.

◆ Draw 1.5 cc of air into the syringe; then reattach the syringe to the hub.

◆ Watching the monitor, inject the air through the hub slowly and smoothly.

◆ When you see a wedge tracing on the monitor, immediately stop inflating the balloon. Never inflate beyond the volume needed to obtain a wedge tracing.

◆ Take the pressure reading at end expiration.

◆ Note the amount of air needed to change the pulmonary artery tracing to a wedge tracing (normally, 1.25 to 1.5 cc).

TROUBLESHOOTER *If a wedge tracing appears with an injection of less than 1.25 cc, suspect that the catheter has migrated into a more distal branch and requires repositioning.*

WARNING *If the balloon is in a more distal branch, the tracings may move up the oscilloscope, indicating that the catheter tip is recording balloon pressure rather than PAWP. This may lead to pulmonary artery rupture.*

◆ Detach the syringe from the balloon inflation port, and allow the balloon to deflate on its own.

◆ Observe the waveform tracing, and make sure the tracing returns from the wedge tracing to the normal pulmonary artery tracing.

REMOVING THE CATHETER

◆ Inspect the chest X-ray for signs of catheter kinking or knotting.

◆ Obtain baseline vital signs and note the ECG pattern.

◆ Place the head of the bed flat, unless ordered otherwise.

◆ If the catheter was inserted using a superior approach, turn the patient's head to the side opposite the insertion site.

◆ Remove the dressing.

◆ Remove the sutures securing the catheter.

◆ You may turn stopcocks on to the distal port if you wish to observe waveforms. However, use caution because this may cause an air embolism.

◆ After verifying that the balloon is deflated, the practitioner withdraws the catheter slowly and smoothly.

◆ If there's resistance, stop withdrawal.

◆ Watch the ECG monitor for arrhythmias.

◆ If the introducer is removed, apply pressure to the site, and check it frequently for signs of bleeding.

◆ Dress the site as necessary.

◆ If the introducer is left in place, observe the diaphragm for blood backflow, which verifies the integrity of the hemostasis valve.

◆ Return equipment to the appropriate location.

◆ Turn off the bedside pressure modules, but leave the ECG module on.

◆ Reassure the patient and his family that he'll be observed closely.

◆ Make sure the patient understands that the catheter was removed because his condition has improved and he no longer needs it.

◆ Advise the patient to use caution when moving in bed.

◆ Never leave the balloon inflated; it may cause pulmonary infarction.

◆ To determine if the balloon is inflated, check the monitor for a wedge tracing, which indicates inflation.

◆ A pulmonary artery tracing confirms balloon deflation.

◆ Never inflate the balloon with more than the recommended air volume; overinflation may cause loss of elasticity or balloon rupture.

◆ With appropriate inflation volume, the balloon floats easily through the heart chambers and rests in the main branch of the pulmonary artery, producing accurate waveforms.

◆ Never inflate the balloon with fluid because it may not be able to be retrieved from inside the balloon, preventing deflation.

◆ Be aware that the catheter may slip back into the right ventricle.

◆ Check the monitor for a right ventricular waveform to detect ventricle irritation promptly.

◆ To minimize valvular trauma, make sure the balloon is deflated when the catheter is withdrawn from the pulmonary artery to the right ventricle or from the right ventricle to the right atrium.

◆ Change the dressing whenever it's moist or every 24 to 48 hours per facility policy; initial and date the dressings when changed.

◆ Change the catheter every 72 hours.

◆ Change the pressure tubing every 48 hours.

◆ Change the flush solution every 24 hours.

COMPLICATIONS

◆ Pulmonary artery perforation or rupture
◆ Pulmonary infarction
◆ Catheter knotting
◆ Local or systemic infection
◆ Cardiac arrhythmias
◆ Heparin-induced thrombocytopenia
◆ Catheter dislodgement

PATIENT TEACHING

◆ Explain all procedures to the patient to lessen anxiety.
◆ Tell the patient and family that the pressure waveform on the monitor may "move around," usually as a result of artifact.

DOCUMENTATION

◆ Record the date and time of catheter insertion.
◆ Note the practitioner who performed the procedure.
◆ Document the catheter insertion site.
◆ Record pressure waveforms and values for various heart chambers.
◆ Note the balloon inflation volume required to obtain a wedge tracing.
◆ Document arrhythmias that occurred during or after procedure.
◆ Record the type of flush solution used and its heparin concentration.
◆ Note the type of dressing applied.
◆ Document the patient's tolerance of the procedure.
◆ After catheter removal, document the patient's tolerance of the procedure, and note any problems encountered.

SELECTED REFERENCES

Bakker, R. "The Evidence-Based Character of the Pulmonary Artery Catheter (in Cardiac Patients)," *European Journal of Cardiovascular Nursing* 3(2):165-71, July 2004.

Bossert, T., et al. "Swan-Ganz Catheter-Induced Severe Complications in Cardiac Surgery: Right Ventricular Perforation, Knotting, and Rupture of a Pulmonary Artery," *Journal of Cardiac Surgery* 21(3):292-95, May-June 2006.

Harvey, S., et al. "Assessment of the Clinical Effectiveness of Pulmonary Artery Catheters in Management of Patients in Intensive Care (PAC-Man): A Randomised Controlled Trial," *Lancet* 366(9484):472-77, August 2005.

Pulse assessment

DESCRIPTION

- Pulse taking that determines rate (number of beats per minute), rhythm (pattern or regularity of the beats), and volume (amount of blood pumped with each beat).
- In adults and children older than age 3, the radial artery in the wrist is the most common palpation site.
- In infants and children younger than age 3, a stethoscope is used to listen to the heart itself (apical pulse) rather than palpating a pulse. (See *Pulse points.*)

- An apical-radial pulse is taken by simultaneously counting apical and radial beats: the first by auscultation at the apex of the heart, the second by palpation at the radial artery.
- Some heartbeats detected at the apex can't be detected at peripheral sites. When this occurs, the apical pulse rate is higher than the radial; the difference is the pulse deficit.
- If the pulse is faint or weak, a Doppler ultrasound blood flow detector may be used if available.

CONTRAINDICATIONS

- None known

EQUIPMENT

Watch with second hand ◆ stethoscope (for auscultating apical pulse) ◆ Doppler ultrasound ◆ flow detector ◆ alcohol pad

PREPARATION

- Assemble all equipment at the patient's bedside.
- Check Doppler for charged batteries.

KEY STEPS

- Wash your hands.
- Tell the patient you intend to take his pulse.
- Make sure the patient is comfortable and calm.

TAKING A RADIAL PULSE

- Position the patient: sitting or supine, arm at side or across chest.
- Gently press your index, middle, and ring fingers on the radial artery, inside his wrist. Don't use your thumb.
- Count the beats for 60 seconds or count for 30 seconds and multiply by 2.
- While counting the rate, assess pulse rhythm and volume.
- Repeat the count if there's an irregularity. Note if it occurs in a pattern or randomly.
- If you're still in doubt, take an apical pulse. (See *Identifying pulse patterns.*)

TAKING AN APICAL PULSE

- Place the patient in a supine position, and drape him.
- Warm the diaphragm or bell of the stethoscope in your hand.
- The bell transmits low-pitched sounds more effectively than the diaphragm.
- Place the diaphragm or bell of the stethoscope over the apex of the heart.
- Insert the earpieces.
- Count for 60 seconds; note rhythm, volume, and intensity.

Pulse points

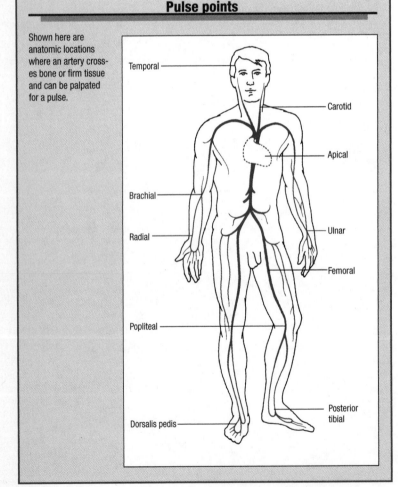

Shown here are anatomic locations where an artery crosses bone or firm tissue and can be palpated for a pulse.

Temporal

Carotid

Apical

Brachial

Radial

Ulnar

Femoral

Popliteal

Dorsalis pedis

Posterior tibial

TAKING AN APICAL-RADIAL PULSE

◆ Two nurses work together to obtain the apical-radial pulse.
◆ One palpates the radial pulse while the other auscultates the apical pulse with a stethoscope.
◆ The same watch must be used.
◆ Help the patient to a supine position, and drape him if necessary.
◆ Locate the apical and radial pulses.
◆ Begin counting at the same time for 60 seconds.

SPECIAL CONSIDERATIONS

◆ Take an apical pulse when the peripheral pulse is irregular.
◆ Use a Doppler ultrasound blood flow detector if the pulse is faint.
◆ For a one-person reading of an apical-radial pulse, hold the stethoscope in place with the hand that holds the watch while palpating the radial pulse with the other hand.

COMPLICATIONS
◆ None known

PATIENT TEACHING

◆ Teach the patient how to obtain a radial pulse if he's taking medication that controls his heart rate.

DOCUMENTATION

◆ Record the pulse rate, rhythm, volume, and time of measurement.
◆ When recording the apical pulse, include intensity of heart sounds.
◆ Chart apical-radial pulse by the pulse site: A/R pulse of 80/76.

SELECTED REFERENCES

Castledine, G. "The Importance of Measuring and Recording Vital Signs Correctly," *British Journal of Nursing* 15(5):285, March 2006.
Trim, J. "Monitoring Pulse," *Nursing Times* 101(21):30-31, May 2005.
White, J., et al. "Parents Measuring Pulses: An Observational Study," *Archives of Disease in Childhood* 89(3):274-75, March 2004.

Identifying pulse patterns

TYPE	RATE	RHYTHM (PER 3 SECONDS)	CAUSES AND RISK FACTORS
Normal	60 to 80 beats/minute; in neonates, 120 to 140 beats/minute	● ● ● ●	◆Varies with such factors as age, physical activity, and sex (men usually have lower pulse rates than women)
Tachycardia	More than 100 beats/minute	●●●●●●●	◆Accompanies stimulation of the sympathetic nervous system by emotional stress, such as anger, fear, or anxiety, or by the use of certain drugs such as caffeine ◆May result from exercise and from certain health conditions, such as heart failure, anemia, and fever (which increases oxygen requirements and, therefore, pulse rate)
Bradycardia	Less than 60 beats/minute	● ● ●	◆Accompanies stimulation of the parasympathetic nervous system by drug use, especially cardiac glycosides, and such conditions as cerebral hemorrhage and heart block ◆May be present in fit athletes
Irregular	Uneven time intervals between beats (for example, periods of regular rhythm interrupted by pauses or premature beats)	●●●● ●●●	◆May indicate cardiac irritability, hypoxia, digoxin toxicity, potassium imbalance or, sometimes, more serious arrhythmias if premature beats occur frequently ◆Occasional premature beats are normal

Pulse oximetry

DESCRIPTION

◆ Noninvasive technique is used to intermittently or continuously monitor arterial oxygen saturation (Sao_2).
◆ A photodetector slipped over the finger measures transmitted light as it passes through the vascular bed, detects the relative amount of color absorbed by arterial blood, and calculates exact mixed venous oxygen saturation without interference from surrounding venous blood, skin, connective tissue, or bone.
◆ With an ear probe, oximetry works by monitoring transmission of light waves through the vascular bed of a patient's earlobe. Results are inaccurate if the patient's earlobe is poorly perfused, as from low cardiac output. (See *How oximetry works*.)

CONTRAINDICATIONS

◆ None known

Oximeter ◆ finger or ear probe ◆ alcohol pads ◆ nail polish remover if necessary

PREPARATION

◆ Review manufacturer's instructions for assembly.

◆ Explain the procedure to the patient.

USING A FINGER PROBE

◆ Select a finger (usually index finger) for the test.
◆ Remove false fingernails and nail polish from the test finger.
◆ Place the transducer (photodetector) probe over the patient's finger so the light beams and sensors oppose each other.
◆ Trim long fingernails or position the probe perpendicular to the finger.
◆ Position the patient's hand at heart level.

AGE FACTOR *If testing a neonate or small infant, wrap the probe around the foot so the light beams and detectors oppose each other. For a large infant, use a probe that fits on the great toe and secure it to the foot.*

◆ Turn on the power switch. If the device is working properly, a beep will sound, a display will light momentarily, and the pulse searchlight will flash.
◆ After four to six heartbeats, the pulse amplitude indicator will begin tracking the pulse.

USING AN EAR PROBE

◆ Using an alcohol pad, massage the patient's earlobe for 10 to 20 seconds.
◆ Mild erythema indicates adequate vascularization.
◆ Securely attach the ear probe to the patient's earlobe or pinna.
◆ Use the ear probe stabilizer for prolonged or exercise testing.
◆ After a few seconds, a saturation reading and pulse waveform will appear on the oximeter's screen.
◆ Leave the ear probe in place for 3 or more minutes.
◆ After the procedure, remove the probe, turn off and unplug the unit, and clean the probe by gently rubbing it with an alcohol pad.

How oximetry works

The pulse oximeter allows noninvasive monitoring of a patient's arterial oxygen saturation (Sao_2) levels by measuring absorption (amplitude) of light waves as they pass through areas of the body that are highly perfused by arterial blood. Oximetry also monitors pulse rate and amplitude.

Light-emitting diodes in a transducer (photodetector) attached to the patient's body (shown at right on index finger) send red and infrared light beams through tissue. The photodetector records the relative amount of each color absorbed by arterial blood and transmits the data to a monitor, which displays the information with each heartbeat. If the Sao_2 level or pulse rate varies from preset limits, the monitor triggers visual and audible alarms.

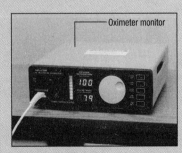

Oximeter monitor

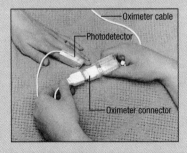

Oximeter cable

Photodetector

Oximeter connector

SPECIAL CONSIDERATIONS

◆ The pulse rate on the oximeter should correspond to the patient's actual pulse. If it doesn't, assess the patient, check the oximeter, and reposition the probe.
◆ Factors that interfere with accuracy include:
– elevated bilirubin level
– elevated carboxyhemoglobin or methemoglobin levels
– lipid emulsions and dyes
– excessive light
– excessive patient movement
– excessive ear pigment
– hypothermia
– hypotension
– vasoconstriction.
◆ Use the bridge of the nose if the patient has compromised circulation in his extremities.
◆ If Sao_2 is used to guide weaning the patient from forced inspiratory oxygen, obtain arterial blood gas analysis occasionally to correlate pulse oximetry readings with arterial oxygen saturation levels in the blood.

◆ If an automatic blood pressure cuff is used on the same extremity used for measuring Sao_2, the cuff will interfere with Sao_2 readings during inflation.
◆ In a patient with continuous pulse oximetry monitoring, move the probe every 2 hours to decrease risk of damage to the digits.
◆ If light is a problem, cover the probes.
◆ If patient movement is a problem, move the probe or select a different probe.
◆ If ear pigment is a problem, reposition the probe, revascularize the site, or use a finger probe. (See *Diagnosing pulse oximeter problems*.)
◆ Normal Sao_2 levels for pulse oximetry are 95% to 100% for adults and 93.8% to 100% by 1 hour after birth for healthy, full-term neonates.
◆ Lower levels may indicate hypoxemia that warrants intervention.
◆ Notify the practitioner of any significant change in the patient's condition.

COMPLICATIONS
◆ None known

PATIENT TEACHING

◆ Explain the reason for use of the device.
◆ Explain that the values displayed may be affected by movement and position of the sensor.
◆ Explain the alarm system and possible causes of false alarm.

DOCUMENTATION

◆ Note the procedure, date, time, oxygen saturation, and actions taken.
◆ Record the reading on appropriate flowcharts if indicated.

SELECTED REFERENCES
Allen, K. "Principles and Limitations of Pulse Oximetry in Patient Monitoring," *Nursing Times* 100(41):34-37, October 2004.

Cooper, R. "Using Finger-Toe Pulse Oximetry to Assess Arterial Blood Flow," *Nursing Times* 101(46):47-49, November 2005.

Giuliano, K.K., and Higgins, T.L. "New-Generation Pulse Oximetry in the Care of Critically Ill Patients," *American Journal of Critical Care* 14(1):26-37, January 2005.

Giuliano, K.K., and Liu, L.M. "Knowledge of Pulse Oximetry Among Critical Care Nurses," *Dimensions of Critical Care Nursing* 25(1):44-49, January-February 2006.

McMorrow, R.C., and Mythen, M.G. "Pulse Oximetry," *Current Opinion in Critical Care* 12(3):269-71, June 2006.

 TROUBLESHOOTER

Diagnosing pulse oximeter problems

To maintain continuous display of arterial oxygen saturation levels, keep the monitoring site clean and dry. Make sure the skin doesn't become irritated from adhesives used to keep disposable probes in place. Change the site if this happens. Disposable probes that irritate skin can also be replaced with nondisposable models.

Another common problem with pulse oximeters is failure of the device to obtain a signal. If this happens, first check the patient's vital signs. If they're sufficient to produce a signal, check for the following problems.

POOR CONNECTION

Check that the sensors are properly aligned. Make sure wires are intact and securely fastened and the pulse oximeter is plugged into a power source.

INADEQUATE OR INTERMITTENT BLOOD FLOW TO SITE

Check the patient's pulse rate and capillary refill time, and take corrective action if blood flow to the site is decreased. Loosen any restraints, remove tight-fitting clothes, remove blood pressure cuff if one is present, and check arterial and I.V. lines. If none of these interventions work, you may need to find an alternate site. Finding a site with proper circulation may also prove challenging when a patient is receiving vasoconstrictive drugs.

EQUIPMENT MALFUNCTIONS

Remove the pulse oximeter from the patient, set the alarm limits according to your facility's policies, and try the instrument on yourself or another healthy person. This will tell you if the equipment is working correctly.

Radiation implant therapy

OVERVIEW

DESCRIPTION

◆ Also called *brachytherapy,* implants of radioactive isotopes (encapsulated in seeds, needles, or sutures) deliver ionizing radiation within a body cavity or interstitially to a tumor site.

◆ It can deliver a continuous radiation dose over several hours or days to a specific site while minimizing exposure to adjacent tissues.

◆ Implants may be permanent or temporary.

◆ Isotopes, such as cesium 137, gold 198, iodine 125, iridium 192, palladium 103, and phosphorus 32, are used to treat cancers.

◆ Common implant sites include the brain, breast, cervix, endometrium, lung, neck, oral cavity, prostate, and vagina.

◆ Implant therapy is commonly combined with external radiation therapy for increased effectiveness.

◆ The patient is usually placed in a private room (with its own bathroom) located as far away from high-traffic areas as practical.

◆ If monitoring shows increased radiation hazard, adjacent rooms and hallways may also need to be restricted.

◆ Consult your facility's radiation safety policy for specific guidelines.

CONTRAINDICATIONS

◆ Pregnancy and patients trying to conceive

EQUIPMENT

Film badge or pocket dosimeter ◆ RADIATION PRECAUTION sign for door ◆ RADIATION PRECAUTION warning labels ◆ masking tape ◆ lead-lined container ◆ long-handled forceps ◆ lead shield and lead strip (optional)

IMPLANTS INSERTED IN THE ORAL CAVITY OR NECK
Emergency tracheotomy tray

IMPLANTS INSERTED IN THE ANAL CAVITY OR VAGINA
Male T-binder ◆ two sanitary napkins with safety pins

PREPARATION

◆ Place the lead-lined container and long-handled forceps in a corner of the patient's room.

◆ Mark a "safe line" on the floor with masking tape 6′ (1.8 m) from the patient's bed.

◆ Place a portable lead shield in the room to use when providing care.

◆ Place an emergency tracheotomy tray in the room if an implant will be inserted in the oral cavity or neck.

KEY STEPS

◆ Confirm the patient's identity using two patient identifiers according to facility policy.

◆ Explain the treatment and its goals to the patient.

◆ Review radiation safety procedures, visitation policies, potential adverse effects, and interventions. Also review long-term concerns and home care issues.

◆ Place the RADIATION PRECAUTION sign on the door.

◆ Check to see that informed consent has been obtained.

◆ Perform all laboratory tests before beginning treatment.

◆ A badged technician should obtain specimens during treatment.

◆ Use a RADIATION PRECAUTION label on the specimen tube.

◆ Alert laboratory personnel before bringing it.

◆ Ask the radiation oncology department how to transport specimens safely.

◆ Affix a RADIATION PRECAUTION label to the patient's wristband.

◆ Affix RADIATION PRECAUTION warning labels to the patient's chart and the Kardex to ensure staff awareness of patient's radioactive status.

◆ Wear a film badge or dosimeter at waist level during the entire shift. Turn in the radiation badge monthly.

◆ Pocket dosimeters measure immediate exposures, aren't part of the permanent exposure record, and are used to make sure that nurses receive the lowest possible exposure.

◆ Each nurse must have a personal, nontransferable film or ring badge that documents cumulative lifetime radiation exposure.

◆ Allow only badged primary caregivers into the patient's room.

◆ To minimize exposure to radiation, use the three principles of time, distance, and shielding.

◆ Provide essential nursing care only; omit bed baths.

- Dressing changes over an implanted area must be supervised by the radiation technician or another designated caregiver.
- Before discharge, a patient's temporary implant must be removed and properly stored by the radiation oncology department.
- A patient with a permanent implant may not be released until his radioactivity level becomes less than 5 millirems/hour at 3.3′ (1 m).

SPECIAL CONSIDERATIONS

- Anyone pregnant or trying to conceive or father a child must avoid patients receiving radiation implant therapy.
- Notify the receiving department if the patient must be moved.
- Clear the route of equipment and people.
- Secure and lock the elevator.
- Two badged caregivers should transport the patient.
- If the patient is delayed, stand as far away as possible.
- Staff from the radiation oncology department monitors the patient's room daily.
- Disposables must be monitored and removed per facility policy.
- If a code is called on a patient with an implant, notify the code team and the radiation oncology department.
- Cover the implant site with a strip of lead shielding.
- Monitor anything that leaves the room for radiation.
- The primary care nurse must remain in the room (as far away from the patient as possible) to act as a resource for the patient and provide film badges or dosimeters to code team members.
- If an implant becomes dislodged, notify the radiation oncology department staff and follow their instructions.
- Typically, the dislodged implant is collected with long-handled forceps and placed in a lead-shielded canister.

- If a patient with an implant dies on the unit, notify the radiation oncology department so they can remove a temporary implant and store it properly.
- If the implant is permanent, radiation oncology staff members determine which precautions to follow before postmortem care can be provided and before the body can be moved to the morgue.

COMPLICATIONS

- Dislodgment of the radiation source or applicator
- Tissue fibrosis
- Xerostomia
- Radiation pneumonitis
- Muscle atrophy
- Sterility
- Vaginal dryness or stenosis
- Fistulas
- Hypothyroidism
- Altered bowel habits
- Infection
- Airway obstruction
- Diarrhea
- Cystitis
- Myelosuppression
- Neurotoxicity
- Secondary cancers

PATIENT TEACHING

- Provide the patient and family with radiation oncology department contact information.
- Tell the patient who has had a cervical implant to expect slight to moderate vaginal bleeding after being discharged. This flow normally changes color from pink to brown to white.
- Instruct the patient to notify the practitioner if bleeding increases, persists for more than 48 hours, or has a foul odor.
- Caution the patient to avoid sexual intercourse and the use of tampons until after her follow-up visit (about 6 weeks after discharge).

- Instruct the patient to take showers rather than baths for 2 weeks, to avoid douching unless allowed by the practitioner, and to avoid activities that cause abdominal strain for 6 weeks.
- Refer the patient for sexual or psychological counseling if needed.

DOCUMENTATION

- Record radiation precautions taken during treatment.
- Note adverse effects of therapy.
- Document patient and family teaching given and their responses.
- Record the patient's tolerance of isolation procedures.
- Note the family's compliance with procedures.
- Document referrals to local cancer services.

SELECTED REFERENCES

Colella, J., et al. "Prostate HDR Radiation Therapy: A Comparative Study Evaluating the Effectiveness of Pain Management with Peripheral PCA vs. PCEA," *Urologic Nursing* 26(1):57-61, February 2006.

Hancock, C.M., and Burrow, M.A. "The Role of Radiation Therapy in the Treatment of Central Nervous System Tumors," *Seminars in Oncology Nursing* 20(4):253-59, November 2004.

Warnock, C. "Patients' Experiences of Intracavity Brachytherapy Treatment for Gynaecological Cancer," *European Journal of Oncology Nursing* 9(1):44-55, March 2005.

Zeroski, D., et al. "Factors Affecting Patient Selection for Prostate Brachytherapy: What Nurses Should Know," *Clinical Journal of Oncology Nursing* 9(5):553-60, October 2005.

Radiation therapy, external

DESCRIPTION
- About 60% of patients with cancer are treated with external radiation therapy.
- Also called *radiotherapy*, treatment delivers radiation — X-rays or gamma rays — directly to the cancer site.
- Doses are based on the type, stage, and location of the tumor as well as on the patient's size, condition, and overall treatment goals.
- Doses are given in increments, usually three to five times per week, until the total dose is reached.
- Goals include cure, control, or palliation.
- Radiation is delivered by machines that aim a concentrated beam of high-energy particles (photons and gamma rays) at the target site.
- Two types of machines are commonly used — units containing cobalt or cesium as radioactive sources for gamma rays, and linear accelerators that use electricity to produce X-rays.
- Linear accelerators produce high energy with great penetrating ability.
- Orthovoltage machines produce less powerful electron beams that may be used for superficial tumors.
- Radiation therapy may be augmented by chemotherapy, brachytherapy (radiation implant therapy), or surgery, as needed.

CONTRAINDICATIONS
- None known

Radiation therapy machine

- Confirm the patient's identity using two patient identifiers according to facility policy.
- Explain the treatment to the patient and his family.
- Review the treatment goals.
- Discuss adverse effects as well as interventions to minimize them.
- Discuss possible long-term complications and treatment issues.
- Educate the patient and his family about local cancer services.
- Make sure that informed consent has been obtained.
- Report recent laboratory and imaging results to the radiation oncology staff.
- Transport the patient to the radiation oncology department.
- Simulation (treatment planning) takes place before treatment; it includes mapping the target area and marking it.
- Duration and frequency of treatments are determined based on body size, portal size, the extent and location of the cancer, and treatment goals.
- The patient is positioned on the treatment table.
- Treatments last from a few seconds to a few minutes.
- Reassure the patient that he won't feel anything and that he won't be radioactive after the procedure.
- After treatment, the patient may return home or to his room.

SPECIAL CONSIDERATIONS

- ◆ The full benefit may not occur for weeks or months.
- ◆ Adverse effects arise and diminish gradually after treatments; they may be acute, subacute chronic, or long term.
- ◆ Adverse effects are localized. Their severity depends on the total radiation dosage, organ sensitivity, and the patient's overall condition.
- ◆ Common acute and subacute adverse effects include altered skin integrity, altered GI and genitourinary function, altered fertility and sexual function, altered bone marrow production, fatigue, and alopecia.

COMPLICATIONS

- ◆ Long-term complications may include:
- – radiation pneumonitis
- – neuropathy
- – skin and muscle atrophy
- – telangiectasia
- – fistulas
- – altered endocrine function
- – secondary cancers.
- ◆ Other complications include:
- – headache
- – alopecia
- – xerostomia
- – dysphagia
- – stomatitis
- – altered skin integrity (wet or dry desquamation)
- – nausea
- – vomiting
- – heartburn
- – diarrhea
- – cystitis
- – fatigue.

PATIENT TEACHING

- ◆ Instruct the patient and his family on proper skin care and how to manage possible adverse effects.
- ◆ Instruct the patient to report any long-term adverse effects.
- ◆ Instruct the patient to leave target area markings intact.
- ◆ Emphasize the importance of keeping follow-up appointments with the practitioner.
- ◆ Refer the patient to a support group.

DOCUMENTATION

- ◆ Record radiation precautions taken during treatment.
- ◆ Note interventions used and the patient's response to them.
- ◆ Document grading of adverse effects.
- ◆ Record teaching given to the patient and family and their responses.
- ◆ Document the patient's tolerance of isolation procedures.
- ◆ Record the family's compliance with the procedures.
- ◆ Note discharge plans and teaching.
- ◆ Record referrals to local cancer services.

SELECTED REFERENCES

Cady, J. "Navigating External Beam Radiation Therapy for Head and Neck Cancer," *Clinical Journal of Oncology Nursing* 9(3):362-66, June 2005.

Horiot, J.C. "Prophylaxis Versus Treatment: Is There a Better Way to Manage Radiotherapy-Induced Nausea and Vomiting?" *International Journal of Radiation Oncology, Biology, Physics* 60(4):1018-25, November 2004.

Seegenschmiedt, H. "Management of Skin and Related Reactions to Radiotherapy," *Frontiers of Radiation Therapy and Oncology* 39:102-19, 2006.

Radioactive iodine therapy

OVERVIEW

DESCRIPTION

- Usually administered orally, the isotope is used to treat postoperative residual cancer, recurrent disease, inoperable primary thyroid tumors, invasion of the thyroid capsule, or thyroid ablation as well as cancers that have metastasized to cervical or mediastinal lymph nodes or other distant sites.
- Because radioactive iodine (^{131}I) is absorbed systemically, all body secretions, especially urine, must be considered radioactive.
- For ^{131}I treatments, the patient is usually placed in a private room (with its own bathroom) located as far away from high-traffic areas as practical.
- Adjacent rooms and hallways may also need to be restricted.
- Consult your facility's radiation safety policy for specific guidelines.
- Most patients receive this treatment on an outpatient basis and are sent home with appropriate home care instructions.

CONTRAINDICATIONS

- Allergies to iodine
- Pregnancy
- Patients trying to conceive

EQUIPMENT

Film badges ◆ pocket dosimeters or ring badges ◆ RADIATION PRECAUTION sign for door ◆ RADIATION PRECAUTION warning labels ◆ waterproof gowns ◆ clear and red plastic bags for contaminated articles ◆ plastic wrap ◆ absorbent plastic-lined pads ◆ masking tape ◆ radioresistant gloves ◆ trash cans ◆ emergency tracheotomy tray ◆ portable lead shield (optional)

PREPARATION

- Assemble all necessary equipment in the patient's room.
- Keep an emergency tracheotomy tray just outside the room.

- Place the RADIATION PRECAUTION sign on the door.
- Affix RADIATION PRECAUTION warning labels to the patient's chart and drug administration record.
- Place an absorbent plastic-lined pad on the bathroom floor and under the sink.
- If the patient's room is carpeted, cover it with a pad.
- Place an additional pad over the bedside table.
- Secure plastic wrap over the telephone, television controls, bed controls, mattress, call button, and toilet.
- Line trash cans with two clear bags inserted inside an outer red bag.
- Monitor all objects before they leave the room.
- Use disposable utensils and containers for food and beverages.

KEY STEPS

- Confirm the patient's identity using two patient identifiers according to facility policy.
- Review the procedure and treatment goals with the patient and his family.
- Review radiation safety procedures, visitation, potential adverse effects, interventions, and home care procedures.
- Verify that informed consent has been obtained.
- Check for allergies to iodine.
- Review the drug history for thyroid-containing or thyroid-altering drugs or lithium carbonate, which may increase ^{131}I uptake.
- Review the patient's health history for vomiting, diarrhea, productive cough, and sinus drainage.
- Remove dentures to avoid contaminating them and reduce radioactive secretions. Replace them 48 hours after treatment.
- Affix a RADIATION PRECAUTION label to the patient's wristband.
- Encourage use of the toilet rather than a bedpan or urinal and to flush it three times after each use to reduce radiation levels.

- Tell the patient to remain in his room except for tests or procedures. Allow him to ambulate.
- Instruct the patient to increase his fluid intake to 3 qt (3 L) daily.
- Encourage the patient to chew or suck on hard candy to reduce dry mouth.
- Make sure that all laboratory tests are performed before treatment.
- If required, the badged laboratory technician obtains the specimen, labels the collection tube with a RADIATION PRECAUTION label, and alerts laboratory personnel before transporting it.
- If urine tests are needed, ask the radiation oncology department or laboratory technician how to transport the specimens safely.
- Wear a film badge or dosimeter at waist level.
- Turn in the radiation badge monthly or per facility protocol.
- Record your exposures accurately.
- Pocket dosimeters measure immediate exposures and may not be part of the permanent exposure record. They help to make sure that nurses receive the lowest possible exposure.
- Each nurse must have a nontransferable film or ring badge.
- Only primary caregivers are badged and allowed into the room.
- Wear gloves when touching the patient or objects in his room.
- Wear a waterproof gown and gloves when handling body secretions.
- Allow visitors to stay no more than 30 minutes every 24 hours.
- Stress that no visitors will be allowed who are pregnant or trying to conceive or father a child.
- Restrict direct contact to no more than 30 minutes or 20 millirems per day.

AGE FACTOR *Visitors younger than age 18 aren't allowed in the patient's room.*

- If the patient is receiving 200 millicuries of ^{131}I, remain with him only 2 to 4 minutes and stand no closer than 12″ (30.5 cm) away.
- Give essential nursing care only; omit bed baths.

- If the patient vomits or urinates on the floor, notify the nuclear medicine department. Use nondisposable radioresistant gloves when cleaning the floor.
- After cleanup, wash your gloved hands, remove the gloves and leave them in the room, and then rewash your hands.
- Notify the receiving department if the patient must be moved.
- Clear the route of equipment and people.
- Secure and lock the elevator.
- Two badged caregivers should transport the patient.
- If the patient is delayed, stand as far away as possible.
- Staff from the radiation oncology department rather than housekeeping clean the room.
- Staff from the radiation oncology department monitor the patient's room daily.
- Disposables must be monitored and removed per facility policy.
- At discharge, schedule the patient for a follow-up examination.
- Arrange for a whole-body scan about 7 to 10 days after ^{131}I treatment.
- Provide information on community support services.

SPECIAL CONSIDERATIONS

- In lower doses, ^{131}I may also be used to treat hyperthyroidism.
- Anyone pregnant or trying to conceive or father a child must avoid patients receiving radioactive iodine therapy.
- If a code is called on a patient undergoing ^{131}I therapy, notify the code team of the patient's radioactive status, and exclude any team member who's pregnant or trying to conceive or father a child.
- Notify the radiation oncology department.
- Don't allow anything out of the room until it's monitored.
- The primary care nurse must remain in the room (as far as possible from the patient) to act as a resource person and provide film badges or dosimeters to code team members.
- If the patient dies, notify the radiology safety officer, who can advise on postmortem care.

COMPLICATIONS
- Myelosuppression
- Radiation pulmonary fibrosis
- Nausea
- Vomiting
- Headache
- Radiation thyroiditis
- Fever
- Sialadenitis
- Pain and swelling at metastatic sites

PATIENT TEACHING

- Instruct the patient to report long-term adverse reactions.
- Review signs and symptoms of hypothyroidism and hyperthyroidism.
- Ask the patient to report signs and symptoms of thyroid cancer, such as enlarged lymph nodes, dyspnea, bone pain, nausea, vomiting, and abdominal discomfort.
- Although the patient's radiation level at discharge may be safe, suggest that he take precautions during the first week, such as using separate eating utensils, sleeping in a separate bedroom, and avoiding body contact.
- Sexual intercourse may be resumed 1 week after ^{131}I treatment; however, urge a female patient to avoid pregnancy for 6 months after treatment.
- Tell a male patient to avoid impregnating his partner for 3 months after treatment.

DOCUMENTATION

- Record radiation precautions taken during treatment.
- Note teaching given to the patient and his family.
- Document the patient's tolerance of and his family's compliance with isolation procedures.
- Record referrals made to local cancer counseling services.

SELECTED REFERENCES
Brans, B., et al. "Clinical Applications of Newer Radionuclide Therapies," *European Journal of Cancer* 42(8):994-1003, May 2006.

Chaukar, D.A., et al. "Pediatric Thyroid Cancer," *Journal of Surgical Oncology* 92(2):130-33, November 2005.

Liu, Y.Y., et al. "Lithium as Adjuvant to Radioiodine Therapy in Differentiated Thyroid Carcinoma: Clinical and In Vitro Studies," *Clinical Endocrinology* 64(6):617-24, June 2006.

Miller, R.W., and Zanzonico, P.B. "Radioiodine Fallout and Breast-Feeding," *Radiation Research* 164(3):339-40, September 2005.

Rectal suppository or ointment administration

OVERVIEW

DESCRIPTION
Suppositories
- A rectal suppository is a small, solid, medicated mass that's made with a cocoa butter or glycerin base. It's usually cone shaped.
- It may be inserted to stimulate peristalsis and defecation or relieve pain, vomiting, and local irritation.
- Rectal suppositories commonly contain drugs that reduce fever, induce relaxation, interact poorly with digestive enzymes, or have a taste too offensive for oral use.
- Rectal suppositories melt at body temperature and are absorbed slowly.

Ointments
- An ointment is a semisolid drug used to produce local effects that may be applied externally to the anus or internally to the rectum.
- Rectal ointments commonly contain drugs that reduce inflammation or relieve pain and itching.

CONTRAINDICATIONS
- Cardiac arrhythmias
- Recent rectal or prostate surgery

EQUIPMENT

Rectal suppository or tube of ointment ◆ ointment applicator ◆ patient's drug record and chart ◆ gloves ◆ water-soluble lubricant ◆ 4″ × 4″ gauze pads ◆ bedpan (optional)

PREPARATION
- Store rectal suppositories in the refrigerator until needed.
- If softened, hold the suppository (in its wrapper) under cold running water.

KEY STEPS

- Verify the order, comparing the label on the package with the order.
- Read the label before you open the wrapper and as you remove the drug.
- If your facility uses a bar code system, scan your I.D. badge, the patient's bracelet, and the bar code on the drug's wrapper.
- Check the expiration date.
- Wash your hands with warm soap and water.
- Confirm the patient's identity using two patient identifiers according to facility policy.
- Explain the purpose and procedure to the patient.
- Provide privacy.

INSERTING A RECTAL SUPPOSITORY
- Place the patient on his left side in Sims' position.
- Drape him with bedcovers to expose only the buttocks.
- Put on gloves.
- Remove the suppository from its wrapper, and lubricate it with water-soluble lubricant.
- Lift the patient's upper buttock with your nondominant hand to expose the anus.
- Instruct the patient to take several deep breaths through his mouth to help relax the anal sphincters and reduce anxiety or discomfort during insertion.
- Using the index finger of your dominant hand, insert the suppository — tapered end first — about 3″ (7.5 cm), until you feel it pass the internal anal sphincter. (See *How to administer a rectal suppository or ointment*.)
- Encourage the patient to lie quietly and retain the suppository for the appropriate length of time.
- Remove and discard your gloves.

APPLYING RECTAL OINTMENT
♦ Put on gloves.
♦ Apply external drug with gloves or a gauze pad.
♦ To apply internally, attach the applicator to the tube of ointment and coat with water-soluble lubricant.
♦ Squeeze a small amount of ointment from the tube to gauge needed pressure.
♦ Lift the patient's upper buttock with your nondominant hand to expose the anus.
♦ Instruct the patient to take several deep breaths through his mouth to relax the anal sphincters and reduce anxiety or discomfort during insertion.
♦ After insertion, slowly squeeze about 1″ (2.5 cm) of ointment. Remove the applicator.
♦ Place a folded 4″ × 4″ gauze pad between the patient's buttocks to absorb excess ointment.
♦ Detach the applicator from the tube, and recap the tube.
♦ Clean the applicator thoroughly with soap and warm water.

SPECIAL CONSIDERATIONS

♦ To relieve constipation, insert a suppository 30 minutes before mealtime.
♦ Insert a medicated retention suppository between meals.
♦ Place the call button in easy reach and watch for the signal.

COMPLICATIONS
♦ None known

PATIENT TEACHING

♦ Explain the procedure to the patient.
♦ Instruct the patient to retain the suppository.
♦ Tell the patient that the suppository may discolor his next bowel movement.

DOCUMENTATION

♦ Record administration time and dose.
♦ Note the patient's response to the procedure.

SELECTED REFERENCES
El-Kamel, A., and El-Khatib, M. "Thermally Reversible In Situ Gelling Carbamazepine Liquid Suppository," *Drug Delivery* 13(2):143-48, March-April 2006.
Hidaka, N., et al. "Effect of Simultaneous Insertion of Oleaginous Base on the Absorption and on the Anticonvulsant Effect of Diazepam Suppository," *Biological & Pharmaceutical Bulletin* 29(4):705-708, April 2006.
Zweig, S.B., et al. "Rectal Administration of Propylthiouracil in Suppository Form in Patients with Thyrotoxicosis and Critical Illness: Case Report and Review of Literature," *Endocrine Practice* 12(1):43-47, January-February 2006.

How to administer a rectal suppository or ointment

When inserting a suppository, direct its tapered end toward the side of the rectum so that it contacts the membranes to encourage absorption of the medication.

When applying a rectal ointment internally, be sure to lubricate the applicator to minimize pain on insertion. Then direct the applicator tip toward the patient's umbilicus.

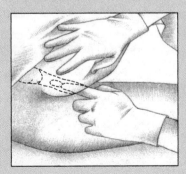
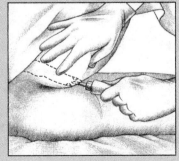

Rectal tube insertion and removal

DESCRIPTION

- Inserting a rectal tube may relieve the discomfort of distention and flatus.
- Decreased motility may result from various medical or surgical conditions; certain medications, such as atropine sulfate; or even swallowed air.

CONTRAINDICATIONS

- Recent rectal or prostate surgery
- Recent myocardial infarction
- Diseases of the rectal mucosa

Stethoscope ◆ linen-saver pads ◆ drape ◆ water-soluble lubricant ◆ commercial kit or #22 to #32 French rectal tube of soft rubber or plastic ◆ container (emesis basin, plastic bag, or water bottle with vent) ◆ tape ◆ gloves

PREPARATION

- Bring all equipment to the patient's bedside, provide privacy, and wash your hands.

- Confirm the patient's identity using two patient identifiers according to facility policy.
- Explain the procedure and encourage the patient to relax.
- Check for abdominal distention. Using the stethoscope, auscultate for bowel sounds.
- Place the linen-saver pads under the patient's buttocks to absorb drainage that may leak from the tube.
- Position the patient in the left-lateral Sims' position to facilitate rectal tube insertion.
- Put on gloves.
- Drape the patient's exposed buttocks.
- Lubricate the rectal tube tip with water-soluble lubricant to ease insertion and prevent rectal irritation.
- Lift the patient's right buttock to expose the anus.
- Insert the rectal tube tip into the anus, advancing the tube 2″ to 4″ (5 to 10 cm) into the rectum. Direct the tube toward the umbilicus along the anatomic course of the large intestine.
- As you insert the tube, tell the patient to breathe slowly and deeply, or suggest that he bear down as he would for a bowel movement to relax the anal sphincter and ease insertion.
- Using tape, secure the rectal tube to the buttocks. Then attach the tube to the container to collect possible leakage.
- Remove the tube after 15 to 20 minutes. If the patient reports continued discomfort or if gas wasn't expelled, you can repeat the procedure in 2 or 3 hours, if ordered.
- Clean the patient, and replace soiled linens and the linen-saver pad. Make sure that the patient feels as comfortable as possible. Again, check for abdominal distention and listen for bowel sounds.
- If you plan to reuse the equipment, clean it and store it in the bedside cabinet; otherwise, discard the tube.

SPECIAL CONSIDERATIONS

◆ Fastening a plastic bag (like a balloon) to the external end of the tube lets you observe gas expulsion. Leaving a rectal tube in place indefinitely does little to promote peristalsis, can reduce sphincter responsiveness, and may lead to permanent sphincter damage or pressure necrosis of the mucosa.

◆ Repeat insertion periodically to stimulate GI activity. If the tube fails to relieve distention, notify the practitioner.

COMPLICATIONS

◆ None known

PATIENT TEACHING

◆ Inform the patient about each step and offer reassurance during the procedure to encourage cooperation and promote relaxation.

DOCUMENTATION

◆ Record the date and time that you inserted the tube. Note the amount, color, and consistency of any evacuated matter.

◆ Describe the patient's abdomen — hard, distended, soft, or drumlike on percussion.

◆ Note bowel sounds before and after insertion.

SELECTED REFERENCES

Chaitowitz, I.M., et al. "Rectal Guiding Tube to Facilitate Distal Colonic Stent Insertion," *Australasian Radiology* 50(3):275-77, June 2006.

Gurjar, S.V., et al. "The Use of Rectal Tubes in UK and Ireland," *Colorectal Disease Supplement* 7(Suppl 1):135-36, July 2005.

Nozu, T., et al. "Repetitive Rectal Painful Distention Induces Rectal Hypersensitivity in Patients with Irritable Bowel Syndrome," *Journal of Gastroenterology* 41(3):217-22, March 2006.

Respiration assessment

DESCRIPTION

◆ External respiration (breathing) is accomplished by the diaphragm and chest muscles and delivers oxygen to the lower respiratory tract and alveoli.
◆ There are four measures of respiration: rate, rhythm, depth, and sound, which reflect the body's metabolic state, diaphragm and chest-muscle condition, and airway patency.

– The rate is recorded as the number of cycles (with inspiration and expiration comprising one cycle) per minute.
– The rhythm is recorded as the regularity of these cycles.
– The depth is recorded as the volume of air inhaled and exhaled with each respiration.
– Sound is recorded as the audible digression from normal, effortless breathing.

CONTRAINDICATIONS
◆ None known

EQUIPMENT

Watch with second hand

Identifying respiratory patterns

This chart shows several common types of irregular respiratory patterns and their possible causes. It's important to assess the patient for the underlying cause and effect on the patient.

TYPE	CHARACTERISTICS	PATTERN	POSSIBLE CAUSES
Apnea	Periodic absence of breathing		◆ Mechanical airway obstruction ◆ Conditions affecting the brain's respiratory center in the lateral medulla oblongata
Apneustic breathing	Prolonged, gasping inspiration followed by extremely short, inefficient expiration		◆ Lesions of the respiratory center
Bradypnea	Slow, regular respirations of equal depth		◆ Normal pattern during sleep ◆ Conditions affecting the respiratory center: tumors, metabolic disorders, respiratory decompensation, and use of opiates or alcohol
Cheyne-Stokes respirations	Fast, deep respirations of 30 to 170 seconds punctuated by periods of apnea lasting 20 to 60 seconds		◆ Increased intracranial pressure, severe heart failure, renal failure, meningitis, drug overdose, and cerebral anoxia
Eupnea	Normal rate and rhythm		◆ Normal respiration
Kussmaul's respirations	Fast (over 20 breaths/minute), deep (resembling sighs), labored respirations without pause		◆ Renal failure and metabolic acidosis, particularly diabetic ketoacidosis
Tachypnea	Rapid respirations; rate rises with body temperature — about 4 breaths/minute for every degree Fahrenheit above normal		◆ Pneumonia, compensatory respiratory alkalosis, respiratory insufficiency, lesions of the respiratory center, and salicylate poisoning

---

KEY STEPS

- Assess respirations immediately after taking the patient's pulse.
- Keep your fingertips over the radial artery, but count respirations.
- Observe the rise and fall of the patient's chest.
- Alternatively, position the patient's opposite arm across his chest and count respirations by feeling its rise and fall.
- Count respirations for 30 seconds and multiply by two. Count for 60 seconds if respirations are irregular.
- Monitor and record stertor, stridor, wheezing, and expiratory grunts.

   AGE FACTOR When listening for stridor in infants and children with croup, also observe for sternal, substernal, or intercostal retractions.

- Wheezing is caused by partial obstruction in the smaller bronchi and bronchioles.

   AGE FACTOR In infants, an expiratory grunt indicates imminent respiratory distress.

   AGE FACTOR In older patients, an expiratory grunt may result from partial airway obstruction or neuromuscular reflex.

- Watch the patient's chest movements and listen to his breathing to determine the rhythm and sound of respirations. (See *Identifying respiratory patterns.*)
- Use a stethoscope to detect crackles and rhonchi or the lack of sound.
- Observe the depth of respirations (shallow or deep).
- Observe for accessory muscle use, indicating weakness of the diaphragm and external intercostal muscles.

SPECIAL CONSIDERATIONS

- Respiratory rates less than 8 or more than 40 breaths/minute are usually considered abnormal.
- Report the sudden onset of such rates promptly.
- Observe the patient for signs of dyspnea.
- Note bluish discoloration in the nail beds, lips, under the tongue, in the buccal mucosa, or in the conjunctiva.
- Consider personal and family history.
- Inquire about the patient's smoking history.

   AGE FACTOR A child's respiratory rate may double in response to exercise, illness, or emotion. Normally, the rate for a neonate is 30 to 80 breaths/minute; for a toddler, 20 to 40; and for a child of school age and older, 15 to 25. Children usually reach the adult rate (12 to 20) at about age 15.

COMPLICATIONS

- Dyspnea

PATIENT TEACHING

- Encourage the patient to relax but avoid explaining the procedure because this might alter his breathing pattern.

DOCUMENTATION

- Note the rate, depth, rhythm, and sound of the patient's respirations.

SELECTED REFERENCES

Castledine, G. "The Importance of Measuring and Recording Vital Signs Correctly," *British Journal of Nursing* 15(5): 285, March 2006.

Hogan, J. "Why Don't Nurses Monitor the Respiratory Rates of Patients?" *British Journal of Nursing* 15(9):489-92, May 2006.

Lovett, P.B., et al. "The Vexatious Vital: Neither Clinical Measurements by Nurses nor an Electronic Monitor Provides Accurate Measurements of Respiratory Rate in Triage," *Annals of Emergency Medicine* 45(1):68-76, January 2005.

Trim, J. "Respirations," *Nursing Times* 101(22):30-1, May-June 2005.

Restraint application

DESCRIPTION

- Soft restraints limit movement to prevent a confused, disoriented, or combative patient from injuring himself or others.
- They should be used only when less restrictive measures have proven ineffective.
- Vest and belt restraints, used to prevent falls from a bed or a chair, permit full movement of the arms and legs.
- Limb restraints, used to prevent the removal of supportive equipment, such as I.V. lines, indwelling catheters, and nasogastric tubes, allow only slight limb motion.
- Mitts prevent removal of supportive equipment, keep the patient from scratching rashes or sores, and prevent a combative patient from injuring himself or others.
- Body restraints, used to control the combative or hysterical patient, immobilize all or most of the body.
- When soft restraints aren't sufficient and sedation is dangerous or ineffective, leather restraints can be used.
- Depending on the patient's behavior, leather restraints may be applied to all limbs (four-point restraints) or to one arm and one leg (two-point restraints). Duration of such restraint is governed by state law and facility policy.

CONTRAINDICATIONS

- None known

WARNING *Restraints can cause skin irritation and restrict blood flow; don't apply over wounds or I.V. catheters.*

WARNING *Use restraints cautiously in seizure-prone patients and those with heart failure or respiratory disorders.*

EQUIPMENT

SOFT RESTRAINTS

Restraint (vest, limb, mitt, belt, or body, as needed) ◆ gauze pads, if needed ◆ restraint flow sheet

LEATHER RESTRAINTS

Two wrist and two ankle leather restraints ◆ four straps ◆ key ◆ large gauze pads to cushion each extremity ◆ restraint flow sheet

PREPARATION

- Choose the correct size restraints.
- For leather restraints, unlock straps and check that the key fits.

KEY STEPS

- Obtain a practitioner's order for restraint.
- The order must be time limited: 4 hours for adults, 2 hours for patients ages 9 to 17, and 1 hour for patients younger than age 9.
- The practitioner must see and evaluate the patient within 1 hour after initiation of restraint use.
- The original order expires in 24 hours.
- A practitioner must see and evaluate the patient before a new order can be issued.
- Obtain adequate assistance before entering the patient's room.
- Assure the patient that restraints are being used to protect him.
- Confirm the patient's identity using two patient identifiers according to facility policy.

APPLYING A VEST RESTRAINT

- Put the patient in a sitting position if his condition permits.
- Slip the vest over his gown. Crisscross the cloth flaps at the front, placing the V-shaped opening at the patient's throat.
- Pass the tab on one flap through the slot on the opposite flap.
- Adjust the vest for comfort. Avoid wrapping too tightly.

- Tie restraints securely and out of the patient's reach.
- Use a bow or a knot that can be released quickly.
- Leave 1″ or 2″ (2.5 to 5 cm) of slack in the straps to allow room for movement.
- Stay alert for signs of respiratory distress.
- Make sure that the vest hasn't tightened with the patient's movement.
- Loosen the vest frequently so the patient can stretch, turn, and breathe deeply.

APPLYING A LIMB RESTRAINT

- Wrap the patient's wrist or ankle with gauze pads to reduce friction.
- Wrap the restraint around the gauze pads.
- Pass the strap on the narrow end of the restraint through the slot in the broad end and adjust for a snug fit or fasten the buckle or Velcro cuffs to fit the restraint.
- Avoid applying the restraint too tightly. Tie the restraint as above.
- Monitor the patient for signs of impaired circulation.
- Release the restraint every 2 hours.

APPLYING A MITT RESTRAINT

- Wash and dry the patient's hands.
- Place a rolled up washcloth or gauze pad in the patient's palm.
- Have him form a loose fist, pull the mitt over it, and secure it.
- To restrict arm movement, attach the strap to the mitt and tie it.
- Check hand movement and skin color frequently.
- Remove mitts every 2 hours to stimulate circulation, and perform passive range-of-motion (ROM) exercises.

APPLYING A BELT RESTRAINT

- Center the flannel pad of the belt on the bed.
- Wrap the short strap of the belt around the bed frame and fasten it under the bed.
- Position the patient on the pad.
- Have the patient roll to one side. Guide the long strap around his waist and through the slot in the pad.

- Wrap the long strap around the bed frame and fasten it under the bed.
- Check that the belt is comfortable, yet secure.

APPLYING A BODY (POSEY NET) RESTRAINT

- Place the restraint flat on the bed, with arm and wrist cuffs facing down and the V at the head of the bed.
- Place the patient in the prone position on top of the restraint.
- Lift the V over the patient's head. Thread the chest belt through one of the loops in the V to ensure a snug fit.
- Secure straps around the patient's chest, thighs, and legs.
- Turn the patient on his back.
- Secure the straps to the bed frame.
- Secure the straps around the patient's arms and wrists.

APPLYING LEATHER RESTRAINTS

- Place the patient supine, holding each arm and leg securely.
- Immobilize the patient's arms and legs at the joints — knee, ankle, shoulder, and wrist.
- Apply pads to wrists and ankles to reduce friction.
- Wrap the restraint around the gauze pads.
- Insert the metal loop through the hole that gives the best fit.
- Apply the restraints securely, but not too tightly.
- Thread the strap through the metal loop on the restraint, close the metal loop, and secure the strap to the bed frame, out of the patient's reach.
- Flex the patient's arm or leg slightly before locking the restraint.
- Place the key in an accessible location at the nurses' station.
- Provide emotional support and reassess the need for continued use.
- Check the patient's vital signs at least every 2 hours.
- Remove or loosen restraints one at a time, every hour, to perform passive ROM exercises.
- Watch for signs of impaired peripheral circulation.
- To unlock the restraint, insert the key into the metal loop, opposite the locking button.

SPECIAL CONSIDERATIONS

- Know your facility's policy and your state's regulations regarding restraints.
- Modify the care plan to reflect restraint use.
- If a patient is at high risk for aspiration, restrain him on his side.
- Never secure all four restraints to one side of the bed.
- Have a coworker assist when loosening restraints.
- For a two-point restraint, restrain one arm and the opposite leg.
- Don't apply a limb restraint above an I.V. line.
- Never secure restraints to the side rails.
- Never secure restraints to the bed frame if the patient's position is to be changed.
- Don't restrain a patient in the prone position.
- Nutrition, elimination, and positioning of a restrained patient are the staff's responsibility.
- Reposition the patient regularly. Massage and pad bony prominences.
- Continually monitor the patient. Release the restraints, as ordered.
- Assess the patient's pulse and skin condition, and perform ROM exercises.
- Maintain hourly notes on the restraint flow sheet.
- For children, who typically are too small for standard restraints, use a child restraint.

COMPLICATIONS

- Reduced circulation
- Impaired respiration
- Skin breakdown
- Pneumonia, urine retention, constipation, or sensory deprivation from immobility
- Injuries from biting, kicking, scratching, or head butting

PATIENT TEACHING

- Explain the need for restraints and how they'll be applied, as appropriate.

DOCUMENTATION

- Record behavior that necessitated restraints.
- Note when restraints were applied and removed.
- Document the type of restraints used.
- Record hourly notations on the restraint flow sheet.
- Note the patient's vital signs, skin condition, respiratory status, peripheral circulation, and mental status.

SELECTED REFERENCES

Cheung, P.P., and Yam, B.M. "Patient Autonomy in Physical Restraint," *Journal of Clinical Nursing* 14(Suppl 1):34-40, March 2005.

Kwok, T., et al. "Does Access to Bed-Chair Pressure Sensors Reduce Physical Restraint Use in the Rehabilitative Care Setting?" *Journal of Clinical Nursing* 15(5):581-87, May 2006.

Martin, B., and Mathisen, L. "Use of Physical Restraints in Adult Critical Care: A Bicultural Study," *American Journal of Critical Care* 14(2):133-42, March 2005.

Wang, W.W., and Moyle, W. "Physical Restraint Use on People with Dementia: A Review of the Literature," *Australian Journal of Advanced Nursing* 22(4): 46-52, June-August 2005.

Rotation beds

DESCRIPTION

- Rotation beds promote postural drainage and peristalsis and help prevent complications of immobility.
- The bed rotates from side to side in a cradlelike motion, achieving a maximum elevation of 62 degrees and full side-to-side turning about every 4½ minutes.
- The bed holds the patient motionless; this is helpful for patients with spinal cord injury, multiple trauma, stroke, multiple sclerosis, coma, severe burns, hypostatic pneumonia, atelectasis, or other unilateral lung involvement causing poor ventilation and perfusion.
- Different models of the Roto Rest bed can accommodate cervical traction devices and tongs; provide access to perineal, cervical, and thoracic areas; and have arm and leg hatches that fold down to allow range-of-motion (ROM) exercises.
- Other features include variable angles of rotation, a fan, access for X-rays, and supports and clips for chest tubes, catheters, and drains.
- Patient transfer and positioning on the bed should be performed by at least two persons to ensure safety.

CONTRAINDICATIONS

- Severe claustrophobia
- Unstable cervical fracture without neurologic deficit

EQUIPMENT

Rotation bed with appropriate accessories ◆ pillowcases or linen-saver pads ◆ flat sheet or padding

PREPARATION

- Inspect the bed and run it through a complete cycle.
- Check the tightness of the set screws if using the Mark I model.
- Remove the counterbalance weights from the keel and place them in the base frame's storage area.

- Release the connecting arm by pulling down on the cam handle and depressing the lower side of the footboard.
- Lock the table in the horizontal position and place all side supports in the extreme lateral position by loosening the cam handles on the underside of the table.
- Slide the supports off the bed.
- Remove the knee packs.
- Remove the abductor packs by depressing and sliding them toward the head of the bed.
- Loosen the foot and knee assemblies by lifting the cam handle at its base, and then slide them to the foot of the bed.
- Loosen the shoulder clamp assembly and knobs.
- Swing the shoulder clamps to a vertical position and retighten.
- If using the Mark I model, remove the cervical, thoracic, and perineal packs; cover with pillowcases or linen-saver pads, smooth all wrinkles, and replace the packs.
- If using the Mark III model, remove the perineal pack, cover, and replace.
- Cover the upper half of the bed with padding or a sheet.
- Install disposable foam cushions for the patient's head, shoulders, and feet.

KEY STEPS

- Explain and demonstrate the bed's operation.
- Reassure the patient that the bed will hold him securely.
- Before positioning the patient on the bed, make sure that it's turned off.
- Place and lock the bed in a horizontal position, out of gear.
- Latch all hatches and lock the wheels.
- Obtain assistance and transfer the patient.
- Move him gently to the center of the bed.
- Smooth the pillowcase or linen-saver pad beneath his hips.
- Place tubes through the appropriate notches in the hatches.

- Make sure that traction weights hang freely.
- Insert the thoracic side supports in their posts.
- Adjust the patient's longitudinal position to allow a 1″ (2.5 cm) space between the axillae and the supports.
- Push the supports against his chest and lock cam arms securely.
- Place disposable supports under his legs.
- Install and adjust foot supports to normal anatomic position.
- Place the abductor packs in the appropriate supports, allowing a 6″ (15 cm) space between the packs and the patient's groin.
- Tighten knobs on the bed's underside at the base of the support tubes.
- Install leg side supports snugly against the patient's hips.
- Tighten the cam arms.
- Position the knee assemblies slightly above his knees and tighten the cam arms.
- Place your hand on the patient's knee and move the knee pack until it rests lightly on the top of your hand. Repeat for the other knee.
- Loosen retaining rings on the crossbar, and slide the head and shoulder assembly laterally.
- Carefully lower head and shoulder assembly into place and slide it to touch the patient's head.
- Place your hand on the patient's shoulder, and move the shoulder pack until it touches your hand. Tighten it in place. Repeat for the other shoulder.
- Leave 1″ clearance between the shoulders and the packs.
- Place the head pack close to, but not touching, the patient's ears.
- Tighten the head and shoulder assembly securely.
- Position restraining rings next to the shoulder assembly bracket and tighten them.
- Place the patient's arms on the disposable supports.
- Install the side arm supports and secure the safety straps, placing one across the shoulder assembly and the other over the thoracic supports.

BALANCING THE BED

◆ Place one hand on the footboard to prevent the bed from turning rapidly if it's unbalanced.
◆ Remove the locking pin.
◆ If the bed rotates to one side, reposition the patient in its center.
◆ If it tilts to the right, turn it slightly to the left and slide the packs on the right side toward the patient.
◆ If it tilts to the left, reverse the process.
◆ If a large imbalance exists, adjust the packs on both sides.
◆ After the patient is centered, slowly turn the bed to the 62-degree position.
◆ Measure the space between the chest, hip, and thighs and the inside of the packs.
◆ If this space exceeds ½″ (1.3 cm) for the Mark III model or 1″ (2.5 cm) for the Mark I, return the bed to the horizontal position, lock it in place, and slide the packs inward on both sides.
◆ If the space appears too tight, proceed as above but slide both packs outward.
◆ Excessively loose packs cause the patient to slide from side to side.
◆ Overly tight packs can place pressure on the patient during turning.
◆ After adjusting the packs, balance the bed.
◆ If using the Mark III model bed and the patient weighs more than 160 lb (72.6 kg), the bed may become top-heavy. To correct this, place counterbalance weights in the appropriate slots in the keel of the bed.
◆ If you're using the Mark I model, it may be necessary to add weights for the patient weighing less than 160 lb.

INITIATING AUTOMATIC BED ROTATION

◆ Make sure that all packs are securely in place.
◆ Hold the footboard firmly; remove the locking pin to start the bed's motor. The bed will continue to rotate until the pin is reinserted.
◆ Raise the connecting arm cam handle until the connecting assembly snaps into place, locking the bed into automatic rotation.

◆ Remain with the patient to evaluate his comfort and safety.

SPECIAL CONSIDERATIONS

◆ For cardiac arrest, perform cardiopulmonary resuscitation after taking the bed out of gear, locking it in the horizontal position, removing the side arm support and the thoracic pack, lifting the shoulder assembly, and dropping the arm pack.
◆ If the electricity fails, lock the bed in the horizontal or lateral position and rotate it manually every 30 minutes to prevent pressure ulcers.
◆ If cervical traction causes the patient to slide upward, place the bed in reverse Trendelenburg's position.
◆ If the patient slides toward the foot of the bed, use Trendelenburg's position.
◆ Lock the bed in the extreme lateral position for access to the back of the head, thorax, and buttocks through the appropriate hatches.
◆ Clean and rinse the mattress and nondisposable packs during patient care.
◆ When replacing the packs and hatches, take care not to pinch the patient's skin between the packs.
◆ Expect increased drainage from pressure ulcers for the first few days.
◆ Perform or schedule daily ROM exercises.
◆ Drop the arm hatch for shoulder rotation.
◆ Remove the thoracic packs for shoulder abduction.
◆ Drop the leg hatch and remove leg and knee packs for hip rotation and full leg motion.
◆ For female patients, tape an indwelling urinary catheter to the thigh before bringing it through the perineal hatch.
◆ For the male patient with spinal cord lesions, tape the catheter to the abdomen and then to the thigh to facilitate gravity drainage.
◆ Hang the drainage bag on the clips provided.
◆ If the patient has a tracheal or endotracheal tube and is on mechanical

ventilation, attach the tube support bracket between the cervical pack and the arm packs.
◆ Tape the connecting T-tubing to the support and run it beside the patient's head and off the center of the table to help prevent reflux of condensation.
◆ For a patient with pulmonary congestion or pneumonia, suction secretions more often during the first 12 to 24 hours.
◆ A vibrating unit is available for use under the thoracic hatch of the Mark I to help mobilize pulmonary secretions more quickly.

COMPLICATIONS

◆ Pressure ulcers
◆ Claustrophobia

PATIENT TEACHING

◆ Explain why the bed is being used and demonstrate how it works.
◆ Tell the patient to report discomfort.

DOCUMENTATION

◆ Record changes in the patient's condition.
◆ Document the patient's response to therapy.
◆ Note turning times and ongoing care on the flowchart.

SELECTED REFERENCES

Anderson, C., and Rappl, L. "Lateral Rotation Mattresses for Wound Healing," *Ostomy/Wound Management* 50(4): 50-54, 56, 58 passim, April 2004.
Russell, T., and Logsdon, A. "Pressure Ulcers and Lateral Rotation Beds: A Case Study," *Journal of Wound, Ostomy, and Continence Nursing* 30(3):143-45, May 2003.
Washington, G.T., and Macnee, C.L. "Evaluation of Outcomes: The Effects of Continuous Lateral Rotational Therapy," *Journal of Nursing Care Quality* 20(3):273-82, July-September 2005.

Seizure management

DESCRIPTION

◆ Partial seizures are usually unilateral, involving a localized or focal area of the brain; generalized seizures involve the entire brain.
◆ Nursing care aims to protect the patient from injury and prevent serious complications.
◆ Care includes observing seizure characteristics to help determine the area of the brain involved.
◆ Predisposing conditions include metabolic abnormalities (hypocalcemia, hypoglycemia, pyridoxine deficiency), brain tumors or other space-occupying lesions, infections (meningitis, encephalitis, brain abscess), traumatic injury (especially if the dura mater was penetrated), toxins (mercury, lead, carbon monoxide), genetic abnormalities (tuberous sclerosis, phenylketonuria), perinatal injuries, drug or alcohol withdrawl, or stroke.
◆ Patients at risk need precautionary measures to help prevent injury if a seizure occurs.

CONTRAINDICATIONS

◆ None known

Oral airway ◆ suction equipment ◆ side rail pads ◆ seizure activity record ◆ I.V. line ◆ normal saline solution ◆ oxygen ◆ endotracheal intubation equipment

◆ If the patient experiences an aura, help him into bed, raise the side rails, and adjust the bed flat.
◆ If he's away from his room, lower him to the floor and place a pillow, blanket, or other soft material under his head to keep it from hitting the floor.
◆ Stay with the patient and be ready to intervene if complications develop.
◆ Provide privacy, if possible.
◆ If the patient is in the beginning of the tonic phase of the seizure, you may insert an oral airway into his mouth.
◆ If an oral airway isn't available, don't try to hold his mouth open or place your hands inside because you may be bitten.
◆ After the patient's jaw becomes rigid, don't force the airway into place. Wait until the seizure subsides before inserting an airway.
◆ Move hard or sharp objects out of the patient's way and loosen his clothing.
◆ Don't forcibly restrain the patient or restrict his movements.
◆ Continually assess the patient during the seizure.
◆ If this is the patient's first seizure, notify the practitioner immediately.
◆ If the patient has had seizures before, notify the practitioner only if the seizure activity is prolonged or if the patient fails to regain consciousness.
◆ If ordered, establish an I.V. line and infuse normal saline solution at a keep-vein-open rate.
◆ If the seizure is prolonged and the patient becomes hypoxemic, administer oxygen as ordered.
◆ For a patient known to be diabetic, administer 50 ml of dextrose 50% in water by I.V. push, as ordered.
◆ For a patient known to be an alcoholic, a 100-mg bolus of thiamine may be ordered to stop the seizure.
◆ After the seizure, turn the patient on his side and apply suction, if necessary, to remove secretions or vomitus.
◆ Insert an oral airway if needed.
◆ Check for injuries.

- Reorient and reassure the patient as necessary.
- When the patient is comfortable and safe, document what happened during the seizure.
- Place side rail pads on the bed.
- Monitor the patient's vital signs and mental status every 15 to 20 minutes for 2 hours.
- Ask the patient about his aura and activities preceding the seizure.

SPECIAL CONSIDERATIONS

- Because a seizure commonly indicates an underlying disorder, such as meningitis, or a metabolic or electrolyte imbalance, a complete diagnostic workup is ordered if the cause of the seizure isn't evident. This is especially important for instances of status epilepticus. (See *Understanding status epilepticus*.)

COMPLICATIONS

- Injury
- Respiratory difficulty
- Decreased mental capacity
- Aspiration
- Airway obstruction
- Hypoxemia
- Postictal period of decreased mental status lasting 30 minutes to 24 hours

PATIENT TEACHING

- If the patient hasn't had a seizure before, explain what has happened.
- Answer any questions as best as you can or convey them to the practitioner.
- Teach about any medications that may be prescribed and any adverse reactions and what to report to the practitioner.

DOCUMENTATION

- Note seizure precautions needed and provided.
- Record the date and time the seizure began, its duration, and precipitating factors.
- Note any sensation that may be considered an aura. Have the patient describe it.
- Document involuntary behavior that occurred at the onset.
- Record where movement began and body parts involved.
- Note the progression or pattern to the activity.
- Document eye movement and changes in pupil size, shape, equality, or reaction to light.
- Record if the patient's teeth were clenched or open.
- Note incontinence, vomiting, or salivation.
- Document the patient's response to the seizure.
- Record drugs administered, interventions, complications, and post-seizure mental status.

SELECTED REFERENCES

Crawford, P. "Best Practice Guidelines for the Management of Women with Epilepsy," *Epilepsia* 46(Suppl 9):117-24, 2005.

Cross, C. "Seizures. Regaining Control," *RN* 67(12):44-50, December 2004.

Hayes, C. "Clinical Skills: Practical Guide for Managing Adults with Epilepsy," *British Journal of Nursing* 13(7):380-87, April 2004.

Huying, F., et al. "Antiepileptic Drug Use in Nursing Home Residents: A Cross-Sectional, Regional Study," *Seizure* 15(3):194-97, April 2006.

Self-catheterization

DESCRIPTION
- Self-catheterization provides routine bladder drainage for a patient with impaired or absent bladder function.
- The procedure requires thorough and careful teaching by the nurse.
- The patient will probably use clean technique at home, but must use sterile technique in the facility because of the increased risk of infection.

CONTRAINDICATIONS
- None known

Rubber catheter ◆ washcloth ◆ soap and water ◆ small packet of water-soluble lubricant ◆ plastic storage bag ◆ paper towels ◆ cornstarch ◆ plastic sheets ◆ gooseneck lamp ◆ catheterization record ◆ mirror ◆ drainage container (optional)

PREPARATION
- Instruct the patient to keep a supply of catheters at home and to use each catheter only once before cleaning it.
- Advise him to wash the used catheter in warm, soapy water, rinse it inside and out, and then dry it with a clean towel and store it in a plastic bag until the next time it's needed.
- Because catheters become brittle with repeated use, tell the patient to check them often and to order a new supply well in advance.

FEMALE PATIENTS
- Demonstrate and explain to the female patient that she should separate the labial folds as widely as possible with the fingers of her nondominant hand to obtain a full view of the urinary meatus.
- She may need to use a mirror to visualize the meatus.
- Ask if she's right- or left-handed and then tell her which her nondominant hand is.
- While holding her labia open with the nondominant hand, she should use the dominant hand to wash the perineal area thoroughly with a soapy washcloth, using downward strokes.
- Tell her to rinse the area with the washcloth, using downward strokes as well.
- Show her how to squeeze some lubricant onto the first 3″ (7.5 cm) of the catheter and then how to insert it. (See *Teaching self-catheterization*.)
- When the urine stops draining, tell her to remove the catheter slowly, get dressed, and wash the catheter with warm, soapy water.
- She should rinse it inside and out and dry it with a paper towel.

MALE PATIENTS
- Tell a male patient to wash and rinse the end of his penis thoroughly with soap and water, pulling back the foreskin if appropriate.
- He should keep the foreskin pulled back during the procedure.
- Show him how to squeeze lubricant onto a paper towel and have him roll the first 7″ to 10″ (18 to 25.5 cm) of the catheter in the lubricant.
- Tell him to use a lot of lubricant to make the procedure more comfortable; show him how to insert the catheter.
- When the urine stops draining, tell him to remove the catheter slowly and, if necessary, pull the foreskin forward again.
- Have him get dressed and wash and dry the catheter as described above.

Teaching self-catheterization

Teach a woman to hold the catheter in her dominant hand as if it were a pencil or dart, about ½″ (1 cm) from its tip. Keeping the labial folds separated, she should slowly insert the lubricated catheter about 3″ (7.5 cm) into the urethra. Tell her to press down with her abdominal muscles to empty the bladder, allowing all urine to drain through the catheter and into the toilet or drainage container.

Teach a man to hold his penis in his nondominant hand, at a right angle to his body. He should hold the catheter in his dominant hand as if it were a pencil or dart and slowly insert it 7″ to 10″ (18 to 25.5 cm) into the urethra until urine begins flowing. Then he should gently advance the catheter about 1″ (2.5 cm) farther, allowing all urine to drain into the toilet or drainage container.

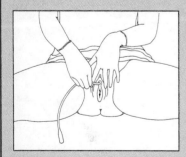
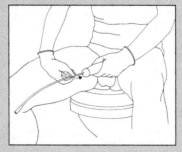

SPECIAL CONSIDERATIONS

◆ Self-catheterization usually occurs every 4 to 6 hours around the clock (or more often at first).
◆ For home use, washing with soapy water provides sufficient safeguard against spreading infection.
◆ For managing incontinence, the practitioner or a home health care nurse can help develop a plan such as more frequent catheterizations.

COMPLICATIONS

◆ Urinary tract infection
◆ Urine leakage
◆ Injury to the urethral or bladder mucosa

PATIENT TEACHING

◆ Explain that timing of catheterization is critical to prevent overdistention of the bladder, which can lead to infection.
◆ Teach female patients the body parts involved in self-catheterization — labia majora, labia minora, vagina, and urinary meatus.
◆ Stress the importance of taking drugs as ordered.
◆ Advise the patient to avoid calcium- and phosphorus-rich foods, as ordered, to reduce the chance of renal calculus formation.
◆ Stress the importance of regulating fluid intake, as ordered, to prevent incontinence while maintaining adequate hydration.
◆ Explain that incontinent episodes may occur occasionally.
◆ After an incontinent episode, tell the patient to wash with soap and water, pat dry with a towel, and expose the skin to the air until dry.
◆ Instruct the patient to reduce urine odor by putting cornstarch on the skin. Bedding and furniture can be protected by covering them with rubber or plastic sheets and then covering the rubber or plastic with fabric.

DOCUMENTATION

◆ Record the dates and times of catheterization.
◆ Note the character of urine (color, odor, clarity, presence of particles or blood).
◆ Document the amount of urine (for example, increase, decrease, or no change) and problems encountered during the procedure.
◆ Note whether the patient has difficulty performing a return demonstration.

SELECTED REFERENCES

Ghandi, S., et al. "Foley versus Intermittent Self-Catheterization after Transvaginal Sling Surgery: Which Works Best?" *Urology* 64(1):53-57, July 2004.

Robinson, J. "Intermittent Self-Catheterization: Principles and Practice," *British Journal of Community Nursing* 11(4):144, 146, 148 passim, April 2006.

To, H.C., et al. "Factors Affecting Success in Learning Clean Intermittent Self-Catheterization," *International Journal of Urology* 11(Suppl 1):A72, October 2004.

Williams, M.E. "How Do We Teach Clean Intermittent Self-Catheterization Using Touch Technique?" *Rehabilitation Nursing* 30(5):171-72, September-October 2005.

Sequential compression therapy

OVERVIEW

DESCRIPTION

- Sequential compression therapy is a safe, effective, noninvasive means of preventing deep vein thrombosis (DVT) in surgical patients at high risk for DVT.
- It massages the legs in a wavelike, milking motion that promotes blood flow and deters thrombosis.
- Sequential compression therapy counteracts blood stasis and coagulation changes — two of the three major factors that promote DVT.
- It reduces stasis by increasing peak blood flow velocity, helping to empty the femoral vein's valve cusps of pooled or static blood.
- The compressions cause an anticlotting effect by increasing fibrinolytic activity, which stimulates the release of a plasminogen activator.
- It typically complements other preventive measures, such as antiembolism stockings and anticoagulant medications.
- Sequential compression sleeves and antiembolism stockings are commonly used preoperatively and postoperatively to prevent blood clots that tend to form during surgery.
- Preventive measures are continued for as long as the patient remains at risk.

CONTRAINDICATIONS

- Acute DVT or DVT diagnosed within the past 6 months
- Severe arteriosclerosis
- Other ischemic vascular disease
- Massive leg edema resulting from pulmonary edema or heart failure
- Dermatitis
- Vein ligation
- Gangrene
- Recent skin grafting

EQUIPMENT

Measuring tape ◆ sizing chart for the brand of sleeves you're using ◆ pair of compression sleeves in correct size ◆ connecting tubing ◆ compression controller

PREPARATION

- Confirm the patient's identity using two patient identifiers according to facility policy.
- Explain the procedure to the patient.
- Wash your hands.
- To determine the proper size of sleeve, measure the circumference of the upper thigh (as shown below).

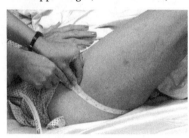

- Hold the tape snugly, but not tightly, under the patient's thigh at the gluteal furrow.
- Find the patient's thigh measurement on the sizing chart and locate the corresponding size of the compression sleeve.
- Remove the compression sleeves from the package and unfold them.
- Lay the unfolded sleeves on a flat surface with the cotton lining facing up (as shown below).

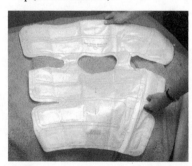

- Position the sleeve at the appropriate ankle or knee landmark.

KEY STEPS

APPLYING THE SLEEVES

- Place the patient's leg on the sleeve lining; position the back of the knee over the popliteal opening.
- Make sure that the back of the ankle is over the ankle marking.
- Starting at the side opposite the clear plastic tubing, wrap the sleeve snugly around the patient's leg.
- Fasten the sleeve securely with the Velcro fasteners starting at the ankle and then moving to the calf and thigh.
- Check the fit by inserting two fingers between the sleeve and the patient's leg at the knee opening.
- Using the same procedure, apply the second sleeve (as shown below).

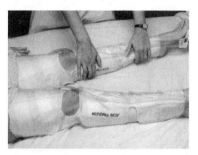

OPERATING THE SYSTEM

- Connect both sleeves to the tubing leading to the controller.
- Line up the blue arrows on the sleeve connector with the arrows on the tubing connectors and push the ends together firmly.
- Listen for a click, signaling a firm connection. Make sure that the tubing isn't kinked.
- Plug the compression controller into the proper wall outlet. Turn the controller on.
- The controller automatically sets the compression sleeve pressure at 45 mm Hg, which is the midpoint of the normal range (35 to 55 mm Hg).
- Observe the patient to see how well he tolerates therapy.
- The green light on the AUDIBLE ALARM key should be lit.

- The compression sleeves should function continuously (24 hours daily) until the patient is fully ambulatory.
- Check sleeves once each shift to ensure proper fit and inflation.

REMOVING THE SLEEVES
- You may remove the sleeves when the patient is walking, bathing, or leaving the room for tests or other procedures. Reapply them immediately after these activities.
- To disconnect the sleeves from the tubing, depress the latches on each side of the connectors and pull the connectors apart.
- Store the tubing and compression controller according to facility protocol.

SPECIAL CONSIDERATIONS

- The compression controller has a mechanism to cool the patient.
- If a malfunction triggers the instrument's alarm, you'll hear beeping. The system shuts off whenever the alarm is activated.

COMPLICATIONS
- Pronounced leg deformity

PATIENT TEACHING

- Explain how sequential compression therapy helps prevent DVT.
- Show the patient how a sequential compression device is applied.
- Tell the patient what signs and symptoms of DVT and pulmonary embolism to report.

DOCUMENTATION

- Record the date and time the device was applied.
- Note the type of sleeve used (knee- or thigh-length).
- Document the patient's response to and understanding of the procedure.
- Record maximum sequential compression device inflation pressure and the patient's blood pressure.
- Note the reason for removing the sequential compression device along with the length of time it was removed.
- Document the status of the alarm and cooling settings.
- Record the sleeve cooling mode status.
- Document the proper application of sleeves.
- Document assessments of skin and circulation of lower extremities, including distal pulses.
- Provide rationale if only one leg sleeve is applied.

SELECTED REFERENCES
Bonner, L. "The Prevention and Treatment of Deep Vein Thrombosis," *Nursing Times* 100(29):38-42, July 2004.

Hums, W., and Blostein, P. "A Comparative Approach to Deep Vein Thrombosis Risk Assessment," *Journal of Trauma Nursing* 13(1):28-30, January-March 2006.

Kakkos, S.K., et al. "Comparison of Two Intermittent Pneumatic Compression Systems. A Hemodynamic Study," *International Angiology* 24(4):330-35, December 2005.

Kakkos, S.K., et al. "The Efficacy of a New Portable Sequential Compression Device (SCD Express) in Preventing Venous Stasis," *Journal of Vascular Surgery* 42(2):296-303, August 2005.

Sitz bath

DESCRIPTION

- A sitz bath involves immersing the pelvic area in warm or hot water.
- It's used to relieve discomfort, especially after perineal or rectal surgery or childbirth.
- It promotes wound healing by cleaning the perineum and anus, increasing circulation, and reducing inflammation.
- It helps relax local muscles.
- It requires frequent checks of water temperature to ensure therapeutic effects, correct draping of the patient during the bath, and prompt dressing afterward to prevent vasoconstriction.

CONTRAINDICATIONS

- Symptomatic hypotension

A disposable sitz bath kit is available for single-patient use. It includes a plastic basin that fits over a commode and an irrigation bag with tubing and clamp.

Sitz tub ◆ portable sitz bath, or regular bathtub ◆ bath mat ◆ rubber mat ◆ bath (utility) thermometer ◆ two bath blankets ◆ towels ◆ patient gown ◆ gloves, if the patient has an open lesion or has been incontinent ◆ footstool ◆ overbed table ◆ I.V. pole (to hold irrigation bag) ◆ wheelchair or cart ◆ dressings ◆ rubber ring

PREPARATION

- Make sure that the tub is clean and disinfected or use a disposable one.
- Position the bath mat next to the bathtub, sitz tub, or commode.
- Place the rubber ring on the bottom of the tub to serve as a seat for the patient. Cover the ring with a towel for comfort.
- Keeping the patient elevated improves water flow over the wound site and avoids unnecessary pressure on tender tissues.
- If you're using a commercial kit, open the package and familiarize yourself with the equipment.
- Fill the sitz tub or bathtub one-third to one-half full.
- Use warm water (94° to 98° F [34.4° to 36.7° C]) for relaxation or wound cleaning and healing and hot water (110° to 115° F [43.3° to 46.1° C]) for heat application.
- Run the water slightly warmer than desired because it will cool while the patient prepares for the bath. Measure the water temperature using the bath thermometer.
- If you're using a commercial kit, fill the basin to the specified line with water at the prescribed temperature. Place the basin under the commode seat, clamp the irrigation tubing to block water flow, and fill the irrigation bag with water of the same temperature as that in the basin.
- To create flow pressure, hang the bag above the patient's head on a hook, towel rack, or I.V. pole.

- Check the practitioner's order and assess the patient's condition.
- Confirm the patient's identity using two patient identifiers according to facility policy.
- Explain the procedure to the patient.

  ● **WARNING** *Instruct the patient to rise slowly after a sitz bath to prevent dizziness and loss of balance.*
- Wash your hands thoroughly and put on gloves.
- Have the patient void.
- Assist the patient to the bath area, provide privacy, and make sure that the area is warm and free from drafts.
- Help the patient undress, as needed.
- Remove and dispose of soiled dressings. If a dressing adheres to a wound, allow it to soak off in the tub.
- Assist the patient into the tub or onto the commode, as needed.
- Instruct him to use the safety rail for balance.
- Explain that the sensation may be unpleasant initially because the wound area is tender. Assure him that the warm water will relieve discomfort.
- Place a small stool under the patient's feet for comfort.
- Place a folded towel against the patient's lower back to prevent discomfort and promote correct body alignment.
- Drape the patient's shoulders and knees with bath blankets to avoid chills that cause vasoconstriction.
- If you're using the sitz bath kit, open the clamp on the irrigation tubing to allow a stream of water to flow continuously over the wound site.
- Refill the bag with water of the correct temperature as needed.
- Encourage the patient to regulate the flow himself.
- Place the patient's overbed table in front of him to provide support and comfort.
- Check water temperature frequently with the bath thermometer. If temperature drops significantly, add warm water.

- To prevent dizziness and loss of balance, help the patient to stand slowly.
- Instruct the patient to hold the safety rail while he runs warm water into the tub.
- Help the patient sit down again to resume the bath; if necessary, stay with the patient during the bath. Tell the patient how to use the call button if you must leave.
- Check the patient's color and general condition frequently.

⚠ **WARNING** *If the patient complains of feeling weak, faint, or nauseated or shows signs of cardiovascular distress, discontinue the bath, check the patient's pulse and blood pressure, assist him back to bed using a wheelchair or cart, and notify the practitioner.*

- After 15 to 20 minutes, tell the patient to use the safety rail for balance, and help him to stand slowly to prevent dizziness.
- If necessary, help the patient dry himself.
- Redress the wound as needed, provide a clean gown, and assist the patient in dressing and returning to bed or back to his room.
- Dispose of soiled materials properly.
- Empty, clean, and disinfect the sitz tub.
- Return the commercial kit to the patient's bedside for later use.

SPECIAL CONSIDERATIONS

- Use a regular bathtub only if a special sitz tub, portable sitz bath, or commercial sitz bath kit is unavailable.
- Because the application of heat to the extremities causes vasodilation and draws blood away from the perineal area, a regular bathtub is less effective for local treatment than a sitz device.
- Check the patient's pulse before, during, and after the bath to help detect vasodilation that could make him feel faint when he stands up.
- Tell the patient not to touch an open wound because of the risk of infection.

COMPLICATIONS

- Weakness or faintness
- Irregular or accelerated pulse
- Possible wound contamination and infection

PATIENT TEACHING

- Tell the patient about the therapeutic effects of a sitz bath.
- Explain how the procedure is performed.
- Advise the patient of proper water temperature.
- Discuss signs and symptoms to report immediately.
- Teach the patient how to use the call button for assistance.
- Instruct the patient to wait for assistance after the procedure and to rise slowly.
- Tell the patient how to perform the procedure at home.

DOCUMENTATION

- Record the date, time, duration, and temperature of the bath.
- Document wound condition before and after treatment — color, odor, and amount of drainage.
- Note complications.
- Record the patient's response to treatment.

SELECTED REFERENCES

Kahraman, A., et al. "Perianal Burn as a Complication of Hemorrhoid Treatment Caused by Hot Water Sitz Bath," *Burns* 30(8):868-70, December 2004.

Leeds, A. "The Art of the Sitz Bath," *Midwifery Today with International Midwife* (65):25-26, Spring 2003.

Tejirian, T., and Abbas, M.A. "Sitz Bath: Where Is the Evidence? Scientific Basis of a Common Practice," *Diseases of the Colon and Rectum* 48(12):2336-40, December 2005.

Skin biopsy

OVERVIEW

DESCRIPTION
- One of three techniques may be used for a skin biopsy — shave biopsy, punch biopsy, or excisional biopsy.
- A shave biopsy cuts the lesion above the skin line, which allows further biopsy of the site.
- A punch biopsy removes an oval core from the center of the lesion.
- An excisional biopsy removes the entire lesion; it's indicated for rapidly expanding lesions.
- Excisional biopsy is used for sclerotic, bullous, or atrophic lesions and for examination of the border of a lesion surrounding normal skin.
- Fully developed, rather than early stage lesions, should be selected.

CONTRAINDICATIONS
- None known

EQUIPMENT

Gloves ◆ #15 scalpel for shave or excisional biopsy ◆ local anesthetic ◆ specimen bottle containing 10% formaldehyde solution ◆ 4-0 sutures for punch or excisional biopsy ◆ adhesive bandage ◆ forceps ◆ adhesive strips ◆ sterile labels ◆ sterile marker

KEY STEPS

- Confirm the patient's identity using two patient identifiers according to facility policy.
- Explain to the patient that the biopsy provides a skin sample for microscopic study.
- Describe the procedure, tell the patient who will perform it, and answer any questions.
- Inform the patient that he need not restrict food or fluids.
- Tell him that he'll receive a local anesthetic for pain.
- Inform him that the biopsy will take about 15 minutes.
- Tell him that the test results are usually available in 1 day.
- Have the patient or an appropriate family member sign the consent form.
- Check the patient's history for hypersensitivity to the local anesthetic.
- Position the patient comfortably.
- Label all medication syringes, medication containers, and all solution containers on and off the sterile field.
- Clean the biopsy site before the local anesthetic is administered.

SHAVE BIOPSY
- Use a #15 scalpel to cut the protruding growth off at the skin line.
- Immediately place the specimen in a properly labeled bottle containing 10% formaldehyde solution.
- Apply pressure to the area to stop bleeding.
- Apply an adhesive bandage.

PUNCH BIOPSY
- Pull the skin taut surrounding the lesion.
- Firmly introduce the punch into the lesion and rotate to obtain the specimen.
- Lift the plug with forceps or a needle.
- Sever as deeply into the fat layer as possible.
- Place the specimen in a properly labeled specimen bottle containing 10% formaldehyde solution or in a sterile container if indicated.

- Close the wound.
  - For a 3-mm punch, use an adhesive bandage.
  - For a 4-mm punch, use one suture.
  - For a 6-mm punch, use two sutures.

EXCISIONAL BIOPSY
- Use a #15 scalpel to excise the lesion.
- Make the incision as wide and deep as necessary.
- Remove the tissue specimen and place it immediately in a properly labeled specimen bottle containing 10% formaldehyde solution.
- Apply pressure to the site to stop bleeding.
- Close the wound using a 4-0 suture.
- For a large incision, a skin graft may be required.
- For a small incision, adhesive strips may be applied.
- Check the biopsy site for bleeding.
- Send the specimen to the laboratory immediately.
- Administer analgesics to the patient as needed.

SPECIAL CONSIDERATIONS

- Normal skin consists of squamous epithelium (epidermis) and fibrous connective tissue (dermis).
- Histologic examination of the tissue specimen may reveal a benign or malignant lesion.
- Benign growths include cysts, seborrheic keratoses, warts, pigmented nevi (moles), keloids, dermatofibromas, and neurofibromas.
- Malignant tumors include basal cell carcinoma, squamous cell carcinoma, and malignant melanoma.
- Characteristics of malignant lesions include change in color, size, or appearance or have failed to heal properly after injury.

COMPLICATIONS
- Bleeding
- Infection of surrounding tissue

PATIENT TEACHING

- Advise a patient going home with sutures to keep the area clean and as dry as possible.
- Tell the patient that facial sutures will be removed in 3 to 5 days and trunk sutures removed in 7 to 14 days.
- If adhesive strips were used, tell the patient to leave them in place for 14 to 21 days.

DOCUMENTATION

- Note the time the specimen was obtained.
- Record the location where the specimen was obtained.
- Document the appearance of the specimen and the biopsy site.
- Record whether bleeding occurred at the biopsy site.

SELECTED REFERENCES

Colyar, M. "Skin Biopsy Techniques," *Advance for Nurse Practitioners* 13(1): 25-26, January 2005.

Giuseppe, L. "Skin Biopsy in the Diagnosis of Peripheral Neuropathies," *Practical Neurology* 5(2):92-99, April 2005.

Godsell, G.A. "The Development of the Nurse Biopsy Role," *British Journal of Nursing* 14(13):690-92, July 2005.

Palotas, A., et al. "New Chapter in Skin Biopsy: Diagnostic Tool for Neurodegenerative Disorders," *Experimental Dermatology* 13(9):589, September 2004.

Skin graft care

DESCRIPTION

- Healthy skin taken from the patient (autograft) or a donor (allograft) is applied to a part of the patient's body to resurface an area damaged by burns, traumatic injury, or surgery.
- The size and depth of burns determine whether grafting is required.
- Effort is made to cover all wounds within 2 weeks.
- Care procedures for an autograft or allograft are essentially the same; however, an autograft requires care for two sites — the graft site and the donor site.
- The graft may be one of several types — split-thickness, full-thickness, or pedicle-flap.
- Successful grafting depends on clean wound granulation with adequate vascularization, complete contact of the graft with the wound bed, aseptic technique to prevent infection, adequate graft immobilization, and skilled care.
- Grafting usually occurs after wound debridement.
- With enzymatic debridement, grafting may be performed 5 to 7 days after debridement is complete.
- With surgical debridement, grafting can occur on the same day as surgery.
- Depending on facility policy, a physician or a specially trained nurse may change graft dressings.
- The dressings usually stay in place for 3 to 5 days after surgery.

CONTRAINDICATIONS

- None known

Ordered analgesic ✦ clean and sterile gloves ✦ sterile gown ✦ cap ✦ mask ✦ sterile forceps ✦ sterile scissors ✦ sterile scalpel ✦ sterile 4″ × 4″ gauze pads ✦ Xeroflo gauze ✦ elastic gauze dressing ✦ warm, normal saline solution ✦ moisturizing cream ✦ topical drug (micronized silver sulfadiazine cream) ✦ sterile, cotton-tipped applicators (optional)

PREPARATION

- Assemble equipment on the dressing cart.

- Confirm the patient's identity using two patient identifiers according to facility policy.
- Explain the procedure to the patient and provide privacy.
- Administer an analgesic, as ordered, 20 to 30 minutes before procedure.
- Give an I.V. analgesic immediately before the procedure.
- Wash your hands.
- Put on a sterile gown and clean mask, cap, and gloves.
- Gently lift off all outer dressings.
- Soak the middle dressings with warm, normal saline solution.
- Remove these carefully and slowly to avoid disturbing the graft.
- Leave the Xeroflo intact to avoid dislodging the graft.
- Remove and discard the clean gloves, wash your hands, and put on the sterile gloves.
- Assess the condition of the graft.
- Notify the practitioner if purulent drainage is present.
- Remove the Xeroflo with sterile forceps, and gently clean the area.
- If necessary, soak the Xeroflo with warm, normal saline solution to ease removal.
- Inspect an allograft for signs of rejection, such as infection and delayed healing.
- Inspect a sheet graft frequently for blebs; if ordered, evacuate them carefully with a sterile scalpel. (See *Evacuating fluid from a sheet graft.*)
- Apply topical drug if ordered.
- Place fresh Xeroflo over the site to promote wound healing and prevent infection. Use sterile scissors to cut the appropriate size.
- Cover with 4″ × 4″ gauze pads and an elastic gauze dressing.
- Clean any completely healed areas.
- Apply moisturizing cream to keep skin pliable and minimize scarring.

♦ To avoid dislodging the graft, hydrotherapy is usually discontinued for 3 to 4 days after grafting.
♦ Avoid using a blood pressure cuff over the graft.
♦ Don't tug or pull dressings during dressing changes.
♦ Keep the patient from lying on the graft.
♦ If the graft dislodges, apply sterile skin compresses to keep the area moist until the surgeon reapplies the graft.
♦ If the graft is on an arm or a leg, elevate the affected extremity to reduce postoperative edema.
♦ Check for bleeding and signs of neurovascular impairment, such as increasing pain, numbness or tingling, coolness, and pallor.

COMPLICATIONS
♦ Graft failure resulting in:
– Traumatic injury
– Hematoma or seroma formation
– Infection
– Inadequate graft bed
– Rejection
– Compromised nutritional status

♦ Teach the patient how to apply moisturizing cream.
♦ Tell the patient to use sunscreen containing titanium dioxide or oxybenzone with a sun protection factor of 20 or higher on all grafted areas.

Evacuating fluid from a sheet graft

When small pockets of fluid (blebs) accumulate beneath a sheet graft, evacuate the fluid using sterile, cotton-tipped applicators. First, carefully perforate the center of the bleb with the scalpel.

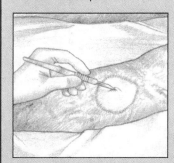

Gently express the fluid with the cotton-tipped applicators. Never express fluid by rolling the bleb to the edge of the graft. This disturbs healing in other areas.

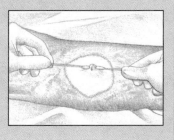

♦ Record the time and date of dressing changes.
♦ Note drugs used.
♦ Document the patient's response to drugs.
♦ Record the condition of the graft.
♦ Note signs of infection or rejection.
♦ Document additional treatment.
♦ Record the patient's reaction to the graft.

SELECTED REFERENCES
Beldon, P. "Comparison of Four Different Dressings on Donor Site Wounds," *British Journal of Nursing* 13(6 Suppl): S38-45, March 2004.
Kairinos, N. "A Short Report on the Prevention of Slippage in Donor Site Dressings," *Journal of Wound Care* 14(1):18, January 2005.
McPhee, H. "Using an Adhesive Retention Tape on Split Skin Graft Donor Areas," *Nursing Times* 101(16):57-58, April 2005.
Shaaban, H. "The Proximal Phalanx: Another Option to Harvest a Skin Graft for Skin Defects on the Fingers," *Plastic & Reconstructive Surgery* 117(6):2104-105, May 2006.

Skin preparation, preoperative

DESCRIPTION

◆ Skin preparation reduces the risk of infection at the incision site.
◆ It doesn't duplicate or replace full sterile preparation that immediately precedes surgery.
◆ The area of preparation always exceeds that of the expected incision to help minimize microorganisms in the adjacent areas and allow surgical draping without contamination.
◆ The procedure may involve a bath, shower, or local scrub with an antiseptic detergent solution.

CONTRAINDICATIONS

◆ None known

EQUIPMENT

Antiseptic soap solution ◆ tap water ◆ bath blanket ◆ two clean basins ◆ linen-saver pad ◆ adjustable light ◆ scissors ◆ cotton-tipped applicators ◆ acetone or nail polish remover ◆ orangewood stick ◆ trash bag ◆ towel ◆ gloves ◆ 4″ × 4″ gauze pads and electric clippers (optional)

PREPARATION

◆ Using warm tap water, dilute the antiseptic soap solution in one basin for washing.
◆ Pour plain warm water into the second basin for rinsing.

KEY STEPS

◆ Check the practitioner's order.
◆ Confirm the patient's identity using two patient identifiers according to facility policy.
◆ Explain the procedure to the patient, and provide privacy.
◆ Wash your hands and put on gloves.
◆ Put the patient in a comfortable position and drape him with the bath blanket.
◆ Expose the preparation area, which commonly extends 12″ (30.5 cm) in each direction from the expected incision site.
◆ To ensure privacy and avoid chilling, expose only one small area at a time while performing skin preparation.
◆ Position a linen-saver pad beneath the patient.
◆ Adjust the light to illuminate the preparation area.
◆ Assess the patient's skin condition in the preparation area and report any rash, abrasion, or laceration to the practitioner.
◆ A break in the skin increases the risk of infection and could cause cancellation of planned surgery.
◆ Have the patient remove all jewelry on or near the operative site.
◆ Begin removing hair from the preparation area by clipping long hairs with scissors.
◆ Perform the procedure as near to the time of surgery as possible.
◆ Proceed with a 10-minute scrub.
◆ Wash the area with a gauze pad dipped in the antiseptic soap.
◆ Using a circular motion, start at the expected incision site and work outward, pulling loose skin taut.
◆ Apply light friction while washing to improve the antiseptic effect.
◆ Carefully clean skin folds and crevices; scrub the perineal area last if it's part of the preparation area.
◆ Replace the gauze pad as necessary.
◆ Use cotton-tipped applicators to clean the umbilicus, if needed.
◆ Dry the area with a clean towel and remove the linen-saver pad.
◆ Use an orangewood stick to clean under nails.

- Remove nail polish to see nail bed color to determine adequate oxygenation.
- Place a probe on the nail to measure oxygen saturation.
- Give the patient special instructions for care of the prepared area, and remind him to keep the area clean for surgery.
- Make sure that the patient is comfortable.
- Properly dispose of solutions and the trash bag.
- Dispose of soiled equipment.

SPECIAL CONSIDERATIONS

- Never shave eyebrows to avoid unsightly regrowth.
- If required, prepare the patient's scalp, put hair in a plastic or paper bag, and store it with the patient's possessions.

COMPLICATIONS
- Rashes
- Nicks
- Lacerations and abrasions (most common), increasing the risk of postoperative infection

PATIENT TEACHING

- Explain the procedure to the patient.
- Explain the reason for a preoperative hair clipping.

DOCUMENTATION

- Record the date, time, and area of preparation.
- Note the patient's skin condition before and after preparation.
- Document complications.
- Record the patient's tolerance of the procedure.
- Prepare an incident report if required for nicks, lacerations, or abrasions.

SELECTED REFERENCES
Hulse, N., and Paul, A.S. "Warm Povidone-Iodine for Surgical Skin Preparation," *Annals of the Royal College of Surgeons of England* 87(6):47, November 2005.

Keblish, D.J., et al. "Preoperative Skin Preparation of the Foot and Ankle: Bristles and Alcohol are Better," *Journal of Bone and Joint Surgery* 87(5): 986-92, May 2005.

Lee, J.T. "Preoperative Skin Preparation," *Journal of the American College of Surgeons* 202(5):853, May 2006.

McGrath, D.R., and McCrory, D. "An Audit of Pre-operative Skin Preparation Methods," *Annals of the Royal College of Surgeons of England* 87(5):366-68, September 2005.

Paulson, D.S. "Efficacy of Preoperative Antimicrobial Skin Preparation Solutions on Biofilm Bacteria," *AORN Journal* 81(3):492-501, March 2005.

Skin staple and clip removal

OVERVIEW

DESCRIPTION

◆ Staples or clips may be used instead of standard sutures as a quicker way to close lacerations or surgical wounds.

◆ They're used as substitute for surface sutures when cosmetic results aren't a prime consideration.

◆ Proper placement of staples and clips distributes tension evenly along the suture line, minimizes tissue trauma and compression, promotes healing, and minimizes scarring.

◆ They're made from surgical stainless steel, minimizing tissue reaction.

◆ They're removed by physicians and, in some facilities, by qualified nurses.

CONTRAINDICATIONS

◆ Wound location requiring cosmetically superior results

◆ Incision site that makes it impossible to maintain minimum of 5-mm distance between staple and underlying bone, vessels, or internal organs

EQUIPMENT

Waterproof trash bag ◆ adjustable light ◆ clean gloves ◆ sterile gloves, if needed ◆ sterile gauze pads ◆ sterile staple or clip extractor ◆ povidone-iodine solution or other antiseptic cleaning agent ◆ sterile cotton-tipped applicators ◆ compound benzoin tincture or other skin protectant ◆ butterfly closures or adhesive strips (optional)

PREPARATION

◆ Assemble the equipment in the patient's room.

◆ Check the expiration date on each sterile package and inspect for tears.

◆ Open the waterproof trash bag and place it near the patient's bed.

◆ Position the bag to avoid reaching across the sterile field.

◆ Form a cuff by turning down the top of the bag to provide a wide opening.

KEY STEPS

◆ Check for patient allergies, especially to adhesive tape and povidone-iodine or other topical solutions or drugs.

◆ Confirm the patient's identity using two patient identifiers according to facility policy.

◆ Explain the procedure to the patient and provide privacy.

◆ Tell him that he may feel a slight pulling or tickling sensation, but little discomfort, during staple removal.

◆ Reassure him that because his incision is healing properly, removing the supporting staples or clips won't weaken the incision line.

◆ Position him to promote comfort and avoid undue tension on the incision. Have him recline to avoid nausea or dizziness.

◆ Adjust the light to shine directly on the incision.

◆ Wash your hands.

◆ Put on clean gloves and carefully remove the dressing, if present.

◆ Discard the dressing and gloves in the waterproof trash bag.

◆ Assess the patient's incision.

◆ Notify the practitioner of gaping, drainage, inflammation, and other signs of infection.

◆ Establish a sterile work area.

◆ Open the package containing the sterile staple or clip extractor.

◆ Put on sterile gloves.

◆ Remove surface encrustations by gently wiping the incision with sterile gauze pads soaked in an antiseptic cleaning agent or with sterile cotton-tipped applicators.

◆ Starting at one end of the incision, remove the staple or clip. (See *Removing a staple.*)

◆ Hold the extractor over the trash bag, and release the handle to discard the staple or clip.

◆ Repeat the procedure for each staple or clip.

◆ Apply a sterile gauze dressing, if needed.

◆ Discard your gloves.

◆ Make sure that the patient is comfortable.

◆ Inform the patient that he may shower in 1 or 2 days if the incision is dry and healing well.

◆ Properly dispose of solutions, soiled supplies, and the trash bag, and clean soiled equipment.

Removing a staple

Position the extractor's lower jaws beneath the span of the first staple, as shown below.

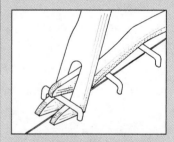

Squeeze the handles until they're completely closed, and then lift the staple away from the skin, as shown below. The extractor changes the shape of the staple and pulls the prongs out of the intradermal tissue.

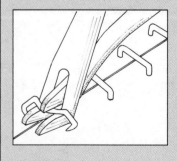

SPECIAL CONSIDERATIONS

◆ Only remove skin staples and clips by yourself if policy allows.
◆ When removing a staple or clip, place the extractor's jaws carefully between the patient's skin and the staple or clip.
◆ Staples or clips placed too deeply or left in place too long may resist removal. If extraction is difficult, notify the practitioner.
◆ If the wound dehisces after staples or clips are removed, apply butterfly adhesive strips or adhesive strips to approximate and support the edges, and call the practitioner immediately.
◆ Butterfly strips or adhesive strips may be applied after removing staples or clips (even if the wound is healing normally) to give added support and prevent lateral tension from forming a wide scar. (See *Types of adhesive skin closures*.)
◆ Use a small amount of compound benzoin tincture or other skin protectant to ensure adherence.
◆ Leave the strips in place for 3 to 5 days.

COMPLICATIONS
◆ None known

PATIENT TEACHING

◆ Teach the patient how to remove the dressing and care for the wound after staple removal.
◆ Instruct the patient to call the practitioner immediately if wound discharge or other abnormal change occurs.
◆ Tell the patient that the redness surrounding the incision should gradually disappear and that, after a few weeks, only a thin line should show.

DOCUMENTATION

◆ Record the date and time of staple or clip removal.
◆ Note the number of staples or clips removed.
◆ Document the appearance of the incision and dressings or butterfly strips applied.
◆ Record signs of wound complications.
◆ Note the patient's tolerance of the procedure.

SELECTED REFERENCES

Alexander, G., and Al-Rasheed, A.A. "Skin Staple Removal by Artery Forceps: A Hazardous Practice?" *Burns* 31(1):116, February 2005.

Holzheimer, R.G. "Adverse Events of Sutures: Possible Interactions of Biomaterials?" *European Journal of Medical Research* 10(12):521-26, December 2005.

Pullen, R.L. Jr. "Removing Sutures and Staples," *Nursing* 33(10):18, October 2003.

Types of adhesive skin closures

Adhesive strips are used as a primary means of keeping a wound closed after suture removal. They're made of thin strips of sterile, nonwoven, porous fabric tape.

Butterfly closures consist of sterile, waterproof adhesive strips. A narrow, nonadhesive "bridge" connects the two expanded adhesive portions. These strips are used to close small wounds and to assist healing after suture removal.

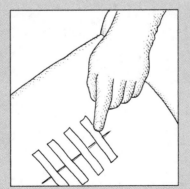
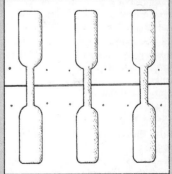

Skull tong care

DESCRIPTION

- Skeletal traction with skull tongs immobilizes the cervical spine.
- Skull tongs are applied after a fracture or dislocation, invasion by tumor or infection, or surgery.
- Three types of skull tongs are commonly used — Crutchfield, Gardner-Wells, and Vinke. (See *Types of skull tongs*.)
- Crutchfield tongs are applied by incising the skin with a scalpel, drilling a hole in the exposed skull, and inserting the pins into the hole. Gardner-Wells and Vinke tongs are less invasive.
- When in place, traction is created by extending a rope from the center of the tongs over a pulley and attaching weights to it.
- The weights are adjusted, with the help of X-ray monitoring, to establish reduction and maintain alignment.
- Meticulous pin-site care is required three times per day.
- Frequent observation of the traction apparatus is required to make sure that it's working properly.

CONTRAINDICATIONS

- None known

EQUIPMENT

Three sterile specimen containers ◆ one bottle each of ordered cleaning solution ◆ normal saline solution ◆ povidone-iodine solution ◆ sterile, cotton-tipped applicators, sandbags, or cervical collar (hard or soft) ◆ fine mesh gauze strips ◆ 4″ × 4″ gauze pads ◆ sterile gloves ◆ sterile basin ◆ sterile scissors ◆ sterile labels ◆ sterile marker ◆ hair clippers ◆ turning frame, antibacterial ointment (optional)

PREPARATION

- Bring the equipment to the patient's room.
- Place the sterile specimen containers on the bedside table.

- Fill one with a small amount of cleaning solution, one with normal saline solution, and one with povidone-iodine solution.
- Label all medication syringes, medication containers, and all solution containers on and off the sterile field.
- Set out the cotton-tipped applicators.
- Keep the sandbags or cervical collar handy for emergency immobilization of the head and neck.

KEY STEPS

- Confirm the patient's identity using two patient identifiers according to facility policy.
- Explain the procedure to the patient.
- Wash your hands.
- Inform the patient that pin sites usually feel tender for several days after the tongs are applied.
- Tell him that he'll also feel some muscular discomfort in the injured area.
- Before providing care, observe each pin site carefully for signs of infection — loose pins, swelling or redness, or purulent drainage.

- Use hair clippers to trim the patient's hair around the pin sites.
- Put on gloves.
- Wipe pin sites with a cotton-tipped applicator dipped in cleaning solution.
- Repeat with a fresh applicator, as needed, for thorough cleaning.
- Use a separate applicator for each site to avoid cross-contamination.
- Wipe the sites with normal saline solution to remove excess cleaning solution.
- Wipe with povidone-iodine to provide asepsis at the site and prevent infection.
- After providing care, discard all pin-site cleaning materials.
- Apply a povidone-iodine wrap, as ordered, for infected pin sites.
- Obtain strips of fine mesh gauze or cut a 4″ × 4″ gauze pad into strips (using sterile scissors and wearing sterile gloves).
- Soak the strips in a sterile basin of povidone-iodine solution or normal saline solution, and squeeze out excess solution.
- Wrap one strip securely around each pin site.

Types of skull tongs

Skull (or cervical) tongs consist of a stainless steel body with a pin at the end of each arm. Each pin is about ⅛″ (0.5 cm) in diameter with a sharp tip.

On Crutchfield tongs, pins are placed about 5″ (12.5 cm) apart in line with the long axis of the cervical spine.

On Gardner-Wells tongs, pins are farther apart. They're inserted slightly above the patient's ears.

On Vinke tongs, pins are placed at the parietal bones, near the widest transverse diameter of the skull, about 1″ (2.5 cm) above the helix.

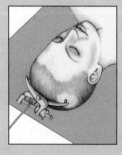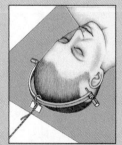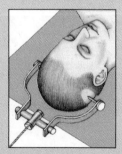

- Leave the strip in place to dry until you provide care again.
- Removing the dried strip aids in debridement and helps clear infection.
- Check the traction apparatus — rope, weights, pulleys — at the start of each shift, every 4 hours, and as necessary.
- Make sure that the rope hangs freely.

SPECIAL CONSIDERATIONS

- Antibacterial ointment for pin-site care may be ordered instead of povidone-iodine solution.
- To remove old ointment, wrap a cotton-tipped applicator with a $4'' \times 4''$ gauze pad, moisten with cleaning solution, and gently clean each site.
- Keep a box of sterile gauze pads at the patient's bedside.
- Osteoporosis can cause skull pins to slip or pull out, which requires immediate attention to prevent further injury.
- Watch for signs and symptoms of loose pins, such as persistent pain or tenderness at pin sites, redness, drainage, or patient reports of feeling or hearing the pins move.
- If you suspect a pin has loosened or slipped, notify the practitioner.
- Await the practitioner's examination before turning the patient.
- If the pins pull out, immobilize the patient's head and neck with sandbags or apply a cervical collar, and carefully remove the traction weights.
- Apply manual traction to the patient's head by placing your hands on each side of the mandible and pulling gently, while maintaining proper alignment.
- After you stabilize the alignment, have someone send for the practitioner immediately.
- Remain calm and reassure the patient.
- When traction is reestablished, take the patient's neurologic vital signs.

WARNING *Never add or subtract weights to the traction apparatus without an order from the practitioner. Improper procedure can result in neurologic impairment to the patient.*

- Take the patient's neurologic vital signs at the beginning of each shift, every 4 hours, and as necessary.
- Carefully assess cranial nerve function, which may be impaired by pin placement.
- Note asymmetry, deviation, or atrophy.
- Review the patient's chart to determine baseline neurologic vital signs and those immediately after tongs were applied.
- Monitor respirations closely and keep suction equipment handy.
- Injury to the cervical spine may affect respiration, so stay alert for signs of respiratory distress.
- Patients with skull tongs may be placed on a turning frame to facilitate turning without disrupting vertebral alignment. Establish a turning schedule to help prevent complications of immobility.
- Never remove a patient from the bed or turning frame when transporting him.

COMPLICATIONS
- Infection
- Excessive traction force

PATIENT TEACHING

- Explain how skull tong care is performed to lessen the patient's anxiety.
- Tell the patient that pin sites may feel tender for several days after tongs are applied.
- Inform the patient about signs and symptoms of complications, such as pain at the pin sites or hearing or feeling the pins move, and to notify the practitioner or nurse if these occur.
- Teach the patient how to turn and reposition with skull tongs in place.
- Reassure the patient that he'll be closely monitored.

DOCUMENTATION

- Record the date, time, and type of pin-site care.
- Note the patient's response to the procedure.
- Document signs of infection.
- Record whether weights were added or removed.
- Note the patient's neurologic vital signs and respiratory status.
- Record the turning schedule.

SELECTED REFERENCES
Awasthy, N., and Chand, K. "Intracranial Bleed Complicating the Use of Crutchfield Tongs," *Journal of Neurosurgical Sciences* 50(1):13-15, March 2006.

Davis, P. "Skeletal Pin Traction: Guidelines on Postoperative Care and Support," *Nursing Times* 99(21):46-48, May-June 2003.

Holmes, S.B., et al. "Skeletal Pin Site Care: National Association of Orthopaedic Nurses Guidelines for Orthopaedic Nursing," *Orthopaedic Nursing* 24(2): 99-107, March-April 2005.

Malomo, A.O., et al. "Conservative Management of Third Trimester Cervical Spinal Cord Injury Using Gardner-Wells Tongs Traction," *Nigerian Journal of Clinical Practice* 8(1):46-50, June 2005.

Sling (triangular) application

OVERVIEW

DESCRIPTION
◆ A sling is made from a triangular piece of muslin, canvas, or cotton to support and immobilize an injured arm, wrist, or hand due to fracture or dislocation or to support a muscle sprain.
◆ It facilitates healing.
◆ It can support the weight of a splint or help secure dressings.

CONTRAINDICATIONS
◆ None known

EQUIPMENT

Triangular bandage or commercial sling ◆ gauze (for padding) ◆ safety pins (tape for children younger than age 7)

KEY STEPS

◆ Confirm the patient's identity using two patient identifiers according to facility policy.
◆ Explain the procedure to the patient.
◆ Wash your hands.

AGE FACTOR *If the patient is a child, fold the bandage in half to make a smaller triangle. Then follow the regular steps for making a sling.*

◆ If you anticipate prolonged use of a sling, pad the area under the knot with gauze to prevent skin irritation. (See *Making a sling.*)
◆ Place the sling outside the shirt collar to reduce direct pressure on the neck and shoulder.
◆ If the arm requires complete immobilization, apply a swathe after placing the arm in a sling. (See *Applying a swathe.*)
◆ Check the sling frequently for proper position, and assess the patient's comfort and circulation to the fingers.

AGE FACTOR *For a child younger than age 7, use tape instead of a pin to secure a triangular sling to avoid the chance of an injury.*

Making a sling

Place the apex of a triangular bandage behind the patient's elbow on the injured side.

Hold one end of the bandage so it extends up toward the patient's neck on the uninjured side and let the other end hang straight down. The bandage's long side should parallel the midline of his body.

Loop the top corner of the bandage over the shoulder on the uninjured side and around the back of the patient's neck. Then bring the lower end of the bandage over the flexed forearm and up to the shoulder on the injured side.

Adjust the bandage so the forearm and upper arm form an angle slightly less than 90 degrees to increase venous return from the hand and forearm and facilitate drainage from swelling. Tie the two ends at the side of his neck, rather than at the back, to prevent neck flexion and avoid irritation and pressure over a cervical vertebra.

Carefully secure the sling with a safety pin or tape above and behind the elbow.

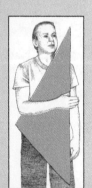
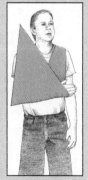
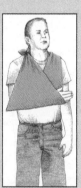
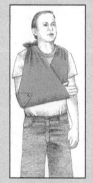

◆ Provide an extra triangular bandage before patient discharge.

COMPLICATIONS
◆ Axillary and cervical skin breakdown
◆ Irritation and infection

◆ Teach the patient and a family member or friend how to change the sling and apply a swathe, if necessary.
◆ Instruct the patient that a soiled sling can cause irritation and infection.
◆ Teach the patient how to check for axillary and cervical skin breakdown.

◆ Record the date, time, and location of sling application.
◆ Note the patient's tolerance of the procedure.
◆ Document the patient's neurovascular status, noting color and temperature.

SELECTED REFERENCES
Foongchomcheay, A., et al. "Use of Devices to Prevent Subluxation of the Shoulder after Stroke," *Physiotherapy Research International* 10(3):134-45, 2005.

Murrell, G.A. "Treatment of Shoulder Dislocation: Is a Sling Appropriate?" *Medical Journal of Australia* 179(7):370-71, October 2003.

Richard, R., et al. "The Use of Figure-of-8 Sling for Treatment of Axillary Contractures," *Burns* 31(7):940, November 2005.

Applying a swathe

Wrap a folded triangular bandage or wide elastic bandage around the patient's upper torso and the upper arm on the injured side. Don't cover the uninjured arm. Make the swathe just tight enough to secure the injured arm to the body. Tie or pin the ends of the bandage just in front of the axilla on the uninjured side.

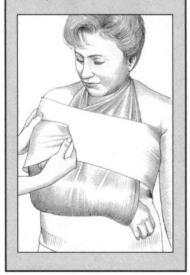

Soaks

DESCRIPTION

◆ Soaks involve the immersion of a body part in warm water or a medicated solution.

◆ They help soften exudate, facilitate debridement, enhance suppuration, clean wounds or burns, rehydrate wounds, apply a drug to infected areas, and increase local blood supply and circulation.

◆ Soaks are most commonly applied with clean tap water and clean technique.

◆ Sterile solutions and equipment are required for treating wounds, burns, and other skin breaks.

CONTRAINDICATIONS

◆ None known

Basin, or arm or foot tub ◆ bath (utility) thermometer ◆ tap water or prescribed solution ◆ cup ◆ pitcher ◆ linen-saver pad ◆ overbed table ◆ footstool ◆ pillows ◆ towels ◆ gauze pads and other dressing materials ◆ clean and sterile gloves, if necessary

PREPARATION

◆ Clean and disinfect the basin or tub.

◆ Run hot tap water into a pitcher or heat the prescribed solution to within the prescribed range (typically 105° to 110° F [40.6° to 43.3° C]).

◆ Measure the water or solution temperature with a bath thermometer.

◆ If you're preparing the soak outside the patient's room, heat the liquid slightly above the correct temperature to allow for cooling during transport.

◆ If the solution for a medicated soak isn't premixed, prepare the solution and heat it.

◆ Check the practitioner's order.

◆ Confirm the patient's identity using two patient identifiers according to facility policy.

◆ Assess the patient's condition and explain the procedure.

◆ Check his history for previous allergic reaction to the medicated solution.

◆ Provide privacy and wash your hands.

◆ If the soak basin or tub will be placed in bed, make sure that the bed is flat.

◆ For an arm soak, have the patient sit erect.

◆ For a leg or foot soak, ask him to lie down and bend the appropriate knee.

◆ For a foot soak in the sitting position, let him sit on the edge of the bed or transfer him to a chair.

◆ Place a linen-saver pad under the treatment site and cover the pad with a towel to absorb spillage.

◆ Expose the treatment site.

◆ Put on gloves.

◆ Remove and dispose of soiled dressings.

◆ If a dressing is encrusted and stuck to the wound, leave it in place and proceed with the soak; you can remove the dressing several minutes later when it has begun to soak free.

◆ Position the soak basin under the treatment site on the bed, overbed table, footstool, or floor.

◆ Pour the heated liquid into the soak basin or tub.

◆ Lower the arm or leg into the basin gradually to allow adjustment to the temperature change.

◆ Make sure that the soak solution covers the treatment site.

◆ Support other body parts with pillows or towels to prevent discomfort and muscle strain.

◆ Make the patient comfortable and ensure proper body alignment.

◆ Check the temperature of the soak solution every 5 minutes; if the temperature drops below the prescribed range, remove some of the cooled solution with a cup.

- Lift the patient's arm or leg from the basin to avoid burns, and add hot water or solution to the basin. Mix the liquid thoroughly, and then check the temperature.
- If the temperature is within the prescribed range, lower the patient's affected part back into the basin.
- Observe the patient for signs of tissue intolerance, such as extreme redness at the treatment site, excessive drainage, bleeding, and maceration.
- If such signs develop or if the patient complains of pain, discontinue the treatment and notify the practitioner.
- After 15 to 20 minutes, or as ordered, lift the patient's arm or leg from the basin and remove the basin.
- Dry the arm or leg thoroughly with a towel without touching wounds.
- While the skin is hydrated from the soak, use gauze pads to remove loose scales or crusts.
- Observe the treatment area for general appearance, degree of swelling, debridement, suppuration, and healing.
- Put on sterile gloves and redress the wound, if appropriate.
- Remove the towel and linen-saver pad, and make the patient comfortable.
- Discard the soak solution and soiled materials properly.
- Clean and disinfect the basin.
- Remove and discard your gloves.
- Store the equipment in the patient's room if the treatment is to be repeated; otherwise, return it to central supply.

SPECIAL CONSIDERATIONS

- Use a whirlpool or Hubbard tank if large areas, especially burns, are to be treated.

COMPLICATIONS
- None known

PATIENT TEACHING

- Explain the procedure and answer the patient's questions, as needed.

DOCUMENTATION

- Record the date, time, and duration of the soak.
- Note the treatment site, the solution, and its temperature.
- Document skin and wound appearance before, during, and after treatment, and the patient's tolerance of the treatment.

SELECTED REFERENCES

Gutman, A.B., et al. "Soak and Smear: A Standard Technique Revisited," *Archives of Dermatology* 141(12):1556-59, December 2005.

Visscher, M.O., et al. "Effect of Soaking and Natural Moisturizing Factor on Stratum Corneum Water-Handling Properties," *Journal of Cosmetic Science* 54(3):289-300, May-June 2003.

Spiritual care

DESCRIPTION

◆ Religious beliefs can influence recovery rates, attitudes toward treatment, and overall response to hospitalization.

◆ In certain religious groups, beliefs can preclude diagnostic tests and therapeutic treatments, require dietary restrictions, and prohibit organ donation and artificial life support. (See *Beliefs and practices of selected religions*.)

◆ Effective patient care requires recognition of and respect for the patient's religious beliefs.

◆ Recognizing beliefs and the need for spiritual care may require close attention to nonverbal cues or seemingly casual remarks that express spiritual concerns.

◆ Respecting beliefs may require setting aside your own beliefs.

◆ Providing spiritual care may require contacting an appropriate member of the clergy, gathering equipment needed to help the clergy perform rites and administer sacraments, and preparing the patient for a visit with clergy.

CONTRAINDICATIONS

◆ None known

Clean towels (one or two) ◆ teaspoon or 1-oz (30-ml) medicine cup (for baptism) ◆ container of water (for emergency baptism) ◆ other supplies specific to the patient's religious affiliation

Some facilities provide baptismal trays. The clergy member may bring holy water, holy oil, or other religious articles to minister to the patient.

PREPARATION

Baptism

◆ Cover a small table with a clean towel.

◆ Fold a second towel and place it on the table.

◆ Place the teaspoon or medicine cup on the table.

Communion and anointment

◆ Cover the bedside stand with a clean towel.

◆ Check the patient's admission record to determine his religious affiliation. He may claim no religious beliefs, but may still wish to speak with a clergy member; watch and listen carefully for subtle expressions of this desire.

◆ Confirm the patient's identity using two patient identifiers according to facility policy.

◆ Evaluate the patient's behavior for signs of loneliness, anxiety, or fear.

◆ Help the patient who feels acutely distressed because of his inability to participate in religious observances to verbalize his concerns.

◆ Refrain from imposing your beliefs.

◆ If the patient requests, arrange a visit by an appropriate clergy member.

◆ If the patient faces medical procedures with important medical or spiritual implications (for example, abortion, amputation, transfusion), try to assess the patient's spiritual attitude.

◆ Try to determine attitudes toward the importance of laying on of hands, confession, communion, observance of holy days, and restrictions in diet or physical appearance.

◆ Help the patient continue his normal religious practices to reduce the stress of hospitalization.

◆ If the patient is pregnant, find out her beliefs concerning infant baptism and circumcision, and comply with them after delivery.

◆ If a neonate is in critical condition, call the parents and a designated clergy member immediately.

◆ In an extreme emergency, you can perform a Roman Catholic baptism, as appropriate, using a container of any available water. Sprinkle a few drops of water over the infant's head while saying, "(name of child), I baptize you in the name of the Father, the Son, and the Holy Spirit. Amen."

◆ If you do so, be sure to notify the priest because this sacrament must be administered only once.

Beliefs and practices of selected religions

A patient's religious beliefs can affect his attitudes toward illness and traditional medicine. By trying to accommodate the patient's religious beliefs and practices in your care plan, you can increase his willingness to learn and comply with treatment regimens. Because religious beliefs may vary within particular sects, individual practices may differ from those described here.

RELIGION	BIRTH AND DEATH RITUALS	DIETARY RESTRICTIONS	PRACTICES IN HEALTH CRISIS
Adventist	None (baptism of adults only)	Alcohol, coffee, tea, narcotics, stimulants; in many groups, meat also prohibited	Communion and baptism are performed. Some members believe in divine healing, anointing with oil, and prayer. Some regard Saturday as the Sabbath.
Baptist	At birth, none (baptism of believers only); before death, counseling by clergy member and prayer	Alcohol; in some groups, coffee and tea also prohibited	Some believe in healing by laying on of hands. Resistance to medical therapy is occasionally approved.
Christian Scientist	At birth, none; before death, counseling by a Christian Science practitioner	Alcohol, coffee, and tobacco prohibited	Many members refuse all treatment, including drugs, biopsies, physical examination, and blood transfusions, and permit vaccination only when required by law. Alteration of thoughts is believed to cure illness. Hypnotism and psychotherapy are prohibited. (Christian Scientist nurses and nursing homes honor these beliefs.)
Church of Christ	None (baptism at age 8 or older)	Alcohol discouraged	Communion, anointing with oil, laying on of hands, and counseling by a minister are performed. The sick are anointed.
Eastern Orthodox	At birth, baptism and confirmation; before death, last rites (For members of the Russian Orthodox Church, the arms are crossed after death, the fingers are set in a cross, and the unembalmed body is clothed in natural fiber.)	For members of the Russian Orthodox Church and usually the Greek Orthodox Church, no meat or dairy products on Wednesday, Friday, and during Lent	The sick are anointed. For members of the Russian Orthodox Church, a cross necklace is replaced immediately after surgery and shaving of male patients is prohibited, except in preparation for surgery. For members of the Greek Orthodox Church, communion and Sacrament of Holy Unction are given.
Episcopal	At birth, baptism; before death, occasional last rites	For some members, abstention from meat on Friday, fasting before communion (which may be daily)	Communion, prayer, and counseling are performed by a minister.
Jehovah's Witness	None	Abstention from foods to which blood has been added	Typically, no blood transfusions are permitted; a court order may be required for an emergency transfusion.
Judaism	Ritual circumcision on eighth day after birth; burial of dead fetus; ritual washing of dead; burial (including organs and other body tissues) occurs as soon as possible; no autopsy or embalming	For Orthodox and Conservative Jews, kosher dietary laws (for example, pork and shellfish prohibited); for Reform Jews, usually no restrictions	Donation or transplantation of organs requires rabbinical consultation. For Orthodox and Conservative Jews, medical procedures may be prohibited on the Sabbath — from sundown Friday to sundown Saturday — and special holidays.
Lutheran	Baptism usually performed 6 to 8 weeks after birth	None	Communion, prayer, and counseling are performed by a minister.
Mormon	At birth, none (baptism at age 8 or older); before death, baptism and gospel preaching	Alcohol, tobacco, tea, and coffee prohibited; meat intake limited	They believe in divine healing through the laying on of hands; communion on Sunday; some members may refuse medical treatment. Many wear a special undergarment.

(continued)

(continued)

- If a Jewish woman delivers a male infant prematurely or by cesarean birth, ask her whether she plans to observe the rite of circumcision (bris), performed on the eighth day after birth.
- For a bris, ensure privacy and, if requested, sterilize the instruments.
- If the patient requests communion, prepare him for it before the clergy member arrives.
- Place him in Fowler's or semi-Fowler's position (if permitted), tuck a clean towel under his chin, and straighten the bed linens.
- If a terminally ill patient requests the Sacrament of the Sick (Last Rites) or special treatment of his body after death, call an appropriate clergy member.

- For the Roman Catholic patient, call a Roman Catholic priest to administer the sacrament even if the patient is unresponsive or comatose.
- To prepare the patient for this sacrament, uncover his arms and fold back the top linens to expose his feet.
- After the clergy member anoints the patient's forehead, eyes, nose, mouth, hands, and feet, straighten and retuck the bed linens.

SPECIAL CONSIDERATIONS

- Handle the patient's religious articles carefully.
- Become familiar with religious resources in your facility.
- Some facilities employ one or more clergy members who counsel patients and staff and link patients to other pastoral resources.
- If the patient tries to convert you to his personal beliefs, tell him that you respect his beliefs but are content with your own.
- Avoid attempts to convert the patient to your personal beliefs.

COMPLICATIONS
- None known

Beliefs and practices of selected religions *(continued)*

RELIGION	BIRTH AND DEATH RITUALS	DIETARY RESTRICTIONS	PRACTICES IN HEALTH CRISIS
Muslim	If spontaneous abortion occurs before 130 days, fetus treated as discarded tissue; after 130 days, as a human being (Before death, confession of sins with family present; after death, only relatives or friends may touch the body.)	Pork prohibited; daylight fasting during ninth month of Islamic calendar	Faith healing is for the patient's morale only; conservative members reject medical therapy.
Orthodox Presbyterian	Infant baptism; scripture reading and prayer before death	None	Communion, prayer, and counseling are performed by a minister.
Pentecostal Assembly of God, Foursquare Church	None (baptism only after age of accountability)	Abstention from alcohol, tobacco, meat slaughtered by strangling, any food to which blood has been added and, sometimes, pork	Belief in divine healing through prayer, anointing with oil, and laying on of hands is practiced.
Roman Catholic	Infant baptism, including baptism of an aborted fetus without signs of clinical death (tissue necrosis); before death, anointing of the sick	Fasting or abstention from meat on Ash Wednesday and on Fridays during Lent; practice usually waived for the hospitalized	Major amputated limb (sometimes) is buried in consecrated ground; donation or transplantation of organs allowed if the benefit to the recipient outweighs the potential harm to the donor. Sacraments of the Sick are also performed when patients are ill, not just before death. Sometimes it's performed shortly after admission.
United Methodist	None (baptism of children and adults only)	None	Communion is ministered before surgery or a similar crisis; donation of body parts is encouraged.

PATIENT TEACHING

◆ Tell the patient about any spiritual resources available at your facility.

DOCUMENTATION

◆ After a baptism, attach a baptismal form to the patient's record and send a copy to the appropriate clergy.
◆ Record the rites of circumcision, as appropriate.
◆ Document the performance of last rites in red on the Kardex so it won't be repeated.

SELECTED REFERENCES

Cavendish, R., et al. "Patients' Perceptions of Spirituality and the Nurse as a Spiritual Care Provider," *Holistic Nursing Practice* 20(1):41-47, January-February 2006.

Kilpatrick, S.D., et al. "A Review of Spiritual and Religious Measures in Nursing Research Journals: 1995-1999," *Journal of Religion and Health* 44(1):55-66, Spring 2005.

Mattison, D. "The Forgotten Spirit: Integration of Spirituality in Health Care," *Nephrology News & Issues* 20(2):30-32, February 2006.

Speck, P. "The Evidence Base for Spiritual Care," *Nursing Management* 12(6): 28-31, October 2005.

Tanyi, R.A. "Spirituality and Family Nursing: Spiritual Assessment and Interventions for Families," *Journal of Advanced Nursing* 53(3):287-94, February 2006.

Splints

OVERVIEW

DESCRIPTION

◆ A splint is used to immobilize the site of an injury.

◆ It alleviates pain and allows proper alignment during healing, minimizing possible complications.

◆ In multiple serious injuries, it allows caretakers to move the patient without risking further damage to bones, muscles, nerves, blood vessels, and skin.

◆ It may be applied to immobilize a simple or compound fracture, a dislocation, or a subluxation.

◆ During an emergency, an injury suspected of being a fracture, dislocation, or subluxation should be splinted.

CONTRAINDICATIONS

◆ Traction splints in upper extremity injuries or open fractures

EQUIPMENT

Rigid splint ◆ Velcro support splint ◆ spine board or traction splint bindings ◆ padding ◆ sandbags or rolled towels or clothing strips ◆ sterile compress ◆ ice bag ◆ roller gauze (optional)

PREPARATION

◆ Consult the manufacturer's instructions before applying a splint.

◆ In an emergency, a long, sturdy object (tree limb, mop handle, broom, rolled magazine) can be used as a rigid splint. A door can be used as a spine board.

◆ An inflatable semirigid splint, called an air splint, can sometimes be used to secure an injured extremity. (See *Using an air splint*.)

◆ Velcro straps, 2″ roller gauze, or 2″ cloth strips can be used as bindings.

◆ Avoid using twine or rope, which can restrict circulation.

Using an air splint

In an emergency, an air splint (shown below) can be applied to immobilize a fracture or control bleeding, especially from a forearm or lower leg. This compact splint is made of double-walled plastic and provides gentle, diffuse pressure over an injured area.

The splint is wrapped around the affected extremity, secured with Velcro or other strips, and inflated. The fit should be snug enough to immobilize the extremity without impairing circulation.

An air splint may control bleeding better than a local pressure bandage. Its clear plastic construction simplifies inspection of the affected site for bleeding, pallor, or cyanosis. It also allows the patient to be moved without causing further damage.

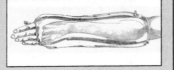

KEY STEPS

◆ Obtain a history of the injury and inspect for swelling, obvious deformities, bleeding, discoloration, and evidence of fracture or dislocation.

◆ Ask the patient if he can move the injured area; compare it with the uninjured extremity.

◆ Remove or cut away clothing from the injury site and palpate the injured area.

◆ Check neurovascular integrity distal to the site.

◆ If an obvious bone misalignment causes the patient acute distress or severe neurovascular problems, align the extremity in its normal anatomic position. Stop if this causes further neurovascular deterioration.

◆ To avoid damaging displaced vessels and nerves, don't try to straighten a dislocation.

◆ Don't attempt reduction of a contaminated bone end because this may cause additional laceration of soft tissues, vessels, and nerves as well as gross contamination of deep tissues.

◆ Apply a sterile compress to an open wound.

◆ Choose a splint that will immobilize the joints above and below the fracture.

◆ Pad the splint as necessary to protect bony prominences.

APPLYING A RIGID SPLINT

◆ Support the injured extremity above and below the fracture site while applying firm, gentle traction.

◆ Place the splint under, beside, or on top of the extremity.

◆ Apply the bindings to secure the splint, but don't obstruct circulation.

◆ If the neurovascular status of the extremity is impaired by bindings, reapply them.

APPLYING A SPINE BOARD

◆ Pad the spine board.

◆ Pay special attention to areas that support the lumbar region and knees.

- If the patient is supine, place one hand on each side of his head and apply gentle traction to the head and neck. Keep the patient's head aligned with his body.
- Logroll the patient onto his side.
- Slide the spine board under the patient.
- Instruct the assistants to roll the patient onto the board while you maintain traction and alignment.
- If the patient is prone, logroll him onto the board so he ends up in a supine position.
- Use strips of cloth to secure the patient on the spine board and maintain alignment.
- Place sandbags or rolled towels or clothing on both sides of his head to keep his head and neck aligned.

APPLYING A TRACTION SPLINT

- Specialized training is required before applying a traction splint.
- Place the splint beside the injured leg.
- Never use a traction splint on an arm because the major axillary plexus of nerves and blood vessels can't tolerate countertraction.
- Adjust the splint to the correct length, and then open and adjust the Velcro straps.
- Keep the leg motionless while you pad the ankle and foot and fasten the ankle hitch around them. The shoe may stay on.
- Lift and support the leg at the injury site as you apply firm, gentle traction.
- Slide the splint under the leg, pad the groin to avoid excessive pressure on external genitalia, and gently apply the ischial strap.
- Maintain traction.
- Connect the loops of the ankle hitch to the end of the splint.
- Adjust the splint to apply enough traction to secure the leg comfortably in the corrected position.
- Fasten the Velcro support splints to secure the leg closely to the splint.

⚡ **WARNING** *Don't use a traction splint for a severely angulated femur or knee fracture.*

SPECIAL CONSIDERATIONS

- At the scene of an accident, examine the patient completely for injuries.
- Avoid unnecessary movement or manipulation.
- Always consider the possibility of cervical injury in an unconscious patient.
- If possible, apply the splint before repositioning the patient.
- If a rigid splint is needed but one isn't available, use another body part as a splint. To splint a leg in this manner, pad its inner aspect and secure it to the other leg with roller gauze or cloth strips.
- After applying any type of splint, check the patient's vital signs frequently to monitor for shock.
- Monitor the neurovascular status of the fractured limb. Assess skin color and temperature. Check for pain and numbness in the fingers or toes. Check capillary refill and sensation in the affected extremities.
- Numbness or paralysis distal to the injury indicates pressure on nerves.
- Apply ice to the injury.
- Transport the patient as soon as possible to a hospital.
- Don't allow the patient to eat or drink until a practitioner evaluates him.
- Indications for removing a splint include evidence of improper application or vascular impairment.
- Apply gentle traction, and remove the splint carefully under a practitioner's direct supervision.

COMPLICATIONS

- Fat embolism manifested by shortness of breath, agitation, and irrational behavior (typically occurs within 24 to 72 hours of injury or manipulation)

PATIENT TEACHING

- Explain what you're doing, as appropriate, to help lessen the patient's anxiety.

DOCUMENTATION

- Document the circumstances and cause of the injury.
- Record the patient's complaints and whether symptoms are localized.
- Record neurovascular status before and after applying the splint.
- Note the type of wound and the amount and type of drainage.
- Record the time of splint application.
- Document whether bone end slips into surrounding tissue.
- Record if transportation causes a change in the degree of dislocation.

SELECTED REFERENCES

Hobman, J.W., and Southern, S.J. "Upper Limb Splints and the Right to Drive — Who Decides?" *British Journal of Plastic Surgery* 57(4):354-57, June 2004.

Miller, N.J., et al. "Improvement in the Emergency Splinting of Fractures after a Simple Educational Exercise," *ANZ Journal of Surgery* 75(9):754-56, September 2005.

Plint, A.C., et al. "A Randomized, Controlled Trial of Removable Splinting versus Casting for Wrist Buckle Fractures in Children," *Pediatrics* 117(3): 691-97, March 2006.

Vehmeyer-Heeman, M., et al. "Axillary Burns: Extended Grafting and Early Splinting Prevents Contractures," *Journal of Burn Care & Rehabilitation* 26(6):539-42, November-December 2005.

Sputum collection

OVERVIEW

DESCRIPTION

◆ Sputum is secreted by mucous membranes lining the bronchioles, bronchi, and trachea; it helps protect the respiratory tract from infection.

◆ When expelled, it carries saliva, nasal and sinus secretions, dead cells, and normal oral bacteria from the respiratory tract.

◆ It may be cultured to identify respiratory pathogens.

◆ Expectoration is the usual method of sputum specimen collection.

◆ Expectoration may require ultrasonic nebulization, hydration, or chest percussion and postural drainage.

◆ Less common methods include tracheal suctioning and bronchoscopy.

CONTRAINDICATIONS

◆ Performed within 1 hour of eating
◆ Esophageal varices
◆ Nausea
◆ Facial or basilar skull fractures
◆ Laryngospasm
◆ Bronchospasm

EQUIPMENT

Commercial suction kits include all equipment except the suction machine and an in-line specimen container.

EXPECTORATION

Sterile specimen container with tight-fitting cap ◆ gloves ◆ label ◆ laboratory request form ◆ aerosol (10% sodium chloride, propylene glycol, acetylcysteine, or sterile or distilled water)

TRACHEAL SUCTIONING

#12 to #14 French sterile suction catheter ◆ water-soluble lubricant ◆ laboratory request form ◆ sterile gloves ◆ mask ◆ goggles ◆ sterile in-line specimen trap (Lukens trap) ◆ normal saline solution ◆ portable suction machine ◆ oxygen therapy equipment (if wall suction is unavailable)

PREPARATION

◆ Gather the appropriate equipment for the procedure.

KEY STEPS

◆ Confirm the patient's identity using two patient identifiers according to facility policy.

◆ Explain the procedure.

◆ Put on gloves.

◆ Collect the specimen early in the morning by expectoration.

◆ Instruct the patient to sit on a chair or edge of the bed; if he can't sit up, place him in high Fowler's position.

◆ Have him rinse his mouth with water to reduce specimen contamination. Avoid mouthwash and toothpaste; they may affect the mobility of organisms in the sputum sample.

◆ Tell him to cough deeply and expectorate at least 15 ml of sputum directly into the specimen container.

◆ Cap the container and, if necessary, clean its exterior.

◆ Remove and discard your gloves.

◆ Wash your hands.

◆ Label the container with the patient's name, room number, the practitioner's name, date and time of collection, and initial diagnosis. Include on the laboratory request form whether the patient was febrile, taking antibiotics, and whether sputum was induced.

◆ Send the specimen to the laboratory immediately.

COLLECTING BY TRACHEAL SUCTIONING

◆ Collect a specimen by suctioning if the patient can't produce an adequate specimen by coughing.

◆ Explain the suctioning procedure to him.

◆ Tell him that he may cough, gag, or feel short of breath during the procedure.

◆ Check the suction equipment to make sure that it's functioning properly.

◆ Place the patient in high or semi-Fowler's position.

◆ Administer oxygen to the patient before beginning the procedure.

◆ Wash your hands and put on a face mask and goggles.

- Put on sterile gloves; consider one hand sterile and the other hand clean to prevent cross-contamination.
- With your clean hand, connect the suction tubing to the male adapter of the in-line specimen trap.
- Using your sterile gloved hand, attach the sterile suction catheter to the rubber tubing of the trap.
- Tell the patient to tilt his head back slightly.
- Lubricate the catheter with normal saline solution and insert it in the patient's nostril without suction.
- When the catheter reaches the larynx, the patient will cough. As he does, quickly advance the catheter into the trachea.
- Tell him to take several deep breaths through his mouth.
- Apply suction for 5 to 10 seconds but never longer than 15 seconds, which may cause hypoxia.
- If the procedure must be repeated, let the patient rest for four to six breaths.
- When collection is completed, discontinue suction and remove the catheter.
- Administer oxygen.
- Detach the catheter from the in-line trap.
- Gather it in your dominant hand and pull the glove cuff inside out and down around the used catheter to enclose it for disposal.
- Remove and discard the other glove, your mask, and goggles.
- Detach the trap from the tubing connected to the suction machine.
- Seal the trap tightly by connecting the rubber tubing to the male adapter of the trap.
- Label the trap's container as an expectorated specimen.
- Send the specimen to the laboratory immediately with a completed laboratory request form.
- Offer the patient a glass of water or mouthwash.

SPECIAL CONSIDERATIONS

- Tracheal suctioning provides a more reliable diagnostic specimen.
- If tracheal suctioning doesn't produce a sputum specimen, perform chest percussion to loosen and mobilize secretions.
- Position the patient for optimal drainage.
- After 20 to 30 minutes, repeat tracheal suctioning.
- Before sending the specimen to the laboratory, examine it to make sure that it's actually sputum, not saliva, which will produce inaccurate test results.
- Remove the catheter immediately if the patient becomes hypoxic or cyanotic, and administer oxygen.
- Watch for aggravated bronchospasms if using an aerosol with more than 10% sodium chloride or acetylcysteine in patients with asthma or chronic bronchitis.
- Don't use more than 20% propylene glycol with water when inducing a sputum specimen in someone suspected of having tuberculosis. A higher concentration of propylene glycol inhibits growth of the pathogen and alters test results.
- Use 10% to 20% acetylcysteine with water or sodium chloride if propylene glycol isn't available.

COMPLICATIONS
- Tracheal trauma or bleeding
- Vomiting
- Aspiration
- Hypoxemia
- Hypoxia
- Arrhythmias (with presence of cardiac disease, especially when specimen is obtained by suctioning)

PATIENT TEACHING

- Explain and answer questions about the tracheal suctioning procedure to lessen the patient's anxiety and gain cooperation.

DOCUMENTATION

- Note the collection method.
- Record the time and date of collection and how the patient tolerated the procedure.
- Document the color and consistency of the specimen.
- Record proper disposition.

SELECTED REFERENCES

Elkins, M.R., et al. "Effect of Airway Clearance Techniques on the Efficacy of the Sputum Induction Procedure," *European Respiratory Journal* 26(5):904-908, November 2005.

Ko, D.S., et al. "Clinical Implication of Atypical Cells from Sputum in Patients without Lung Cancer," *Respirology* 11(4):462-66, July 2006.

Lumb, R., et al. "An Alternative Method for Sputum Storage and Transport for Mycobacterium Tuberculosis Drug Resistance Surveys," *International Journal of Tuberculosis and Lung Disease* 10(2):172-77, February 2006.

Standard precautions

OVERVIEW

DESCRIPTION
◆ Standard precautions were developed by the Centers for Disease Control and Prevention to provide the best possible protection against the transmission of infection.
◆ All blood, body fluids, tissues, and contact with mucous membranes and broken skin should be handled as if they contain infectious agents, regardless of the patient's diagnosis.
◆ Standard precautions are to be used in conjunction with other transmission-based precautions.
◆ Causative organisms are coughed, talked, or sneezed into air in droplets of moisture; the moisture evaporates, leaving suspended microorganisms to be breathed in.
◆ Airborne precautions are initiated when suspected or known infections spread through the air.
◆ Airborne precautions include placing the infected patient in a negative-pressure isolation room. Respiratory protection should be worn by anyone entering the room.
◆ Droplet precautions are used to protect health care workers and visitors from mucous membrane contact with oral and nasal secretions of the infected patient.
◆ Contact precautions use barrier precautions to interrupt the transmission of specific epidemiologically important organisms by direct or indirect contact.
◆ Each facility must establish an infection control policy that lists specific barrier precautions.

CONTRAINDICATIONS
◆ None known

EQUIPMENT

Gloves ◆ masks ◆ goggles or face shields ◆ gowns or aprons ◆ resuscitation bag ◆ bags for specimens ◆ Environmental Protection Agency (EPA)-registered tuberculocidal disinfectant or diluted bleach solution (diluted 1:10 to 1:100, mixed fresh daily), or both ◆ EPA-registered disinfectant labeled effective against hepatitis B virus (HBV) and human immunodeficiency virus (HIV)

KEY STEPS

◆ Wash your hands immediately if they become contaminated with blood or body fluids, excretions, secretions, or drainage.
◆ Wash your hands before and after patient care and after removing gloves.
◆ An alcohol-based hand rub can be used for routine decontamination if your hands aren't visibly soiled.
◆ Wear gloves if you may come in contact with blood, specimens, tissue, body fluids, secretions or excretions, mucous membranes, broken skin, or contaminated surfaces or objects. (See *Choosing the right glove.*)
◆ Change your gloves and wash your hands between patient contacts.
◆ Wear a fluid-resistant gown, face shield or goggles, and a mask during procedures likely to generate splash-

---

Choosing the right glove

Allergic reactions may result from cumulative exposure to latex gloves and other latex-containing products. Patients may also have latex sensitivity.

Take these steps to protect yourself and your patient from allergic reactions to natural rubber latex:
◆ Use nonlatex (vinyl or synthetic) gloves for activities not likely to involve contact with infectious materials (food preparation, routine cleaning).
◆ Nonlatex gloves can be worn for activities of short duration, even if contact with infectious material is possible.
◆ Use appropriate barrier protection when handling infectious materials. If you choose latex gloves, use powder-free gloves with reduced protein content. Powder in any gloves is very drying to skin and may cause a greater risk of exposure to skin if it's dry and cracked.
◆ After wearing and removing gloves, wash your hands with soap and dry them thoroughly.
◆ When wearing latex gloves, don't use oil-based hand creams or lotions unless they have been shown to maintain glove barrier protection.
◆ Refer to the material safety data sheet for the appropriate glove to wear when handling chemicals.

◆ Learn latex allergy prevention and know the symptoms of latex allergy — skin rashes; hives; flushing; itching; nasal, eye, or sinus symptoms; asthma; and shock.
◆ If you suspect you have a latex sensitivity, use nonlatex gloves, avoid contact with latex-containing products, and consult a practitioner experienced in treating latex allergy. Report problems to your supervisor and follow facility policy for evaluation.

For known latex allergy
If you're allergic to latex:
◆ Avoid contact with latex and other products that contain latex.
◆ Avoid areas where you might inhale powder from latex gloves worn by other workers.
◆ Inform your employer and your health care providers.
◆ Wear a medical alert bracelet.
◆ Follow your practitioner's instructions for dealing with latex reactions.
◆ Check packages, trays, and kits for items containing latex. (Products containing natural rubber latex must be labeled clearly on the exterior.)

ing of blood or body fluids (surgery, endoscopic procedures, dialysis, assisting with intubation or manipulation of arterial lines).

◆ Protective clothing, such as shoe covers, may be worn if there may be exposure to large amounts of blood or body fluids (trauma care).

◆ Handle used needles and other sharp instruments carefully. Don't bend, break, reinsert them into their original sheaths, remove needles from syringes, or handle them unnecessarily. Discard them intact immediately after use into a puncture-resistant disposal box.

◆ Use tools to pick up broken glass or other sharp objects.

◆ Use a needleless I.V. system if available.

◆ Immediately notify your employer of all needle-stick or other sharp object injuries, mucosal splashes, or contamination of open wounds or nonintact skin with blood or body fluids.

◆ Properly label all specimens collected from patients and place them in plastic bags at the collection site. Attach requisition slips to the outside of bags.

◆ Place all items that have come in direct contact with the patient's secretions, excretions, blood, drainage, or body fluids in a single impervious bag or container before removal from the room.

◆ Place linens and trash in single bags of sufficient thickness to contain the contents.

◆ While wearing appropriate personal protective equipment, promptly clean all blood and body fluid spills with detergent and water followed by an EPA-registered tuberculocidal disinfectant or diluted bleach solution (diluted 1:10 to 1:100, mixed daily), or both, or an EPA-registered disinfectant labeled effective against HBV and HIV provided that the surface hasn't been contaminated with agents or volumes of or concentrations of agents for which higher-level disinfection is recommended.

◆ Avoid all patient contact if you have an exudative lesion until the condition has resolved and you've been cleared by your employer's health provider.

◆ If you have broken skin on your hands, avoid situations where you may have contact with blood and body fluids (even though gloves could be worn) until the condition has resolved and you've been cleared by your employer's health provider.

SPECIAL CONSIDERATIONS

◆ Hand washing and appropriate use of personal protective equipment should be routine infection control practices.

◆ Keep mouthpieces, resuscitation bags, and other ventilation devices nearby to eliminate the need for emergency mouth-to-mouth resuscitation.

⚫ **WARNING** *You may not know what organisms are present in every clinical situation; use standard precautions for every contact with blood, body fluids, secretions, excretions, drainage, mucous membranes, and nonintact skin.*

◆ Use your judgment in individual cases about when to implement additional isolation precautions, such as airborne, droplet, or contact precautions.

◆ If your work requires you to be exposed to blood, you should receive the HBV vaccine series.

COMPLICATIONS

◆ Exposure to blood-borne diseases or other infections and to the complications they may cause by failing to follow standard precautions

PATIENT TEACHING

◆ Teach the patient about the use of standard precautions, as needed.

DOCUMENTATION

◆ Record special needs for isolation precautions.

◆ Record standard precaution measures taken per facility policy.

SELECTED REFERENCES

Blenkharn, J.I. "Lowering Standards of Clinical Waste Management: Do the Hazardous Waste Regulations Conflict with the CDC's Universal/Standard Precautions?" *Journal of Hospital Infection* 62(4):467-72, April 2006.

Chalmers, C., and Straub, M. "Standard Principles for Preventing and Controlling Infection," *Nursing Standard* 20(23):57-65, February 2006.

Rankin, A., and Kean, L. "Application of Standard Precautions in the Community Setting," *British Journal of Community Nursing* 10(11):503-504, November 2005.

Truong, J., et al. "Young Children's Perceptions of Physicians Wearing Standard Precautions versus Customary Attire," *Pediatric Emergency Care* 22(1):13-17, January 2006.

Stool collection

DESCRIPTION

◆ Stool is collected to determine the presence of blood, ova and parasites, bile, fat, pathogens, or such substances as ingested drugs.

◆ Gross examination of stool characteristics, such as color, consistency, and odor, can reveal such conditions as GI bleeding and steatorrhea.

◆ Stool specimens are collected randomly or for specific periods such as 72 hours.

◆ Because stool specimens can't be obtained on demand, proper collection requires careful instructions to the patient to ensure an uncontaminated specimen.

CONTRAINDICATIONS

◆ None known

EQUIPMENT

Specimen container with lid ◆ gloves ◆ two tongue blades ◆ paper towel ◆ bedpan or portable commode ◆ two patient-care reminders (for timed specimens) ◆ laboratory request form ◆ enema (optional)

KEY STEPS

◆ Confirm the patient's identity using two patient identifiers according to facility policy.

◆ Explain the procedure to the patient and his family, if possible, to ensure their cooperation and prevent inadvertent disposal of timed stool specimens.

COLLECTING A RANDOM SPECIMEN

◆ Tell the patient to notify you when he has the urge to defecate.

◆ Have him defecate into a clean, dry bedpan or commode.

◆ Instruct him not to contaminate the specimen with urine or toilet tissue because urine inhibits fecal bacterial growth and toilet tissue contains bismuth, which interferes with test results.

◆ Put on gloves.

◆ Using a tongue blade, transfer the most representative stool specimen from the bedpan to the container, and cap the container. If the patient passes blood, mucus, or pus with the stool, be sure to include this with the specimen.

◆ Wrap the tongue blade in a paper towel and discard it.

◆ Remove and discard your gloves, and wash your hands thoroughly to prevent cross-contamination.

COLLECTING A TIMED SPECIMEN

◆ Place a patient-care reminder stating SAVE ALL STOOL over the patient's bed, in his bathroom, and in the utility room.

◆ After putting on gloves, collect the first specimen, and include this in the total specimen.

◆ Obtain the timed specimen as you would a random specimen, but remember to transfer all stool to the specimen container.

◆ If stool must be obtained with an enema, use only tap water or normal saline solution.

- As ordered, send each specimen to the laboratory immediately with a laboratory request form or, if permitted, refrigerate the specimens collected during the test period and send them when collection is complete.
- Remove and discard your gloves.
- Make sure that the patient is comfortable after the procedure and that he has the opportunity to thoroughly clean his hands and perianal area. Perineal care may be necessary in some cases.

SPECIAL CONSIDERATIONS

- Never place a stool specimen in a refrigerator that contains food or medication to prevent contamination.
- Notify the practitioner if the stool specimen looks unusual.

COMPLICATIONS
- None known

PATIENT TEACHING

- For the patient collecting a specimen at home, instruct him to collect it in a clean container with a tight-fitting lid, to wrap the container in a brown paper bag, and to keep it in the refrigerator (separate from any food items) until it can be transported.

DOCUMENTATION

- Record the time of specimen collection and transport to the laboratory.
- Note stool color, odor, and consistency and any unusual characteristics; also note whether the patient had difficulty passing the stool.

SELECTED REFERENCES
Greenwald, B. "A Pilot Study Evaluating Two Alternate Methods of Stool Collection for the Fecal Occult Blood Test," *Medsurg Nursing* 15(2):89-84, April 2006.
Haug, U., and Brenner, H. "New Stool Tests for Colorectal Cancer Screening: A Systematic Review Focusing on Performance Characteristics and Practicalness," *International Journal of Cancer* 117(2):169-76, November 2005.
Mai, V., et al. "Timing in Collection of Stool Samples," *Science* 310(5751): 1118, November 2005.

Straining urine for calculi

DESCRIPTION

- Renal calculi, or kidney stones, may develop anywhere in the urinary tract.
- They may be excreted with urine or become lodged in the urinary tract, causing hematuria, urine retention, renal colic and, possibly, hydronephrosis.
- Ranging in size from microscopic to several centimeters, calculi form in the kidneys when mineral salts — principally calcium oxalate or calcium phosphate — collect around a nucleus of bacterial cells, blood clots, or other particles.
- Other substances involved in calculus formation include uric acid, xanthine, and ammonia.
- Renal calculi result from many causes, including hypercalcemia, which may occur with hyperparathyroidism, excessive dietary intake of calcium, prolonged immobility, abnormal urine pH levels, dehydration, hyperuricemia associated with gout, and some hereditary disorders.
- Most commonly, calculi form as a result of urine stasis stemming from dehydration (which concentrates urine), benign prostatic hyperplasia, neurologic disorders, or urethral strictures.
- Testing for the presence of calculi requires careful straining of all of the patient's urine through a gauze pad or fine-mesh sieve and, at times, quantitative laboratory analysis of questionable specimens.
- Such testing typically continues until the patient passes the calculi or until surgery, as ordered.

CONTRAINDICATIONS

- None known

Fine-mesh sieve or 4″ × 4″ gauze pad ◆ graduated container ◆ urinal or bedpan ◆ gloves ◆ laboratory request form ◆ three patient-care reminders ◆ specimen container (for use if calculi are found)

- Confirm the patient's identity using two patient identifiers according to facility policy.
- Explain the procedure to the patient and his family, if possible, to ensure cooperation and to stress the importance of straining all of the patient's urine.
- Post a patient-care reminder stating STRAIN ALL URINE over the patient's bed, in his bathroom, and on the collection container.
- Tell the patient to notify you after each voiding.
- If a commercial strainer isn't available, unfold a 4″ × 4″ gauze pad, place it over the top of a graduated measuring container, and secure it with a rubber band.
- Put on gloves.
- With the strainer secured over the mouth of the collection container, pour the specimen from the urinal or bedpan into the container.
- If the patient has an indwelling catheter in place, strain all urine from the collection bag before discarding it.
- Examine the strainer for calculi.
- If you detect calculi or if the filter looks questionable, notify the practitioner, place the filtrate in a specimen container, and send it to the laboratory with a laboratory request form.
- If the strainer is intact, rinse it carefully and reuse it. If it has become damaged, discard it and replace it with a new strainer.
- Remove and discard your gloves.

SPECIAL CONSIDERATIONS

◆ Save and send to the laboratory any small or suspicious-looking residue in the specimen container because even tiny calculi can cause hematuria and pain.
◆ Be aware that calculi may appear in various colors, each of which has diagnostic value.

COMPLICATIONS

◆ None known

PATIENT TEACHING

◆ For straining urine at home, teach the patient how to use a strainer and the importance of straining all urine for the prescribed period.

DOCUMENTATION

◆ Chart the time of the specimen collection and transport to the laboratory, if necessary.
◆ Describe any filtrate passed, and note pain or hematuria that occurred during voiding.

SELECTED REFERENCES

Colella, J., et al. "Urolithiasis/Nephrolithiasis: What's It All About?" *Urologic Nursing* 25(6):427-48, 475, 449, December 2005.

Krieg, C. "The Role of Diet in the Prevention of Common Kidney Stones," *Urologic Nursing* 25(6):451-57, December 2005.

Matlaga, B.R., et al. "Changing Composition of Renal Calculi in Patients with Neurogenic Bladder," *Journal of Urology* 175(5):1716-19, May 2006.

ST-segment monitoring

OVERVIEW

DESCRIPTION

◆ ST segments are normally flat or iso-electric and are a sensitive indicator of myocardial damage.
◆ A depressed ST segment may result from cardiac glycosides, myocardial ischemia, or a subendocardial infarction.
◆ An elevated ST segment suggests myocardial infarction.
◆ Monitoring is helpful for patients with acute coronary syndromes and for those who have received thrombolytic therapy or undergone coronary angioplasty.
◆ Monitoring allows early detection of reocclusion and is useful for patients who have had previous episodes of cardiac ischemia without chest pain, have difficulty distinguishing cardiac pain from pain associated with other sources, or have difficulty communicating.
◆ Monitoring allows early identification and intervention to reverse ischemia.

CONTRAINDICATIONS

◆ None known

EQUIPMENT

Electrocardiogram (ECG) electrodes ◆ gauze pads ◆ ECG monitor cable ◆ leadwires ◆ alcohol pads ◆ cardiac monitor programmed for ST-segment monitoring ◆ gloves ◆ indelible ink marker

PREPARATION

◆ Plug the cardiac monitor into an electrical outlet.

KEY STEPS

◆ Confirm the patient's identity using two patient identifiers according to facility policy.
◆ Bring the equipment to the patient's bedside and explain the procedure.
◆ Provide privacy.
◆ Wash your hands and follow standard precautions.
◆ If the patient isn't already on a monitor, turn on the device and attach the cable.
◆ Select the sites for electrode placement and prepare the patient's skin for attachment of electrodes.
◆ Attach the leadwires to electrodes and position them on the patient's skin.
◆ Activate ST-segment monitoring by pressing the MONITORING PROCEDURES key and then the ST key.
◆ Activate individual ST-segment parameters by pressing the ON/OFF parameter key.
◆ Select the appropriate ECG for each ST-segment channel to be monitored by pressing the PARAMETERS key and then the key labeled ECG.
◆ Press the key labeled CHANGE LEAD to select the appropriate lead (usually lead II). Repeat this for all three channels.

Understanding ST-segment changes

Closely monitoring the ST segment can help detect ischemia or injury before infarction develops.

ST-SEGMENT ELEVATION

An ST segment is considered elevated when it's 1 mm or more above the baseline. An elevated ST segment may indicate myocardial injury.

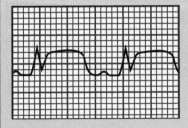

ST-SEGMENT DEPRESSION

An ST segment is considered depressed when it's 0.5 mm or more below the baseline. A depressed ST segment may indicate myocardial ischemia or digoxin toxicity.

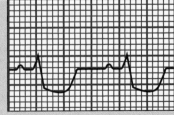

- Adjust the ST-segment measurement points.
- Adjust the baseline for the ST segment by pressing the ISO POINT to move the cursor to the PQ or TP interval.
- Adjust the J point by pressing the key labeled J POINT to move the cursor to the appropriate location.
- Adjust the ST point to 80 msec after the J point.
- Check facility policy for measuring the ST point. Some facilities recommend using 60 msec instead of 80 msec.
- Set the alarm limits for each ST-segment parameter by manipulating the HIGH LIMIT and LOW LIMIT keys.
- Set the ST alarm parameter 1 to 2 mm above and below the patient's baseline ST-segment level, or as ordered by the practitioner, and measure ST-segment changes 60 msec beyond the J point of the ECG.
- Press the key labeled STANDARD DISPLAY to return to the display screen.
- Assess the waveform shown on the monitor.

SPECIAL CONSIDERATIONS

- Abrade the patient's skin gently to ensure electrode adhesion and promote electrical conductivity.
- Because ischemia typically occurs in only one portion of the heart muscle, not all ECG leads detect it.
- Select the most appropriate lead by examining ECG tracings obtained during an ischemic episode.
- The leads showing ischemia are the same leads to use for ST-segment monitoring.
- If monitoring only one lead, choose the lead most likely to show arrhythmias and ST-segment changes.
- Mark the electrode placement with an indelible ink marker.

WARNING *Always give precedence to the lead that shows arrhythmias.*

- When a limit is surpassed for more than 1 minute, visual and audible alarms are commonly activated.
- If the patient isn't being monitored continuously, remove the electrodes, clean the skin, and disconnect the leadwires from the electrodes.
- Evaluate the monitor for ST-segment depression or elevation. (See *Understanding ST-segment changes*.)

COMPLICATIONS
- None known

PATIENT TEACHING

- Explain the monitoring procedure and answer the patient's questions, as necessary.

DOCUMENTATION

- Record the leads being monitored.
- Note ST-segment measurement points.

SELECTED REFERENCES
Chantad, D., et al. "Derived 12-Lead Electrocardiogram in the Assessment of ST-Segment Deviation and Cardiac Rhythm," *Journal of Electrocardiology* 39(1):7-12, January 2006.

Flanders, S.A. "Continuous ST-Segment Monitoring: Raising the Bar," *Critical Care Nursing Clinics of North America* 18(2):169-77, June 2006.

Housholder-Hughes, S.D. "Non-ST-Segment Elevation Acute Coronary Syndromes: Management Strategies for Optimal Outcomes," *Critical Care Nurse* 26(Suppl):8-10, 12, 14 passim, February 2006.

MacLeod, R.S., et al. "Mechanisms of Ischemia-Induced ST-Segment Changes," *Journal of Electrocardiology* 38(4 Suppl):8-13, October 2005.

Stump and prosthesis care

DESCRIPTION

◆ Patient care immediately after limb amputation includes monitoring drainage from the stump, positioning the affected limb, assisting with exercises prescribed by a physical therapist, and wrapping and conditioning the stump.

◆ Postoperative care will vary slightly, depending on the amputation site and whether an elastic bandage or plaster cast is used.

◆ After the stump heals it requires only routine daily care (proper hygiene and continued muscle-strengthening exercises).

◆ A prosthesis must be cleaned and lubricated daily and checked for proper fit.

CONTRAINDICATIONS

◆ None known

POSTOPERATIVE STUMP CARE

Pressure dressing, abdominal (ABD) pad ◆ suction equipment, if ordered ◆ overhead trapeze ◆ 1" adhesive tape ◆ bandage clips or safety pins ◆ sandbags or trochanter roll (for a leg) ◆ elastic stump shrinker or 4" elastic bandage ◆ tourniquet (optional, as last resort to control bleeding)

DAILY STUMP AND PROSTHESIS CARE

Mild soap or alcohol pads ◆ stump socks or athletic tube socks ◆ two washcloths ◆ two towels ◆ appropriate lubricating oil

◆ Confirm the patient's identity using two patient identifiers according to facility policy.

◆ Perform routine postoperative care.

◆ Provide for the patient's comfort, pain management, and safety.

MONITORING STUMP DRAINAGE

◆ Gravity causes fluid to accumulate at the stump. Frequently check the amount of blood and drainage on the dressing.

◆ Notify the practitioner if accumulations of drainage or blood increase rapidly or excessive bleeding occurs.

◆ Apply a pressure dressing or compress to the appropriate pressure points.

◆ Keep a tourniquet available and use it as a last resort.

◆ Tape the ABD pad over the moist part of the dressing to provide a dry area to help prevent bacterial infection.

◆ Monitor the suction drainage equipment and note the amount and type of drainage.

POSITIONING THE EXTREMITY

◆ Elevate the extremity for the first 24 hours.

◆ To prevent contractures, position an arm with the elbow extended and the shoulder abducted.

◆ To correctly position a leg, elevate the foot of the bed slightly and place sandbags or a trochanter roll against the hip to prevent external rotation.

● **WARNING** *Don't place a pillow under the thigh to flex the hip because this can cause hip flexion contracture. For the same reason, tell the patient to avoid prolonged sitting.*

◆ After a below-the-knee amputation, maintain knee extension to prevent hamstring muscle contractures.

◆ After a leg amputation, place the patient on a firm surface in the prone position for at least 2 hours per day, with his legs close together and without pillows under his stomach, hips, knees, or stump, unless this position is contraindicated.

ASSISTING WITH PRESCRIBED EXERCISES

◆ After arm amputation, encourage the patient to exercise the remaining arm to prevent muscle contractures.
◆ Help the patient perform isometric and range-of-motion (ROM) exercises for both shoulders.
◆ After leg amputation, stand behind the patient and, if necessary, support him with your hands at his waist during balancing exercises.
◆ Instruct the patient to exercise the affected and unaffected limbs to maintain muscle tone and increase muscle strength.
◆ The patient with a leg amputation may perform push-ups in the sitting position, arms at his sides, or pull-ups on the overhead trapeze to strengthen his arms, shoulders, and back, in preparation for using crutches.

WRAPPING AND CONDITIONING THE STUMP

◆ If the patient doesn't have a rigid cast, apply an elastic stump shrinker to prevent edema and shape the limb in preparation for the prosthesis.
◆ Wrap the stump so it narrows toward the distal end. (See *Wrapping a stump.*) This promotes comfort when the patient wears the prosthesis.
◆ If an elastic stump shrinker isn't available, you can wrap the stump in a 4″ elastic bandage. Stretch the bandage to about two-thirds its maximum length as you wrap it diagonally around the stump, with the greatest pressure distally.
◆ Make sure that the bandage covers all portions of the stump smoothly because wrinkles or exposed areas encourage skin breakdown.
◆ If the patient experiences throbbing after the stump is wrapped, the bandage may be too tight. Remove the bandage immediately, reapply it less tightly, and check it regularly.
◆ Rewrap the bandage when it begins to bunch up at the end (typically about every 12 hours for a moderately active patient).
◆ After removing the bandage to rewrap it, massage the stump gently,

always pushing toward the suture line rather than away from it.
◆ When healing begins, instruct the patient to push the stump against a pillow.
◆ Have him progress gradually to pushing against harder surfaces.

CARING FOR THE HEALED STUMP

◆ Bathe the stump at the end of the day because the warm water may cause swelling, making reapplication of the prosthesis difficult. Don't soak the stump for long periods.
◆ Don't apply lotion to the stump. This may clog follicles, increasing the risk of infection.
◆ Rub the stump with alcohol daily to toughen the skin and reduce the risk of skin breakdown.
◆ Instruct the patient to watch for and report severe irritation after rubbing the stump with alcohol.
◆ Avoid using powders or lotions, which can soften or irritate the skin.
◆ Inspect the stump for redness, swelling, irritation, and calluses. Report these to the practitioner.
◆ Change and wash the patient's elastic bandages every day to avoid exposing the skin to excessive perspiration.
◆ To shape the stump, have the patient wear an elastic bandage 24 hours per day except while bathing.
◆ To prevent infection, never shave the stump.
◆ Tell the patient to avoid putting weight on the stump, but continue muscle-strengthening exercises.

CARING FOR THE PLASTIC PROSTHESIS

◆ Wipe the plastic socket of the prosthesis with a damp cloth and mild soap or alcohol to prevent bacterial accumulation.
◆ Wipe the insert (if the prosthesis has one) with a dry cloth and dry the prosthesis thoroughly. When possible, allow it to dry overnight.
◆ Maintain and lubricate the prosthesis and check for malfunctions.
◆ Frequently check the condition of a shoe on a foot prosthesis and change it as necessary.

Wrapping a stump

Proper stump care helps protect the limb, reduces swelling, and prepares the limb for a prosthesis. As you perform the procedure, teach it to the patient.

Start by obtaining two 4″ elastic bandages. Center the end of the first 4″ bandage at the top of the patient's thigh. Unroll the bandage downward over the stump and to the back of the leg (as shown below).

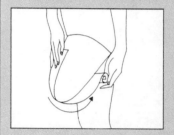

Make three figure-eight turns to adequately cover the ends of the stump. As you wrap, be sure to include the roll of flesh in the groin area. Use enough pressure to ensure that the stump narrows toward the end so that it fits comfortably into the prosthesis.

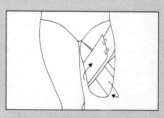

Use the second 4″ bandage to anchor the first bandage around the waist. For a below-the-knee amputation, use the knee to anchor the bandage in place. Secure the bandage with clips, safety pins, or adhesive tape. Check the stump bandage regularly, and rewrap it if it bunches at the end.

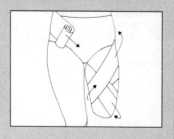

(continued)

APPLYING THE PROSTHESIS

◆ Apply a stump sock, keeping the seams away from bony prominences.
◆ If the prosthesis has an insert, remove it from the socket, place it over the stump, and insert the stump into the prosthesis.
◆ If it has no insert, slide the prosthesis over the stump.
◆ Secure the prosthesis onto the stump according to the manufacturer's directions.

◆ If the patient arrives at the hospital with a traumatic amputation, the amputated part may be saved for possible reimplantation. (See *Caring for an amputated body part.*)
◆ Exercise of the remaining muscles in an amputated limb must begin the day after surgery.
◆ Arm exercises progress from isometrics to assisted ROM to active ROM.
◆ Leg exercises include rising from a chair, balancing on one leg, and ROM exercises of the knees and hips.
◆ For a below-the-knee amputation, you may substitute an athletic tube sock for a stump sock by cutting off the elastic band.
◆ If the patient has a rigid dressing, perform normal cast care.
◆ If the cast slips off, apply an elastic bandage immediately and notify the practitioner because edema will develop rapidly.

COMPLICATIONS

◆ Hemorrhage
◆ Stump infection
◆ Contractures
◆ Swollen or flabby stump
◆ Skin breakdown or irritation
◆ Friction from an irritant in the prosthesis
◆ Sebaceous cyst or boil
◆ Psychological problems
◆ Phantom limb pain

Caring for an amputated body part

After traumatic amputation, a surgeon may be able to reimplant the severed body part through microsurgery. The chance of successful reimplantation is much greater if the amputated part has received proper care (amputated parts should be placed in a clean plastic bag).

If the patient arrives at the hospital with a severed body part, first make sure that bleeding at the amputation site has been controlled. Then follow these guidelines for preserving the body part.

◆ Put on sterile gloves. Place several sterile gauze pads and an appropriate amount of sterile roller gauze in a sterile basin, and pour sterile normal saline or sterile lactated Ringer's solution over them. *Never* use another solution and don't try to scrub or debride the part.
◆ Holding the body part in one gloved hand, carefully pat it dry with sterile gauze. Place saline-soaked gauze pads over the stump, and then wrap the whole body part with saline-soaked roller gauze. Wrap the gauze with a sterile towel, if available. Then, put this package in a watertight container or bag and seal it.
◆ Fill another plastic bag with ice and water and place the part, still in its wa-

tertight container, inside. Seal the outer bag (always protect the part from direct contact with ice — and *never* use dry ice — to prevent irreversible tissue damage, which would make the part unsuitable for reimplantation). Keep this bag ice-cold until reimplantation surgery.
◆ Label the bag with the patient's name, identification number, identification of the amputated part, the hospital identification number, and the date and time when cooling began.
◆ The body part must be wrapped and cooled quickly. Irreversible tissue damage occurs after only 6 hours at ambient temperature. However, hypothermic management seldom preserves tissues for more than 24 hours.

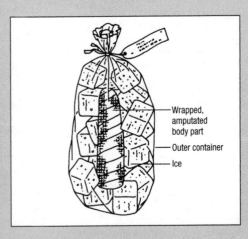

Wrapped, amputated body part

Outer container

Ice

- Teach the patient how to care for the stump and prosthesis. Encourage proper daily stump care.
- Emphasize that proper care of the stump can speed healing.
- Tell the patient to inspect the stump every day, using a mirror.
- Make sure that the patient knows the signs and symptoms that indicate problems in the stump.
- Instruct the patient to call the practitioner if the incision appears to be opening, looks red or swollen, feels warm, is painful to touch, or is seeping drainage.
- Explain to the patient that a 10-lb (4.5-kg) change in body weight will alter stump size and require a new prosthesis socket.
- Tell the patient to massage the stump toward the suture line to mobilize the scar and prevent its adherence to bone.
- Advise the patient to avoid exposing the skin around the stump to excessive perspiration, which can cause irritation.
- Tell the patient to change the elastic bandages or stump socks daily.
- Tell the patient that twitching, spasms, or phantom limb sensations, such as pain, warmth, cold, or itching, may occur as his stump muscles adjust to amputation.
- Discuss measures, such as imagery, biofeedback, or distraction, to relieve phantom limb pain or other sensations.
- Advise the patient to use heat, massage, or gentle pressure for these symptoms.
- If the stump is sensitive to touch, tell the patient to rub it with a dry washcloth for 4 minutes, three times per day.

- Stress the importance of performing prescribed exercises to help minimize complications, maintain muscle strength and tone, prevent contractures, and promote independence.
- Stress the importance of positioning to prevent contractures and edema.

- Record the date, time, and specific procedures of postoperative care.
- Note the amount and type of drainage and the condition of the dressing.
- Document the need for dressing reinforcement.
- Record the appearance and condition of the suture line and surrounding tissue.
- Note pain assessment.
- Record signs of skin irritation or infection, such as redness or tenderness.
- Record complications and the nursing actions taken.
- Note the patient's tolerance of exercises, progress in caring for the stump or prosthesis, and psychological reaction to the amputation.

SELECTED REFERENCES

Back-Pettersson, S., and Bjorkelund, C. "Care of Elderly Lower Limb Amputees, as Described in Medical and Nursing Records," *Scandinavian Journal of Caring Sciences* 19(4):337-43, December 2005.

Gleaves, J.R., and Eldridge, K. "Silicone Sheeting as an Alternative to Elastic Bandages in Dressing Lower Extremity Amputations," *Ostomy/Wound Management* 50(9):8, 10, September 2004.

Hayes, D. "How to Wrap an Above-the-Knee Amputation Stump," *Nursing* 33(1):70, January 2003.

Laskowski-Jones, L. "First Aid for Amputation," *Nursing* 36(4):50-52, April 2006.

Subcutaneous injection

OVERVIEW

DESCRIPTION

◆ When injected into the adipose (fatty) tissue beneath the skin, a drug moves into the bloodstream more rapidly than if given by mouth.
◆ A subcutaneous (subQ) injection allows slower, more sustained drug administration than an I.M. injection.
◆ SubQ injection causes minimal tissue trauma and carries little risk of striking large blood vessels and nerves.
◆ Drugs recommended for subQ injection, absorbed mainly through capillaries, include nonirritating aqueous solutions and suspensions contained in 0.5 to 2 ml of fluid.
◆ Heparin and insulin are usually administered subcutaneously.
◆ Drugs and solutions for subQ injection are injected through a relatively short needle, using meticulous sterile technique. (See *Locating subcutaneous injection sites*.)

CONTRAINDICATIONS

◆ Sites that are inflamed, edematous, scarred, or covered by a mole, birthmark, or other lesion
◆ Impaired coagulation mechanisms

EQUIPMENT

Prescribed drug ◆ patient's drug record and chart ◆ 25G to 27G ⅝" to ½" needle ◆ gloves ◆ 1- to 3-ml syringe ◆ alcohol pads ◆ filter needle ◆ insulin syringe ◆ insulin pump ◆ antiseptic cleaning agent (optional)

PREPARATION

◆ Verify the order on the patient's drug record.
◆ Note whether the patient has allergies, especially before the first dose.
◆ Inspect the drug to make sure that it isn't abnormally discolored or cloudy and doesn't contain precipitates.
◆ Wash your hands.
◆ Choose equipment appropriate to the prescribed drug and injection site, and make sure that it works properly.
◆ Check the drug label against the patient's drug record.
◆ Read the label again as you draw up the drug for injection.

SINGLE-DOSE AMPULES

◆ Wrap an alcohol pad around the ampule's neck and snap off the top, directing the force away from your body.
◆ Attach a filter needle to the needle and withdraw the drug.
◆ Keep the needle's bevel tip below the level of the solution.
◆ Tap the syringe to clear air.
◆ Cover the needle with the needle sheath.
◆ Before discarding the ampule, check the drug label against the patient's drug record.
◆ Discard the filter needle and the ampule.
◆ Attach the appropriate needle to the syringe.

SINGLE-DOSE OR MULTIDOSE VIALS

◆ Reconstitute powdered drugs according to instructions.
◆ Make sure that all crystals have dissolved in the solution.
◆ Warm the vial by rolling it between your palms to help the drug dissolve faster.
◆ Clean the vial's rubber stopper with an alcohol pad.
◆ Pull the syringe plunger back until the volume of air in the syringe equals the volume of drug to be withdrawn from the vial.
◆ Without inverting the vial, insert the needle into the vial.
◆ Inject the air, invert the vial, and keep the needle's bevel tip below the level of the solution as you withdraw the prescribed amount of drug.
◆ Cover the needle with the needle sheath.
◆ Tap the syringe to clear air.
◆ Check the drug label against the patient's drug record before discarding the single-dose vial or returning the multidose vial to the shelf.

KEY STEPS

◆ Confirm the patient's identity using two patient identifiers according to facility policy and explain the procedure.
◆ Provide privacy.
◆ Select an appropriate injection site.
◆ Rotate sites according to a schedule for repeated injections.
◆ Put on gloves.
◆ Position the patient and expose the injection site.
◆ Clean the injection site with an alcohol pad, beginning at the center of the site and moving outward in a circular motion.
◆ Allow the skin to dry before injecting the drug to avoid a stinging sensation caused by introducing alcohol into subcutaneous tissues.
◆ Loosen the protective needle sheath.
◆ With your nondominant hand, grasp the skin around the injection site firmly to elevate the subcutaneous tissue and form a 1" (2.5-cm) fat fold.
◆ Holding the syringe in your dominant hand, insert the loosened needle sheath between the fourth and fifth fingers of your other hand while still pinching the skin around the injection site.
◆ Pull back the syringe with your dominant hand to uncover the needle by grasping the syringe like a pencil.
◆ Don't touch the needle.
◆ Position the needle with its bevel up.
◆ Tell the patient that he'll feel a needle prick.
◆ Release the patient's skin to avoid injecting the drug into compressed tissue and irritating nerve fibers.
◆ Pull back the plunger slightly to check for blood return.
◆ Don't aspirate for blood return when giving insulin or heparin. It isn't necessary with insulin and may cause a hematoma with heparin.
◆ If none appears, begin injecting the drug slowly.
◆ If blood appears upon aspiration, withdraw the needle, prepare another syringe, and repeat the procedure.

- After injection, remove the needle gently but quickly at the same angle used for insertion.
- Cover the site with an alcohol pad and massage (unless contraindicated, as with heparin or insulin) to distribute the drug and facilitate absorption.
- Remove the alcohol pad.
- Check the injection site for bleeding and bruising.
- Dispose of injection equipment according to facility policy.
- To avoid needle-stick injuries, don't resheath the needle.

SPECIAL CONSIDERATIONS

- When using prefilled syringes, adjust the angle and depth of insertion according to needle length.

INSULIN INJECTIONS
- To establish consistent blood insulin levels, rotate insulin injection sites within anatomic regions.
- Preferred insulin injection sites are the arms, abdomen, thighs, and buttocks.
- Make sure that the type of insulin, unit dosage, and syringe are correct.
- When combining insulins in a syringe, make sure that they're compatible.

- Regular insulin can be mixed with all other types.
- Prompt insulin zinc suspension (Semilente insulin) can't be mixed with NPH insulin.
- Follow facility policy regarding which insulin to draw up first.
- Before drawing up insulin suspension, gently roll and invert the bottle.
- Don't shake the bottle because this can cause foam or bubbles to develop in the syringe.
- Before administering insulin, make sure that the patient doesn't already have an insulin pump in place.

HEPARIN INJECTIONS
- The preferred site for a heparin injection is the lower abdominal fat pad, 2″ (5 cm) beneath the umbilicus, between the right and left iliac crests.
- Using this area reduces the risk of local capillary bleeding.
- Always rotate the sites from one side to the other.
- Inject the drug slowly into the fat pad.
- Leave the needle in place for 10 seconds after injection, and then withdraw it.
- Don't administer injections within 2″ of a scar, a bruise, or the umbilicus.
- Don't aspirate to check for blood return because this can cause bleeding into the tissues at the site.

- Don't rub or massage the site after the injection because this can cause localized minute hemorrhages or bruises.
- If the patient bruises easily, apply ice to the site for the first 5 minutes after the injection to minimize local hemorrhage, and then apply pressure.

COMPLICATIONS
- Concentrated or irritating solutions causing sterile abscesses
- Repeated injections in the same site causing lipodystrophy

PATIENT TEACHING

- Explain the procedure to the patient to lessen his anxiety.
- If the patient will be giving himself subQ injections at home, teach him the proper method.

DOCUMENTATION

- Record the time and date of the injection.
- Note the drug and dose administered.
- Document the injection site and route.
- Record the patient's response to the treatment.

SELECTED REFERENCES

Meece, J. "Dispelling Myths and Removing Barriers about Insulin in Type 2 Diabetes," *Diabetes Education* 32(1 Suppl):9S-18S, January-February 2006.

Mikhail, N.E. "Is Exenatide a Useful Edition to Diabetes Therapy?" *Endocrine Practice* 12(3):307-14, May-June 2006.

Prettyman, J. "Subcutaneous or Intramuscular? Confronting a Parenteral Administration Dilemma," *Medsurg Nursing* 14(2):93-99, April 2005.

Rushing, J. "How to Administer a Subcutaneous Injection," *Nursing* 34(6):32, June 2004.

Locating subcutaneous injection sites

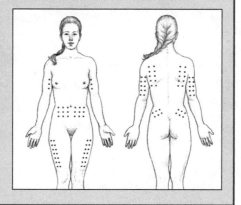

Subcutaneous (subQ) injection sites (indicated by dotted areas) include the fat pads on the abdomen, upper hips, upper back, and lateral upper arms and thighs. For subQ injections administered repeatedly, such as insulin, rotate sites.

When returning to an area, choose a new site in that area. Preferred injection sites for insulin are the arms, abdomen, thighs, and buttocks. The preferred injection site for heparin is the lower abdominal fat pad, just below the umbilicus.

Surgical site verification

DESCRIPTION

- Wrong site surgery is a general term that refers to a surgical procedure performed on the wrong patient, wrong body part, or wrong side of the body.
- A procedure may be performed on the wrong site in the operating room or in settings outside of the operating room, such as in ambulatory care or interventional radiology.
- Several factors may increase the risk of a procedure being performed on the wrong site, including inadequate patient assessment, inadequate medical record review, inaccurate communication among health team members, multiple surgeons involved in the procedure, failure to include the patient in the site identification process, and relying solely on the practitioner for site identification.
- Because serious consequences may result from a surgery performed on the wrong site, the nurse must confirm that the correct site has been identified before surgery begins.

CONTRAINDICATIONS

- None known

Surgical consent ◆ medical record ◆ procedure schedule ◆ hypoallergenic, nonlatex permanent marker

- Confirm the patient's identity using two patient identifiers according to facility policy.
- Before the procedure, check the chart for documentation and compare the information using the history and physical examination form, nursing assessment, preprocedure checklist, signed informed consent with the exact procedure site identified, procedure schedule, and the patient's verbal confirmation of the correct site.
- After verbally confirming the site with the patient, the person performing the procedure or another member of the surgical team who's fully informed about the patient and the intended procedure, marks the site. The mark needs to be placed so that it's visible after the patient is prepped and draped.
- Make sure that the surgical team (that is, the surgeon, operating room or procedure staff, and anesthesia personnel) takes a "time-out" before the surgery begins to identify the patient and verify the correct procedure and correct site.

SPECIAL CONSIDERATIONS

◆ If the patient's condition prevents him from verifying the correct site, the surgeon will identify and mark the site using the medical history and physical examination forms, signed surgical consent form, preprocedure verification checklist, surgical procedure schedule, X-rays, and other diagnostic imaging studies.

COMPLICATIONS
◆ None known

PATIENT TEACHING

◆ Explain to the patient the need for verifying the surgical site.

DOCUMENTATION

◆ Complete the preprocedure checklist used by your facility.
◆ Verify that the patient's or family member's verbalization of the procedure and correct site coincides with the informed consent and the practitioner's order sheet.
◆ Document that you confirmed the patient's identity using two patient identifiers according to facility policy.
◆ Verify that the procedure schedule coincides with the practitioner's order sheet.
◆ Document the ordered diagnostic tests and test results, noting any abnormal values.

SELECTED REFERENCES
Hainsworth, T. "The NPSA Recommendations to Promote Correct-Site Surgery," *Nursing Times* 101(12):28-29, March 2005.
Kwaan, M.R., et al. "Incidence, Patterns, and Prevention of Wrong-Site Surgery," *Archives of Surgery* 141(4):353-57, April 2006.
Rusynko, B., and Perry-Ewald, J. "Keeping Patients Safe — Procedure and Site Verification and Preprocedure Pause," *AORN Journal* 79(4):787-93, 796, April 2004.

Suture removal

DESCRIPTION

- The goal is to remove skin sutures from a healed wound without damaging newly formed tissue.
- Timing depends on the shape, size, and location of the sutured incision; the absence of inflammation, drainage, and infection; and the patient's general condition.
- If sufficiently healed, sutures are removed 7 to 10 days after insertion.
- Techniques for removal depend on the method of suturing.
- Sterile procedures are required.
- Sutures are usually removed by the physician. Nurses may remove sutures based on facility policy and the practitioner's orders.

CONTRAINDICATIONS

- Insufficient wound healing

Waterproof trash bag ◆ adjustable light ◆ clean gloves, if the wound is dressed ◆ sterile forceps or sterile hemostat ◆ normal saline solution ◆ sterile gauze pads ◆ antiseptic cleaning agent ◆ sterile curve-tipped suture scissors ◆ povidone-iodine pads ◆ adhesive butterfly strips or adhesive strips, compound benzoin tincture or other skin protectant (optional)

Prepackaged, sterile suture-removal trays are available.

PREPARATION

- Assemble equipment in the patient's room.
- Check the expiration date on each sterile package and inspect for tears.
- Open the waterproof trash bag, and place it near the patient's bed to avoid reaching across the sterile field or suture line when disposing of soiled articles.
- Turn down the top of the trash bag to provide a wide opening and prevent contamination of instruments or gloves by touching the bag's edge.

- Check the practitioner's order to confirm details of the procedure.
- Check patient allergies, especially to adhesive tape, povidone-iodine, or other topical solutions or drugs.
- Confirm the patient's identity using two patient identifiers according to facility policy.
- Explain the procedure to the patient.
- Assure him that the procedure is usually painless, but he may feel a tickling sensation; reassure him that removing sutures won't weaken the incision.
- Provide privacy.
- Position the patient so he's comfortable without placing undue tension on the suture line.
- To avoid nausea or dizziness, have the patient recline.
- Adjust the light so it shines directly on the suture line.
- Wash your hands.
- Put on clean gloves to remove the dressing, if present.
- Discard the dressing and gloves in the waterproof trash bag.
- Observe the wound for gaping, drainage, inflammation, signs of infection, or embedded sutures.
- Notify the practitioner if the wound has failed to heal properly.
- Absence of a healing ridge under the suture line 5 to 7 days after the incision indicates that continued support and protection are needed.
- Establish a sterile work area with needed equipment and supplies.
- Put on sterile gloves.
- Open the sterile suture removal tray if you're using one.
- Using sterile technique, clean the suture line, which moistens the sutures to ease removal.
- Soften them further, if needed, with normal saline solution.
- Proceed according to the type of suture you're removing.
- The visible part of a suture is contaminated; cut sutures at the skin surface on one side.
- Lift and pull the visible end off the skin.

- If ordered, remove every other suture to maintain support for the incision, and then go back and remove remaining sutures.
- After suture removal, wipe the incision with gauze pads soaked in an antiseptic cleaning agent or with a povidone-iodine pad.
- Apply a light sterile gauze dressing, if needed.
- Discard your gloves.
- Make sure that the patient is comfortable.
- According to the practitioner's preference, inform the patient that he may shower in 1 or 2 days if the incision is dry and heals well.
- Properly dispose of the solutions and trash bag; clean or dispose of soiled equipment and supplies.

SPECIAL CONSIDERATIONS

- Check the practitioner's order for the time of suture removal.
- A typical guideline follows for suture removal:
  – head and neck — 3 to 5 days after insertion
  – chest and abdomen — 5 to 7 days after insertion
  – lower extremities — 7 to 10 days after insertion.
- For interrupted sutures or an incompletely healed suture line, remove only those sutures specified by the practitioner.
- Some sutures may be left in place for 1 to 2 days to support the suture line.
- If retention and regular sutures are in place, check the practitioner's order for the removal sequence.
- Retention sutures usually remain in place for 14 to 21 days.
- Retention sutures give added support to obese or slow-healing patients.
- Carefully clean the suture line before removing mattress sutures to decrease the risk of infection when the visible, contaminated part of the stitch is too small to cut twice for sterile removal and must be pulled through the tissue.
- After removing mattress sutures, monitor the suture line for subsequent infection.
- If the wound dehisces during suture removal, apply butterfly adhesive strips or adhesive strips to support and approximate the edges.
- Call the practitioner immediately to repair the wound.
- Apply butterfly adhesive strips or adhesive strips after suture removal for added support of the incision line and prevention of wide scar formation.
- Use compound benzoin tincture or other skin protectant to ensure adherence.
- Leave strips in place for 3 to 5 days.

COMPLICATIONS
- Dehiscence
- Infection

PATIENT TEACHING

- Before discharge, teach the patient how to remove the dressing and care for the wound.
- Instruct the patient to call the practitioner immediately if wound discharge or other abnormal change occurs.
- Tell the patient that the redness surrounding the incision should gradually disappear with only a thin line remaining after a few weeks.

DOCUMENTATION

- Record the date and time of suture removal.
- Note the type and number of sutures and the appearance of the suture line.
- Record signs of wound complications.
- Note dressings or butterfly strips applied.
- Document the patient's tolerance of the procedure.

SELECTED REFERENCES

Adams, B., et al. "Frequency of Use of Suturing and Repair Techniques Preferred by Dermatologic Surgeons," *Dermatologic Surgery* 32(5):682-89, May 2006.

Clark, A. "Understanding the Principles of Suturing Minor Skin Lesions," *Nursing Times* 100(29):32-34, July 2004.

Pullen, R.L. Jr. "Removing Sutures and Staples," *Nursing* 33(10):18, October 2003.

Swab specimens

OVERVIEW

DESCRIPTION

◆ Specimens are collected to identify pathogens or asymptomatic carriers of certain easily transmitted disease organisms.
◆ Pathogen identification with minimal contamination depends on correct collection and handling.
◆ Collection involves sampling inflamed tissues and exudates.
◆ Typical sources include the throat, nasopharynx, wounds, eye, ear, or rectum.
◆ Sterile swabs of cotton or other absorbent material are used.
◆ Swab type depends on the part of the body that's affected.
◆ After obtaining a specimen, the swab is immediately placed in a sterile tube.
◆ The sterile tubes contain either a transport medium or inert gas.

CONTRAINDICATIONS

◆ None known

EQUIPMENT

THROAT SPECIMEN

Gloves ◆ tongue blade ◆ penlight ◆ sterile, cotton-tipped swab ◆ sterile culture tube with transport medium (or commercial collection kit) ◆ label ◆ laboratory request form

NASOPHARYNGEAL SPECIMEN

Gloves ◆ penlight ◆ sterile, flexible, cotton-tipped swab ◆ tongue blade ◆ sterile culture tube with transport medium ◆ label ◆ laboratory request form ◆ small open-ended Pyrex tube or nasal speculum (optional)

WOUND SPECIMEN

Sterile gloves ◆ sterile forceps ◆ alcohol or povidone-iodine pads ◆ sterile swabs ◆ sterile culture tube with transport medium (or commercial collection kit for aerobic culture) ◆ labels ◆ special anaerobic culture tube containing carbon dioxide or nitrogen ◆ fresh dressings for the wound ◆ laboratory request form

EAR SPECIMEN

Gloves ◆ normal saline solution ◆ two 2″ × 2″ gauze pads ◆ sterile swabs ◆ sterile culture tube with transport medium ◆ label ◆ 10-ml syringe and 22G 1″ needle (for tympanocentesis) ◆ laboratory request form

EYE SPECIMEN

Sterile gloves ◆ sterile normal saline solution ◆ two 2″ × 2″ gauze pads ◆ sterile swabs ◆ sterile wire culture loop (for corneal scraping) ◆ sterile culture tube with transport medium ◆ label ◆ laboratory request form

RECTAL SPECIMEN

Gloves ◆ soap and water ◆ washcloth ◆ sterile swab ◆ normal saline solution ◆ sterile culture tube with transport medium ◆ label ◆ laboratory request form

KEY STEPS

COLLECTING A THROAT SPECIMEN

◆ Confirm the patient's identity using two patient identifiers according to facility policy.
◆ Tell the patient that he may gag during the swabbing, but that the procedure probably takes less than 1 minute.
◆ Instruct him to sit erect at the edge of the bed or in a chair, facing you.
◆ Wash your hands and put on gloves.
◆ Ask the patient to tilt his head back.
◆ Depress his tongue with the tongue blade.
◆ Illuminate his throat with the penlight to check for inflamed areas.
◆ If he starts to gag, withdraw the tongue blade and tell him to breathe deeply.
◆ When he's relaxed, reinsert the tongue blade but not as deeply as before.
◆ Using the cotton-tipped wire swab, wipe the tonsillar areas from side to side, including inflamed or purulent sites.
◆ Don't touch the tongue, cheeks, or teeth with the swab.
◆ Withdraw the swab and immediately place it in the culture tube.
◆ When using a commercial kit, crush a culture medium ampule at the bottom of the tube. Push the swab into the medium to keep it moist.
◆ Remove and discard your gloves and wash your hands.
◆ Label the specimen with the patient's name and room number, the practitioner's name, and the date, time, and site of collection.
◆ Indicate on the laboratory request form whether a specific organism is strongly suspected.
◆ *Corynebacterium diphtheriae* requires two swabs and a special growth medium.
◆ *Bordetella pertussis* requires a nasopharyngeal culture and a special growth medium.
◆ *Neisseria meningitides* requires enriched selective media.

- Immediately send the specimen to the laboratory.

COLLECTING A NASOPHARYNGEAL SPECIMEN
- Confirm the patient's identity using two patient identifiers according to facility policy.
- Tell the patient that he may gag or feel the urge to sneeze during the swabbing but that the procedure takes less than 1 minute.
- Have him sit erect at the edge of the bed or on a chair, facing you.
- Wash your hands and put on gloves.
- Ask him to blow his nose to clear his nasal passages.
- Check his nostrils for patency with a penlight.
- Tell him to occlude one nostril and then the other as he exhales.
- Listen for the more patent nostril and insert the swab into it.
- If the nostril is narrow, use a nasal speculum for better access.
- Ask the patient to cough to bring organisms to the nasopharynx.
- While it's still in the package, bend the sterile swab in a curve.
- Open the package without contaminating the swab.
- Ask the patient to tilt his head back.
- Gently pass the swab into the more patent nostril, 3" to 4" (7.5 to 10 cm) into the nasopharynx.
- Keep the swab near the septum and floor of the nose.
- Rotate the swab quickly and remove it. (See *Obtaining a nasopharyngeal specimen*.)
- Alternatively, depress the patient's tongue with a tongue blade.
- Pass the bent swab up behind the uvula.
- Rotate the swab and withdraw it.
- Remove the cap from the culture tube.
- Insert the swab and break off the contaminated end.
- Close the tube tightly.
- Remove and discard your gloves and wash your hands.
- Label the specimen for culture and complete a laboratory request form.
- Immediately send the specimen to the laboratory.

- If the specimen is obtained to isolate a possible virus, check with the laboratory for the recommended collection technique.

COLLECTING A WOUND SPECIMEN
- Confirm the patient's identity using two patient identifiers according to facility policy.
- Wash your hands.
- Prepare a sterile field and put on sterile gloves.
- Remove the dressing with sterile forceps to expose the wound.
- Dispose of the soiled dressings properly.
- Clean the area around the wound with alcohol or povidone-iodine, and allow the area to dry.
- For an aerobic culture, use a sterile, cotton-tipped swab to collect as much exudate as possible, or insert the swab deeply into the wound and rotate it.
- Remove the swab from the wound.
- Immediately place it in the aerobic culture tube and label it.
- Immediately send it to the laboratory with a completed laboratory request form.

Obtaining a nasopharyngeal specimen

After you've passed the swab into the nasopharynx, quickly rotate the swab to collect the specimen. Then remove the swab, taking care not to injure the nasal mucous membrane.

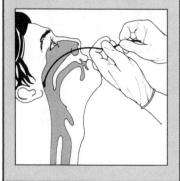

- Never collect exudate from the skin and insert the same swab into the wound.
- For an anaerobic culture, insert the sterile, cotton-tipped swab deeply into the wound and rotate it. (See *Anaerobic specimen collection*, page 482, and *Culturing a wound*, page 483.)
- Remove it and immediately place it in the anaerobic culture tube.
- Alternative method: Insert a sterile 10-ml syringe without a needle into the wound, and aspirate 1 to 5 ml of exudate into the syringe.
- Attach the 21G needle to the syringe, and immediately inject the aspirate into the anaerobic culture tube.
- If an anaerobic culture tube is unavailable, obtain a rubber stopper, attach the needle to the syringe, and gently push all the air out of the syringe.
- Stick the needle tip into the rubber stopper.
- Remove and discard your gloves.
- Immediately send the syringe of aspirate to the laboratory with a completed laboratory request form.
- Put on sterile gloves.
- Apply a new dressing to the wound.

COLLECTING AN EAR SPECIMEN
- Confirm the patient's identity using two patient identifiers according to facility policy.
- Wash your hands and put on gloves.
- Gently clean excess debris from the patient's ear with normal saline solution and gauze pads.
- Insert the sterile swab into the ear canal.
- Rotate it gently along the walls of the canal to avoid damaging the eardrum.
- Withdraw the swab.
- Avoid touching other surfaces to prevent contamination.
- Place the swab in the culture tube with transport medium.
- Remove and discard your gloves and wash your hands.
- Label the specimen for culture.

(continued)

◆ Complete a laboratory request form and immediately send the specimen to the laboratory.

COLLECTING A MIDDLE EAR SPECIMEN

◆ Confirm the patient's identity using two patient identifiers according to facility policy.
◆ Wash your hands and put on gloves.
◆ Clean the outer ear with normal saline solution and gauze pads.
◆ Remove and discard your gloves.
◆ The practitioner punctures the eardrum with a needle and aspirates fluid into the syringe.
◆ Label the container.
◆ Complete a laboratory request form and immediately send the specimen to the laboratory.

COLLECTING AN EYE SPECIMEN

◆ Confirm the patient's identity using two patient identifiers according to facility policy.
◆ Wash your hands and put on sterile gloves.
◆ Gently clean excess debris from outside the eye with normal saline solution and gauze pads.
◆ Wipe from the inner to the outer canthus.
◆ Retract the lower eyelid to expose the conjunctival sac, and gently rub the sterile swab over the conjunctiva.
◆ Take care not to touch other surfaces.
◆ Hold the swab parallel to the eye to prevent corneal irritation or trauma due to sudden movement.
◆ A corneal scraping is performed by the practitioner, using a wire culture loop.
◆ Immediately place the swab or wire loop in the culture tube with transport medium.
◆ Remove and discard your gloves and wash your hands.
◆ Label the specimen for culture.
◆ Complete a laboratory request form and immediately send the specimen to the laboratory.

COLLECTING A RECTAL SPECIMEN

◆ Confirm the patient's identity using two patient identifiers according to facility policy.
◆ Wash your hands and put on gloves.
◆ Clean around the patient's anus with a washcloth and soap and water.
◆ Moisten the swab with normal saline solution or sterile broth medium.

◆ Insert the swab through the anus and advance it about ⅜″ (1 cm) for infants or 1½″ (4 cm) for adults.
◆ While withdrawing the swab, gently rotate it against the walls of the lower rectum to sample a large area of the rectal mucosa.
◆ Place the swab in a culture tube with transport medium.
◆ Remove and discard your gloves and wash your hands.
◆ Label the specimen for culture.
◆ Complete a laboratory request form and immediately send the specimen to the laboratory.

Anaerobic specimen collection

Because most anaerobes die when exposed to oxygen, they must be transported in tubes filled with carbon dioxide or nitrogen. The anaerobic specimen collector shown here includes a rubber-stoppered tube filled with carbon dioxide, a small inner tube, and a swab attached to a plastic plunger.

Before specimen collection, the small inner tube containing the swab is held in place with the rubber stopper (as shown on the left). After collecting the specimen, quickly replace the swab in the inner tube and depress the plunger to separate the inner tube from the stopper (as shown on the right), forcing it into the larger tube and exposing the specimen to a carbon dioxide-rich environment.

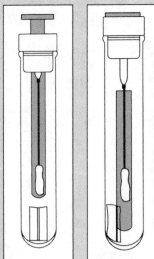

BEFORE   **AFTER**

- Ideally, a specimen should be collected before the patient has received antibiotic therapy.
- After obtaining the specimen, give antibiotics as prescribed.
- Note recent antibiotic therapy on the laboratory request form.
- Don't clean a perineal wound with alcohol because this could irritate sensitive tissues. Make sure that antiseptic doesn't enter the wound.
- For an eye specimen: Don't use an antiseptic before culturing to avoid irritating the eye and inhibiting organism growth in the culture.
- When collecting an eye specimen in a child or an uncooperative adult, restrain the patient's head to prevent eye trauma resulting from sudden movement.

COMPLICATIONS

- None known

- Explain the procedure to the patient and answer questions, as needed.

- Record the time, date, and site of specimen collection.
- Note recent or current antibiotic therapy.
- Document whether the specimen has an unusual appearance or odor.

SELECTED REFERENCES

Ekanayaka, M., et al. "Is it Cost Effective to do Routine Pharyngeal Swabs for Chlamydia Trachomatis in Patients Who Practice Unprotected Oral Sex?" *Sexually Transmitted Infections* 82(Suppl 2):A4, June 2006.

Humair, J.P., et al. "Management of Acute Pharyngitis in Adults: Reliability of Rapid Streptococcal Tests and Clinical Findings," *Archives of Internal Medicine* 166(6):640-44, March 2006.

Kessler, L., et al. "Comparison of Microbiological Results of Needle Puncture vs. Superficial Swab in Infected Diabetic Foot Ulcer with Osteomyelitis," *Diabetic Medicine* 23(1):99-102, January 2006.

Lampinen, T.M., et al. "Illustrated Instructions for Self-Collection of Anorectal Swab Specimens and Their Adequacy for Cytological Examination," *Sexually Transmitted Diseases* 33(6):386-88, June 2006.

Tanaka, K., et al. "The Cytopathological Comparison of the Uterine Cervical Smear Obtained by Cotton-Swab and Cervix-Brush," *Cytopathology* 16(Suppl S2):59, October 2005.

Culturing a wound

Insert the culture swab into the wound to obtain a sample (as shown).

Temperature assessment

OVERVIEW

DESCRIPTION

◆ Body temperature represents balance between heat produced by metabolism, muscular activity, and other factors and heat lost through the skin, lungs, and body wastes.

◆ A stable temperature pattern promotes proper function of cells, tissues, and organs. A change in pattern usually signals onset of illness.

◆ Normal temperature is highest in neonates and lowest in elderly persons.

◆ Gender, age, emotional conditions, and environment influence temperature.

◆ Women normally have higher temperatures than men, especially during ovulation.

◆ Heightened emotions raise temperature; depressed emotions lower it.

◆ Hot external environments raise temperature; cold environments lower it.

◆ Temperature can be measured with electronic digital thermometers. (See *Electronic and tympanic thermometers.*)

◆ Oral temperature in adults normally ranges from 97° to 99.5° F (36.1° to 37.5° C)

◆ Rectal temperature is the most accurate reading; in adults it's usually 1° F (0.6° C) higher than oral.

◆ Axillary temperature is least accurate; in adults, it reads 1° to 2° F (0.6° to 1.1° C) lower than oral or rectal.

◆ Tympanic temperature reads 0.5° to 1° F (0.3° to 0.6° C) higher than rectal.

◆ Temperature normally fluctuates with rest and activity.

◆ Highest readings occur between 4 p.m. and 8 p.m.; lowest readings occur between 4 and 5 a.m.

CONTRAINDICATIONS

◆ Oral measurement in unconscious, disoriented, or seizure-prone patients

◆ Oral measurement in young children and infants and those who mouth-breathe

◆ Rectal measurement in patients with diarrhea, recent rectal or prostatic surgery, injury, or recent myocardial infarction

EQUIPMENT

Electronic thermometer, chemical-dot thermometer, or tympanic thermometer ◆ water-soluble lubricant or petroleum jelly (for rectal temperature) ◆ gloves (for rectal temperature) ◆ facial tissue ◆ disposable thermometer sheath or probe cover (except for chemical thermometer) ◆ alcohol pad

PREPARATION

◆ If you use an electronic thermometer, make sure it's been recharged.

KEY STEPS

◆ Confirm the patient's identity using two patient identifiers according to facility policy.

◆ Explain the procedure to the patient.

◆ Wash your hands.

◆ Wait 15 minutes before taking an oral temperature if the patient has had hot or cold liquids, chewed gum, or smoked recently.

USING AN ELECTRONIC THERMOMETER

◆ Insert the probe into a disposable probe cover.

◆ Lubricate the probe cover if taking a rectal temperature to reduce friction and ease insertion.

◆ Leave the probe in place until the maximum temperature appears on the digital display.

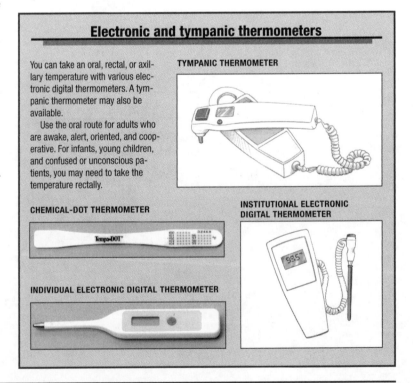

Electronic and tympanic thermometers

You can take an oral, rectal, or axillary temperature with various electronic digital thermometers. A tympanic thermometer may also be available.

Use the oral route for adults who are awake, alert, oriented, and cooperative. For infants, young children, and confused or unconscious patients, you may need to take the temperature rectally.

TYMPANIC THERMOMETER

CHEMICAL-DOT THERMOMETER

INSTITUTIONAL ELECTRONIC DIGITAL THERMOMETER

INDIVIDUAL ELECTRONIC DIGITAL THERMOMETER

USING A TYMPANIC THERMOMETER

- Make sure the lens under the probe is clean and shiny.
- Attach a disposable probe cover.
- Stabilize the patient's head.
- Gently pull the ear straight back (for children up to age 1) or up and back (for children age 1 and older to adults).
- Insert the thermometer until the ear canal is sealed.
- The thermometer should be inserted toward the tympanic membrane in the same way an otoscope is inserted.
- Press the activation button and hold for 1 second.
- The temperature will appear on the display.

AGE FACTOR *For infants under age 3 months, take three readings and use the highest.*

TAKING AN ORAL TEMPERATURE

- Place thermometer tip under the patient's tongue, as far back as possible on either side of the frenulum linguae to promote contact with superficial blood vessels and contribute to an accurate reading.
- Instruct the patient to close his lips.
- Insert a chemical-dot thermometer 45 seconds.
- Electronic thermometer: wait until the maximum temperature is displayed; note the temperature, then remove and discard probe cover.
- Chemical-dot thermometer: read the temperature as the last dye dot that has changed color (fired); discard thermometer and dispenser case.

TAKING A RECTAL TEMPERATURE

- Position the patient on his side with his top leg flexed.
- Drape him to provide privacy; fold back the bed linens to expose the anus.
- Squeeze the lubricant onto a facial tissue to prevent contamination of the lubricant supply.
- Put on gloves.

- Lubricate about ½″ (1.5 cm) of the thermometer tip for an infant, 1″ (2.5 cm) for a child, and about 1½″ (4 cm) for an adult.
- Lubrication reduces friction and eases insertion (may be unnecessary when using prelubricated disposable rectal sheaths).
- Lift the patient's upper buttock and insert thermometer about ½″ (1.5 cm) for an infant or 1½″ (4 cm) for an adult.
- Gently direct the thermometer along the rectal wall toward the umbilicus.
- This avoids perforating the anus or rectum and ensures an accurate reading.
- Hold the electronic thermometer until the maximum temperature is displayed.
- Holding the thermometer prevents damage to rectal tissues caused by displacement or loss of the thermometer into the rectum.
- Carefully remove the thermometer, wiping it as necessary.
- Wipe the patient's anal area to remove lubricant or stool.
- Remove and dispose of the rectal sheath.
- Remove and discard your gloves and wash your hands.

TAKING AN AXILLARY TEMPERATURE

- Position the patient with the axilla exposed.
- Pat the axilla dry (moisture conducts heat); avoid harsh rubbing, which generates heat.
- Ask the patient to reach across his chest and grasp his opposite shoulder, lifting his elbow.
- Position the thermometer in the center of the axilla, with the tip pointing toward his head.
- Tell the patient to continue grasping his shoulder and lower his elbow, holding it against his chest.
- Remove the thermometer when it displays the maximum temperature.
- Axillary temperature takes longer to register than oral or rectal temperature because the thermometer isn't enclosed in a body cavity.

SPECIAL CONSIDERATIONS

- Avoid taking rectal temperatures in patients with recent myocardial infarction; anal manipulation may stimulate the vagus nerve, causing bradycardia or another rhythm disturbance.
- To avoid variations, use the same thermometer for repeated temperature taking.
- Store chemical-dot thermometers in a cool area.
- An oral temperature can be taken when the patient is receiving nasal oxygen, which only raises oral temperature by about 0.3° F (0.2° C).

COMPLICATIONS
- None known

PATIENT TEACHING

- Explain the procedure to the patient as needed.

DOCUMENTATION

- Record the time, route, and temperature.

SELECTED REFERENCES
Farnell, S., et al. "Temperature Measurement: Comparison of Non-invasive Methods Used in Adult Critical Care," *Journal of Clinical Nursing* 14(5):632-39, May 2005.

Smith, J.J., et al. "Temperature — The Forgotten Vital Sign," *Accident and Emergency Nursing* 13(4):247-50, October 2005.

Stanhope, N. "Temperature Measurement in the Phase I PACU," *Journal of Perianesthesia Nursing* 21(1):27-33, February 2006.

Sund-Levander, M., et al. "Errors in Body Temperature Assessment Related to Individual Variation, Measuring Technique and Equipment," *International Journal of Nursing Practice* 10(5):216-23, October 2004.

Thompson, H.J. "Fever: A Concept Analysis," *Journal of Advanced Nursing* 51(5):484-92, September 2005.

Therapeutic bath

OVERVIEW

DESCRIPTION

- A therapeutic bath combines water and additives to soothe and relax the patient, clean the skin, relieve inflammation and pruritus, and soften and remove crusts, scales, debris, and old drugs.
- A balneotherapy bath, used primarily for antipruritic and emollient actions, also constricts surface blood vessels and has an anti-inflammatory effect.
- Oatmeal powder, soluble cornstarch, or soybean complex may be added to create a colloid bath, which has a soothing effect on generalized itching.
- Oil baths are useful for lubricating dry skin and easing eczematous eruptions.
- Sodium bicarbonate produces an alkaline bath that has a cooling effect and helps relieve pruritus.
- A medicated tar bath may be used to treat psoriasis. The film of tar left on the skin works in combination with ultraviolet light to inhibit the rapid cell turnover characteristic of psoriasis. (See *Comparing therapeutic baths*.)
- A bedridden patient may benefit from a local soak with the therapeutic additive instead of a therapeutic tub bath.

CONTRAINDICATIONS

- None known

EQUIPMENT

Bathtub ◆ bath mat ◆ rubber mat ◆ bath thermometer ◆ therapeutic additive ◆ measuring device ◆ colander or sieve for oatmeal powder ◆ two washcloths ◆ two towels ◆ patient gown or loose-fitting cotton pajamas ◆ lubricating cream or ointment, if ordered

PREPARATION

- Assemble supplies and draw the bath before bringing the patient to the bath area to prevent chilling him.
- Make sure the tub is clean and disinfected; a patient with broken skin is particularly vulnerable to infection.
- Place the bath mat next to the tub and the rubber mat on the bottom of the tub to prevent falls; the therapeutic additive may make the tub exceptionally slippery.
- Fill the tub with 6″ to 8″ (15 to 20 cm) of water at 95° to 100° F (35° to 37.8° C).
- The treatment's purpose and type of additive used will determine water temperature. Cool to lukewarm water is used for relieving pruritus and when adding tar or starch. Warm baths soothe, but water warmer than 100° F causes vasodilation, which could aggravate pruritus.
- Measure the correct amount of therapeutic additive, according to the practitioner's order or package instructions.
- As the tub is filling, thoroughly mix the additive in the water.
- Add most substances directly to the water, but place oatmeal powder in a sieve or colander under the tub faucet to help it dissolve.
- Begin with 2 tbs of oatmeal powder; then add more powder or water as needed to regulate the thickness of the oatmeal bath.
- When giving a tar bath, wear a plastic apron or protective gown because tar preparations stain clothing.

KEY STEPS

- Check the practitioner's order, and assess the patient's condition.
- Confirm the patient's identity using two patient identifiers according to facility policy.
- Explain the procedure and have the patient void.
- Wash your hands, take the patient to the bath area, and close the door.
- Check water temperature and help the patient undress and get in the tub.
- Advise him to use the safety rails to prevent falls.
- Tell the patient that the bath may feel unpleasant at first because the skin is irritated, but assure the patient that the solution will soon coat and soothe the skin.
- Ask the patient to stretch out in the tub and submerge up to the chin.
- If the patient is capable, offer a washcloth to apply the bath solution to the face and other body areas not immersed, if these areas require treatment.

⚡ **WARNING** *When giving a tar bath, tell the patient not to get the bath solution in his eyes because tar is an eye irritant.*

- To prevent further irritation, warn the patient against scrubbing the skin.
- Add warm water to the bath as needed to maintain a comfortable temperature.
- Allow the patient to soak for 15 to 30 minutes.
- If you stay with the patient, pull the curtain to provide privacy and avoid drafts.
- If you must leave the room, show the patient how to use the call button.
- After the bath, help the patient from the tub and help pat dry with towels.

⚡ **WARNING** *Don't rub the skin. Rubbing removes some solutes and oils clinging to the skin and produces friction, thereby worsening pruritus.*

- Apply lubricating cream or ointment, if ordered, to help hold water in the newly hydrated skin.
- Provide a fresh gown or loose-fitting cotton pajamas.
- Advise the patient to avoid wearing pajamas, underwear, or other clothing that isn't cotton and loose fitting. Tight clothing and scratchy or synthetic materials can aggravate skin conditions by causing friction and increasing perspiration.
- Escort the patient to his room and make sure he's comfortable.
- Drain the bath water, clean and disinfect the tub, and dispose of soiled materials properly.
- If you've given an oatmeal powder bath, drain and rinse the tub immediately or the powder will cake, making later removal difficult.

SPECIAL CONSIDERATIONS

- Because pruritus seems worse at night, give a therapeutic bath before bedtime, unless ordered otherwise, to promote restful sleep.
- Because the patient with a skin disorder may be self-conscious, maintain eye contact during conversation and avoid staring at his skin. Also avoid nonverbal expressions and gestures that show revulsion.
- Allow the patient to talk about his condition and how it affects his self-esteem.
- Refrain from using soap during a therapeutic bath because its drying effect counteracts the bath emollient.
- A patient with skin breakdown chills easily, so protect him from drafts. After the bath, avoid covering or dressing him too warmly because perspiration aggravates pruritus. Instruct the patient not to scratch his skin to prevent excoriation and infection.
- If the patient is confined to bed, place the therapeutic additive in a basin of water at 95° to 100° F (35° to 37.8° C) and apply it with a washcloth, using light, gentle strokes.

COMPLICATIONS
- None known

PATIENT TEACHING

- Instruct the patient to bathe only as often as prescribed. Excessive bathing can dry skin.
- Advise the patient to buy commercial bath oil. Salad or cooking oils may give clothes an unpleasant odor and mineral oil mixes poorly with water.
- Tell the patient to follow manufacturer's instructions for commercially prepared colloid preparations.
- Teach the patient how to make a colloid oatmeal bath at home by putting one-half cup of raw oatmeal into a blender and blending at medium-high speed until the material has the consistency of flour, then sifting it to remove unground pieces.

DOCUMENTATION

- Record the date, time, and duration of the bath.
- Note the water temperature, type and amount of additive, skin appearance before and after the bath, the patient's tolerance of the treatment, and the bath's effectiveness.

SELECTED REFERENCES
Bettzuege-Pfaff, B.I., and Melzer, A. "Treating Dry Skin and Pruritus with a Bath Oil Containing Soya Oil and Lauromacrogols," *Current Medical Research and Opinion* 21(11):1735-39, November 2005.

Ciardullo, A.V. "Calendula and Thermal Baths for Treating a High-Grade Iatrogenic Disability," *Journal of Alternative and Complementary Medicine* 11(5): 787, October 2005.

Roebuck, H.L. "For Pruritus, Combination Therapy Works Best," *Nurse Practitioner* 31(3):12-13, March 2006.

Wallengren, J. "Prurigo: Diagnosis and Management," *American Journal of Clinical Dermatology* 5(2):85-95, 2004.

Comparing therapeutic baths

TYPE	AGENTS	PURPOSE
Antibacterial	- Acetic acid - Potassium permanganate - Povidone-iodine	Used to treat infected eczema, dirty ulcerations, furunculosis, and pemphigus
Colloidal	- Aveeno colloidal oatmeal - Aveeno colloidal oatmeal, oilated - Starch and baking soda	Used to relieve pruritus and to soothe irritated skin; indicated for an irritated or oozing condition such as atopic eczema
Emollient	- Bath oils - Mineral oil	Used to clean and hydrate the skin; indicated for a dry skin condition
Tar	- Bath oils with tar - Coal tar concentrate	Used to treat scaly dermatoses, sometimes in combination with ultraviolet light therapy; loosens scales and relieves pruritus

Thoracentesis

DESCRIPTION

- Thoracentesis relieves pulmonary compression and respiratory distress by removing accumulated air or fluid from the pleural space, which has resulted from injury or a condition such as tuberculosis or cancer.
- It provides a specimen of pleural fluid or tissue for analysis.
- It also allows instillation of chemotherapeutic agents or other drugs into the pleural space.

CONTRAINDICATIONS

- Bleeding disorders

EQUIPMENT

Most facilities use a prepackaged thoracentesis tray.

Sterile gloves ◆ sterile drapes ◆ 70% isopropyl alcohol or povidone-iodine solution ◆ 1% or 2% lidocaine ◆ 5-ml syringe with 21G and 25G needles for anesthetic injection ◆ 17G thoracentesis needle for aspiration ◆ 50-ml syringe ◆ three-way stopcock and tubing ◆ sterile specimen containers ◆ sterile hemostat ◆ sterile 4″ × 4″ gauze pads ◆ adhesive tape ◆ sphygmomanometer ◆ gloves ◆ stethoscope ◆ laboratory request slips ◆ drainage bottles ◆ hair clipping supplies ◆ biopsy needle ◆ prescribed sedative with 3-ml syringe and 21G needle ◆ drainage bottles (if the practitioner expects a large amount of drainage) ◆ Teflon catheter (optional)

PREPARATION

- Assemble all equipment at the patient's bedside or treatment area.
- Check expiration date on each sterile package, and inspect for tears.
- Prepare laboratory request form, listing current antibiotics (this will be considered in analyzing the specimens).
- Make sure the patient signs a consent form; note drug allergies, especially to the local anesthetic.
- Have chest X-rays available.

KEY STEPS

- Confirm the patient's identity using two patient identifiers according to facility policy.
- Explain the procedure to the patient. Inform him that he may feel discomfort and a sensation of pressure during needle insertion.
- Provide privacy and emotional support.
- Wash your hands.
- Give the prescribed sedative as ordered.
- Obtain baseline vital signs, and assess respiratory function.
- Position the patient on the edge of the bed with his legs supported and head and folded arms resting on a pillow on the overbed table; alternatively, have him straddle a chair backward and rest his head and folded arms on the back of the chair.
- If he can't sit, turn him on the unaffected side with the arm of the affected side raised above his head.
- Elevate the head of the bed 30 to 45 degrees, if not contraindicated. Proper positioning stretches the chest or back and allows easier access to intercostal spaces.
- Remind the patient not to cough, breathe deeply, or move suddenly during the procedure to avoid puncture of the visceral pleura or lung.

⚡ **WARNING** *If the patient coughs, the practitioner will briefly halt the procedure and withdraw the needle slightly to prevent puncture.*

- Expose the patient's entire chest or back and clip hair from the aspiration site, as ordered.
- Wash your hands again before touching the sterile equipment.
- Using sterile technique, open the thoracentesis tray and assist the practitioner as necessary in disinfecting the site.
- If an ampule of local anesthetic isn't included in the sterile tray and a multidose vial of local anesthetic is to be used, assist the practitioner by wiping the rubber stopper with an alcohol pad and holding the inverted vial while the practitioner withdraws the anesthetic solution.
- After draping the patient and injecting the local anesthetic, the practitioner attaches a three-way stopcock with tubing to the aspirating needle and turns the stopcock to prevent air from entering the pleural space through the needle.
- Attach the other end of the tubing to the drainage bottle.

Performing needle thoracentesis

For a patient with life-threatening tension pneumothorax, needle thoracentesis temporarily relieves pleural pressure until a practitioner can insert a chest tube.

HOW NEEDLE THORACENTESIS WORKS

A needle attached to a flutter valve is inserted into the affected pleural space. (If no flutter valve is available, one can be made from a perforated finger cot or glove attached with a rubber band.) When the patient exhales, trapped air escapes via the flutter valve instead of being retained under pressure. The flutter valve also prevents more air from entering the involved lung during inhalation.

HOW TO PERFORM THE PROCEDURE

You may need to assist the practitioner in performing the procedure. Here's how to proceed:

- Clean the skin around the second intercostal space at the midclavicular line with povidone-iodine solution. Use a circular motion, starting at the center and working outward.
- The practitioner inserts a sterile 16G (or larger) needle over the superior portion of the rib and through the tissue covering the pleural cavity. The vein, artery, and nerve lie behind the rib's inferior border.
- Listen for a hissing sound. This signals the needle's entry into the pleural cavity.
- If a flutter valve is used, it's secured to the needle. The arrow on the valve indicates the direction of airflow. A sterile glove is placed on the distal end of the valve to collect drainage.
- The needle is left in place until a chest tube can be inserted.

- The practitioner inserts the needle into the pleural space and attaches a 50-ml syringe to the needle's stopcock.
- A hemostat may be used to hold the needle in place and prevent pleural tear or lung puncture. Alternatively, the practitioner may introduce a Teflon catheter into the needle, remove the needle, and attach a stopcock and syringe or drainage tubing to the catheter to reduce risk of pleural puncture by the needle. (See *Performing needle thoracentesis.*)
- Check vital signs regularly during the procedure.

  WARNING *Watch for signs of distress, such as pallor, vertigo, faintness, weak and rapid pulse, decreased blood pressure, dyspnea, tachypnea, diaphoresis, chest pain, blood-tinged mucus, and excessive coughing. Alert the practitioner; these signs may indicate hypovolemic shock, tension pneumothorax, or other complications.*

- Put on gloves and assist the practitioner as necessary in specimen collection, fluid drainage, and dressing the site.
- After the practitioner withdraws the needle or catheter, apply pressure to the puncture site, using a sterile $4'' \times 4''$ gauze pad. Apply a new sterile gauze pad and secure with tape.
- Place the patient in a comfortable position, take his vital signs, and assess his respiratory status.
- Label the specimens properly and send them to the laboratory.
- Discard of disposable equipment. Clean nondisposable items, and return them for sterilization.
- Check vital signs and dressing for drainage every 15 minutes for 1 hour. Continue to assess vital signs and respiratory status as indicated by condition.

SPECIAL CONSIDERATIONS

- If more than 500 ml of fluid have been removed try to keep the patient off the affected side.
- To prevent pulmonary edema and hypovolemic shock after thoracentesis, remove fluid slowly (no more than 1,000 ml of fluid during the first 30 minutes). Removing fluid increases negative intrapleural pressure, which can lead to edema if the lung doesn't reexpand to fill the space.
- Pleuritic or shoulder pain may indicate pleural irritation by the needle point.
- A chest X-ray is usually ordered after the procedure to detect pneumothorax and evaluate the results of the procedure.

COMPLICATIONS

- Pneumothorax (possibly leading to mediastinal shift and requiring chest tube insertion) if needle punctures lung and allows air to enter pleural cavity
- Pyogenic infection from contamination
- Pain
- Cough
- Anxiety
- Dry taps
- Subcutaneous hematoma

PATIENT TEACHING

- Explain the procedure and keep the patient informed of each step.
- Watch for signs of anxiety and provide reassurance as necessary.

DOCUMENTATION

- Record the date and time of thoracentesis.
- Note location of the puncture site.
- Document volume and description (such as color, viscosity, and odor) of fluid withdrawn.
- Record specimens sent to the laboratory.
- Note vital signs and respiratory assessment before, during, and after procedure.
- Document postprocedural tests such as chest X-ray.
- Record complications and nursing actions taken.
- Note the patient's reaction to the procedure.

SELECTED REFERENCES

Aelony, Y. "Thoracentesis Without Ultrasonic Guidance: Infrequent Complications When Performed by an Experienced Pulmonologist," *Journal of Bronchology* 12(4):200-02, October 2005.

Doelken, P., et al. "Pleural Manometry: Technique and Clinical Implications," *Chest* 126(6):1764-69, December 2004.

Garg, P., et al. "Re-expansion Pulmonary Edema: A Potentially Fatal Complication of Thoracentesis," *Journal of General Internal Medicine* 21 (Suppl. 4):264, April 2006.

Giacomini, M., et al. "How to Avoid and Manage a Pneumothorax," *Journal of Vascular Access* 7(1):7-14, January-March 2006.

Suddaby, E.C., and Schiller, S. "Management of Chylothorax in Children," *Pediatric Nursing* 30(4):290-95, July-August 2004.

Thoracic drainage

DESCRIPTION

- Thoracic drainage uses gravity and, possibly, suction to restore negative pressure and remove material that collects in the pleural cavity.
- A disposable drainage system combines drainage collection, a water seal, and suction control into a single unit.
- The underwater seal in the drainage system allows air and fluid to escape from the pleural cavity but doesn't allow air to reenter.
- The procedure removes accumulated air, fluids (blood, pus, chyle, and serous fluids), or solids (blood clots) from the pleural cavity.
- It restores negative pressure in the pleural cavity and reexpands a partially or totally collapsed lung.

CONTRAINDICATIONS

- None known

EQUIPMENT

Thoracic drainage system (Pleur-evac, Argyle, Ohio, or Thora-Klex system, which can function as a gravity draining system or be connected to suction to enhance chest drainage) ◆ sterile distilled water ◆ adhesive tape ◆ sterile clear plastic tubing ◆ bottle or system rack ◆ two rubber-tipped Kelly clamps ◆ sterile 50-ml catheter-tip syringe ◆ suction source, if ordered ◆ rubber band or safety pin

PREPARATION

- Check the practitioner's order to determine type of drainage system to be used and specific procedural details.
- Collect the appropriate equipment and take to the patient's bedside.

KEY STEPS

- Confirm the patient's identity using two patient identifiers according to facility policy.
- Explain the procedure and wash your hands.
- Maintain sterile technique throughout procedure and when you make changes in the system or alter connections.
- Open the packaged system and place it on the floor in the rack supplied by the manufacturer.
- After the system is prepared, hang it from the side of the bed.
- Remove the plastic connector from the short tube attached to the water-seal chamber.
- Using a 50-ml catheter-tip syringe, instill sterile distilled water into the water-seal chamber until it reaches the 2-cm mark or the mark specified by the manufacturer.
- Water may need to be added to help detect air leaks.
- Replace the plastic connector.
- If suction is ordered, remove the cap (also called the *muffler* or *atmosphere vent cover*) on the suction-control chamber to open the vent.
- Next, instill sterile distilled water until it reaches the 20-cm mark or the ordered level, and recap the suction-control chamber.
- Using the long tube, connect the patient's chest tube to the closed drainage collection chamber and secure the connection with tape.
- Connect the short tube on the drainage system to the suction source, and turn on the suction.
- Gentle bubbling should begin in the suction chamber, indicating that the correct suction level has been reached.
- Note the character, consistency, and amount of drainage in the drainage collection chamber.
- Mark the drainage level in the drainage collection chamber by noting the time and date at the drainage level on the chamber every 8 hours (or more often if there's a large amount of drainage).
- Check the water level in the water-seal chamber every 8 hours. If necessary, carefully add sterile distilled water until the level reaches the 2-cm mark indicated on the water-seal chamber of the commercial system.
- Check for fluctuation in the water-seal chamber as he breathes.
- Normal fluctuations of 2″ to 4″ (about 5 to 10 cm) reflect pressure changes in the pleural space during respiration.
- To check for fluctuation with a suction system, momentarily disconnect the suction system so the air vent is opened, and observe for fluctuation.
- Check for intermittent bubbling in the water-seal chamber. This usually occurs when the system is removing air from the pleural cavity. If bubbling isn't readily apparent during quiet breathing, have the patient take a deep breath or cough. Absence of bubbling indicates that the pleural space has sealed.
- Check the water level in the suction-control chamber.
- Detach the chamber or bottle from the suction source; when bubbling ceases, observe the water level. If needed, add sterile distilled water to bring the level to the 20-cm line or as ordered.
- Check for gentle bubbling in the suction control chamber because it indicates that the proper suction level has been reached. Vigorous bubbling in this chamber increases the rate of water evaporation. Periodically check that the air vent in the system is working properly.

⚡ **WARNING** *Occlusion of the air vent results in a buildup of pressure in the system that could cause the patient to develop a tension pneumothorax.*

- Coil the system's tubing and secure it to the edge of the bed.
- Be sure tubing remains at the level of the patient. Avoid creating dependent loops, kinks, or pressure on the tubing. Avoid lifting the drainage system above the patient's chest because fluid may flow back into the pleural space.
- Be sure to keep two rubber-tipped clamps at the bedside to clamp the chest tube if the commercially prepared system cracks or to locate an air leak in the system.
- Encourage the patient to cough frequently and breathe deeply.

◆ Instruct him to sit upright and to splint the insertion site while coughing to minimize pain.
◆ Check the rate and quality of respirations and auscultate the patient's lungs periodically to assess air exchange in the affected lung. Diminished or absent breath sounds may indicate that the lung hasn't reexpanded.

WARNING *Tell the patient to report breathing difficulty immediately. Notify the practitioner immediately if the patient develops cyanosis, rapid or shallow breathing, subcutaneous emphysema, chest pain, or excessive bleeding.*

◆ When clots are visible, you may be able to milk the tubing, depending on your facility's policy. Milk tubing in direction of the drainage chamber as needed.
◆ Check the chest tube dressing at least every 8 hours.

WARNING *Palpate the area surrounding the dressing for crepitus or subcutaneous emphysema, which indicates that air is leaking into the subcutaneous tissue surrounding the insertion site.*

◆ Change the dressing if necessary, according to policy.
◆ Encourage active or passive range-of-motion (ROM) exercises for the patient's arm or the affected side if he's been splinting the arm.
◆ Give ordered pain drug as needed for comfort and to help with deep breathing, coughing, and ROM exercises.
◆ Remind the ambulatory patient to keep the drainage system below chest level and be careful not to disconnect the tubing to maintain the water seal.

SPECIAL CONSIDERATIONS

◆ Instruct staff and visitors to avoid touching the equipment to prevent complications from separated connections.
◆ If excessive continuous bubbling is present in the water-seal chamber, especially if suction is being used,

rule out a leak in the drainage system.
◆ Try to locate the leak by clamping the tube momentarily at various points along its length.
◆ Begin clamping at the tube's proximal end and work down toward the drainage system; pay special attention to the seal around the connections.

TROUBLESHOOTER *If a connection is loose, push it back together and tape it securely. Bubbling will stop when a clamp is placed between the air leak and the water seal.*

TROUBLESHOOTER *If you clamp along the tube's entire length and bubbling doesn't stop, the drainage unit may be cracked and need replacement.*

◆ If the drainage collection chamber fills, replace it. Double-clamp the tube close to the insertion site (use two clamps facing in opposite directions), exchange the system, remove the clamps, and retape the connection.

WARNING *Never leave tubes clamped for more than 1 minute to prevent a tension pneumothorax, which may occur when air and fluid are kept from escaping.*

TROUBLESHOOTER *If the system cracks, clamp the chest tube momentarily with the two rubber-tipped clamps at the bedside (placed there at the time of tube insertion). Place the clamps close to each other near the insertion site; they should face in opposite directions to provide a more complete seal.*

Observe the patient for altered respirations while the tube is clamped. Replace the damaged equipment. (Prepare the new unit before clamping.)

◆ Instead of clamping the tube, you may submerge the distal end of the tube in a container of normal saline solution to create a temporary water seal while you replace the drainage system. Check facility policy for the proper procedure.

COMPLICATIONS
◆ Tension pneumothorax

PATIENT TEACHING

◆ Explain the procedure to the patient.
◆ Encourage the patient to cough frequently and breathe deeply to help drain the pleural space and expand the lungs.
◆ Instruct the patient to sit upright for optimal lung expansion and to splint the insertion site while coughing to minimize pain.
◆ Tell the patient to report breathing difficulty immediately.
◆ Remind the ambulatory patient to keep the drainage system below chest level and to be careful not to disconnect the tubing to maintain the water seal.

DOCUMENTATION

◆ Note date and time thoracic drainage began.
◆ Document type of system used.
◆ Record amount of suction applied to pleural cavity.
◆ Note presence or absence of bubbling or fluctuation in the water-seal chamber.
◆ Record initial amount and type of drainage, and document the patient's respiratory status.
◆ Note the frequency of system inspection, and record how often chest tubes were milked.
◆ Document amount, color, and consistency of drainage; note condition of the chest dressings.
◆ Record pain drugs given.
◆ Document complications and nursing actions taken.

SELECTED REFERENCES
Bruce, E.A., et al. "Chest Drain Removal Pain and Its Management: A Literature Review," *Journal of Clinical Nursing* 15(2):145-54, February 2006.
Carroll, P. "Keeping Up with Mobile Chest Drains," *RN* 68(10):26-31, October 2005.
Roman, M., and Mercado, D. "Review of Chest Tube Use," *Medsurg Nursing* 15(1):41-43, February 2006.

Thoracic electrical bioimpedance monitoring

OVERVIEW

DESCRIPTION

- The procedure is a noninvasive alternative for tracking hemodynamic status, providing information about a patient's cardiac index, preload, afterload, contractility, cardiac output, and blood flow.
- It eliminates the risk of infection, bleeding, pneumothorax, emboli, and arrhythmias associated with traditional invasive monitoring.
- Electrodes are placed on the patient's thorax to send harmless low-level electricity through the body and detect return electrical signals (interruptions in the electrical flow), which come from changes in the volume and velocity of blood as it flows through the aorta.
- A bioimpedance monitor interprets the signals as a waveform.
- Cardiac output is computed from the heart rate on the electrocardiogram (ECG) monitor and the stroke volume calculated by the thoracic fluid content.
- Accuracy of monitoring is comparable to thermodilution.
- The monitor updates information every second to tenth heartbeat.

CONTRAINDICATIONS

- None known

EQUIPMENT

Thoracic electrical bioimpedance unit ◆ patient harness with color-coded leadwires ◆ connecting cable ◆ four sets of thoracic electrical bioimpedance electrodes ◆ three ECG electrodes ◆ $3'' \times 3''$ or $4'' \times 4''$ gauze pads ◆ tape measure ◆ gloves

PREPARATION

- Confirm the patient's identity using two patient identifiers according to facility policy.
- Explain the procedure to the patient.
- Wash your hands and put on gloves.
- Plug the thoracic electrical bioimpedance unit into a power supply.
- Press the POWER button: the initial display screen will appear.
- Press the RUN key on the display screen: the patient data screen will appear.
- Enter patient data by pressing each patient data block on the screen. When you select METRIC or ENGLISH for numbers, MALE or FEMALE, and ADULT or PED-NEO, a dot will appear beside your choice.
- To enter data for identification number, thoracic length, height, and weight, press the block that identifies the index you wish to include. Afterward, the numeric keypad screen will appear.
- Enter the actual value for the chosen index by pressing the smaller blocks on the keypad; then press ENTER to return to the patient data screen. Repeat for each index needed.
- Next, press the block on the patient data screen to call up the waveform screen to monitor patient status.
- The waveform screen displays ECG and a pulmonary artery pressure waveform as well as six parameters that you choose by pressing PARAMETERS.
- When the parameter screen appears, press the blocks labeled with the parameters you wish to display on the waveform screen.
- Press the block at the bottom of the parameter screen to return to the waveform screen. All of the selected parameters will now appear on the waveform screen.

KEY STEPS

- Assist the patient onto his back; provide privacy and expose his chest.
- Wet $4'' \times 4''$ or $3'' \times 3''$ gauze pads with warm water and clean the skin on each side of the patient's neck from the base to 2" (5 cm) above the base. Clean the skin on both sides of his chest at the midaxillary line directly across the xiphoid process.
- Clean at least two fingerbreadths above and below the site.
- Place one electrode set vertically at the neck base below the ear with the arrow end (containing the round electrode) pointing down.
- Place the bar electrode at least 2" (5 cm) above the round electrode.
- If the two electrodes are an attached set, place the bar electrode directly above the round one.
- Place the second set of electrodes on the opposite side of the neck in line with the ear and about 180 degrees from the first set.
- Place the remaining two sets of electrodes on either side of the patient's chest.
- To determine the correct location, draw a line with your finger from the xiphoid process to the midaxillary line on one side of the chest. This is the site for the first chest electrode.
- Place the round electrode here with the arrow pointing up.
- Place the second (bar) electrode at least 2" (5 cm) below the first. Alternatively, if you're using an attached set of electrodes, place the bar electrode directly below the round one.
- Place the final set of electrodes on the midaxillary line directly opposite the first set of electrodes.
- Attach ECG electrodes and try different lead selections until you obtain a consistent QRS signal.

WARNING *Don't remove the patient from the primary monitor. The regular system must be maintained to ensure monitoring at the central station and to keep the alarms intact.*

◆ Attach the leadwires of the bioimpedance harness to the thoracic electrical bioimpedance electrodes and the ECG electrodes.
◆ Attach the harness cable to the cable from the bioimpedance monitor.
◆ Measure the distance between the round electrode on one side of the patient's neck and the round electrode on the same side of the chest. This distance (thorax length) is the numeric value required by the monitor's computer to calculate accurate stroke volume.
◆ Call up the patient data screen and enter this value; then return to the waveform screen.

SPECIAL CONSIDERATIONS

◆ Baseline bioimpedance values may be reduced in patients who have conditions characterized by increased fluid in the chest, such as pulmonary edema and pleural effusion.
◆ Bioimpedance values may be lower than thermodilution values in patients with tachycardia and other arrhythmias.

TROUBLESHOOTER *If you fail to get a clear waveform, place the bar electrode on each side of the patient's forehead, which increases the distance between the electrodes and usually improves the waveform quality.*

COMPLICATIONS
◆ None known

PATIENT TEACHING

◆ Explain the procedure to the patient as needed.

DOCUMENTATION

◆ Note the waveforms and values on the monitor and document the values by pressing PRINT on the waveform screen.
◆ Place the printed strip on the patient's chart.

SELECTED REFERENCES

Bougault, V., et al. "Does Thoracic Bioimpedance Accurately Determine Cardiac Output in COPD Patients during Maximal or Intermittent Exercise?" *Chest* 127(4):1122-31, April 2005.

Fortin, J., et al. "Non-Invasive Beat-to-Beat Cardiac Output Monitoring by an Improved Method of Transthoracic Bioimpedance Measurement," *Computers in Biology and Medicine* 36(11):1185-1203, November 2006.

Shochat, M., et al. "Internal Thoracic Impedance Monitoring: A Novel Method for the Preclinical Detection of Acute Heart Failure," *Cardiovascular Revascularization Medicine* 7(1):41-45, January-March 2006.

Topical drug application

OVERVIEW

DESCRIPTION

- Lotions, pastes, ointments, creams, powders, shampoos, and aerosol sprays are applied directly to skin surface.
- Topical drugs are absorbed through the epidermal layer into the dermis; extent of absorption depends on the vascularity of the region.
- Nitroglycerin, fentanyl, nicotine, and certain supplemental hormone replacements are used for systemic effects; most other topical drugs are used for local effects.
- Ointments have a fatty base, which is an ideal vehicle for such drugs as antimicrobials and antiseptics.
- Ointments should be applied two to three times a day to achieve therapeutic effect.

CONTRAINDICATIONS

- Broken skin
- Scarring

EQUIPMENT

Patient's drug record and chart ◆ prescribed drug ◆ gloves ◆ sterile tongue blades ◆ sterile 4″ × 4″ gauze pads ◆ transparent semipermeable dressing ◆ adhesive tape ◆ solvent (such as cottonseed oil)

KEY STEPS

- Verify the order on the patient's drug record by checking against the practitioner's order on the chart; make sure the label on the drug agrees with the drug order.
- Read the label again before you open the container and as you remove the drug from the container.
- Check the expiration date.
- Confirm the patient's identity using two patient identifiers according to facility policy.
- Provide privacy and explain the procedure.
- Wash your hands and put a glove on your dominant hand.
- Use gloves on both hands if exposure to body fluids is likely.
- Help the patient find a comfortable position and expose the area to be treated.
- Make sure the skin or mucous membrane is intact (unless the drug has been ordered to treat a skin lesion, such as an ulcer). Applying drug to broken or abraded skin may cause unwanted systemic absorption and result in irritation.
- If necessary, clean the skin of debris, including crusts, epidermal scales, and old drug. Change the glove if it becomes soiled.
- Open the container. Place the lid or cap upside down to prevent contamination of the inside surface.
- Remove a tongue blade from its sterile wrapper, and cover one end with drug from the tube or jar; transfer the drug from the tongue blade to your gloved hand.
- Apply the drug to the affected area with long, smooth strokes that follow the direction of hair growth.
- This technique avoids forcing drug into hair follicles, which can cause irritation and lead to folliculitis. Avoid excessive pressure when applying the drug, which could abrade the skin.
- To prevent contamination of the drug, use a new tongue blade each time you remove drug from the container.

REMOVING OINTMENT

- Wash your hands and put on gloves.
- Rub solvent on the gloves and apply it liberally to the treated area in the direction of hair growth. Alternatively, saturate a sterile gauze pad with solvent and use the pad to gently remove the ointment.
- Remove excess oil by gently wiping the area with a sterile gauze pad.
- Don't rub too hard when removing the drug; you could irritate the skin.

APPLYING OTHER TOPICAL DRUGS

- To apply shampoos, follow package directions. (See *Using medicated shampoos.*)
- To apply aerosol sprays, shake the container, if indicated, to completely mix the drug.
- Hold the container 6″ to 12″ (15 to 30 cm) from the skin, or follow manufacturer's recommendation. Spray a thin film of drug evenly over the treatment area.
- To apply powders, dry the skin surface, making sure to spread skin folds where moisture collects.
- Apply a thin layer of powder over the treatment area.
- To protect applied drugs and prevent them from soiling the patient's clothes, tape an appropriate sized sterile gauze pad or a transparent semipermeable dressing over the treated area.

WARNING *With certain drugs (such as topical steroids), semipermeable dressings may be contraindicated. Check drug information and cautions.*

- If you're applying a topical drug to the patient's hands or feet, cover the site with white cotton gloves for the hands or terrycloth scuffs for the feet.

AGE FACTOR *In children, where appropriate, topical drugs (such as steroids) should be covered only loosely with a diaper. Don't use plastic pants.*

- Assess the patient's skin for signs of irritation, allergic reaction, or breakdown.

SPECIAL CONSIDERATIONS

⚡ **WARNING** *Never apply drug without first removing previous applications to prevent skin irritation from accumulation of drug.*

◆ Wear gloves to prevent absorption by your own skin. If the patient has an infectious condition, use sterile gloves and dispose of old dressings according to facility policy.
◆ Don't apply ointments to mucous membranes as liberally as you would to skin; mucous membranes are usually moist and absorb ointment more quickly than skin.
◆ Don't apply too much ointment; it may cause irritation and discomfort, stain clothing and bedding, and make removal difficult.
◆ Never apply ointment to the eyelids or ear canal unless ordered. The ointment may congeal and occlude the tear duct or ear canal.
◆ Inspect the treated area frequently for adverse effects such as signs of allergic reaction.

COMPLICATIONS
◆ Skin irritation
◆ Rash
◆ Allergic reaction

PATIENT TEACHING

◆ Provide patient teaching for home use, as necessary.

Using medicated shampoos

Medicated shampoos include keratolytic and cytostatic agents, coal tar preparations, and lindane (gamma benzene hexachloride) solutions. They're used to treat such conditions as dandruff, psoriasis, and head lice, but are contraindicated in patients with broken or abraded skin.

Application instructions vary among brands; check the label on the shampoo before starting the procedure. Keep shampoo away from the patient's eyes; if any gets in his eyes, irrigate promptly with water. Selenium sulfide, used in cytostatic agents, is extremely toxic if ingested.

To apply a medicated shampoo:
◆ Prepare the patient.
◆ Shake the shampoo bottle well to mix solution.
◆ Wet the patient's hair and wring out excess water.
◆ Apply shampoo as directed on the label.
◆ Work into a lather, adding water as necessary. Part the hair and work the shampoo into the scalp; don't use your fingernails.
◆ Leave the shampoo on the scalp and hair as long as instructed, then rinse thoroughly.
◆ Towel-dry the patient's hair. After the hair is dry, comb or brush it.
◆ Use a fine-tooth comb to remove nits if necessary.

DOCUMENTATION

◆ Note drug and record the time, date and site of application.
◆ Document condition of the patient's skin at the time of application.
◆ Note subsequent effects of the drug.

SELECTED REFERENCES

Davies, E.H., and Molloy, A. "Comparison of Ethyl Chloride Spray with Topical Anaesthetic in Children Experiencing Venipuncture," *Paediatric Nursing* 18(3):39-43, April 2006.

Dunning, G. "The Choice, Application and Review of Topical Treatments for Skin Conditions," *Nursing Times* 101(4):55-56, January 2005.

Peters, J. "Exploring the Use of Emollient Therapy in Dermatological Nursing," *British Journal of Nursing* 14(9):494-502, May 2005.

Rudy, S.J., and Parham-Vetter, P.C. "Percutaneous Absorption of Topically Applied Medication," *Dermatology Nursing* 15(2):145-46, 150-52, April 2003.

Total parenteral nutrition

OVERVIEW

DESCRIPTION
- Total parenteral nutrition (TPN) refers to any nutrient solution, including lipids, given through a central venous line.
- Typically prescribed for anyone who can't absorb nutrients though the GI tract for more than 10 days.
- The solution contains protein, carbohydrates, electrolytes, vitamins, and trace minerals. A lipid emulsion provides the necessary fat.
- Most common delivery route for TPN is through a central venous catheter (CVC) into the superior vena cava.

CONTRAINDICATIONS
- Normally functioning GI tract
- Normal function to resume within 10 days
- Poor prognosis

EQUIPMENT

Bag or bottle of prescribed parenteral nutrition solution ◆ sterile I.V. tubing with attached extension tubing ◆ 0.22-micron filter (or 1.2-micron filter if solution contains lipids or albumin) ◆ reflux valve ◆ time tape ◆ alcohol pads ◆ electronic infusion pump ◆ portable glucose monitor ◆ scale ◆ intake and output record ◆ sterile gloves ◆ mask (optional)

PREPARATION
- Prepare the solution, patient, and equipment.
- Remove the solution from the refrigerator at least 1 hour before use to avoid pain, hypothermia, venous spasm, or venous constriction from chilled solution.
- Check the solution against the practitioner's order for correct patient name, expiration date, and formula components.
- Observe the container for cracks and the solution for cloudiness, turbidity, and particles; if present, return the solution to the pharmacy.
- If giving a total nutrient admixture solution, look for a brown layer on the solution, which indicates that the lipid emulsion has "cracked," or separated from the solution. If you see a brown layer, return the solution to the pharmacy.
- Confirm the patient's identity using two patient identifiers according to facility policy, and verify matching name on the solution container.
- Explain the procedure to the patient.
- Put on gloves and, if specified by policy, a mask. Throughout the procedure, use strict aseptic technique.
- In sequence, connect the pump tubing, the micron filter with attached extension tubing (if the tubing doesn't contain an in-line filter), and the reflux valve.
- Insert the filter as close to the catheter site as possible.
- If the tubing doesn't have luer-lock connections, tape all connections to prevent separation, which could lead to air embolism, exsanguination, and sepsis.
- Squeeze the I.V. drip chamber and, holding the drip chamber upright, insert the tubing spike into the I.V. bag or bottle.
- Release the drip chamber, and prime the tubing.
- Invert the filter at the distal end of the tubing; open the roller clamp; let solution fill the tubing and the filter. Tap it to dislodge air bubbles in the Y-ports.
- If indicated, attach a time tape to the parenteral nutrition container.
- Record the date and time you hung the fluid, and initial the parenteral nutrition solution container.
- Attach the setup to the infusion pump, and prepare it according to manufacturer's instructions. Remove and discard gloves.
- With the patient supine, flush the catheter with normal saline solution, according to facility policy; put on gloves and clean the catheter injection cap with an alcohol pad.

KEY STEPS

- If the container of parenteral nutrition solution is attached to a central venous line, clamp the central venous line before disconnecting it to prevent air from entering the catheter.
- If a clamp isn't available, have the patient perform Valsalva's maneuver just as you change the tubing, if possible. If he's being mechanically ventilated, change I.V. tubing right after the machine delivers a breath at peak inspiration. These measures increase intrathoracic pressure and prevent air embolism.
- Using aseptic technique, attach tubing to the designated luer-locking port.
- After connecting the tubing, remove the clamp, if applicable.
- Set the infusion pump at the ordered flow rate, and start the infusion.
- Check to make sure the catheter junction is secure; tag tubing with date and time of change.
- Because parenteral nutrition solution often contains a large amount of glucose, start the infusion slowly.
- Parenteral nutrition is usually initiated at a rate of 40 to 50 ml/hour; then advanced by 25 ml/hour every 6 hours (as tolerated) until the desired infusion rate is achieved.
- If the glucose concentration is low, initiate the rate necessary to infuse the complete 24-hour volume and discontinue the solution without tapering.
- A parenteral nutrition solution container can hang for 24 hours.

CHANGING SOLUTIONS
- Prepare the new solution and I.V. tubing as described earlier. Put on gloves.
- Remove the protective caps from the solution containers; wipe the tops of containers with alcohol pads; turn off the infusion pump and close the flow clamps.
- Using strict aseptic technique, remove the spike from the solution container that's hanging and insert it into the new container.
- Hang the new container and tubing alongside the old. Turn on the infu-

sion pump, set the flow rate, and open the flow clamp completely.

◆ If attaching the solution to a peripheral line, examine the skin above the insertion site for redness and warmth and assess for pain.

⚡ **WARNING** *If you suspect phlebitis, remove the existing I.V. line and start a line in a different vein. Insert a new line if the I.V. catheter has been in place for 72 hours or more to reduce risk of phlebitis and infiltration.*

◆ Turn off the infusion pump, and close the flow clamp on the old tubing.

◆ Disconnect the tubing from the catheter hub, and connect new tubing.

◆ Open the flow clamp on the new container to a moderately slow rate.

◆ Remove the old tubing from the infusion pump, and insert the new tubing according to manufacturer's instructions.

◆ Turn on the infusion pump, set it to the desired flow rate, and open the flow clamp completely. Remove the old equipment and dispose of it properly.

SPECIAL CONSIDERATIONS

◆ Always infuse a parenteral nutrition solution at a constant rate without interruption to avoid blood glucose fluctuations. If the infusion slows, consult the practitioner before changing the infusion rate.

◆ Monitor vital signs every 4 hours or more often if necessary. Watch for increased temperature, an early sign of catheter-related sepsis.

◆ Check the patient's glucose every 6 hours. Some patients may require supplementary insulin, either subcutaneously or added to the solution.

◆ Record daily intake and output accurately, specifying volume and type of each fluid, and calculate daily caloric intake.

◆ Monitor results of routine laboratory tests; report abnormal findings to the practitioner.

◆ Such tests typically include measurement of:

– electrolytes, calcium, urea nitrogen, creatinine, and glucose levels at least three times weekly

– magnesium and phosphorus levels twice weekly

– liver function studies, complete blood count and differential, and albumin and transferrin levels, urine nitrogen balance, and creatinine-height index studies weekly

– zinc level at the start of parenteral nutrition therapy.

◆ The practitioner may also order prealbumin, total lymphocyte count, fatty acid-phospholipid fraction, amino acid levels, skin testing, and expired gas analysis.

◆ Weigh the patient each morning and suspect fluid imbalance if he gains more than 1 lb (0.5 kg) daily.

◆ Change the dressing over the catheter according to facility policy or whenever the dressing becomes wet, soiled, or nonocclusive.

◆ Always use strict aseptic technique. When performing dressing changes, watch for signs of phlebitis and catheter retraction from the vein. Measure the catheter length from the insertion site to the hub for verification.

◆ Change tubing and filters every 24 hours or according to facility policy.

◆ Monitor the catheter site for swelling, which may indicate infiltration. Extravasation of parenteral nutrition solution can lead to tissue necrosis.

◆ Don't use a single-lumen CVC to infuse blood or blood products, give a bolus injection, give simultaneous I.V. solutions, measure central venous pressure, or draw blood for laboratory tests.

◆ Provide regular mouth care.

◆ Provide emotional support; patients commonly associate eating with positive feelings and become disturbed when they can't eat.

COMPLICATIONS

◆ Catheter-related sepsis (most serious)

◆ Thrombosis

◆ Sepsis

◆ Air embolism

◆ Extravasation causing necrosis and sloughing of epidermis and dermis

PATIENT TEACHING

◆ Explain that long-term parenteral nutrition may be given at home and reduces need for long hospitalizations.

◆ Meet before discharge to make sure that the patient knows how to perform the administration procedure and how to handle complications.

◆ Teach the patient about potential adverse effects and complications.

◆ Encourage the patient to inspect his mouth regularly for signs of parotitis, glossitis, and oral lesions.

◆ Explain that fewer bowel movements may occur while the patient is receiving therapy.

◆ Encourage the patient to remain physically active to help the body use nutrients more fully.

DOCUMENTATION

◆ Record the times of dressing, filter, and solution changes.

◆ Note the condition of catheter insertion site.

◆ Document observations of the patient's condition.

◆ Record complications and interventions.

SELECTED REFERENCES

Driscoll, D.F. "Stability and Compatibility Assessment Techniques for Total Parenteral Nutrition Admixtures: Setting the Bar According to Pharmacopeial Standards," *Current Opinion in Clinical Nutrition & Metabolic Care* 8(3): 297-303, May 2005.

Hamilton, H. "Complications Associated with Venous Access Devices: Part One," *Nursing Standard* 20(26):43-50, March 2006.

Muhlebach, S. "Practical Aspects of Multichamber Bags for Total Parenteral Nutrition," *Current Opinion in Clinical Nutrition & Metabolic Care* 8(3):291-95, May 2005.

Total parenteral nutrition monitoring

OVERVIEW

DESCRIPTION

- Total parenteral nutrition (TPN) therapy causes marked changes in fluid and electrolyte status and in glucose, amino acid, mineral, and vitamin levels.
- TPN requires careful monitoring because the patient is typically in a protein-wasting state.
- If adverse reactions or complications occur, the regimen can be changed as needed.
- Assessment of nutritional status includes a physical examination, anthropometric measurements, biochemical determinations, and tests of cell-mediated immunity.
- Because TPN solution is high in glucose content, the infusion must start slowly to allow pancreatic beta cells to adapt by increasing insulin output.
- Within the first 3 to 5 days, the typical adult patient can tolerate 3 L of solution daily without adverse reactions.
- Lipid emulsions also require monitoring.

CONTRAINDICATIONS

- None known

EQUIPMENT

TPN solution and administration equipment ◆ blood glucose meter ◆ stethoscope ◆ sphygmomanometer ◆ watch with second hand ◆ scale ◆ input and output chart ◆ time tape ◆ additional equipment for nutritional assessment, as ordered

PREPARATION

- Attach a time tape to the TPN container to allow approximate measurement of fluid intake.
- Make sure each bag or bottle has a label listing expiration date, glucose concentration, and total volume of solution.
- If the bag or bottle is damaged and you don't have an immediate replacement, hang a bag of dextrose 10% in water until a new container is ready.

KEY STEPS

- Confirm the patient's identity using two patient identifiers according to facility policy.
- Explain the procedure to the patient.
- Record the patient's vital signs every 4 hours or more often if necessary; increased temperature is an early signs of catheter-related sepsis.
- Perform I.V. site care and dressing changes at least three times per week (once per week for transparent semipermeable dressings) or whenever the dressing becomes wet, soiled, or nonocclusive.
- Use strict aseptic technique and physically assess the patient daily. If ordered, measure arm circumference and skinfold thickness over the triceps.
- Weigh the patient at the same time each morning (after voiding), in similar clothing, on the same scale. Compare data with fluid intake and output record.

- Weight gain, particularly early in treatment, may indicate fluid overload rather than increasing fat and protein stores. The patient shouldn't gain more than 3 lb (1.4 kg) a week; a gain of 1 lb (0.5 kg) a week is a reasonable goal for most patients.
- Suspect fluid imbalance if he gains more than 1 lb daily; assess for peripheral and pulmonary edema.
- Monitor for signs and symptoms of glucose metabolism disturbance, fluid and electrolyte imbalances, and nutritional aberrations.
- Some patients may require supplemental insulin for the duration of TPN; the pharmacy usually adds insulin directly to the TPN solution.
- Monitor levels daily for electrolytes and twice per week for albumin. As the patient's condition stabilizes, these values won't need monitoring as closely.
- In a severely dehydrated patient, albumin levels may drop initially as treatment restores hydration.
- If magnesium and calcium have been added to the TPN solution, the dosage may need adjusted to maintain normal levels. Assess for magnesium and calcium imbalances.
- Monitor glucose levels every 6 hours initially, then once per day; stay alert for signs and symptoms of hyperglycemia, such as thirst and polyuria.
- Periodically confirm blood glucose meter readings with laboratory tests.
- Check renal function by monitoring blood urea nitrogen and creatinine levels; increases may indicate excess amino acid intake.
- Assess nitrogen balance with 24-hour urine collection; assess liver function by monitoring liver enzyme, bilirubin, triglyceride, and cholesterol levels.
- Abnormal values may indicate an intolerance or excess of lipid emulsions or problems with metabolizing the protein or glucose in the TPN formula.
- Change the I.V. administration set according to facility policy. Use aseptic technique and coordinate the change with a solution change.

- The tubing, injection caps, stop-cocks, catheter, and patient's skin are potential sources of microbial contamination. The catheter hub, where most manipulations take place, is especially vulnerable.
- Many facilities require changing I.V. administration sets every 24 hours; some now wait 48 to 72 hours. Because risk of contamination is high with TPN, facilities should routinely evaluate protocols based on quality-control findings.
- Monitor for inflammation, infection, fever, or sepsis. Microbial contamination of the venous access device is the usual cause. Watch for redness and drainage at the venous access site.
- While weaning the patient from TPN, document his dietary intake and work with the nutritionist to determine the total calorie and protein intake.
- Instruct other health care staff caring for the patient to record food intake.
- Use percentages of food consumed ("ate 50% of a baked potato") instead of subjective descriptions ("had a good appetite") for a more accurate account of intake.
- Provide emotional support; patients often associate eating with positive feelings and become disturbed when eating is prohibited.
- Provide frequent mouth care, and keep the patient active to enable him to use nutrients more fully.
- When discontinuing TPN, decrease the infusion rate slowly, depending on the patient's current glucose intake, to minimize risk of hyperinsulinemia and resulting hypoglycemia.
- Weaning usually takes place over 24 to 48 hours but can be completed in 4 to 6 hours if the patient receives sufficient oral or I.V. carbohydrates.

SPECIAL CONSIDERATIONS

- Always maintain strict aseptic technique when handling equipment.
- Because the TPN solution serves as a medium for bacterial growth and the central venous line provides systemic access, there are risks of infection and sepsis.
- When using a filter, position it as close to the access site as possible. Check the filter's porosity and pounds-per-square-inch (psi) capacity to make sure it exceeds the number of psi exerted by the infusion pump.
- Don't allow TPN solutions to hang for more than 24 hours.
- Be careful when using the TPN line for other functions. If using a single-lumen catheter, don't use the line to infuse blood or blood products, to give a bolus injection, to give simultaneous I.V. solutions, to measure pressure, or to draw blood for laboratory tests.

⚡ **WARNING** *Never add drug to a TPN solution container. Don't use a three-way stopcock, if possible, because add-on devices increase the risk of infection.*

- For a severely malnourished patient, starting TPN may spark "refeeding syndrome" (a rapid drop in potassium, magnesium, and phosphorus levels).
- To avoid compromising cardiac function, initiate feeding slowly and monitor blood values closely until they stabilize.

COMPLICATIONS
- Catheter-, metabolic-, and mechanical-related

PATIENT TEACHING

- Explain the procedure to the patient to lessen anxiety and gain cooperation.
- Tell the patient to inform you if any unusual sensations occur during the infusion.

DOCUMENTATION

- Record serial monitoring indexes on the appropriate flowchart to determine the patient's progress and response.
- Note abnormal, adverse, or altered responses.

SELECTED REFERENCES
Fox, V.J., et al. "Nutritional Support in the Critically Injured," *Critical Care Nursing Clinics of North America* 16(4):559-69, December 2004.

Guenter, P., et al. "The Impact of Nursing Practice on the History and Effectiveness of Total Parenteral Nutrition," *Journal of Parenteral and Enteral Nutrition* 28(1):54-59, January-February 2004.

Naylor, C.J., et al. "Does a Multidisciplinary Total Parenteral Nutrition Team Improve Patient Outcomes? A Systematic Review," *Journal of Parenteral and Enteral Nutrition* 28(4):251-58, July-August 2004.

Scolapio, J.S. "A Review of the Trends in the Use of Enteral and Parenteral Nutrition Support," *Journal of Clinical Gastroenterology* 38(5):403-407, May-June 2004.

Tracheal cuff pressure measurement

DESCRIPTION

- A tracheal cuff provides a closed system for mechanical ventilation, allowing a desired tidal volume to be delivered to the patient's lungs.
- To function properly, it must exert enough pressure on the tracheal wall to seal the airway without compromising the blood supply to the tracheal mucosa.
- The ideal pressure (minimal occlusive volume) is the lowest amount needed to seal the airway.
- Many authorities recommend maintaining a cuff pressure lower than venous perfusion pressure — about 16 to 24 cm H_2O (more than 24 cm H_2O may exceed venous perfusion pressure). Actual cuff pressure will vary.
- To keep pressure within safe limits, measure minimal occlusive volume at least once each shift or as directed by facility policy.
- Cuff pressure can be measured by a respiratory therapist or by the nurse.

CONTRAINDICATIONS

- None known

10-ml syringe ◆ three-way stopcock ◆ cuff pressure ◆ manometer ◆ stethoscope ◆ suction equipment ◆ gloves

PREPARATION

- Assemble all equipment at the patient's bedside.
- If measuring with a blood pressure manometer, attach the syringe to one stopcock port, then attach the tubing from the manometer to another port of the stopcock.
- Turn off the stopcock port where you'll be connecting the pilot balloon cuff so air can't escape from the cuff.
- Use the syringe to instill air into the manometer tubing until the pressure reading reaches 10 mm Hg. This will prevent sudden cuff deflation when you open the stopcock to the cuff and the manometer.

- Confirm the patient's identity using two patient identifiers according to facility policy.
- Explain the procedure to the patient.
- Put on gloves and suction the endotracheal or tracheostomy tube and the patient's oropharynx to remove accumulated secretions above the cuff.
- Attach the cuff pressure manometer to the pilot balloon port.
- Place the diaphragm of the stethoscope over the trachea and listen for an air leak (as shown below).

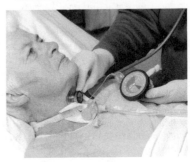

- A smooth, hollow sound indicates a sealed airway; a loud gurgle indicates an air leak.
- If you don't hear an air leak, press the red button under the dial of the cuff pressure manometer to slowly release air from the balloon on the tracheal tube (as shown below).

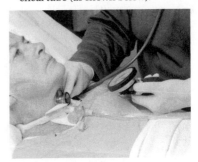

- Auscultate for an air leak.

◆ When you hear an air leak, release the red button and gently squeeze the handle of the cuff pressure manometer to inflate the cuff (as shown below). Continue to add air to the cuff until you no longer hear an air leak.

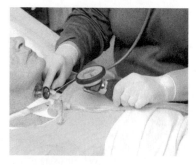

◆ When the air leak ceases, read the dial on the cuff pressure manometer (as shown below).

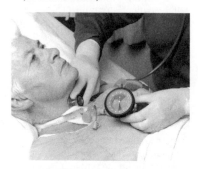

◆ This is the minimal pressure required to effectively occlude the trachea around the tracheal tube. In many cases, this pressure will fall within the green area (16 to 24 cm H_2O) on the manometer dial.
◆ Disconnect the cuff pressure manometer from the pilot balloon port. Document the pressure value.

SPECIAL CONSIDERATIONS

◆ Measure cuff pressure at least every 8 hours to avoid overinflation.
◆ Some patients require less pressure, but others — such as those with tracheal malacia (an abnormal softening of the tracheal tissue) — require more pressure.
◆ Maintaining cuff pressure at the lowest possible level will minimize cuff-related problems.
◆ When measuring cuff pressure, keep the connection between the measuring device and the pilot balloon port tight to avoid an air leak that could compromise cuff pressure.
◆ If using a stopcock, don't leave the manometer in the OFF position because air will leak from the cuff if the syringe accidentally comes off.
◆ Note the volume of air needed to inflate the cuff.

WARNING *A gradual increase in volume indicates tracheal dilation or erosion. A sudden increase in volume indicates rupture of the cuff and requires immediate reintubation if the patient is being ventilated.*

COMPLICATIONS

◆ Aspiration of upper airway secretions
◆ Underventilation
◆ Coughing spasms

PATIENT TEACHING

◆ Explain the procedure to the patient as needed.

DOCUMENTATION

◆ Record the date and time of the procedure.
◆ Note cuff pressure.
◆ Document the total amount of air in the cuff after the procedure.
◆ Record complications and nursing actions taken.
◆ Note the patient's tolerance of the procedure.

SELECTED REFERENCES

Galinski, M., et al. "Intracuff Pressure of Endotracheal Tubes in the Management of Airway Emergencies: The Need for Pressure Monitoring," *Annals of Emergency Medicine* 47(6):545-47, June 2006.
Hoffman, R.J., et al. "Experienced Emergency Medicine Physicians Cannot Safely Inflate or Estimate Endotracheal Tube Cuff Pressure Using Standard Techniques," *American Journal of Emergency Medicine* 24(2):139-43, March 2006.
Stewart, S.L., et al. "A Comparison of Endotracheal Tube Cuff Pressures Using Estimation Techniques and Direct Intracuff Measurement," *AANA Journal* 71(6):443-47, December 2003.
Young, P.J., et al. "A Low-Volume, Low-Pressure Tracheal Tube Cuff Reduces Pulmonary Aspiration," *Critical Care Medicine* 34(3):632-39, March 2006.

Tracheal suction

DESCRIPTION

- Tracheal suction involves removal of secretions from the trachea or bronchi by means of a catheter inserted through the mouth or nose, tracheal stoma, a tracheostomy tube, or an endotracheal (ET) tube.
- Suction stimulates the cough reflex and helps maintain a patent airway; it's done as frequently as condition warrants and calls for strict aseptic technique.

CONTRAINDICATIONS

- None known

EQUIPMENT

Oxygen source (wall or portable unit, and handheld resuscitation bag with a mask ◆ 15-mm adapter or a positive end-expiratory pressure [PEEP] valve, if indicated) ◆ wall or portable suction apparatus ◆ collection container ◆ connecting tube ◆ suction catheter kit or a sterile suction catheter, one sterile glove, one clean glove, goggles, and a disposable sterile solution container ◆ 1 L bottle of sterile water or normal saline solution ◆ sterile water-soluble lubricant (for nasal insertion) ◆ syringe for deflating cuff of ET or tracheostomy tube ◆ waterproof trash bag ◆ sterile towel (optional)

PREPARATION

- Choose a suction catheter of appropriate size; diameter should be no larger than one-half the inside diameter of the tracheostomy or ET tube to minimize hypoxia during suctioning. (A #12 or #14 French catheter may be used for an 8-mm or larger tube.)
- Place the suction apparatus on the overbed table or bedside stand.
- Attach the collection container to the suction unit and the connecting tube to the collection container.
- Label and date the normal saline solution or sterile water.
- Open the waterproof trash bag.

KEY STEPS

- Obtain a practitioner's order, if required.
- Confirm the patient's identity using two patient identifiers according to facility policy.
- Assess the patient's vital signs, breath sounds, and appearance to establish a baseline.
- Review arterial blood gas values and oxygen saturation levels if available.
- Evaluate the patient's ability to cough and deep breathe.
- If performing nasotracheal suctioning, check for a deviated septum, nasal polyps, nasal obstruction, nasal trauma, epistaxis, or mucosal swelling.
- Wash your hands and put on protective equipment.
- Unless contraindicated, put the patient in semi-Fowler's or high Fowler's position.
- Remove the top from the normal saline solution or water bottle, and open the package containing the sterile solution container.
- Using strict aseptic technique, open the suction catheter kit and put on gloves.
- If using individual supplies, open the suction catheter and the gloves, placing the nonsterile glove on your nondominant hand, then the sterile glove on your dominant hand.
- Using your nondominant (nonsterile) hand, pour the normal saline solution or sterile water into the solution container.
- Place a small amount of water-soluble lubricant on the sterile area to facilitate passage of the catheter during nasotracheal suctioning.
- Place a sterile towel over the patient's chest to provide an additional sterile area.
- Using your dominant (sterile) hand, remove the catheter from its wrapper. Keep it coiled so it can't touch a nonsterile object. Using your other hand to manipulate the connecting tubing, attach the catheter to the tubing.

- Using your nondominant hand, set the suction pressure according to facility policy; typically between 80 and 120 mm Hg. Occlude the suction port to assess suction pressure.
- Dip the catheter tip in saline solution to lubricate the outside of the catheter.
- With the catheter tip in the sterile solution, occlude the control valve with the thumb of your nondominant hand. Suction a small amount of solution through the catheter to lubricate the inside and ease passage of secretions.
- For nasal insertion, lubricate the tip of the catheter with the sterile, water-soluble lubricant.
- If the patient isn't intubated or is intubated but not receiving oxygen, instruct him to take three to six deep breaths to minimize or prevent hypoxia during suctioning.
- If the patient isn't intubated but is receiving oxygen, evaluate his need for preoxygenation. If indicated, instruct him to take three to six deep breaths while using his supplemental oxygen.
- The patient may leave his nasal cannula in one nostril or keep the oxygen mask over his mouth.
- If he's being mechanically ventilated, preoxygenate him using either a handheld resuscitation bag or the sigh mode on the ventilator.
- To use the resuscitation bag, set the oxygen flow meter at 15 L/minute, disconnect the patient from the ventilator, and deliver three to six breaths with the resuscitation bag.
- If the patient is being maintained on PEEP, use a resuscitation bag with a PEEP valve.
- To preoxygenate using the ventilator, first adjust the fraction of inspired oxygen (FIO_2) and tidal volume according to facility policy and patient need. Then, use either the sigh mode or manually deliver three to six breaths.

NASOTRACHEAL INSERTION IN A NONINTUBATED PATIENT

◆ Disconnect the oxygen from the patient, if applicable.
◆ Using your nondominant hand, raise the tip of the patient's nose.
◆ Insert the catheter into his nostril while rolling it between your fingers.
◆ As he inhales, quickly advance the catheter as far as possible.

⬛ **WARNING** *To avoid oxygen loss and tissue trauma, don't apply suction during insertion.*

◆ If the patient coughs as the catheter passes through the larynx, briefly hold the catheter still, then resume advancement when the patient inhales.

INSERTION IN AN INTUBATED PATIENT

◆ If you're using a closed system, the closed tracheal suctioning technique may be used.
◆ Using your nonsterile hand, disconnect the patient from the ventilator.
◆ Using your sterile hand, insert the suction catheter into the artificial airway.
◆ Advance the catheter, without applying suction, until you meet resistance.
◆ If the patient coughs, pause; then resume advancement.

SUCTIONING THE PATIENT

◆ After inserting the catheter, apply suction intermittently by removing and replacing the thumb of your nondominant hand over the control valve.
◆ Simultaneously use your dominant hand to withdraw the catheter as you roll it between your thumb and forefinger to prevent tissue damage.

⬛ **WARNING** *To prevent hypoxia, never suction more than 10 seconds at a time.*

◆ If the patient is intubated, use your nondominant hand to stabilize the tip of the ET tube as you withdraw the catheter.
◆ If applicable, resume oxygen delivery to hyperoxygenate the patient's lungs before continuing, to prevent or relieve hypoxia.

◆ Allow him to rest a few minutes before the next suctioning.
◆ Encourage the patient to cough between suctioning attempts.
◆ If secretions are thick, clear the catheter periodically by dipping the tip in the normal saline solution and applying suction.
◆ Watch for color variations.
◆ When sputum contains blood, note whether it's streaked or well mixed.
◆ If arrhythmias occur, stop suctioning and ventilate the patient.

AFTER SUCTIONING

◆ Hyperoxygenate the patient maintained on a ventilator with the handheld resuscitation bag or by using the ventilator's sigh mode.
◆ Readjust the FIO_2 and, for ventilated patients, the tidal volume to ordered settings.
◆ After suctioning the lower airway, assess the need for upper airway suctioning.
◆ If the cuff of the ET or tracheostomy tube is inflated, suction the upper airway before deflating the cuff with a syringe.

⬛ **WARNING** *Always change the catheter and sterile glove before resuctioning the lower airway to avoid introducing microorganisms into the lower airway.*

◆ Clear connecting tubing by aspirating the remaining normal saline solution or water.
◆ Discard your gloves and the catheter in the waterproof trash bag and wash your hands.
◆ Auscultate the lungs bilaterally and take vital signs, if indicated, to assess the procedure's effectiveness.

SPECIAL CONSIDERATIONS

◆ Raising the patient's nose into the sniffing position helps align the larynx and pharynx.
◆ Using an angled catheter may help you guide the catheter into the left mainstem bronchus.

COMPLICATIONS

◆ Anxiety that alters respiratory patterns
◆ Tracheal or bronchial trauma
◆ Hypoxemia, dyspnea, arrhythmias, hypertension, or hypotension especially in patients with compromised cardiovascular or pulmonary status
◆ Increased intracranial pressure (ICP) in patients who already have increased ICP
◆ Laryngospasm or bronchospasm

PATIENT TEACHING

◆ Explain the procedure and provide reassurance even if the patient is unresponsive, to minimize anxiety, promote relaxation, and decrease oxygen demand.
◆ Tell the patient that suctioning usually causes transient coughing or gagging, but that coughing will help remove secretions.

DOCUMENTATION

◆ Record the date, time, technique and reason for procedure.
◆ Document the amount, color, consistency, and odor of secretions.
◆ Record complications and nursing actions taken.
◆ Note pertinent data regarding patient's subjective response to procedure.

SELECTED REFERENCES

Bourgault, A.M., et al. "Effects of Endotracheal Tube Suctioning on Arterial Oxygen Tension and Heart Rate Variability," *Biological Research for Nursing* 7(4):268-78, April 2006.

Pruitt, B., and Jacobs, M. "Clearing away Pulmonary Secretions," *Nursing* 35(7): 36-41, July 2005.

Tracheostomy and ventilator speaking valve

DESCRIPTION

◆ The patient with a tracheostomy tube can't speak because the cuffed tracheostomy tube that directs air into the lungs expels air through the tracheostomy tube rather than the vocal cords, mouth, and nose.

◆ A positive-closure, one-way speaking valve opens upon inspiration and closes after expiration, redirecting exhaled air around the tube, through the vocal cords, allowing the patient to speak.

◆ To function safely, the tracheostomy cuff must be completely deflated to enable the patient to exhale, or the tracheostomy tube must be cuffless.

◆ Both valves fit the 15-mm hub of adult, pediatric, and neonatal tracheostomy tubes and can be used by patients on or off the ventilator.

◆ Short- and long-term adult, pediatric, and infant tracheostomy and ventilator-dependent patients may benefit from the use of a speaking valve.

◆ A speech-language pathologist should assess cognitive, language, and oral motor function and may evaluate swallowing status and risk for aspiration.

◆ A practitioner's order is required for placement of the Passey-Muir valve (PMV) and sometimes for cuff deflation.

CONTRAINDICATIONS

◆ Severe tracheal or laryngeal stenosis
◆ Laryngectomy
◆ Excessive oral secretions
◆ Unconscious patients or those at risk for gross aspiration

Appropriate size ventilator speaking valve ◆ gloves ◆ suction equipment ◆ 10-ml Luer-lock syringe ◆ instruction booklet

◆ Confirm the patient's identity using two patient identifiers according to facility policy.

◆ Elevate the head of the patient's bed about 45 degrees.

◆ The tracheostomy cuff must be completely deflated before valve is placed.

◆ Put on gloves and deflate the cuff slowly so the patient can get used to using his upper airways again. Attach a 10-ml syringe to the tracheostomy tube's pilot balloon and remove the air until air can no longer be extracted and a vacuum is created.

◆ Suction the trachea and oral cavity, as needed.

◆ Hold the valve between your fingers. For a patient who isn't ventilator-dependent, attach the valve to the hub of the existing tracheostomy hub with a quarter-turn twist.

◆ After the valve is in place, encourage the patient to relax and concentrate on exhaling through his mouth and nose.

◆ Have him count aloud to 10, or speak, as he becomes comfortable breathing with the valve in place. The speech-language pathologist can facilitate voice production and speech.

◆ The aqua-colored PMV 007 is more convenient for ventilator-dependent patients because it's tapered to fit into disposable ventilator tubing. Insert the PMV into the end of the wide-mouth, short flex tubing.

◆ Connect the other end of the short flex tubing to the ventilator tubing.

◆ Then attach the PMV (connected to the short flex tubing) and the ventilator tubing to the closed-suction system.

◆ The PMV can also be attached between the swivel adapter and the short flex tubing and ventilator tubing.

- Post cuff-deflation warning signs in the room and label the tracheostomy pilot balloon to remind health care providers to reinflate the pilot balloon after removing the PMV.
- Gently twist the PMV to remove it; restore the original setup, then return ventilator settings to original levels and reinflate the pilot balloon cuff. Always remember to reinflate the tracheostomy cuff after removing the PMV.

SPECIAL CONSIDERATIONS

- For maximum airflow around the tube, the tube shouldn't be larger than two-thirds the size of the tracheal lumen.
- Never place the PMV on the tracheostomy tube before deflating the cuff; the patient won't be able to breathe.
- The nurse and respiratory therapist are responsible for monitoring the patient's response to the PMV by evaluating blood pressure, heart rate, and respiratory status.
- Ensure that the patient is involved in the decision to use the ventilator speaking valve; make sure he understands how it functions and what to expect.
- If he's anxious, especially during cuff deflation, he may be unwilling to use the valve; provide emotional support.
- If he can't tolerate the valve initially; troubleshoot to determine the cause.

  TROUBLESHOOTER *To correct, try repositioning the patient, using a smaller tracheostomy tube, changing to a cuffless tube, or correcting airway obstruction. Some patients have to build tolerance, wearing the valve a few minutes at a time at first.*

- If repeated trials fail, the speech-language pathologist should assess the patient for other communication options.

  WARNING *Remove the PMV if the patient shows signs of distress: significant change in blood pressure or heart rate, increased respiratory rate, dyspnea, diaphoresis, anxiety, uncontrollable coughing, or arterial oxygen saturation less than 90%. Reassess him before trying the valve again.*

COMPLICATIONS
- None known

PATIENT TEACHING

- Explain the procedure to the patient. Provide written instructions, as needed.
- If this is the patient's first experience using a ventilator speaking valve, an initial trial should be coordinated with the respiratory therapist and speech-language pathologist.

DOCUMENTATION

- Note the patient's response to the procedure.
- Record how long the PMV has been in place.
- Document respiratory and hemodynamic status.
- Record secretion management.
- Note ability to vocalize.

SELECTED REFERENCES
Bier, J., et al. "Giving your Patient a Voice with a Tracheostomy Speaking Valve," *Nursing* 34 Suppl:16-18, October 2004.

Fukumoto, M., et al. "Ventilator Weaning Using a Fenestrated Tracheostomy Tube with a Speaking Valve," *Critical Care and Resuscitation* 8(2):117-19, June 2006.

Hess, D.R. "Facilitating Speech in the Patient with a Tracheostomy," *Respiratory Care* 50(4):519-25, April 2005.

Hull, E.M., et al. "Tracheostomy Speaking Valves for Children: Tolerance and Clinical Benefits," *Pediatric Rehabilitation* 8(3):214-19, July-September 2005.

Tracheostomy care

DESCRIPTION

- Tracheostomy care is required to ensure airway patency by keeping the tube free of mucus buildup, to maintain mucous membrane and skin integrity, prevent infection, and provide psychological support.
- It should be performed using aseptic technique until the stoma has healed.
- For recent tracheotomies, use sterile gloves for all manipulations at the site. After the stoma has healed, clean gloves may be substituted for sterile ones.
- Patient may have one of three types of tracheostomy tube: uncuffed, cuffed, or fenestrated. Selection depends on the patient's condition and practitioner's preference.
- An uncuffed plastic or metal tube allows air to flow freely around the tracheostomy tube and through the larynx, reducing risk of tracheal damage.
- A plastic cuffed tube is disposable. The cuff and the tube won't separate inside the trachea because the cuff is bonded to the tube; it doesn't require periodic deflating to lower pressure because cuff pressure is low and evenly distributed against the tracheal wall, reducing the risk of tracheal damage.
- A plastic fenestrated tube permits speech through the upper airway when the external opening is capped and the cuff is deflated. It also allows easy removal of the inner cannula for cleaning, but may become occluded.

CONTRAINDICATIONS

- None known

EQUIPMENT

ASEPTIC STOMA AND OUTER-CANNULA CARE

Waterproof trash bag ◆ two sterile solution containers ◆ sterile normal saline solution ◆ hydrogen peroxide ◆ sterile cotton-tipped applicators ◆ sterile 4″ × 4″ gauze pads ◆ sterile gloves ◆ prepackaged sterile tracheostomy dressing (or 4″ × 4″ gauze pad) ◆ supplies for suctioning and mouth care ◆ water-soluble lubricant or topical antibiotic cream ◆ materials for cuff procedures and changing tracheostomy ties (see below)

ASEPTIC INNER-CANNULA CARE

All preceding equipment plus a prepackaged commercial tracheostomy care set, or sterile forceps ◆ sterile nylon brush ◆ sterile 6″ (15-cm) pipe cleaners ◆ clean gloves ◆ a third sterile solution container ◆ disposable temporary inner cannula (for a patient on a ventilator)

CHANGING TRACHEOSTOMY TIES

30″ (76.2-cm) length of tracheostomy twill tape ◆ bandage scissors ◆ sterile gloves ◆ hemostat

EMERGENCY TRACHEOSTOMY TUBE REPLACEMENT

Sterile tracheal dilator or sterile hemostat ◆ sterile obturator that fits the tracheostomy tube ◆ extra, appropriate-sized, sterile tracheostomy tube and obturator ◆ suction equipment and supplies

CUFF PROCEDURES

5- or 10-ml syringe ◆ padded hemostat ◆ stethoscope

PREPARATION

- Wash your hands and assemble equipment and supplies in patient's room.
- Check the expiration date on each sterile package and inspect for tears.
- Place the open waterproof trash bag next to you to avoid reaching across the sterile field or the patient's stoma when discarding soiled items.
- Establish a sterile field near his bed and place equipment and supplies on it.
- Pour normal saline solution, hydrogen peroxide, or a mixture of equal parts of both solutions into one of the sterile solution containers; pour normal saline solution into the second sterile container for rinsing.
- For inner-cannula care, use a third sterile solution container to hold the gauze pads and cotton-tipped applicators saturated with cleaning solution.
- If replacing the disposable inner cannula, open the package containing the new inner cannula while maintaining sterile technique.
- Obtain or prepare new tracheostomy ties, if indicated.
- Keep supplies in full view for easy emergency access. Consider taping a wrapped, sterile tracheostomy tube to the head of the bed for emergencies.

- Confirm the patient's identity using two patient identifiers according to facility policy.
- Assess the patient's condition to determine need for care.
- Explain the procedure, even if the patient is unresponsive. Provide privacy.
- Place the patient in semi-Fowler's position, unless contraindicated, to decrease abdominal pressure on the diaphragm and promote lung expansion.
- Remove humidification or ventilation device.
- Using sterile technique, suction the entire length of the tracheostomy tube to clear the airway of secretions that may hinder oxygenation.
- Reconnect the patient to the humidifier or ventilator, if necessary.

CLEANING A STOMA AND OUTER CANNULA

- Put on sterile gloves if you aren't already wearing them.
- With your dominant hand, saturate a sterile gauze pad or cotton-tipped applicator with the cleaning solution.
- Squeeze out excess liquid to prevent accidental aspiration.
- Wipe the patient's neck under the tracheostomy tube flanges and twill tapes.
- Saturate a second pad or applicator, and wipe until the skin surrounding the tracheostomy is cleaned. Use additional pads or cotton-tipped applicators to clean the stoma site and the tube's flanges.

⚡ **WARNING** *Wipe only once with each pad or applicator to prevent contamination of a clean area.*

- Rinse debris and peroxide (if used) with one or more sterile 4″ × 4″ gauze pads dampened in normal saline solution.
- Dry the area thoroughly with additional sterile gauze pads; then apply a new sterile tracheostomy dressing. Remove and discard your gloves.

CLEANING A NONDISPOSABLE INNER CANNULA

- Put on sterile gloves. Using your nondominant hand, remove and discard the patient's tracheostomy dressing.
- With the same hand, disconnect the ventilator or humidification device, and unlock the tracheostomy tube's inner cannula by rotating it counterclockwise.
- Place the inner cannula in the container of hydrogen peroxide.
- Working quickly, use your dominant hand to scrub the cannula with the sterile nylon brush.
- If the brush doesn't slide easily into the cannula, then use a sterile pipe cleaner.
- Immerse the cannula in the container of normal saline solution, and agitate it for about 10 seconds to rinse it.
- Inspect the cannula for cleanliness. Repeat the cleaning process if necessary.
- If it's clean, tap it against the inside edge of the sterile container to remove excess liquid and prevent aspiration.

⚡ **WARNING** *Don't dry the outer surface; a film of moisture acts as a lubricant during insertion.*

- Reinsert the inner cannula into the patient's tracheostomy tube.
- Lock it in place and make sure it's positioned securely. Reconnect the mechanical ventilator. Apply a new sterile tracheostomy dressing.
- If the patient can't tolerate being disconnected from the ventilator for the time it takes to clean the inner cannula, replace the existing inner cannula with a clean one and reattach the mechanical ventilator. Then clean the cannula just removed and store it in a sterile container for the next time.

CARING FOR A DISPOSABLE INNER CANNULA

- Put on clean gloves. Using your dominant hand, remove the inner cannula.
- After evaluating the secretions in the cannula, discard it properly.

- Pick up the new inner cannula, touching only the outer locking portion. Insert the cannula into the tracheostomy and, following manufacturer's instructions, lock it securely.

CHANGING TRACHEOSTOMY TIES

- Get help from another nurse or a respiratory therapist to avoid accidental tube expulsion. Patient movement or coughing can dislodge the tube.
- Wash your hands and put on sterile gloves if you aren't already wearing them.
- If you aren't using commercially packaged tracheostomy ties, prepare new ties from a 30″ (76.2 cm) length of twill tape by folding one end back 1″ (2.5 cm) on itself, then, with bandage scissors, cutting a ½″ (1.5-cm) slit down the center of the tape from the folded edge.
- Prepare the other end of the tape the same way.
- Hold both ends together and cut the resulting circle of tape so one piece is about 10″ (25.5 cm) long and the other is about 20″ (51 cm) long.
- Assist the patient into semi-Fowler's position, if possible.
- After your assistant puts on gloves, instruct her to hold the tracheostomy tube in place to prevent expulsion during replacement of the ties. (If performing without assistance, fasten the clean ties in place before removing the old ties to prevent tube expulsion.)
- With the assistant's gloved fingers holding the tracheostomy tube in place, cut the soiled tracheostomy ties with bandage scissors or untie them and discard.

⚡ **WARNING** *Be careful not to cut the tube of the pilot balloon.*

- Thread the slit end of one new tie a short distance through the eye of one tracheostomy tube flange from the underside; use the hemostat, if needed, to pull the tie through. Thread the other end of the tie completely through the slit end and pull it taut so it loops firmly through the flange. This avoids knots that can cause throat discomfort, tissue irritation, pressure, and necrosis.

(continued)

- Fasten the second tie to the opposite flange in the same manner.
- Instruct the patient to flex his neck while you bring the ties around to the side, and tie them together with a square knot. Flexion produces the same neck circumference as coughing and helps prevent an overly tight tie.
- Have your assistant place one finger under the tapes as you tie them to ensure they're tight enough to avoid slippage but loose enough to prevent choking or jugular vein constriction.
- Placing the closure on the side allows easy access and prevents pressure necrosis at the back of the neck when the patient is recumbent.
- After securing the ties, cut off excess tape with scissors and have your assistant release the tracheostomy tube.
- Make sure the patient is comfortable and can reach the call button easily.

⚡ **WARNING** *Check tracheostomy-tie tension frequently on patients with traumatic injury, radical neck dissection, or cardiac failure because neck diameter can increase from swelling and cause constriction; also check neonatal or restless patients frequently because ties can loosen and cause tube dislodgment.*

CONCLUDING TRACHEOSTOMY CARE

- Replace the humidification device.
- Provide oral care as needed because the oral cavity can become dry and malodorous or develop sores from encrusted secretions.
- Observe soiled dressings and suctioned secretions for amount, color, consistency, and odor. Properly clean or dispose of equipment, supplies, solutions, and trash. Remove and discard your gloves.
- Make sure the patient is comfortable and can reach the call button easily.
- Make sure necessary supplies are readily available at the bedside.
- Repeat the procedure at least once every 8 hours, or as needed.

- Change the dressing as often as necessary regardless of whether you perform the entire cleaning procedure. A wet dressing with exudate or secretions predisposes the patient to skin excoriation, breakdown, and infection.

DEFLATING AND INFLATING A TRACHEOSTOMY CUFF

- Read the cuff manufacturer's instructions; cuff types and procedures vary.
- Assess the patient's condition, explain the procedure, and reassure him.
- Wash your hands.
- Help the patient into semi-Fowler's position, if possible, or place him in a supine position so secretions above the cuff site will be pushed up into his mouth if he's receiving positive-pressure ventilation.
- Suction the oropharyngeal cavity to prevent pooled secretions from descending into the trachea after cuff deflation.
- Release the padded hemostat clamping the cuff inflation tubing, if a hemostat is present.
- Insert a 5- or 10-ml syringe into the cuff pilot balloon and slowly withdraw all air from the cuff. Leave syringe attached to tubing for cuff reinflation.
- Slow deflation allows positive lung pressure to push secretions upward from the bronchi. Cuff deflation may also stimulate the cough reflex, producing additional secretions.
- Remove the ventilation device and suction the lower airway through the existing tube to remove all secretions.
- Reconnect the patient to the ventilation device.
- Maintain cuff deflation for the prescribed time.
- Observe for adequate ventilation, and suction as necessary.
- If the patient has difficulty breathing, reinflate the cuff immediately by depressing the syringe plunger very slowly.
- Use a stethoscope to listen over the trachea for the air leak, then inject as little air as necessary to achieve an adequate tracheal seal.

- When inflating the cuff, you may use the minimal-leak technique or the minimal occlusive volume technique to help gauge the proper inflation point.
- If inflating the cuff using cuff pressure measurement, don't exceed 25 mm Hg.

⚡ **WARNING** *Recommended cuff pressure is about 18 mm Hg. If pressure exceeds 25 mm Hg, notify the practitioner. You may need to change to a larger size tube, use higher inflation pressures, or permit a larger air leak.*

- After you've inflated the cuff, if the tubing doesn't have a one-way valve at the end, clamp the inflation line with a padded hemostat and remove the syringe.
- Check for a minimal-leak cuff seal. You shouldn't feel air coming from the patient's mouth, nose, or tracheostomy site, and a conscious patient shouldn't be able to speak.
- Be alert for air leaks from the cuff itself.

⚡ **WARNING** *Suspect a leak if injection of air fails to inflate the cuff or increase cuff pressure, if you're unable to inject the amount of air you withdrew, if the patient can speak, if ventilation fails to maintain adequate respiratory movement with pressures or volumes previously considered adequate, or if air escapes during the ventilator's inspiratory cycle.*

- Note the exact amount of air used to inflate the cuff to detect tracheal malacia if more air is consistently needed.
- Make sure the patient is comfortable and can easily reach the call button and communication aids.
- Properly clean or dispose of equipment, supplies, and trash according to facility policy.
- Replenish used supplies, and make sure all necessary emergency supplies are at the bedside.

- Keep appropriate equipment at the patient's bedside for immediate use in an emergency.
- Consult the practitioner about first-aid measures you can use for your tracheostomy patient should an emergency occur.

⚡ **WARNING** *Follow facility policy if a tracheostomy tube is expelled or the outer cannula becomes blocked. If breathing is obstructed, call the appropriate code and provide manual resuscitation with a handheld resuscitation bag or reconnect the patient to the ventilator. Don't remove the tracheostomy tube; the airway may close completely. Use caution when reinserting, to avoid tracheal trauma, perforation, compression, and asphyxiation.*

- Don't change the tracheostomy ties unnecessarily during the immediate postoperative period before the stoma track is well formed (usually 4 days) to avoid accidental dislodgment and expulsion of the tube. Unless secretions or drainage are a problem, ties can be changed once per day.
- Don't change a single-cannula tracheostomy tube or the outer cannula of a double-cannula tube. Because of the risk of tracheal complications, the practitioner usually changes the cannula; the frequency depends on the patient's condition.
- If the patient's neck or stoma is excoriated or infected, apply a water-soluble lubricant or topical antibiotic cream as ordered. Don't use a powder or oil-based substance on or around a stoma; aspiration can cause infection and abscess.
- Replace all equipment regularly (including solutions) to reduce risk of nosocomial infections.

COMPLICATIONS

- Hemorrhage at the operative site, causing drowning
- Bleeding or edema in tracheal tissue, causing airway obstruction
- Aspiration of secretions
- Introduction of air into pleural cavity, causing pneumothorax
- Hypoxia or acidosis, triggering cardiac arrest
- Introduction of air into surrounding tissues, causing subcutaneous emphysema
- Secretions under dressings and twill tape, causing skin excoriation and infection
- Hardened mucus or a slipped cuff occluding cannula opening and obstruct airway
- Tube displacement stimulating cough reflex if the tip rests on the carina, or causing blood vessel erosion and hemorrhage
- Tracheal erosion and necrosis

PATIENT TEACHING

- For discharge with a tracheostomy, start self-care teaching as soon as the patient is receptive.
- Teach the patient how to change and clean the tube.
- For discharge with suction equipment, make sure the patient and family are knowledgeable and comfortable about using the equipment.

DOCUMENTATION

- Record the date, time, and type of procedure.
- Note the amount, consistency, color, and odor of secretions.
- Document stoma and skin condition.
- Record the patient's respiratory status.
- Note change of the tracheostomy tube by the practitioner.
- Record the duration of cuff deflation.
- Document the amount of cuff inflation.
- Record the cuff pressure readings and specific body position.
- Note complications and nursing actions taken.
- Document patient or family teaching and their understanding.
- Record the patient's tolerance of the treatment.

SELECTED REFERENCES

Edgtton-Winn, M., and Wright, K. "Tracheostomy: A Guide to Nursing Care," *Australian Nursing Journal* 13(5):17-20, November 2005.

Lewis, T., and Oliver, G. "Improving Tracheostomy Care for Ward Patients," *Nursing Standard* 19(19):33-37, January 2005.

Roman, M. "Tracheostomy Tubes," *Medsurg Nursing* 14(2):143-45, April 2005.

Russell, C. "Providing the Nurse with a Guide to Tracheostomy Care and Management," *British Journal of Nursing* 14(8):428-33, April 2005.

St. John, R.E., and Malen, J.F. "Contemporary Issues in Adult Tracheostomy Management," *Critical Care Nursing Clinics of North America* 16(3):413-30, ix-x, September 2004.

Wilson, M. "Tracheostomy Management," *Paediatric Nursing* 17(3):38-43, April 2005.

Tracheotomy

DESCRIPTION

- Tracheotomy involves surgical creation of an external opening (tracheostomy) into the trachea and insertion of an indwelling tube to maintain airway patency.
- If all other attempts to establish an airway have failed, a practitioner may perform a tracheotomy at the patient's bedside.
- Tracheotomy may be necessary when an airway obstruction results from laryngeal edema, foreign-body obstruction, or a tumor.
- An emergency tracheotomy may be performed when endotracheal (ET) intubation is contraindicated.
- Use of a cuffed tracheostomy tube:
  - provides and maintains a patent airway
  - prevents an unconscious or paralyzed patient from aspirating food or secretions
  - allows removal of tracheobronchial secretions from a patient unable to cough
  - replaces an ET tube
  - permits use of positive-pressure ventilation.
- When laryngectomy accompanies a tracheostomy, a laryngectomy tube may be inserted by the practitioner; the trachea is sutured to the skin surface.
- With laryngectomy, accidental tube expulsion doesn't precipitate immediate closure of the tracheal opening. Afterward, the patient has a permanent neck stoma that he breathes through.
- Plastic tubes are commonly used in emergencies because they have a universal adapter for respiratory support equipment, such as a mechanical ventilator, and a cuff to allow positive-pressure ventilation.

CONTRAINDICATIONS

- None known

Tracheostomy tube of proper size (usually #13 to #38 French or #00 to #9 Jackson) with obturator ◆ tracheostomy tape ◆ sterile tracheal dilator ◆ vein retractor ◆ sutures and needles ◆ 4″ × 4″ gauze pads ◆ sterile drapes, gloves, mask, and gown ◆ sterile bowls ◆ stethoscope ◆ sterile tracheostomy dressing ◆ pillow ◆ tracheostomy ties ◆ suction apparatus ◆ alcohol pad ◆ povidone-iodine solution ◆ sterile water ◆ 5-ml syringe with 22G needle ◆ local anesthetic such as lidocaine ◆ oxygen therapy device ◆ oxygen source ◆ sterile marker ◆ sterile labels

Emergency equipment to be kept at the bedside includes suctioning equipment, sterile obturator, sterile tracheostomy tube, sterile inner cannula, sterile tracheostomy tube and inner cannula one size smaller than tube in use, sterile tracheal dilator or sterile hemostats.

PREPARATION

- Have one person stay with the patient while another gets necessary equipment.
- Wash your hands; maintaining sterile technique, open the tray and packages containing the solution.
- Take the tracheostomy tube from its container and place it on the sterile field.
- If necessary, set up the suction equipment and make sure it works.
- After the practitioner opens the sterile bowls, pour in the povidone-iodine solution.
- Label all medication syringes, medication containers, and all solution containers on and off the sterile field

- Explain the procedure even if the patient is unresponsive; assess his condition and provide privacy.
- Maintain ventilation until the tracheotomy is performed.
- Wipe the top of the local anesthetic vial with an alcohol pad. Invert the vial so the practitioner can withdraw the anesthetic using the 22G needle attached to the 5-ml syringe.
- Before the practitioner begins, place a pillow under the patient's shoulders and neck and hyperextend his neck.
- Help with tube insertion as needed.
- When the tube is in position, attach it to the appropriate oxygen therapy device, which is connected to an oxygen source.
- Inject air into the distal cuff port to inflate the cuff; auscultate the patient's lungs using a stethoscope.
- The practitioner will suture the corners of the incision and tape the tracheostomy tube.
- Put on sterile gloves.
- Apply the sterile tracheostomy dressing under the tracheostomy tube flange.
- Place the tracheostomy ties through the openings of the tube flanges, and tie them on the side of the patient's neck. This allows easy access and prevents pressure necrosis at the back of the neck.
- Clean or dispose of the used equipment according to facility policy. Replenish supplies as needed.
- Make sure a chest X-ray is ordered to confirm tube placement.

SPECIAL CONSIDERATIONS

- Assess vital signs and respiratory status every 15 minutes for 1 hour, every 30 minutes for 2 hours, then every 2 hours until the patient's condition is stable.
- Monitor for signs of infection.
- Ideally, the tracheotomy should be performed using sterile technique; in an emergency, this may not be possible.
- Make sure the following equipment is always at the bedside:
  - suctioning equipment (he may need his airway cleared at any time)
  - sterile obturator (for reinsertion if the tube is expelled)
  - sterile tracheostomy tube and obturator (the same size as the one used) in case the tube must be replaced quickly
  - spare, sterile inner cannula that can be used if the cannula is expelled
  - sterile tracheostomy tube and obturator one size smaller than the one used, which may be needed if the tube is expelled and the trachea begins to close
  - sterile tracheal dilator or sterile hemostats to maintain an open airway before inserting a new tracheostomy tube.
- Review emergency first-aid measures, and follow facility policy concerning an expelled or blocked tracheostomy tube.

  WARNING *When a blocked tube can't be cleared by suctioning or withdrawing the inner cannula, policy may require you to stay with the patient while someone calls the practitioner or appropriate code. Continue trying to ventilate with whatever is available, such as a handheld resuscitation bag. Don't remove the tracheostomy tube entirely; the airway may close completely.*

- Use extreme caution if you try to reinsert an expelled tracheostomy tube, to avoid tracheal trauma, perforation, compression, and asphyxiation.

COMPLICATIONS

- Airway obstruction from improper tube placement
- Hemorrhage
- Edema
- Perforated esophagus
- Subcutaneous or mediastinal emphysema
- Aspiration of secretions
- Tracheal necrosis from cuff pressure
- Infection
- Lacerations of arteries, veins, or nerves

PATIENT TEACHING

- Explain the procedure even if the patient is unresponsive.

DOCUMENTATION

- Note the reason for the procedure.
- Record the date and time it took place.
- Document the patient's respiratory status before and after procedure.
- Record complications and nursing actions taken.
- Note the amount of cuff pressure.
- Document respiratory therapy initiated after the procedure.
- Note the patient's response to respiratory therapy.

SELECTED REFERENCES

Carron, M.A., et al. "Airway Obstruction by Granulation Tissue within a Fenestrated Tracheotomy Tube: Case Report," *Ear, Nose, & Throat Journal* 85(1):54-55, January 2006.

Sisk, E.A., et al. "Tracheotomy in Very Low Birth Weight Neonates: Indications and Outcomes," *Laryngoscope* 116(6): 928-33, June 2006.

Tykocinski, M., et al. "Airway Fire During Tracheotomy," *ANZ Journal of Surgery* 76(3):195-97, March 2006.

Wootten, C.T., et al. "Tracheotomy in the First Year of Life: Outcomes in Term Infants, the Vanderbilt Experience," *Otolaryngology — Head and Neck Surgery* 134(3):365-69, March 2006.

Transabdominal tube feeding and care

OVERVIEW

DESCRIPTION

- To access the stomach, duodenum, or jejunum, the practitioner may place a tube through the patient's abdominal wall, either surgically or percutaneously.
- During intra-abdominal surgery, a gastrostomy or jejunostomy tube is usually inserted.
- Procedure may be used for feeding during immediate postoperative period or may provide long-term enteral access, depending on type of surgery.
- Feedings may begin after 24 hours (or when peristalsis resumes).
- Eventually, a tube may need replacement; the practitioner may recommend a similar tube, such as an indwelling urinary catheter or a mushroom catheter, or a gastrostomy button.

CONTRAINDICATIONS

- Obstruction, such as esophageal stricture or duodenal blockage
- Previous gastric surgery
- Morbid obesity
- Ascites

EQUIPMENT

FEEDING

Feeding formula ◆ large-bulb or catheter-tip syringe ◆ 120 ml of water ◆ 4″ × 4″ gauze pads ◆ soap ◆ skin protectant ◆ hypoallergenic tape ◆ gravity-drip administration bags ◆ mouthwash, toothpaste, or mild salt solution ◆ stethoscope ◆ gloves ◆ enteral infusion pump (optional)

DECOMPRESSION

Suction apparatus with tubing and straight drainage collection set

PREPARATION

- Always check the expiration date on commercially prepared feeding formulas.
- If the formula has been prepared by the dietitian or pharmacist, check preparation time and date.
- Discard opened formula more than 1 day old.
- Commercially prepared administration sets and enteral pumps allow continuous formula administration.
- Place the desired amount of formula into the gavage container and purge air from the tubing.
- To avoid contamination, hang only a 4- to 6-hour supply of formula at a time.

KEY STEPS

- Provide privacy and wash your hands.
- Confirm the patient's identity using two patient identifiers according to facility policy.
- Explain the procedure to the patient.
- Assess for bowel sounds before feeding; monitor for abdominal distention.
- Ask the patient to sit, or assist him into semi-Fowler's position.
- For an intermittent feeding, have him maintain this position during the feeding and for 30 minutes to 1 hour afterward.
- Put on gloves.
- Before starting feeding, measure residual gastric contents.
- Attach the syringe to the feeding tube and aspirate. If contents measure more than twice the amount infused, hold the feeding and recheck in 1 hour. If residual contents remain too high, notify the practitioner; formula may not be absorbed properly. Residual contents are minimal with percutaneous endoscopic jejunostomy tube feedings.
- Allow 30 ml of water to flow into the feeding tube to establish patency.
- Be sure to give formula at room temperature.

INTERMITTENT FEEDINGS

- Allow gravity to help the formula flow over 30 to 45 minutes.
- Begin intermittent feedings with a low volume (200 ml) daily. According to the patient's tolerance, increase the volume per feeding, as needed, to reach the desired calorie intake.
- When done feeding, flush the feeding tube with 30 to 60 ml of water. This maintains patency and provides hydration. Cap the tube to prevent leakage.
- Rinse the feeding administration set thoroughly with hot water to avoid contaminating subsequent feedings. Allow it to dry between feedings.

CONTINUOUS FEEDINGS

◆ Measure residual gastric contents every 4 hours.
◆ To give the feeding with a pump, set up equipment according to manufacturer's guidelines and fill the feeding bag.
◆ To give the feeding by gravity, fill the container with formula and purge air from the tubing.
◆ Monitor the gravity drip rate or pump infusion rate frequently to ensure accurate delivery.
◆ Flush the feeding tube with 30 to 60 ml of water every 4 hours to maintain patency and provide hydration.
◆ Monitor intake and output to detect fluid or electrolyte imbalances.

DECOMPRESSION

◆ To decompress the stomach, connect the percutaneous endoscopic gastrostomy port to the suction device with tubing or straight gravity drainage tubing.

TUBE EXIT SITE CARE

◆ Provide daily skin care.
◆ Remove the dressing by hand. Never cut the dressing away over the catheter.
◆ At least daily and as needed, clean the skin around the tube's exit site using a 4″ × 4″ gauze pad soaked in prescribed cleaning solution.
◆ When healed, wash the skin around the exit site daily with soap; rinse with water and dry.
◆ Apply skin protectant, if necessary.
◆ Anchor a gastrostomy or jejunostomy tube to the skin with hypoallergenic tape. Coil the tube, if necessary, and tape it to the abdomen.

SPECIAL CONSIDERATIONS

◆ The practitioner may suture the tube in place to prevent leaking of gastric contents.
◆ If the patient vomits or complains of nausea, feeling too full, or regurgitation, stop feeding immediately and assess his condition.

◆ Flush the feeding tube and attempt to restart the feeding again in 1 hour (measure residual gastric contents first). You may have to decrease the volume or rate of feedings.

⚡ **WARNING** *If the patient develops signs of dumping syndrome (such as nausea, vomiting, cramps, pallor, diarrhea), the feedings may have been given too quickly.*

◆ Brush all surfaces of the teeth, gums, and tongue at least twice daily using mouthwash, toothpaste, or mild salt solution.
◆ You can give most tablets and pills through the tube by crushing them and diluting as necessary.

⚡ **WARNING** *Don't crush enteric-coated or sustained-released drugs, which lose their effectiveness when crushed. Drugs should be in liquid form for administration.*

◆ Control diarrhea resulting from dumping syndrome by using continuous pump or gravity-drip infusions, diluting the feeding formula, or adding antidiarrheal drugs.

COMPLICATIONS

◆ Common complications related to transabdominal tubes including:
– GI or other systemic problems
– mechanical malfunction
– metabolic disturbances
– cramping, nausea, vomiting, bloating, and diarrhea
– fat malabsorption
– intestinal atrophy from malnutrition
– constipation from inadequate hydration or insufficient exercise.
◆ Systemic problems possibly caused by:
– pulmonary aspiration
– infection at the tube exit site
– contaminated formula.
◆ Typical mechanical problems, including:
– tube dislodgment, obstruction, or tube migration
– occlusion
– rupture or tube cracking from age, drying, or frequent manipulation.
◆ Vitamin and mineral deficiencies, glucose tolerance, and fluid and electrolyte imbalances that follow bouts of diarrhea or constipation

PATIENT TEACHING

◆ Instruct the patient and family members or other caregivers in all aspects of enteral feedings, including tube maintenance and site care.
◆ Specify signs and symptoms to report to the practitioner, define emergency situations, and review actions to take.

DOCUMENTATION

◆ On the intake and output record, note the date, time, and amount of each feeding and water volume instilled.
◆ Maintain total volumes for nutrients and water separately to allow calculation of nutrient intake.
◆ Document in your notes the type of formula, infusion method, and rate.
◆ Record the patient's tolerance of the procedure and formula.
◆ Document the amount of residual gastric contents.
◆ Record complications and abdominal assessment findings.
◆ Document patient-teaching topics covered.
◆ Note the patient's progress in self-care.

SELECTED REFERENCES

Carey, T.S., et al. "Expectations and Outcomes of Gastric Feeding Tubes," *American Journal of Medicine* 119(6): 527.e11-16, June 2006.
Todd, V., et al. "Percutaneous Endoscopic Gastrostomy (PEG): The Role and Perspective of Nurses," *Journal of Clinical Nursing* 14(2):187-94, February 2005.
Williams, T.A., and Leslie, G.D. "A Review of the Nursing Care of Enteral Feeding Tubes in Critically Ill Adults: Part I," *Intensive & Critical Care Nursing* 20(6): 330-43, December 2004.

Transcranial Doppler monitoring

DESCRIPTION

◆ Transcranial Doppler monitoring is a noninvasive method of monitoring blood flow in the intracranial vessels, specifically the circle of Willis.

◆ It's used in intensive care unit to monitor patients who have experienced cerebrovascular disorders, such as stroke, head trauma, or subarachnoid hemorrhage.

◆ Monitoring helps detect intracranial stenosis, vasospasm, and arteriovenous malformations as well as assess collateral pathways.

◆ It assesses continuous waveform, and can be used in intraoperative monitoring of cerebral circulation, monitoring the effect of intracranial pressure changes on cerebral circulation, and patient response to various drugs.

◆ The procedure is used to evaluate carbon dioxide reactivity, which may be impaired or lost from arterial obstruction or trauma.

◆ It's been used to confirm brain death.

CONTRAINDICATIONS

◆ None known

EQUIPMENT

Transcranial Doppler unit ◆ transducer with an attachment system ◆ terry cloth headband ◆ ultrasonic coupling gel ◆ marker

KEY STEPS

◆ Confirm the patient's identity using two patient identifiers according to facility policy.

◆ Explain the procedure and answer questions.

◆ Place the patient in the proper position (usually supine).

◆ Turn the Doppler unit on and watch as it performs a self-test. The screen should show six parameters: peak (CM/S), mean (CM/S), depth (M/M), delta (%), emboli (AGR), and pulsatility index (PI+).

◆ Enter the patient's name and identification number in the unit; additional information, such as diagnosis or practitioner's name, may also need to be entered.

◆ Indicate the vessel you wish to monitor (usually the right or left middle cerebral artery [MCA]) and set the approximate depth of the vessel within the skull (50 mm for the MCA).

◆ Use the keypad to increase the power level to 100% to initially locate the signal. You can later decrease the level as needed, depending on skull thickness.

◆ Visualize the three windows of the transtemporal access route: posterior, middle, and anterior.

◆ Apply ultrasonic gel at the level of the temporal bone between the tragus of the ear and the end of the eyebrow, over the area of the three windows.

◆ Place a transducer on the posterior window, angling it slightly in an anterior direction, slowly moving in a narrow circle (the "flashlighting" technique).

◆ During flashlighting, slowly move the transducer forward across the temporal area, listening for the audible signal with the highest pitch. This sound corresponds to the highest velocity signal of the vessel you are assessing.

◆ Headphones allow you to better evaluate the audible signal and provide patient privacy.

◆ After locating the highest-pitched signal, draw a circle around the transducer head on the patient's temple.

◆ Note the angle of the transducer so you can duplicate it after the transducer attachment system is in place.

◆ Place the plate of the transducer attachment system over the patient's temporal area, matching the circular opening in the plate exactly with the circle on his head.

◆ Holding the plate in place, encircle his head with the straps attached to the system.

◆ Tighten the straps so the transducer attachment system stays in place.

◆ Fill the circular opening in the plate with the ultrasonic gel.

◆ Place the transducer in the gel-filled opening in the attachment system plate.

◆ Using plastic screws provided, loosely secure the two plates together to hold the transducer in place, while allowing it to rotate for the best angle.

◆ Adjust the position and angle of the transducer until you again hear the highest-pitched audible signal.

◆ On the monitor you should see a clear waveform with a bright white line (an envelope) at its upper edge. The envelope exactly follows the contours of the waveform.

◆ If the envelope doesn't follow the waveform's contours, adjust the GAIN setting.

◆ If the signal is wrapping around the screen, use the SCALE key to increase the scale and the BASELINE key to drop the baseline.

◆ When you have the strongest, highest-pitched signal and the best waveform, lock the transducer in place by tightening the plastic screws. The tightened plates will hold the transducer at the angle you've chosen.

◆ Disconnect the transducer handle.

◆ Place a wide terrycloth headband over the transducer attachment system, and secure it around the patient's head to provide additional stability for the transducer.

◆ You should be able to see a waveform on the monitor and read the numeric values of the peak, mean velocities, and PI+ above the displayed waveform. The shape of the wave form reveals more information. (See *Comparing velocity waveforms*.)

SPECIAL CONSIDERATIONS

♦ Velocity changes in the signal correlate with changes in cerebral blood flow. The parameter that most clearly reflects this change is the mean velocity.
♦ Establish a baseline for the mean velocity; as velocity increases or decreases, the value (%) will change negatively or positively from the baseline.

♦ Emboli appear as high-intensity transients occurring randomly during the cardiac cycle, making a distinctive "clicking," "chirping," or "plunking" sound.
♦ You can set up an emboli counter to count either the total number of emboli aggregates or the rate of embolic events per minute.
♦ Various screens can be stored on the system's hard drive and can be recalled or printed.
♦ Before using, be sure to remove turban head dressings or thick dressings over the test site.

COMPLICATIONS
♦ None known

PATIENT TEACHING

♦ Explain the procedure and answer the patient's questions as thoroughly as possible.

DOCUMENTATION

♦ Record the date and time monitoring began and which artery was monitored.
♦ Document patient teaching as well as his tolerance of the procedure.

SELECTED REFERENCES

Demchuk, A.M., et al. "Transcranial Doppler in Acute Stroke," *Neuroimaging Clinics of North America* 15(3):473-80, August 2005.
Evans, D.H. "Embolus Differentiation Using Multifrequency Transcranial Doppler," *Stroke* 37(7):1641, July 2006.
Kirkness, C.J. "Cerebral Blood Flow Monitoring in Clinical Practice," *AACN Clinical Issues* 16(4):476-87, October-December 2005.
White, H., and Venkatesh, B. "Applications of Transcranial Doppler in the ICU: A Review," *Intensive Care Medicine* 32(7): 981-94, July 2006.

Comparing velocity waveforms

A normal transcranial Doppler signal is typically characterized by mean velocities that fall within the normal reported values. Additional information can be gathered by evaluating the shape of the velocity waveform.

EFFECT OF SIGNIFICANT PROXIMAL VESSEL OBSTRUCTION
A delayed systolic upstroke can be seen in a waveform when significant proximal vessel obstruction is present.

NORMAL

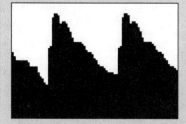

PROXIMAL VESSEL OBSTRUCTION

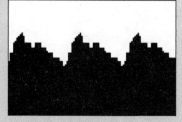

EFFECT OF INCREASED CEREBROVASCULAR RESISTANCE
Changes in cerebrovascular resistance, as occur with increased intracranial pressure, cause a decrease in diastolic flow.

NORMAL

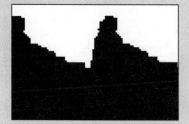

INCREASED RESISTANCE

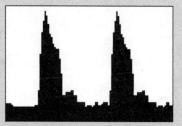

Transcutaneous electrical nerve stimulation

OVERVIEW

DESCRIPTION

- Transcutaneous electrical nerve stimulation (TENS) is based on the gate control theory of pain (painful impulses pass through a "gate" in the brain).
- It's performed with a portable battery-powered device that transmits painless electrical current to peripheral nerves or directly to a painful area over relatively large nerve fibers.
- It effectively alters the patient's perception of pain by blocking painful stimuli traveling over smaller fibers.
- It's used for postoperative patients and those with chronic pain to reduce need for analgesic drugs; it may allow patient to resume normal activities.
- Treatment typically lasts 3 to 5 days.
- Some conditions, such as phantom limb pain, may require continuous stimulation; other conditions, such as a painful arthritic joint, require shorter periods (3 or 4 hours). (See *Uses of TENS.*)

CONTRAINDICATIONS

- Cardiac pacemakers (can interfere with function)
- Pregnancy
- Dementia

⚡ **WARNING** *TENS electrodes shouldn't be placed on the head or neck of a patient with a vascular or seizure disorder.*

EQUIPMENT

Commercial TENS kits are available. They include the stimulator, leadwires, electrodes, spare battery pack, battery recharger, and adhesive patch.

TENS device ◆ alcohol pads ◆ electrodes ◆ electrode gel ◆ warm water and soap ◆ leadwires ◆ charged battery pack ◆ battery recharger ◆ adhesive patch or hypoallergenic tape ◆ hair clippers (optional)

PREPARATION

- Before beginning the procedure, always test the battery pack to make sure it's fully charged.

Uses of TENS

Transcutaneous electrical nerve stimulation (TENS) must be prescribed by a practitioner and is most successful if administered and taught to the patient by a skilled therapist. TENS has been used for temporary relief of acute pain, such as postoperative pain, and for ongoing relief of chronic pain such as sciatica.

Among the types of pain that respond to TENS are:
- arthritis
- bone fracture pain
- bursitis
- cancer-related pain
- lower back pain
- musculoskeletal pain
- myofascial pain
- neuralgia and neuropathy
- phantom limb pain
- postoperative incision pain
- sciatica
- whiplash.

KEY STEPS

- Wash your hands and follow standard precautions.
- Confirm the patient's identity using two patient identifiers according to facility policy.
- Provide privacy and explain the procedure.
- Thoroughly clean the skin where the electrode will be applied with an alcohol pad, then dry.
- If necessary, clip hair at the site where each electrode will be placed.
- Apply electrode gel to the bottom of each electrode.
- Place the ordered number of electrodes on the proper skin area, leaving at least 2″ (5 cm) between them. (See *Positioning TENS electrodes.*)
- Secure electrodes with the adhesive patch or hypoallergenic tape on all sides evenly, so they're firmly attached to the skin.
- Plug the pin connectors into the electrode sockets.
- To protect the cords, hold the connectors — not the cords themselves — during insertion.
- Turn the channel controls to the OFF position or as recommended in the operator's manual.
- Plug the leadwires into the jacks in the control box.
- Turn the amplitude and rate dials slowly, as the manual directs. (The patient should feel a tingling sensation.)
- Adjust the control to the prescribed settings or to settings that are most comfortable. Most patients select stimulation frequencies of 60 to 100 Hz.
- Attach the TENS control box to part of the patient's clothing, such as a belt, pocket, or bra.
- To make sure the device is working effectively, monitor for signs of excessive stimulation, such as muscle twitches, and for signs of inadequate stimulation, signaled by the patient not feeling a mild tingling sensation.

AFTER TRANSCUTANEOUS ELECTRICAL NERVE STIMULATION TREATMENT

◆ Turn off the controls and unplug the electrode leadwires, unless another treatment will be given soon, then leave the electrodes in place.
◆ Clean the electrodes with soap and water, and clean the patient's skin with alcohol pads.
◆ Don't soak the electrodes in alcohol because it will damage the rubber.
◆ Remove the battery pack and replace it with a charged battery pack.
◆ Recharge the used battery pack so it's always ready for use.

SPECIAL CONSIDERATIONS

◆ If you must move electrodes during the procedure, turn off the controls first.
◆ Follow the practitioner's orders regarding electrode placement and control settings.

⚡ **WARNING** *Incorrect placement of electrodes will result in inappropriate pain control. Setting controls too high can cause pain; setting them too low will fail to relieve pain.*

⚡ **WARNING** *Never place the electrodes near the patient's eyes or over the nerves that innervate the carotid sinus or laryngeal or pharyngeal muscles to avoid interference with critical nerve function.*

◆ If TENS is used continuously for postoperative pain, remove the electrodes at least daily to check for skin irritation, provide skin care, and to rotate sites of electrode placement.

COMPLICATIONS
◆ None known

PATIENT TEACHING

◆ If appropriate, let the patient study the operator's manual.
◆ Teach the patient how to place the electrodes properly and how to take care of the TENS unit.

DOCUMENTATION

◆ Record the electrode sites and control settings.
◆ Note patient's tolerance of treatment.
◆ Record the location of pain and how the patient rates his pain using a pain scale.

SELECTED REFERENCES

Kapur, S., et al. "Assessment of the Efficacy of Electronic Nerve Modulation (ENM) in Comparison to TENS in Patients with Chronic Low Back Pain," *Neuromodulation* 9(2):161-62, April 2006.

Khadilkar, A., et al. "Transcutaneous Electrical Nerve Stimulation for the Treatment of Chronic Low Back Pain: A Systematic Review," *Spine* 30(23):2657-66, December 2005.

Limoges, M.F., and Rickabaugh, B. "Evaluation of TENS during Screening Flexible Sigmoidoscopy," *Gastroenterology Nursing* 27(2):61-68, March-April 2004.

Siddle, L. "The Challenge and Management of Phantom Limb Pain after Amputation," *British Journal of Nursing* 13(11):664-67, June 2004.

Positioning TENS electrodes

In transcutaneous electrical nerve stimulation (TENS), electrodes placed around peripheral nerves (or an incisional site) transmit mild electrical pulses to the brain. The current is thought to block pain impulses. The patient can influence the level and frequency of pain relief by adjusting controls on the device.

Typically, electrode placement varies even though patients may have similar complaints. Electrodes can be placed in several ways:
◆ They can cover the painful area or surround it, as with muscle tenderness or spasm or painful joints.

◆ They can "capture" the painful area between electrodes, as with incisional pain.
◆ In peripheral nerve injury, electrodes should be placed proximal to the injury (between the brain and the injury site) to avoid increasing pain.
◆ Placing electrodes in a hypersensitive area can also increase pain.
◆ In an area lacking sensation, electrodes should be placed on adjacent dermatomes.

These illustrations show combinations of electrode placement (colored squares) and areas of nerve stimulation (shaded panels) for lower back and leg pain.

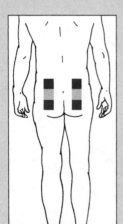 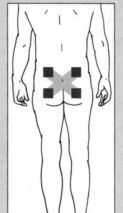 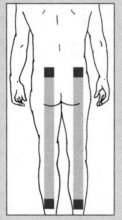

Transdermal drug administration

DESCRIPTION

- An adhesive patch or measured dose of ointment applied to the skin delivers constant, controlled drug directly into the bloodstream for a prolonged systemic effect.
- Drugs available in transdermal form include:
  - nitroglycerin, used to control angina, dilates coronary vessels for up to 4 hours
  - scopolamine, eases motion sickness for up to 72 hours
  - estradiol, provides postmenopausal hormone replacement for up to 1 week
  - clonidine, treats hypertension for 24 hours
  - nicotine, used for smoking cessation, lasts 24 hours
  - fentanyl, a narcotic analgesic used to control chronic pain, lasts up to 72 hours.

CONTRAINDICATIONS

- Skin allergies
- Skin reactions
- Broken or irritated skin (would increase irritation)
- Scarred or callused skin (might impair absorption)

EQUIPMENT

Patient's drug record and chart ◆ gloves ◆ prescribed drug (patch or ointment) ◆ application strip or measuring paper (for nitroglycerin ointment) ◆ adhesive tape ◆ plastic wrap (optional for nitroglycerin ointment) or semipermeable dressing

KEY STEPS

- Verify the order on the patient's drug record by checking it against the practitioner's order.
- Wash your hands and, if necessary, put on gloves.
- Check the label on the drug to make sure you'll be giving the correct drug in the correct dose, and note the expiration date.
- Confirm the patient's identity using two patient identifiers according to facility policy.
- Explain the procedure and provide privacy.
- Remove the previously applied drug.

APPLYING TRANSDERMAL OINTMENT

- Place the prescribed amount of ointment on the application strip or

---

Applying nitroglycerin ointment

Unlike most topical drugs, nitroglycerin ointment is used for its transdermal systemic effect. It's used to dilate veins and arteries to improve cardiac perfusion in a patient with cardiac ischemia or angina pectoris.

Before applying the ointment, take the patient's baseline blood pressure so you can compare it with later readings, and gather your equipment. Nitroglycerin ointment, which is prescribed by the inch, comes with a rectangular piece of ruled paper. Squeeze the prescribed amount of ointment onto the ruled paper (as shown below). Put on gloves, if desired, to avoid contact with the drug. Nitroglycerin ointment also comes in premeasured single-dose packages.

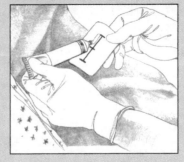

After applying the correct amount of ointment, tape the paper—drug side down—directly to the skin. (Some facilities require you to use the paper to apply the drug to the patient's skin, usually on the chest or arm. Spread a thin layer of the ointment over a 3″ [7.6-cm] area.) For increased absorption, the practitioner may request that you cover the site with plastic wrap or a transparent, semipermeable dressing (as shown below).

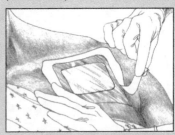

After 5 minutes, record the patient's blood pressure. If it has dropped significantly and he has a headache (from vasodilation of blood vessels in his head), notify the practitioner immediately. He may reduce the dose. If the patient's blood pressure has dropped but he has no symptoms, instruct him to be still until it returns to normal.

---

measuring paper. (See *Applying nitroglycerin ointment*.)

◆ Apply the strip to a dry, hairless area of the body without rubbing ointment into the skin.

◆ Tape the ointment-filled strip to the skin.

◆ If desired, cover the application strip with the plastic wrap, and tape the wrap in place.

APPLYING A TRANSDERMAL PATCH

◆ Open the package and remove the patch.

◆ Without touching the adhesive surface, remove the clear plastic backing.

◆ Apply the patch to a dry, hairless area — behind the ear, for example, as with scopolamine. (See *Applying a transdermal patch*.)

◆ Write the date, time, and your initials on the patch.

AFTER APPLYING TRANSDERMAL DRUGS

◆ Instruct the patient to keep the area around the patch or strip as dry as possible.

◆ If you didn't wear gloves, wash your hands immediately after applying the patch or ointment to avoid absorbing the drug yourself.

SPECIAL CONSIDERATIONS

◆ Reapply daily transdermal drugs at the same time to ensure a continuous effect; alternate application sites to avoid skin irritation.

◆ When applying a scopolamine or fentanyl patch, instruct the patient not to drive or operate machinery until his response to the drug has been determined.

◆ Warn the patient using a clonidine patch to check with his practitioner before taking an over-the-counter cough preparation; such drugs may counteract effects of clonidine.

COMPLICATIONS

◆ Skin irritation, such as pruritus or rash

◆ Headache and orthostatic hypotension (in elderly patients) from nitroglycerin drugs

◆ Dry mouth and drowsiness from scopolamine

◆ Increased risk of endometrial cancer, thromboembolic disease, and birth defects due to estradiol

◆ Severe rebound hypertension, especially if withdrawn suddenly, from clonidine

PATIENT TEACHING

◆ Explain the procedure to the patient who will be applying transdermal drugs at home.

◆ Instruct him how to rotate the application sites to prevent skin irritation.

◆ Instruct him how to remove and discard previous medication patch and to clean the area.

DOCUMENTATION

◆ Record the type and dose of the drug, and the date, time, and site of application.

◆ Note adverse effects and the patient's response to treatment.

SELECTED REFERENCES

McErlane, K. "Keeping Track of the Patch: Transdermal Delivery in Obese Patients," *American Journal of Nursing* 105(6):36-37, June 2005.

Paparella, S. "Transdermal Patches: An Unseen Risk for Harm," *Journal of Emergency Nursing* 31(3):278-81, June 2005.

White, T., et al. "Effect of Oral Versus Transdermal Steroidal Contraceptives on Androgenic Markers," *American Journal of Obstetrics and Gynecology* 192(6):2055-59, June 2005.

Applying a transdermal patch

If the patient will be receiving a drug by transdermal patch, instruct him in its proper use.

◆ Explain that the patch consists of several layers. The layer closest to the skin contains a small amount of drug and allows prompt introduction of the drug into the bloodstream. The next layer controls release of the drug from the main portion of the patch. The third layer contains the main dose of the drug. The outermost layer consists of an aluminized polyester barrier.

◆ Teach the patient to apply the patch to appropriate skin areas, such as on the upper arm or chest or behind the ear. Warn him to avoid touching the gel or surrounding tape. Tell him to use a different site for each application to avoid skin irritation. If necessary, he can clip hair at the site. Tell him to avoid an area that may cause uneven absorption, such as skin folds, scars, and calluses, or irritated or damaged skin areas. Tell him not to apply the disk below the elbow or knee.

◆ Instruct the patient to wash his hands after application to remove residual drug.

◆ Warn him not to get the patch wet and to discard it if it leaks or falls off. Then he should clean the site and apply a new patch at a different site.

◆ Instruct the patient to apply the patch at the same time at the prescribed interval to ensure continuous drug delivery. Bedtime application is ideal for some transdermal drug patches because of reduced body movement. Tell him to apply a new patch about 30 minutes before removing the old one.

Transducer system setup

DESCRIPTION
- The system type used depends on patient needs and practitioner preference.
- Some systems monitor pressure continuously, others monitor pressure intermittently.
- Single-pressure transducers monitor only one type of pressure, such as pulmonary artery pressure (PAP).
- Multiple-pressure transducers can monitor two or more types of pressure, such as PAP and central venous pressure.

CONTRAINDICATIONS
- None known

EQUIPMENT

Bag of heparin flush solution (usually 500 ml normal saline solution with 500 or 1,000 units heparin) ◆ pressure infusion bag ◆ drug-added label ◆ preassembled disposable pressure tubing with flush device and disposable transducer ◆ monitor and monitor cable ◆ I.V. pole with transducer mount ◆ carpenter's level

PREPARATION
- Turn the monitor on and give it time to warm up.
- Gather the equipment you'll need and wash your hands.

KEY STEPS

- Follow facility policy on adding heparin to the flush solution.
- If the patient has a history of bleeding or clotting problems, use heparin with caution. Add the ordered heparin to the solution (usually, 1 or 2 units of heparin/ml of solution) and label the bag.
- Put the pressure module into the monitor, if necessary, connecting the transducer cable to the monitor.
- Remove the preassembled pressure tubing from the package.
- If necessary, connect the pressure tubing to the transducer and tighten all tubing connections.
- Position all stopcocks so the flush solution flows through the entire system.
- Roll the tubing's flow regulator to the OFF position.
- Spike the flush solution bag with the tubing, invert the bag, open the roller clamp, and squeeze all the air through the drip chamber.
- Compress the tubing's drip chamber, filling it no more than halfway with the flush solution.
- Hang the pressure infuser bag on the I.V. pole, then position the flush solution bag inside the pressure infuser bag.
- Open the flow regulator, uncoil the tube if not already done, and remove the protective cap.
- Squeeze the continuous flush device slowly to prime the entire system, including the stopcock ports, with the flush solution.
- As the solution nears the disposable transducer, hold the transducer at a 45-degree angle (as shown) to force solution to flow upward to the transducer. This forces air out of the system.

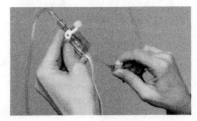

- When the solution nears a stopcock, open the stopcock to air, allowing the solution to flow into the stopcock (as shown).

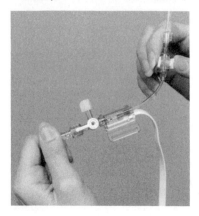

- When the stopcock fills, close it to air and turn it open to the remainder of the tubing. Do this for each stopcock.
- After you've primed the system, replace the protective cap at the tubing end.
- Inflate the pressure infuser bag to 300 mm Hg. This bag keeps the pressure in the arterial line higher than the patient's systolic pressure, preventing blood backflow into the tubing and ensuring a continuous flow rate.

⚡ **WARNING** *Never inflate the pressure infuser bag prior to priming the tubing because this could cause microbubbles.*

- When inflating the pressure bag, don't let the drip chamber completely fill with fluid. Afterward, flush the system again to remove air bubbles.
- Replace the vented caps on the stopcocks with sterile nonvented caps. If you're going to mount the transducer on an I.V. pole, insert the device into its holder.

ZEROING THE SYSTEM

- To ensure accuracy, position the patient and the transducer on the same level each time you zero the transducer or record a pressure. Typically, the patient lies flat in bed, if possible.
- Use the carpenter's level to position the air-reference stopcock or the air-fluid interface of the transducer level with the phlebostatic axis (midway between the posterior chest and sternum at the fourth intercostal space, midaxillary line).
- You may level the air-reference stopcock or the air-fluid interface to the same position as the catheter tip; then turn the stopcock next to the transducer off to the patient and open to air.
- Remove the cap to the stopcock port.
- Place the cap inside an opened sterile gauze package to prevent contamination.
- Now zero the transducer, following manufacturer's directions for zeroing.
- Turn the stopcock on the transducer so that it's closed to air and open to the patient (monitoring position).
- Replace the cap on the stopcock.
- Attach the single-pressure transducer to the patient's catheter to finish assembling the system (as shown below).

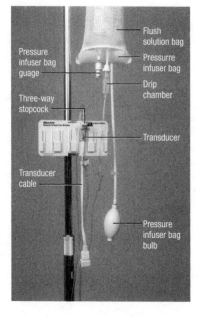

Flush solution bag

Pressure infuser bag guage

Pressurre infuser bag

Three-way stopcock

Drip chamber

Transducer cable

Transducer

Pressure infuser bag bulb

- There are several ways to set up a multiple-pressure transducer system; the easiest is to add to the single-pressure system. Use another bag of heparin flush solution in a second pressure infuser bag. Prime the tubing, mount the second transducer, connect an additional cable to the monitor, and zero the second transducer.
- Alternatively, your facility may use a Y-type tubing setup with two attached pressure transducers, requiring only one bag of heparin flush solution.
- Proceed as you would for a single transducer, with this exception: Prime one branch of the Y-type tubing, then the other; attach two cables to the monitor in the modules for each pressure that you'll be measuring, and zero each transducer.

COMPLICATIONS
- None known

PATIENT TEACHING

No patient teaching is required.

DOCUMENTATION

- Document the patient's position for zeroing so that other health care team members can replicate the placement.

SELECTED REFERENCES

Garretson, S. "Haemodynamic Monitoring: Arterial Catheters," *Nursing Standard* 19(31):55-64, April 2005.
Magder, S. "Central Venous Pressure Monitoring," *Current Opinion In Critical Care* 12(3):219-27, June 2006.

Transfer

DESCRIPTION

- A transfer requires thorough preparation and careful documentation.
- Explain transfer to the patient and his family.
- Discuss his condition and care plan with the receiving unit or facility staff.
- Arrange transportation if necessary.
- Document his condition before and during transfer to ensure continuity of nursing care and legal protection for the transferring facility and its staff.

CONTRAINDICATIONS

- None known

Admission inventory of belongings ◆ patient's chart, drug record, and nursing Kardex ◆ drugs ◆ bag or suitcase ◆ wheelchair or stretcher, as necessary

- Confirm the patient's identity using two patient identifiers according to facility policy.
- Assess the patient's physical condition to determine means of transfer, such as a wheelchair or a stretcher.
- Using the admissions inventory of belongings as a checklist, collect his property.
- Check the patient's room, including closet, tables, and bathroom; if transfer is to another facility, don't forget valuables or personal drugs.
- Gather his drugs from the cart and refrigerator.
- If the patient is being transferred to another unit, send the drugs to the receiving unit. If he's being transferred to another facility, return them to the pharmacy.
- Notify the business office and other departments.
- Notify the dietary department, pharmacy, and facility telephone operator about transfer within the facility.
- Contact the nursing staff on the receiving unit about the patient's condition and drug regimen, and review his nursing care plan to ensure continuity of care.

TRANSFER WITHIN THE FACILITY

- If the patient is transferring from or to an intensive care unit, your facility may require new care orders from his practitioner. If so, review the new orders with the nursing staff at the receiving unit.
- Send his chart, laboratory request slips, Kardex, special equipment, and other required materials to the receiving unit.
- Use a wheelchair to transport the ambulatory patient to the newly assigned room, unless it's on the same unit as his present one, in which case he may walk.
- Use a stretcher to transport a bedridden patient.
- Introduce the patient to the nursing staff at the receiving unit and take him to his room.

◆ Depending on his condition, place the patient in the bed or seat him in a chair.
◆ Introduce the patient to his roommate and tell him about unfamiliar equipment.

TRANSFER TO AN EXTENDED-CARE FACILITY

◆ Make sure the patient's practitioner has written the transfer order on the chart and completed the special transfer form, including diagnosis, care summary, drug regimen, and special care instructions.
◆ Complete the nursing summary, including the patient's assessment, progress, required nursing treatments, and special needs.
◆ Keep one copy of the transfer form and nursing summary with the patient's chart; forward other copies to the receiving facility. Don't send his drugs, Kardex, or chart.
◆ Make sure that the patient's medication list is communicated to the next health care provider.

TRANSFER TO AN ACUTE CARE FACILITY

◆ Make sure the practitioner has written the transfer order on the patient's chart and has completed the transfer form; complete the nursing summary.
◆ Depending on the practitioner's instructions, send one copy of the transfer form and the nursing summary and photocopies of the pertinent excerpts from the patient's chart (such as laboratory test and X-ray results, patient history and physical progress notes, and vital sign records) to the receiving facility with him.
◆ Alternatively, following your facility's policy, substitute a written summary of the patient's condition and facility history for the excerpts from his chart.
◆ Make sure that the patient's medication list is communicated to the next health care provider.

SPECIAL CONSIDERATIONS

◆ If the patient requires an ambulance to take him to another facility, arrange transportation with the social services department.
◆ Assemble necessary equipment to provide care during transport.
◆ Be especially careful that documentation is complete when the patient is transferred to another facility; communication errors can hurt his recovery.
◆ If he's being transferred to a different facility include these patient care measures: airway suctioning, giving prescribed drugs, changing soiled dressing, bathing an incontinent patient, and emptying drainage collection devices.

COMPLICATIONS
◆ None known

PATIENT TEACHING

◆ Explain the transfer to the patient and family.
◆ If the patient is anxious about the transfer or his condition precludes patient teaching, be sure to explain the reason for transfer to family members, especially if the transfer is the result of a serious change in condition.

DOCUMENTATION

◆ Record the time and date of the transfer.
◆ Note the patient's condition during the transfer.
◆ Document the name of the receiving unit or facility.
◆ Note the means of transportation.
◆ Note that the patient's medication list was provide to the next health care facility and provider.

SELECTED REFERENCES

Barry, J. "The HoverMatt System for Patient Transfer: Enhancing Productivity, Efficiency, and Safety," *Journal of Nursing Administration* 36(3):114-17, March 2006.

Enes, S.P., et al. "Discharging Patients from Hospice to Nursing Home: A Retrospective Case Note Review," *International Journal of Palliative Nursing* 10(3):124-30, March 2004.

Midlov, P., et al. "Medication Errors When Transferring Elderly Patients Between Primary Health Care and Hospital Care," *Pharmacy World & Science* 27(2):116-20, April 2005.

Transfer from bed to stretcher

DESCRIPTION

- This procedure requires help of one or more coworkers, depending on patient's size and condition and the primary nurse's physical abilities.
- Techniques include the straight lift, carry lift, lift sheet, and sliding board.
- The straight (patient-assisted) lift is used to move a child, a very light patient, or a patient who can help: Team members place hands and arms under his buttocks and, if necessary, shoulders.
- Other patients may require a four-person straight lift.
- For the carry lift, team members roll the patient onto their upper arms and hold him against their chests.
- For the lift sheet transfer, a sheet is placed under patient and he's lifted or slid onto the stretcher.
- For the sliding-board transfer, two team members slide the patient onto the stretcher.

CONTRAINDICATIONS

- None known

EQUIPMENT

Stretcher ◆ sliding board or lift sheet if necessary

PREPARATION

- Adjust the bed to the same height as the stretcher.

KEY STEPS

- Tell the patient you're going to move him from the bed to the stretcher, and place him in the supine position.
- Ask team members to remove watches and rings to avoid scratching the patient during transfer.
- Remember to use proper body mechanics with all transfers to prevent injury.

FOUR-PERSON STRAIGHT LIFT

- Place the stretcher parallel to the bed, and lock the wheels of both to ensure the patient's safety.
- Stand at the center of the stretcher; have another team member stand at the patient's head. Two other team members stand next to the bed, one at the center and the other at the patient's feet.
- All team members slide arms, palms up, beneath the patient. In this position, you and the team member directly opposite support the patient's buttocks and hips; the team member at the head of the bed supports his head and shoulders; the one at the foot supports his legs and feet.
- On a count of "three," the team members lift the patient several inches, move him onto the stretcher, and slide their arms out from under him.
- Keep movements smooth to minimize patient discomfort and avoid muscle strain to team members.

FOUR-PERSON CARRY LIFT

- Place the stretcher perpendicular to the bed, with its head at the foot of the bed. Lock the bed and stretcher wheels to ensure the patient's safety.
- Raise the bed to a comfortable working height.
- Line up team members on the same side of the bed as the stretcher, with the tallest person at the patient's head and the shortest at his feet. The member at his head is the leader, and gives the lift signals.

- Team members should flex their knees and slide their hands, palms up, under the patient until he rests securely on their upper arms.
- Make sure the patient is supported at the head and shoulders, buttocks and hips, and legs and feet.
- On a count of "three," team members straighten their knees and roll the patient onto his side, against their chests. This reduces strain on the lifters and allows them to hold the patient for several minutes.
- Team members step back, with the member supporting the feet moving the farthest. Team members move forward to the stretcher's edge and, "on three," lower the patient onto the stretcher by bending at the knees and sliding their arms out from under him.

FOUR-PERSON LIFT SHEET TRANSFER

- Position the bed, stretcher, and team members for the straight lift.
- Instruct the team to hold the edges of the sheet under the patient, grasping them close to the patient to obtain a firm grip, provide stability, and make the patient feel stable.
- On a count of "three," the team members lift or slide the patient onto the stretcher in a smooth, continuous motion to avoid muscle strain and minimize patient discomfort.

SLIDING-BOARD TRANSFER

- Place the stretcher parallel to the bed, and lock the wheels of the bed and stretcher to ensure the patient's safety.
- Stand next to the bed, and have a coworker stand next to the stretcher.
- Reach over the patient and pull the far side of the bedsheet toward you to turn him slightly on his side. Your assistant places the sliding board beneath the patient, making sure the board bridges the gap between the stretcher and the bed.

- Ease the patient onto the sliding board and release the sheet. Your assistant grasps the near side of the sheet at the patient's hips and shoulders and pulls the patient onto the stretcher in a smooth, continuous motion; she then reaches over the patient, grasps the far side of the sheet, and logrolls the patient toward her.
- Remove the sliding board as your assistant returns the patient to the supine position.

AFTER ALL TRANSFERS
- Position the patient comfortably on the stretcher, apply safety straps, and raise and secure the side rails.

SPECIAL CONSIDERATIONS

- When transferring an immobile or markedly obese patient from bed to stretcher, first lift and move him, in increments, to the edge of the bed. Rest for a few seconds, repositioning him if necessary, and lift him onto the stretcher.
- If the patient can bear weight on his arms or legs, two or three coworkers can perform this transfer: One supports the buttocks and guides him, another stabilizes the stretcher by leaning over it and guiding him into position, and a third transfers any attached equipment.
- If a team member isn't available to guide equipment, move I.V. lines and other tubing; make sure beforehand that they're out of the way and not going to pull loose or disconnect tubes.
- If the patient is light, three coworkers can perform the carry lift. No matter how many team members are utilized, one must stabilize the patient's head if he can't support it himself, particularly if he has cervical instability or injury, or has undergone surgery.
- Depending on the patient's size and condition, a lift sheet transfer can require two to seven people.

COMPLICATIONS
- None known

PATIENT TEACHING

- Tell the patient you're going to move him from the bed to the stretcher, and place him in the supine position.

DOCUMENTATION

- Record the time and, if necessary, the type of transfer in your notes.
- Complete other required forms, as necessary.

SELECTED REFERENCES
Lloyd, J.D., and Baptiste, A. "Friction-Reducing Devices for Lateral Patient Transfers: A Biomechanical Evaluation," *AAOHN Journal* 54(3):113-19, March 2006.

Pellino, T.A., et al. "The Evaluation of Mechanical Devices for Lateral Transfers on Perceived Exertion and Patient Comfort," *Orthopaedic Nursing* 25(1): 4-10, January-February 2006.

Watson, D. "Planning to Ensure the Safe Transfer of Hospital Patients," *Nursing Times* 102(9):21-22, February-March 2006.

Transfer from bed to wheelchair

OVERVIEW

DESCRIPTION
◆ For the patient with diminished or absent lower-body sensation or one-sided weakness, immobility, or injury, this procedure may initially require partial support to full assistance by at least two persons.
◆ Subsequent transfers may be performed by one nurse, as appropriate.
◆ After transfer, proper positioning helps prevent excessive pressure on bony prominences, which predisposes the patient to skin breakdown.

CONTRAINDICATIONS
◆ None known

EQUIPMENT

Wheelchair with locks (or sturdy chair) ◆ pajama bottoms (or robe) ◆ shoes or slippers with nonslip soles ◆ watch with a second hand ◆ stethoscope ◆ sphygmomanometer ◆ transfer board, if appropriate

KEY STEPS

◆ Confirm the patient's identity using two patient identifiers according to facility policy.
◆ Explain the procedure to the patient and demonstrate his role. Explain how to use a transfer board, if needed. (See *Teaching the patient to use a transfer board*.)

Teaching the patient to use a transfer board

For the patient who can't stand, a transfer board allows safe transfer from bed to wheelchair.
◆ First, explain and demonstrate the procedure. The patient may eventually be able to transfer himself or require minimal help.
◆ Help him put on pajama bottoms or a robe and shoes or slippers.
◆ Lock the bed.
◆ Place the wheelchair angled slightly and facing the foot of the bed. Lock the wheels, and remove the armrest and footrest closest to the patient. Make sure the bed is flat and adjust its height so it's level with the wheelchair seat.
◆ Assist the patient to a sitting position on the edge of the bed, with his feet on the floor. Align the front edge of the wheelchair seat with the back of his knees, as shown below. For safety, an even surface is preferable, but he may find it easier to transfer to a slightly lower surface.

POSITIONING THE BOARD
◆ Have the patient lean away from the wheelchair while you slide one end of the transfer board under him.
◆ Place the other end of the transfer board on the wheelchair seat, and help him return to the upright position.
◆ Stand in front of the patient to prevent him from sliding forward. Tell him to push down with both arms and lift his buttocks up and onto the transfer board. Have him repeat the maneuver, edging along the board, until he's seated in the wheelchair. If he can't use his arms to help, stand in front of him, put your arms around him, and—if he's able—have him put his arms around you. Gradually slide him across the board until he's safely in the chair, as shown below.

ASSISTING THE PATIENT
◆ When the patient is in the chair, fasten a seat belt, if necessary, to prevent falls.
◆ Remove the transfer board, replace the wheelchair armrest and footrest, and reposition him in the chair.

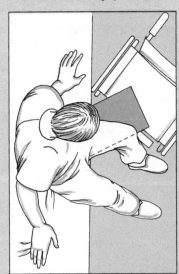

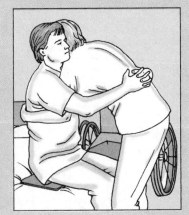

- Use proper body mechanics during the transfer to prevent injury.
- Place the wheelchair parallel to the bed, facing the foot of the bed, and lock its wheels.

  WARNING *Make sure the bed wheels are also locked. Raise the footrests to avoid interfering with the transfer. Be sure the bed is flat and in the lowest position.*
- Check pulse rate and blood pressure with the patient supine to obtain a baseline.
- Help him put on the pajama bottoms and slippers or shoes with nonslip soles to prevent falls.
- Raise the head of the bed and allow the patient to rest briefly to adjust to posture changes.
- Bring him to the dangling position.
- Recheck pulse rate and blood pressure if you suspect cardiovascular instability.

  WARNING *To prevent falls, don't proceed until the patient's pulse rate and blood pressure are stabilized.*
- Tell the patient to move toward the edge of the bed and try to place his feet flat on the floor.
- Stand in front of him, blocking his toes with your feet, and his knees with your knees to prevent his from buckling.
- Flex your knees slightly, place your arms around the patient's waist, and tell him to place his hands on the edge of the bed. To prevent back strain, avoid bending at your waist.
- Ask the patient to push himself off the bed and support as much of his own weight as he can as you straighten your knees and hips, raising him as you straighten your body.
- Supporting him as needed, pivot toward the wheelchair, keeping your knees next to his.
- Have him grasp the farthest armrest of the wheelchair with his closest hand.
- Help him lower himself into the wheelchair by flexing your hips and knees, but not your back.
- Instruct the patient to reach back and grasp the other wheelchair armrest as he sits to avoid abrupt contact with the seat.

- Fasten the seat belt to prevent falls and, if necessary, check the patient's pulse.

  WARNING *If the patient's pulse rate is 20 beats or more above baseline, monitor him closely until it returns to normal; he's experiencing orthostatic hypotension.*
- If the patient can't position himself correctly, help him move his buttocks against the back of the chair so that the ischial tuberosities, not the sacrum, provide the base of support.
- Place the patient's feet flat on the footrests, pointed straight ahead; position his knees and hips with the correct amount of flexion and in appropriate alignment.
- If appropriate, use elevating leg rests to flex his hips at more than 90 degrees; this position relieves pressure on the popliteal space and places more weight on the ischial tuberosities.
- Position the patient's arms on the wheelchair's armrests with shoulders abducted, elbows slightly flexed, forearms pronated, and wrists and hands in the neutral position.
- If necessary, support or elevate his hands and forearms with a pillow to prevent dependent edema.

SPECIAL CONSIDERATIONS

- If the patient starts to fall during transfer, ease him to the closest surface — bed, floor, or chair. Never stretch to finish the transfer.
- If the patient has one-sided weakness, follow the preceding steps, but place the wheelchair on his unaffected side. Tell him to pivot and bear as much weight as possible on the unaffected side.
- Support the affected side because he'll tend to lean to that side. Use pillows to support the hemiplegic patient's affected side to prevent slumping in the wheelchair.

COMPLICATIONS
- None known

PATIENT TEACHING

- Explain the procedure to the patient and demonstrate his role.

DOCUMENTATION

- Record the time of transfer and the extent of assistance in your notes, and note how the patient tolerated the activity.
- Document the length of time the patient was out of bed in the wheelchair and measures taken to relieve pressure from prolonged sitting.

SELECTED REFERENCES
Hagiwara, A., and Kanagawa, K. "Cardiovascular Responses During Bed-to-Wheelchair Transfers in Frail Elderly Who Live at Home," *Geriatrics & Gerontology International* 4(4):215-22, December 2004.

Kjellberg, K., et al. "Patient Safety and Comfort during Transfers in Relation to Nurses' Work Technique," *Journal of Advanced Nursing* 47(3):251-59, August 2004.

Watson, D. "Planning to Ensure the Safe Transfer of Hospital Patients," *Nursing Times* 102(9):21-22, February-March 2006.

Transfer with a hydraulic lift

OVERVIEW

- This procedure allows safe, comfortable transfer between bed and chair.
- It's indicated for the obese or immobile patient for whom manual transfer poses the potential for injury to the nurse or the patient.
- Most models can be operated by one person, but it's better to have two staff members present during transfer to stabilize and support the patient.

CONTRAINDICATIONS

- None known

EQUIPMENT

Hydraulic lift, with sling, chains or straps, and hooks ◆ chair or wheelchair

PREPARATION

- Hydraulic lift models vary in weight capacity. Check the manufacturer's specifications before attempting patient transfer.
- Lock the bed and wheelchair wheels before beginning.

KEY STEPS

- Confirm the patient's identity using two patient identifiers according to facility policy.
- Provide privacy and explain the procedure.
- If the patient has an I.V. line or urinary drainage bag, move it first. Arrange tubing securely to prevent dangling during transfer.
- If urinary drainage bag tubing isn't long enough to permit transfer, clamp the tubing and drainage bag and place it on the patient's abdomen. After the transfer, place the drainage bag in a dependent position and unclamp the tubing.
- Make sure the side rail opposite you is raised and secure; roll the patient toward you onto his side, and raise the side rail.
- Walk to the opposite side of the bed and lower the side rail.
- Place the sling under the patient's buttocks with its lower edge below the greater trochanter.

Using a hydraulic lift

After placing the patient supine in the center of the sling, position the hydraulic lift above him, as shown below. Then attach the chains to the hooks on the sling.

Turn the lift handle clockwise to raise the patient to the sitting position. If he's positioned properly, continue to raise him until he's suspended just above the bed (as shown below).

After positioning the patient above the wheelchair, turn the lift handle counterclockwise to lower him onto the seat (as shown below). When the chains become slack, stop turning and unhook the sling from the lift.

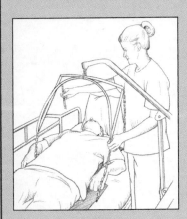

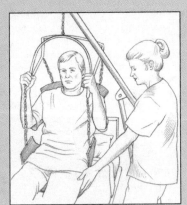

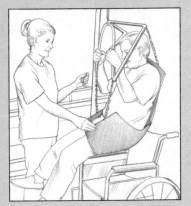

- Fanfold the far side of the sling against the patient's back and buttocks, and roll him toward you onto the sling, and raise the side rail.
- Lower the opposite side rail and slide your hands under the patient, pulling the sling from beneath him and smoothing out all wrinkles. Roll him onto his back and center him on the sling.
- Place the appropriate chair by the head of the bed, facing the foot of the bed.
- Lower the side rail next to the chair, and raise the bed only until the base of the lift can extend under the bed. To avoid alarming and endangering the patient, don't raise the bed completely.
- Set the lift's adjustable base to its widest position to ensure optimal stability.
- Move the lift so that its arm lies perpendicular to the bed, directly over him. (See *Using a hydraulic lift*.)
- Connect one end of the chains (or straps) to the side arms on the lift; connect the other (hooked end) to the sling.

⚡ **WARNING** *Face the hooks away from the patient to prevent them from slipping and to avoid risk of their pointed edges injuring him. To avoid injury, he may place his arms inside or outside the chains (or straps), or grasp them once the slack is gone.*

- Tighten the turnscrew on the lift.
- Depending on the type of lift, pump the handle or turn it clockwise until the patient has assumed a sitting position and his buttocks clear the bed surface by 1″ to 2″ (2.5 to 5 cm).
- Momentarily suspend the patient above the bed until he feels secure in the lift and sees that it can bear his weight.
- Steady the patient as you move the lift or, preferably, have another coworker guide his body while you move the lift. Depending on the type of lift, the arm should now rest in front or to one side of the chair.

- Release the turnscrew and depress the handle or turn it counterclockwise to lower the patient into the chair. While lowering him, push gently on his knees to maintain the correct sitting posture.
- After lowering the patient into the chair, fasten the seat belt to ensure his safety.
- Remove the hooks or straps from the sling, but leave the sling in place under him so you'll be able to transfer him back to the bed from the chair.
- Move the lift away. To return the patient to bed, reverse the procedure.

SPECIAL CONSIDERATIONS

- If the patient has an altered center of gravity (caused by a halo vest or a lower-extremity cast, for example), obtain help from a coworker before transferring with a hydraulic lift.
- If the patient will require use of a hydraulic lift for transfers after discharge, teach his family how to use the device correctly and allow supervised practice.

COMPLICATIONS
- None known

PATIENT TEACHING

- Explain the procedure and answer questions.
- Reassure the patient that the hydraulic lift can safely support his weight and won't tip over.

DOCUMENTATION

- If necessary, record the time of transfer in your notes.

SELECTED REFERENCES

Edlich, R.F., et al. "Prevention of Disabling Back Injuries in Nurses by the Use of Mechanical Patient Lift Systems," *Journal of Long-Term Effects of Medical Implants* 14(6):521-33, 2004.

Keir, P.J., and MacDonell, C.W. "Muscle Activity during Patient Transfers: A Preliminary Study on the Influence of Lift Assists and Experience," *Ergonomics* 47(3):296-306, February 2004.

Watson, D. "Planning to Ensure the Safe Transfer of Hospital Patients," *Nursing Times* 102(9):21-22, February-March 2006.

Transfusion of whole blood and packed cells

DESCRIPTION

◆ Whole blood transfusion replenishes the volume and the oxygen-carrying capacity of the circulatory system by increasing the mass of circulating red blood cells (RBCs).

◆ Transfusing packed RBCs, from which 80% of plasma has been removed, restores only oxygen-carrying capacity.

◆ After plasma is removed, the resulting component has a hematocrit of 65% to 80% and a typical volume of 300 to 350 ml. (Whole blood without plasma removed has a hematocrit of about 38%.)

◆ Each unit of whole blood or RBCs contains enough hemoglobin to raise the hemoglobin concentration in an average-sized adult by 1 g/dl (about 3%).

◆ These blood products are used to treat decreased hemoglobin levels and hematocrit.

◆ Whole blood is usually used when decreased levels result from hemorrhage.

◆ Packed RBCs are used when depressed levels accompany normal blood volume, to avoid possible fluid and circulatory overload.

◆ Both products contain cellular debris, requiring in-line filtration during administration.

◆ Washed packed RBCs (used for patients previously sensitized to transfusions) are rinsed with a special solution that removes white blood cells and platelets, thus decreasing the chance of transfusion reaction.

◆ Depending on facility policy, two nurses may have to identify the patient and blood products before giving a transfusion to prevent errors and potentially fatal reactions.

◆ If the patient is a Jehovah's Witness, special written permission is required.

CONTRAINDICATIONS

◆ Religious practices that may prohibit transfer of blood or blood products

EQUIPMENT

Blood administration set (170 to 260 micron filter and tubing with drip chamber for blood, or combined set) ◆ I.V. pole ◆ gloves ◆ gown ◆ face shield ◆ multiple-lead tubing ◆ whole blood or packed RBCs ◆ 250 ml of normal saline solution ◆ venipuncture equipment, if necessary (should include 20G or larger catheter) ◆ ice bag, warm compresses (optional)

⚡ WARNING *Multiple-lead tubing minimizes the risk of contamination, especially when transfusing multiple units of blood (a straight-line set would require multiple piggybacking). A Y-type set gives the option of adding normal saline solution to packed cells — decreasing their viscosity — if the patient can tolerate the added fluid volume.*

PREPARATION

◆ Straight-line and Y-type blood administration sets are commonly used.

◆ Filters come in mesh and microaggregate types; the latter is preferred, especially when transfusing multiple units of blood.

◆ Highly effective leukocyte removal filters can be used when transfusing blood and packed RBCs; they can postpone sensitization to transfusion therapy.

◆ Give packed RBCs with a Y-type set.

◆ Piggybacking increases the chance of harmful microorganisms entering the tubing because the blood line is connected to the established line.

◆ Avoid obtaining whole blood or packed RBCs until you're ready to begin the transfusion.

◆ Prepare the equipment when you're ready to start the infusion.

KEY STEPS

◆ Confirm the patient's identity using two patient identifiers according to facility policy.

◆ Explain the procedure and make sure the patient signed an informed consent form.

◆ Record the patient's baseline vital signs.

◆ Obtain whole blood or packed RBCs from the blood bank within 30 minutes of starting the transfusion.

◆ Check the expiration date on the blood bag and observe for abnormal color, RBC clumping, gas bubbles, and extraneous material.

◆ Return outdated or abnormal blood to the blood bank.

◆ Compare the name and number on the patient's wristband with those on the blood bag label.

◆ Check the blood bag identification number, ABO blood group, and Rh compatibility.

◆ Compare the patient's blood bank identification number, if present, with the number on the blood bag.

◆ Identification of blood and blood products is performed at the patient's bedside by two licensed professionals, according to policy.

◆ Put on gloves, a gown, and a face shield.

◆ Use a Y-type set; close all the clamps on the set.

◆ Insert the spike of the line you're using for the normal saline solution into the bag of normal saline solution.

◆ Open the port on the blood bag, and insert the spike of the line you're using to give the blood or cellular component into the port.

◆ Hang the bag of normal saline solution and blood or cellular component on the I.V. pole, open the clamp on the line of saline solution, and squeeze the drip chamber until it's one-half full.

◆ Remove the adapter cover at the tip of the blood administration set, open the main flow clamp, and prime the tubing with normal saline solution.

◆ If you're giving packed RBCs with a Y-type set, add normal saline solution to the bag to dilute the cells by closing the clamp between the patient and the drip chamber and opening the clamp from the blood.

◆ Lower the blood bag below the saline container and let 30 to 50 ml of normal saline solution flow into the packed cells.

◆ Close the clamp to the blood bag, rehang the bag, rotate it gently to mix the cells and normal saline solution, and close the clamp to the saline container.

◆ If the patient doesn't have an I.V. line in place, perform a venipuncture, using a 20G or larger-diameter catheter.

◆ Avoid using an existing line if the needle or catheter lumen is smaller than 20G. Central venous access devices may also be used for transfusion therapy.

◆ If giving whole blood, gently invert the bag several times to mix the cells.

◆ Attach the prepared blood administration set to the venipuncture device, and flush it with normal saline solution.

◆ Close the clamp to the normal saline solution, and open the clamp between the blood bag and the patient.

◆ Adjust the flow rate to no greater than 5 ml/minute for the first 15 minutes of the transfusion; remain with him to observe for a possible transfusion reaction.

⚡ **WARNING** *If such signs develop, record vital signs and stop the transfusion. Infuse normal saline solution at a moderately slow infusion rate and notify the practitioner.*

◆ If no signs of a reaction appear within 15 minutes, adjust the flow clamp to the ordered infusion rate. The rate of infusion should be as rapid as his circulatory system can tolerate.

◆ RBC preparations shouldn't remain at room temperature more than 4 hours. If the infusion rate must be so slow that the entire unit can't be infused within 4 hours, divide the unit and keep one portion refrigerated until it's given.

◆ After completing the transfusion, put on gloves and remove and discard the used infusion equipment. Then, reconnect the original I.V. fluid, if necessary, or discontinue the I.V. infusion.

◆ Return the empty blood bag to the blood bank, if facility policy dictates, and discard the tubing and filter. Record the patient's vital signs.

SPECIAL CONSIDERATIONS

◆ Although some microaggregate filters can be used for up to 10 units of blood, always replace the filter and tubing if more than 1 hour elapses between transfusions.

◆ When giving multiple units of blood under pressure, use a blood warmer to prevent hypothermia.

◆ For rapid blood replacement, you may need to use a pressure bag. Be aware that excessive pressure may develop, leading to broken blood vessels and extravasation, with hematoma and hemolysis of the infusing RBCs.

◆ If the transfusion stops, take these steps as needed:

– Check that the I.V. container is at least 3′ (1 m) above the I.V. site.

– Make sure that the flow clamp is open and that blood completely covers the filter. If it doesn't, squeeze the drip chamber until it does.

– Gently rock the bag back and forth to agitate blood cells that may have settled.

– Untape the dressing over the I.V. site to check needle placement. Reposition the needle if necessary.

– Flush the line with normal saline solution and restart the transfusion. Using a Y-type set, close the flow clamp to the patient and lower the blood bag. Next, open the saline clamp and allow some normal saline solution to flow into the blood bag. Rehang the blood bag, open the flow clamp to the patient, and reset the flow rate.

– If a hematoma develops at the I.V. site, immediately stop the infusion and remove the I.V. cannula. Notify the practitioner; ice the site intermittently for 8 hours; then apply warm compresses, according to facility policy.

– If the blood bag empties before the next one arrives, give normal saline solution slowly. If you're using a Y-type set, close the blood-line clamp, open the saline clamp, and let the normal saline solution run slowly until the new blood arrives. Decrease the flow rate or clamp the line before attaching the new unit of blood.

COMPLICATIONS

◆ Transfusion reactions
◆ Infectious disease transmission
◆ Hepatitis C
◆ Circulatory overload
◆ Hemolytic, allergic, febrile, and pyogenic reactions
◆ Coagulation disturbances
◆ Citrate intoxication
◆ Hyperkalemia
◆ Acid-base imbalance
◆ Loss of 2,3-diphosphoglycerate
◆ Ammonia intoxication
◆ Hypothermia

PATIENT TEACHING

◆ Explain the procedure to the patient and answer questions, as needed.

DOCUMENTATION

◆ Record the date and time of transfusion and the patient's vital signs.
◆ Note the type and amount of transfusion product.
◆ Document check of identification data.
◆ Record the patient's response.
◆ Note transfusion reaction and treatment.

SELECTED REFERENCES
Davis, K., et al. "Transfusing Safely: A 2006 Guide for Nurses," *Australian Nursing Journal* 13(6):17-20, December 2005-January 2006.
Hughes, M. "Using Guidelines to Minimise the Hazards of Blood Transfusion," *Nursing Times* 101(4):36, January 2005.
Sandler, S.G., et al. "Bar Code Technology Improves Positive Patient Identification and Transfusion Safety," *Developments in Biologicals* 120:19-24, 2005.

Transfusion reaction management

DESCRIPTION

- Transfusion reaction stems from a major antigen-antibody reaction and can result from a single or massive transfusion of blood or blood products.
- Many reactions occur during transfusion or within 96 hours afterward.
- Transfusion reaction requires immediate recognition and prompt nursing action to prevent further complications or death, particularly if the patient is unconscious or heavily sedated and can't report symptoms. (See *Guide to transfusion reactions.*)

CONTRAINDICATIONS

- None known

Normal saline solution ◆ I.V. administration set ◆ sterile urine specimen container ◆ needle, syringe, and tubes for blood samples ◆ transfusion reaction report form ◆ oxygen ◆ epinephrine ◆ hypothermia blanket ◆ leukocyte removal filter (optional)

- If an adverse reaction is suspected, stop the transfusion and start a normal saline solution infusion (using a new I.V. administration set) at a keep-vein-open rate to maintain venous access. Don't discard the blood bag or administration set.
- Notify the practitioner.
- Monitor vital signs every 15 minutes or as indicated by severity and type of reaction.
- Compare labels on blood containers with corresponding patient identification forms to verify that the transfusion was the correct blood or blood product.
- Notify the blood bank of a possible transfusion reaction and collect blood samples, as ordered.
- Immediately send the samples, transfusion containers (even if empty), and the administration set to the blood bank; they'll test materials to further evaluate the reaction.
- Collect the first posttransfusion urine specimen, mark the collection slip "Possible transfusion reaction," and send it to the laboratory immediately to test for presence of hemoglobin, which indicates a hemolytic reaction.
- Closely monitor intake and output. Note evidence of oliguria or anuria because hemoglobin deposition in the renal tubules can cause renal damage.
- If prescribed, give oxygen, epinephrine, or other drugs and apply a hypothermia blanket to reduce fever.
- Make the patient as comfortable as possible and provide reassurance as necessary.

Guide to transfusion reactions

A patient receiving a transfusion of processed blood products risks certain complications; for example, hemosiderosis and hypothermia. This chart describes *endogenous reactions*—those caused by an antigen-antibody reaction in the recipient, and *exogenous reactions*—those caused by external factors in administered blood.

REACTION AND CAUSES	SIGNS AND SYMPTOMS	NURSING INTERVENTIONS
Endogenous		
Allergic ◆ Allergen in donor blood ◆ Donor blood hypersensitive to certain drugs	◆ Anaphylaxis (chills, facial swelling) ◆ Laryngeal edema ◆ Pruritus, urticaria, wheezing ◆ Fever ◆ Nausea and vomiting	◆ Administer antihistamines as prescribed. ◆ Monitor patient for anaphylactic reaction, and administer epinephrine and corticosteroids if indicated. ◆ As prescribed, premedicate the patient with diphenhydramine before subsequent transfusion.
Bacterial contamination ◆ Organisms that can survive cold, such as *Pseudomonas* and *Staphylococcus*	◆ Chills ◆ Fever ◆ Vomiting ◆ Abdominal cramping ◆ Diarrhea ◆ Shock ◆ Signs of renal failure	◆ Provide broad-spectrum antibiotics, corticosteroids, or epinephrine as prescribed. ◆ Maintain strict blood storage control. ◆ Change blood administration set and filter every 4 hours or after every 2 units. ◆ Infuse each unit of blood over 2 to 4 hours; stop the infusion if the time span exceeds 4 hours. ◆ Maintain sterile technique when administering blood products.
Febrile ◆ Bacterial lipopolysaccharides ◆ Antileukocyte recipient antibodies directed against donor white blood cells	◆ Temperature up to 104° F (40° C) ◆ Chills ◆ Headache ◆ Facial flushing ◆ Palpitations ◆ Cough ◆ Chest tightness ◆ Increased pulse rate ◆ Flank pain	◆ Relieve symptoms with an antipyretic, antihistamine, or meperidine, as prescribed. ◆ If the patient requires further transfusions, use frozen red blood cells (RBCs), add a special leukocyte removal filter to the blood line, or premedicate him with acetaminophen, as prescribed, before starting another transfusion.
Hemolytic ◆ ABO or Rh incompatibility ◆ Intradonor incompatibility ◆ Improper crossmatching ◆ Improperly stored blood	◆ Chest pain ◆ Dyspnea ◆ Facial flushing ◆ Fever ◆ Chills ◆ Shaking ◆ Hypotension ◆ Flank pain ◆ Hemoglobinuria ◆ Oliguria ◆ Bloody oozing at the infusion site or surgical incision site ◆ Burning sensation along vein receiving blood ◆ Shock ◆ Renal failure	◆ Monitor blood pressure. ◆ Manage shock with I.V. fluids, oxygen, epinephrine, a diuretic, and a vasopressor, as prescribed. ◆ Obtain posttransfusion-reaction blood samples and urine specimens for analysis. ◆ Observe for signs of hemorrhage resulting from disseminated intravascular coagulation.
Plasma protein incompatibility ◆ Immunoglobulin-A incompatibility	◆ Abdominal pain and diarrhea ◆ Dyspnea ◆ Chills ◆ Fever ◆ Flushing ◆ Hypotension	◆ Administer oxygen, fluids, epinephrine, or a corticosteroid, as prescribed.

(continued)

REACTION AND CAUSES	SIGNS AND SYMPTOMS	NURSING INTERVENTIONS
Exogenous		
Bleeding tendencies ◆ Low platelet count in stored blood, causing thrombocytopenia	◆ Abnormal bleeding and oozing from a cut ◆ A break in the skin surface or the gums; abnormal bruising and petechiae	◆ Administer platelets, fresh frozen plasma, or cryoprecipitate, as prescribed. ◆ Monitor platelet count.
Circulatory overload ◆ May result from infusing blood too rapidly or in large volumes	◆ Increased plasma volume ◆ Back pain ◆ Chest tightness ◆ Chills ◆ Fever ◆ Dyspnea ◆ Flushed feeling ◆ Headache ◆ Hypertension ◆ Increased central venous pressure and jugular vein pressure	◆ Monitor blood pressure. ◆ Use packed RBCs instead of whole blood. ◆ Administer diuretics, as prescribed.
Elevated blood ammonia level ◆ Increased ammonia level in stored donor blood	◆ Confusion ◆ Forgetfulness ◆ Lethargy	◆ Monitor ammonia level in blood. ◆ Decrease the amount of protein in the patient's diet. ◆ If indicated, give neomycin.
Hemosiderosis ◆ Increased level of hemosiderin (iron-containing pigment) from RBC destruction, especially after many transfusions	◆ Iron plasma level exceeding 200 mg/dl	◆ Perform a phlebotomy to remove excess iron.
Hypocalcemia ◆ Rapidly infused citrate-treated blood causing citrate toxicity; citrate binding with calcium, causing a calcium deficiency, or normal citrate metabolism becoming impeded by hepatic disease	◆ Arrhythmias ◆ Hypotension ◆ Muscle cramps ◆ Nausea ◆ Vomiting ◆ Tingling in fingers	◆ Slow or stop the transfusion, depending on the patient's reaction. Expect a more severe reaction in hypothermic patients or those with elevated potassium levels. ◆ Slowly administer calcium gluconate I.V., if prescribed.
Hypothermia ◆ Rapid infusion of large amounts of cold blood, which decreases body temperature	◆ Chills; shaking; hypotension; arrhythmias, especially bradycardia ◆ Cardiac arrest if core temperature falls below 86° F (30° C)	◆ Stop the transfusion. ◆ Warm him with blankets. ◆ Place him in a warm environment if necessary. ◆ Obtain an electrocardiographic strip. ◆ Warm blood if the transfusion is resumed.
Increased oxygen affinity for hemoglobin ◆ Decreased level of 2,3-diphosphoglycerate in stored blood, causing an increase in the oxygen's hemoglobin affinity; oxygen remaining in the patient's bloodstream and not released into body tissues	◆ Depressed respiratory rate, especially in patients with chronic lung disease	◆ Monitor arterial blood gas values, and provide respiratory support, as needed.

- Treat all transfusion reactions as serious until proven otherwise.
- If the practitioner anticipates a transfusion reaction (as with a leukemia patient), he may order prophylactic treatment with antihistamines or antipyretics to precede blood administration.
- To avoid a possible febrile reaction, the practitioner may order the blood to be washed to remove as many leukocytes as possible, or a leukocyte removal filter may be used during the transfusion.

COMPLICATIONS
- None known

- Advise the patient to report signs and symptoms that may signal an adverse reaction to treatment.
- Explain any procedures or medication administration to the patient.
- Reassure the patient to allay his fears.

- Record the time and date of the transfusion reaction.
- Note the type and amount of infused blood or blood products.
- Document clinical signs of the transfusion reaction in order of occurrence.
- Record vital signs, specimens sent to the laboratory for analysis, treatment given, and the patient's response.
- If required by facility policy, complete the transfusion reaction form.

SELECTED REFERENCES
"Documenting a Transfusion Reaction," *Nursing* 35(3):25, March 2005.

Narvios, A.B., et al. "Underreporting of Minor Transfusion Reactions in Cancer Patients," *Medscape General Medicine* 6(2):17, May 2004.

Sandler, S.G. "How I Manage Patients Suspected of Having Had an IgA Anaphylactic Transfusion Reaction," *Transfusion* 46(1):10-13, January 2006.

Szymanski, I., and Seder, R. "Acute Pancreatitis Associated with Massive Hemolysis Due to a Delayed Hemolytic Transfusion Reaction," *Transfusion* 45(10):1691-92, October 2005.

Guide to transfusion reactions *(continued)*		
REACTION AND CAUSES	**SIGNS AND SYMPTOMS**	**NURSING INTERVENTIONS**
Exogenous (continued)		
Potassium intoxication ◆ An abnormally high level of potassium in stored plasma caused by hemolysis of RBCs	◆ Diarrhea ◆ Intestinal colic ◆ Flaccidity ◆ Muscle twitching ◆ Oliguria ◆ Renal failure ◆ Bradycardia progressing to cardiac arrest ◆ Electrocardiographic changes with tall peaked T waves	◆ Obtain an electrocardiographic strip. ◆ Administer sodium polystyrene sulfonate (Kayexalate) orally or by enema. ◆ Administer dextrose 50% and insulin, bicarbonate, or calcium, as prescribed, to force potassium into cells.

T tube care

DESCRIPTION

- A T tube (also called a *biliary drain-ing tube*) may be placed in the common bile duct after cholecystectomy or choledochostomy.
- The tube facilitates biliary drainage during healing.
- The surgeon inserts the short end (crossbar) into the common bile duct and draws the long end through the incision. The tube is then connected to a closed gravity drainage system.
- Postoperatively, it remains in place between 7 and 14 days.

CONTRAINDICATIONS

- None known

Graduated collection container ♦ small plastic bag ♦ sterile gloves and clean gloves ♦ clamp ♦ sterile 4″×4″ gauze pads ♦ transparent dressings ♦ rubber band ♦ normal saline solution ♦ sterile cleaning solution ♦ two sterile basins ♦ povidone-iodine pads ♦ sterile precut drain dressings ♦ hypoallergenic paper tape ♦ skin protectant, such as petroleum jelly, aluminum-based gel, or zinc oxide ♦ Montgomery straps (optional)

PREPARATION

- Assemble equipment at the bedside.
- Open all sterile equipment. Place one sterile 4″ × 4″ gauze pad in each sterile basin.
- Using sterile technique, pour 50 ml of cleaning solution into one basin and 50 ml of normal saline solution into the other basin.
- Tape a small plastic bag on the table to use for refuse.

- Confirm the patient's identity using two patient identifiers according to facility policy.
- Provide privacy and explain the procedure to the patient.
- Wash your hands.

EMPTYING DRAINAGE

- Put on clean gloves.
- Place the graduated collection container under the outlet valve of the drainage bag. Without contaminating the clamp, valve, or outlet valve, empty the bag's contents completely into the container and reseal the outlet valve.
- Carefully measure and record the character, color, and amount of drainage.
- Discard your gloves.

REDRESSING THE T TUBE

- Wash your hands and put on clean gloves.
- Without dislodging the T tube, remove old dressings, and dispose of them in the small plastic bag. Remove gloves.
- Wash your hands again and put on sterile gloves; follow strict aseptic technique to prevent contamination of the incision.
- Inspect the incision and tube site for signs of infection, including redness,

---

Managing T tube obstruction

If your patient's T tube blocks after chole-cystectomy:

- ♦ Notify the practitioner.
- ♦ Unclamp the T tube (if it was clamped before and after a meal) and connect the tube to a closed gravity-drainage system.
- ♦ Inspect the tube to detect any kinks or obstructions.
- ♦ Prepare for possible T tube irrigation or direct X-ray of the common bile duct (cholangiography). Explain the procedure to lessen anxiety and promote cooperation.
- ♦ Provide encouragement and support.

edema, warmth, tenderness, induration, or skin excoriation. Assess for wound dehiscence or evisceration.

♦ Use sterile cleaning solution as prescribed to clean and remove dried matter or drainage from around the tube. Start at the tube site and gently wipe outward in a continuous motion to prevent recontamination of the incision.

♦ Use normal saline solution to rinse off the prescribed cleaning solution. Dry the area with a sterile 4″ × 4″ gauze pad and discard all used materials.

♦ Using a povidone-iodine pad, wipe the incision site in a circular motion. Allow the area to dry.

♦ Apply a skin protectant (petroleum jelly, zinc oxide, or aluminum-based gel) to prevent injury from draining bile.

♦ Apply a sterile precut drain dressing on each side of the T tube to absorb drainage.

♦ Apply a sterile 4″ × 4″ gauze pad or transparent dressing over the T tube and the drain dressings.

⚡ **WARNING** *Don't kink the tubing, which can block drainage, and don't put the dressing over the open end of the T tube because it connects to the closed drainage system.*

♦ Secure the dressings with the hypoallergenic paper tape or Montgomery straps if necessary.

CLAMPING THE T TUBE

♦ As ordered, occlude the tube lightly with a clamp or wrap a rubber band around the end. Clamping the tube 1 hour before and after meals diverts bile back to the duodenum to aid digestion.

♦ Monitor the patient's response to clamping.

♦ To ensure his comfort and safety, check bile drainage amounts regularly.

⚡ **WARNING** *Report signs of obstructed bile flow, such as chills, fever, tachycardia, nausea, right-upper-quadrant fullness and pain, jaundice, dark foamy urine, and clay-colored stools.*

♦ The T tube usually drains 300 to 500 ml of blood-tinged bile in the first 24 hours after surgery.

⚡ **WARNING** *Report drainage that exceeds 500 ml in the first 24 hours after surgery; if it's 50 ml or less, notify the practitioner; the tube may be obstructed. Drainage typically declines to 200 ml or less after 4 days and the color changes to green-brown. Monitor fluid, electrolyte, and acid-base status.*

♦ To prevent excessive bile loss (over 500 ml in first 24 hours) or backflow contamination, secure the T tube drainage system at abdominal level. Bile will flow into the bag only when biliary pressure increases.

♦ Provide meticulous skin care and frequent dressing changes.

♦ Observe for bile leakage, which may indicate obstruction. (See *Managing T tube obstruction.*)

♦ Assess tube patency and site condition hourly for the first 8 hours, then every 4 hours until the practitioner removes the tube.

♦ Protect the skin edges and avoid excessive taping.

♦ Monitor all urine and stools for color changes. Assess for icteric skin and sclera, which may signal jaundice.

COMPLICATIONS

♦ Obstructed bile flow
♦ Skin excoriation or breakdown
♦ Tube dislodgment
♦ Drainage reflux
♦ Infection

♦ Explain to the patient that loose bowels occur commonly the first few weeks after surgery.

♦ Teach the patient about signs and symptoms of T tube and biliary obstruction and to report them to the practitioner.

♦ Teach the patient how to care for the tube at home.

♦ Caution the patient that bile stains clothing.

♦ Record the date and time of each dressing change.

♦ Note the appearance of the wound and surrounding skin.

♦ Write down the color, character, and volume of bile collected.

♦ Record the color of skin and mucous membranes around the T tube.

♦ Keep a precise record of temperature trends and the amount and frequency of urination and bowel movements.

SELECTED REFERENCES

Angel Mercado, M., et al. "Bile Duct Injuries Related to Misplacement of 'T Tubes'," *Annals of Hepatology* 5(1):44-48, January-March 2006.

Hashimoto, M., et al. "T-Tube Drainage for Biliary Stenosis after Donor Liver Transplantation," *Transplantation* 81(2):293-95, January 2006.

Heikkinen, M., et al. "Removing a Biliary T Tube and Retained Stones by ERCP. A Care Report," *Hepatogastroenterology* 52(66):1666-67, November-December 2005.

Perez, G., et al. "Prospective Randomized Study of T-Tube Versus Biliary Stent for Common Bile Duct Decompression after Open Choledocotomy," *World Journal of Surgery* 29(7):869-72, July 2005.

Tube feedings

DESCRIPTION

- Tube feedings deliver a liquid formula directly to the stomach (known as *gastric gavage*), duodenum, or jejunum.
- They're indicated for the patient who can't eat normally because of dysphagia or oral or esophageal obstruction or injury.
- Tube feedings may be given to an unconscious or intubated patient or to the patient recovering from GI tract surgery who can't eat food by mouth.
- Duodenal or jejunal feedings decrease risk of aspiration because the formula bypasses the pylorus.
- Jejunal feedings reduce pancreatic stimulation; thus, may require an elemental diet.
- They're usually given on an intermittent schedule; patients getting duodenal or jejunal feedings typically better tolerate a continuous slow drip.
- Liquid nutrient solutions come in various formulas for administration through a nasogastric tube, small-bore feeding tube, gastrostomy or jejunostomy tube, percutaneous endoscopic gastrostomy or jejunostomy tube, or gastrostomy feeding button.
- A bulb syringe or large catheter-tip syringe may be substituted for a gavage bag if the patient tolerates a gravity drip infusion.
- The practitioner may order an infusion pump to ensure accurate delivery of the prescribed formula.

CONTRAINDICATIONS

- Absent bowel sounds
- Suspected intestinal obstruction

GASTRIC FEEDINGS

Feeding formula ◆ graduated container ◆ 120 ml of water ◆ gavage bag with tubing and flow regulator clamp ◆ towel or linen-saver pad ◆ 60-ml syringe ◆ pH test strip ◆ adapter to connect gavage tubing to feeding tube ◆ infusion controller and tubing set (optional, for continuous administration)

DUODENAL OR JEJUNAL FEEDINGS

Feeding formula ◆ enteral administration set containing a gavage container, drip chamber, roller clamp or flow regulator, and tube connector ◆ I.V. pole ◆ 60-ml syringe with adapter tip ◆ water ◆ Y connector ◆ pump administration set (optional, for an enteral infusion pump)

NASAL AND ORAL CARE

Cotton-tipped applicators ◆ water-soluble lubricant ◆ oral swabs ◆ petroleum jelly

PREPARATION

- Refrigerate formulas prepared in the dietary department or pharmacy. Refrigerate commercial formulas only after opening them.
- Check the date on all formula containers. Discard expired formula.
- Use powdered formula within 24 hours of mixing.
- Shake the container well to mix thoroughly, and allow the formula to warm to room temperature before giving (never warm it over direct heat or in a microwave; heat may curdle the formula or change its chemical composition). Cold formula can increase the chance of diarrhea.
- Pour 60 ml of water into the graduated container.
- After closing the flow clamp on the administration set, pour the appropriate amount of formula into the gavage bag.
- To prevent bacterial growth, hang no more than a 4 to 6-hour supply at one time.
- Open the flow clamp on the administration set to remove air from the lines. This keeps air from entering the patient's stomach and causing distention.

- Confirm the patient's identity using two patient identifiers according to facility policy.
- Provide privacy and wash your hands.
- Inform the patient that he'll receive nourishment through the tube, and explain the procedure. If possible, give him a schedule of subsequent feedings.
- If the patient has a nasal or oral tube, cover his chest with a towel or linen-saver pad to protect him and the bed linens from spills.
- Assess his abdomen for bowel sounds and distention.

DELIVERING A GASTRIC FEEDING

- Elevate the bed to semi-Fowler's or high Fowler's position to prevent aspiration by gastroesophageal reflux, and to promote digestion.
- Check the feeding tube to be sure it hasn't slipped out since the last feeding.

⚡ **WARNING** *Never give a tube feeding until you're sure the tube is properly positioned in the patient's stomach; otherwise, it could cause formula to enter his lungs.*

- To check tube patency and position, remove the cap or plug from the feeding tube, and attach the syringe.
- Gently aspirate gastric secretions.
- Examine the aspirate and place a small amount on the pH test strip. Proper placement of the gastric tube is likely if the aspirate has a typical gastric fluid appearance (grassy-green, clear and colorless with mucus shreds, or brown) and a pH of 5.0 or less.
- To assess gastric emptying, aspirate and measure residual gastric contents. Hold feedings if residual volume is greater than the predetermined amount specified in the practitioner's order (usually 50 to 100 ml). Reinstill any aspirate obtained.
- Connect the gavage bag tubing to the feeding tube; you may need to use an adapter to connect the two.

- If using a bulb or catheter-tip syringe, remove the bulb or plunger and attach the syringe to the pinched-off feeding tube to prevent excess air from entering the patient's stomach, causing distention.
- If using an infusion controller, thread the tube from the formula container through the controller according to manufacturer's directions.
- Blue food dye can be added to food to quickly identify aspiration.
- Purge the tubing of air and attach it to the feeding tube.
- Open the regulator clamp on the gavage bag tubing and adjust the flow rate appropriately.
- When using a bulb syringe, fill the syringe with formula and release the feeding tube to allow formula to flow through it. The height at which you hold the syringe will determine its flow rate. When the syringe is three-quarters empty, pour more formula into it.
- To prevent air from entering the tube and the patient's stomach, never allow the syringe to empty completely.
- If you're using an infusion controller, set the flow rate according to the manufacturer's directions.
- Always give a tube feeding slowly—typically 200 to 350 ml over 15 to 30 minutes, depending on the patient's tolerance and the practitioner's order—to prevent sudden stomach distention, which can cause nausea, vomiting, cramps, or diarrhea.
- After giving the appropriate amount of formula, flush the tubing by adding about 60 ml of water to the gavage bag or bulb syringe, or manually flush it using a barrel syringe. This maintains the tube's patency by removing excess formula, which could occlude the tube.
- If you're giving a continuous feeding, flush the feeding tube every 4 hours to help prevent tube occlusion. Monitor gastric emptying every 4 hours.
- To discontinue gastric feeding (depending on the equipment), close the regulator clamp on the gavage bag tubing, disconnect the syringe from the feeding tube, or turn off the infusion controller.

- Cover the end of the feeding tube with its plug or cap to prevent leakage and contamination.
- Leave the patient in semi-Fowler's or high Fowler's position for at least 30 minutes.
- Rinse reusable equipment with warm water; dry and store in a convenient place for the next feeding. Change equipment every 24 hours or according to facility policy.

DELIVERING A DUODENAL OR JEJUNAL FEEDING

- Elevate the head of the bed and place the patient in low Fowler's position.
- Open the enteral administration set and hang the gavage container on the I.V. pole.
- If using a nasoduodenal tube, measure its length to check tube placement. Remember, you may not get residual when you aspirate the tube.
- Open the flow clamp and regulate the flow to the desired rate.
- To regulate the rate using a volumetric infusion pump, follow the manufacturer's directions for equipment setup. Most patients receive small amounts at first, with volumes increasing gradually when tolerance is established.
- Flush the tube every 4 hours with water to maintain patency and provide hydration. A needle catheter jejunostomy tube may require flushing every 2 hours to prevent formula buildup inside the tube.
- A Y-connector may be useful for frequent flushing. Attach the continuous feeding to the main port and use the side port for flushes.
- Change equipment every 24 hours or according to facility policy.

(continued)

SPECIAL CONSIDERATIONS

- If the feeding solution doesn't initially flow through a bulb syringe, attach the bulb and squeeze it gently to start the flow; then remove the bulb.
- Never use the bulb to force formula through the tube.
- If the patient becomes nauseated or vomits, stop feeding immediately. He may vomit if his stomach becomes distended from overfeeding or delayed gastric emptying.
- To reduce oropharyngeal discomfort caused by the tube, allow the patient to brush his teeth or care for his dentures regularly, and encourage frequent gargling.
- If he's unconscious, give oral care with wet sponge-tipped swabs every 4 hours. Use petroleum jelly on dry, cracked lips.
- Dry mucous membranes may indicate dehydration, which requires increased fluid intake.
- Clean the patient's nostrils with cotton-tipped applicators, apply lubricant along the mucosa, and assess his skin for signs of breakdown.
- During continuous feedings, assess the patient frequently for abdominal distention. Flush the tubing by adding about 50 ml of water to the gavage bag or bulb syringe. This maintains the tube's patency by removing excess formula, which can occlude the tube.
- If the patient develops diarrhea, give small, frequent, less concentrated feedings, or give bolus feedings over a longer time.
- Make sure the formula isn't cold and proper storage and sanitation practices have been followed.
- Loose stools associated with tube feedings make extra perineal and skin care necessary. Giving paregoric, tincture of opium, or diphenoxylate hydrochloride may improve the condition; changing to a formula with more fiber may eliminate liquid stools. A practitioner's order is required for these interventions.

- If the patient is constipated, the practitioner may increase fruit, vegetable, or sugar content of the formula.
- Assess the patient's hydration status; increase fluid intake as necessary. If the condition persists, give an appropriate drug or enema, as ordered.
- Drugs can be given through the feeding tube; however some drugs may change the osmolarity of the feeding formula and cause diarrhea.
- Except for enteric-coated drugs or time-released drugs, crush tablets or open and dilute capsules in water before giving them. Be sure to flush the tubing afterward to ensure full instillation of drug.

TROUBLESHOOTER *Small-bore feeding tubes may kink, making instillation impossible. Change the patient's position or withdraw the tube a few inches and restart. Never use a guide wire to reposition the tube.*

- Constantly monitor the flow rate of a blended or high-residue formula to determine if the formula is clogging the tubing as it settles. To prevent such clogging, squeeze the bag frequently to agitate the solution.
- Collect blood specimens, as ordered.
- Glycosuria, hyperglycemia, and diuresis can indicate an excessive carbohydrate level, leading to hyperosmotic dehydration, which may be fatal.
- Monitor the patient's blood glucose levels to assess glucose tolerance.
- Also monitor electrolytes, blood urea nitrogen, glucose, and osmolality to determine response to therapy and assess hydration status.
- Check the flow rate hourly to ensure correct infusion. (With an improvised administration set, use a time tape to record the rate because it's difficult to get precise readings from an irrigation container or enema bag.)
- For duodenal or jejunal feeding, most patients tolerate a continuous drip better than bolus feedings, which can cause hyperglycemia and diarrhea.

- Until the patient tolerates the formula, you may need to dilute it to one-half or three-quarters strength to start, and increase it gradually.

⚡ **WARNING** *Patients under stress or receiving steroids may experience a pseudodiabetic state. Assess frequently to determine the need for insulin.*

COMPLICATIONS

- Erosion of esophageal, tracheal, nasal, and oropharyngeal mucosa
- Bloating and retention when using gastric route for frequent or large-volume feedings
- Dehydration, diarrhea, and vomiting, causing metabolic disturbances; cramping and abdominal distention usually indicating intolerance
- Clogged feeding tube when using duodenal or jejunal route
- Metabolic, fluid, and electrolyte abnormalities including hyperglycemia, hyperosmolar dehydration, coma, edema, hypernatremia, and essential fatty acid deficiency
- Dumping syndrome (see *Managing tube feeding problems*)

◆ Teach the patient about the infusion control device to maintain accuracy, use of the syringe or bag and tubing, care of the tube and insertion site, and formula-mixing.

◆ Tell the patient that the formula may be mixed in an electric blender according to package directions.

◆ Tell the patient that formula not used within 24 hours must be discarded. If the formula must hang for more than 8 hours, advise the patient to use a gavage or pump administration set with an ice pouch to decrease the incidence of bacterial growth.

◆ Instruct the patient to use a new bag daily.

◆ Teach family members signs and symptoms to report to the practitioner or home care nurse as well as measures to take in an emergency.

◆ On the intake and output sheet, record the date, volume of formula, and volume of water.

◆ In your notes, record abdominal assessment (including tube exit site, if appropriate); amount of residual gastric contents; verification of tube placement; amount, type, and time of feeding; and tube patency.

◆ Note the patient's tolerance, as well as any nausea, vomiting, cramping, diarrhea, and distention.

◆ Note the result of blood and urine tests, hydration status, and drugs given through the tube.

◆ Record the date and time of administration set changes, oral and nasal hygiene, and results of specimen collections.

SELECTED REFERENCES

Carey, T.S., et al. "Expectations and Outcomes of Gastric Feeding Tubes," *American Journal of Medicine* 119(6): 527.e11-16, June 2006.

Ellett, M.L. "Important Facts About Intestinal Feeding Tube Placement," *Gastroenterology Nursing* 29(2):112-24, March-April 2006.

Ista, E., and Joosten, K. "Nutritional Assessment and Enteral Support of Critically Ill Children," *Critical Care Nursing Clinics of North America* 17(4): 385-93, December 2005.

Metheny, N.A., et al. "Indicators of Tubesite During Feedings," *Journal of Neuroscience Nursing* 37(6):320-25, December 2005.

Managing tube feeding problems

COMPLICATIONS	NURSING INTERVENTIONS
Aspiration of gastric secretions	◆ Discontinue feeding immediately. ◆ Perform tracheal suction of aspirated contents if possible. ◆ Notify the practitioner. Prophylactic antibiotics and chest physiotherapy may be ordered. ◆ Check tube placement before feeding to prevent complication.
Tube obstruction	◆ Flush the tube with warm water. If necessary, replace the tube. ◆ Flush the tube with 50 ml of water after each feeding to remove excess sticky formula, which could occlude the tube.
Oral, nasal, or pharyngeal irritation or necrosis	◆ Provide frequent oral hygiene using mouthwash or oral swabs. Use petroleum jelly on cracked lips. ◆ Change the tube's position. If necessary, replace the tube.
Vomiting, bloating, diarrhea, or cramps	◆ Reduce the flow rate. ◆ Administer prescribed metoclopramide to increase GI motility. ◆ Warm the formula to prevent GI distress. ◆ For 30 minutes after feeding, position the patient on his right side with his head elevated to facilitate gastric emptying. ◆ Notify the practitioner. He may want to reduce the amount of formula being given during each feeding.
Constipation	◆ Provide additional fluids if the patient can tolerate them. ◆ Administer a prescribed bulk-forming laxative. ◆ Increase fruit, vegetable, or sugar content of the feeding, as prescribed by the practitioner.
Electrolyte imbalance	◆ Monitor serum electrolyte levels. ◆ Notify the practitioner. He may want to adjust the formula content to correct the deficiency.
Hyperglycemia	◆ Monitor blood glucose levels. ◆ Notify the practitioner of elevated levels. ◆ Administer insulin if ordered. ◆ The practitioner may adjust the sugar content of the formula.

Turning frames

DESCRIPTION

- A turning frame allows repeated changes between supine and prone positions without disturbing spinal alignment in patients who must remain immobile.
- The patient lies on the anterior frame in the prone position and on the posterior frame in the supine position, secured between both sections, which pivot as one unit.
- The Stryker frame accommodates cervical traction. (See *Operating a Stryker wedge frame.*)
- Another type of frame accommodates cervical and pelvic traction.
- To operate either frame, at least one member of the turning team must have training and experience.

CONTRAINDICATIONS

- Obesity

Turning frames with safety straps ◆ arm boards ◆ special sheets (with ties) for each frame ◆ fresh linens ◆ pillow or sheepskin ◆ hand rolls or cradle boots ◆ footboard

PREPARATION

- Place sheets on the anterior and posterior frames, tying corners to the frame; secure the remainder of each sheet to the nearest fastener.
- Make sure the posterior frame's perineal opening is in the correct position.
- Secure the posterior frame to the bed and lock it in place.
- Turn the bed to check that it's working properly, and lock its wheels.

Operating a Stryker wedge frame

- Obtain the help of a coworker and remove the armboards from the frame.
- Arrange the anterior frame over the patient and lock it at the head end.
- Replace the anterior half of the ring, if removed, and close it over the patient until it locks automatically.
- Place the patient's arms around the anterior frame if he's able to grasp it; otherwise use safety straps to keep his arms in place.
- Pull out the locking pin, release the lock and, with assistance, turn him.
- Always turn the patient in the direction of the narrow wedge to minimize risk of falling.

- Have several coworker's assist with the initial transfer of the patient to the frame.
- Check to see that the posterior frame is locked into position.
- Transfer the patient in the supine position to the posterior frame, maintaining spinal alignment. Attach and adjust the armboards for comfort and support.

WARNING *Make sure the patient's hands are in a functional position to prevent deformity.*

- Support the patient's feet in the correct position with a footboard to prevent footdrop.
- Make sure all tubes are positioned properly to maintain their function.
- Have one or more coworkers assist with turning the patient.
- To turn the patient from supine to prone, remove the top sheet, if present. Place a pillow or sheepskin lengthwise over his legs, chest, or other areas for comfort.
- Detach the arm boards and store them on the shelf under the bed.
- Carefully remove the nuts at both ends of the posterior frame, and position the anterior frame so its face support fits over the patient's face, and its upper portion extends from the shoulders to the symphysis pubis, with the 4″ (10-cm) opening over the perineum.
- Make sure the lower portion of the frame extends to the ankles, allowing the feet to extend over the end of the frame in the prone position. Check that the patient is in proper alignment.
- After adjusting the anterior frame, securely lock it in place at both ends.
- Place the patient's arms at his sides or, if possible, have him grasp the anterior frame for a sense of security during turning.
- Place two or three safety straps around the turning frames to promote safety and to prevent the patient's arms and legs from slipping during turning. If necessary, reposition the I.V. line, indwelling urinary

catheter, or chest tubing appropriately to prevent dislodgment or entanglement during turning.

◆ In wedge-shaped frames, always turn the patient in the direction of the narrow wedge to minimize risk of falling. Tell him which direction he'll be turning.

◆ With one coworker positioned at each end of the bed, simultaneously remove the locking pins and release the bed turning locks.

◆ On a count of three, turn the patient quickly and smoothly, maintaining cervical traction.

◆ Ask extra coworkers to stand beside the frame during the turn to reassure the patient.

◆ Close both locks and replace the pins before releasing your grip on the frame. Then remove the safety straps and the posterior frame.

◆ Position the patient properly and make sure all tubing and equipment are properly positioned.

◆ Replace and adjust the armboards, and change the linens if necessary.

◆ Assess the patient's level of consciousness, mobility, and sensation. Assess his skin for redness or pressure areas, and provide skin care or other prescribed treatments.

◆ Evaluate the patient's tolerance for the prone and supine positions.

◆ Follow the same procedure to return the patient to the supine position.

SPECIAL CONSIDERATIONS

◆ Turn the patient at least every 2 hours. Between turnings, perform appropriate range-of-motion exercises, as ordered.

◆ If the patient finds the prone position uncomfortable, give prescribed analgesics before turning.

◆ If he has skull tongs, turn him cautiously to avoid dislodging them.

◆ If the patient is connected to a mechanical ventilator, disconnect it before turning and reconnect it right afterward.

◆ Hand rolls and cradle boots can be used during turning to help keep the patient's hands and feet comfortable.

◆ Remove the perineal section of the frame for bedpan use, but always replace it immediately afterward to prevent spinal misalignment from inadequate support of the buttocks in the supine position.

◆ Provide appropriate diversion and encourage the patient's family to help counteract boredom.

◆ Adjust the reading board for meals and reading, and provide enough light to prevent eyestrain.

COMPLICATIONS
◆ None known

PATIENT TEACHING

◆ Explain the use of the turning frame to the patient.

◆ Tell the patient he may feel confined and may experience a floating sensation during turning.

◆ Reassure the patient that the frames will hold him securely and that the top frame will be removed after he's turned.

DOCUMENTATION

◆ Record the time of turning and the patient's reaction during turning.

◆ Document treatments given, and your observations of the skin condition.

◆ Note overall status.

SELECTED REFERENCES
Hayes, J.S., and Arriola, T. "Pediatric Spinal Injuries," *Pediatric Nursing* 31(6):464-67, November-December 2005.

Jones, T.S. "A Bolt Out of the Blue: Dealing with the Aftermath of Spinal Cord Injury," *Nursing Made Incredibly Easy!* 3(6):14-15, 17-28, November-December 2005.

Tze, N., et al. "Back Breaking Business: The Implementation of a Spinal Education Program," *Journal of Trauma Nursing* 11(1):25-33, January-March 2004.

Ultraviolet light therapy

DESCRIPTION

◆ Ultraviolet (UV) light causes profound biological changes, including temporary suppression of epidermal basal cell division, followed by later increase in cell turnover, and UV light-induced immune suppression.

◆ Emitted by the sun, the UV spectrum is divided into three bands (UVA, UVB, and UVC); each affects skin differently.

◆ UVA radiation rapidly darkens preformed melanin pigment, may augment UVB in causing sunburn and skin aging, and may induce phototoxicity of some drugs.

◆ The drug methoxsalen, a psoralens agent, creates artificial sensitivity to UVA by binding with the deoxyribonucleic acid in epidermal basal cells.

◆ Treating skin with a photosensitizing agent (such as methoxsalen) and UVA is called *psoralen plus UVA (PUVA) therapy* (or *photochemotherapy*).

◆ Other drugs used in photochemotherapy in combination with PUVA include acitretin (Soriatane), an oral vitamin A derivative, and methotrexate.

◆ UVB radiation causes sunburn and erythema. Topical preparations such as crude coal tar may be used with UVB (known as the *Goeckerman treatment*).

◆ UVC radiation is normally absorbed by the earth's ozone layer and doesn't reach the ground. It kills bacteria and is used in operating-room germicidal lamps.

◆ Psoriasis, mycosis fungoides, atopic dermatitis, and uremic pruritus may respond to therapy that utilizes timed exposure to UV light rays.

◆ Given before a UV light treatment, methoxsalen photosensitizes the skin to enhance therapeutic effect.

CONTRAINDICATIONS

◆ History of photosensitivity diseases, skin cancer, arsenic ingestion, or cataracts or cataract surgery
◆ Current use of photosensitivity-inducing drugs
◆ Previous skin irradiation
◆ Previous ionizing chemotherapy
◆ Photosensitizing or immunosuppressant drugs
◆ Pregnancy

ULTRAVIOLET A RADIATION TREATMENT

Fluorescent black-light lamp ◆ high-intensity UVA fluorescent bulbs

ULTRAVIOLET B RADIATION TREATMENT

Fluorescent sunlamp or hot quartz lamp ◆ sunlamp bulbs

ALL ULTRAVIOLET LIGHT TREATMENTS

Oral or topical phototherapeutic drugs if necessary ◆ body-sized light chamber or smaller light box ◆ dark, polarized goggles ◆ sunscreen if necessary ◆ hospital gown ◆ towels

PREPARATION

◆ The patient may undergo UV light therapy in the hospital, in a practitioner's office, or at home. The light source is a bank of high-intensity fluorescent bulbs. (At home, the patient may use a small fluorescent sunlamp.)

◆ Check the practitioner's orders to confirm the light treatment type and dose. For PUVA, the initial dose is based on the patient's skin type and is increased according to treatment protocol and as tolerated.

◆ The practitioner calculates the UVB dose based on skin type estimation or by determining a minimal erythema dose — the smallest amount of UV light needed to produce mild erythema.

◆ Confirm the patient's identity using two patient identifiers according to facility policy.

◆ Review the patient's health history for contraindications to UV light therapy.

◆ Ask whether he's currently taking photosensitizing drugs, such as anticonvulsants, certain antihypertensives, phenothiazines, salicylates, sulfonamides, tetracyclines, tretinoin, and various cancer drugs.

◆ If the patient will have PUVA therapy, make sure he took methoxsalen (with food) $1\frac{1}{2}$ hours before treatment.

◆ Before therapy, have the patient disrobe and put on a hospital gown.

◆ Have him remove the gown or expose the treatment area when he's in the phototherapy unit. Have him wear goggles to protect his eyes and a sunscreen, towels, or the hospital gown to protect vulnerable skin areas.

⚡ **WARNING** *All male patients receiving PUVA must wear protection over the groin area.*

◆ If the patient is having local UVB treatment, position him at the correct distance from the light source.

◆ For facial treatment with a sunlamp, position his face about 12″ (30.5 cm) from the lamp. For body treatment, position his body about 30″ (76 cm) from either the sunlamp or the hot quartz lamp.

◆ Wear goggles when observing the patient through light-chamber windows.

◆ If the patient must stand for the treatment, ask him to report dizziness.

◆ After delivering the prescribed UVB dose, help the patient out of the unit and instruct him to shield exposed areas of skin from sunlight for 8 hours after therapy.

SPECIAL CONSIDERATIONS

♦ Sunburn can result from prolonged treatment and an inadequate distance between the patient and light sources, from photosensitizing drugs, or from overly sensitive skin.
♦ Prevent eye damage by having the patient use gray or green polarized lenses during UVB therapy or UV-opaque sunglasses during PUVA therapy and for 24 hours after treatment because methoxsalen can cause photosensitivity.
♦ Mild dryness and desquamation will occur in 1 or 2 days.
♦ Before giving methoxsalen or etretinate, check to make sure that baseline liver function studies have been done.

⚡ **WARNING** *Methoxsalen and etretinate are hepatotoxic agents and are never given together. Liver function and blood lipid studies are required before treatment with ac-itretin and at regular intervals during treatment. Liver function studies and a complete blood count are required before and during methotrexate treatment.*

♦ If the practitioner prescribes tar preparations with UVB treatment, watch for signs of sensitivity, such as erythema, pruritus, and eczematous reactions.

COMPLICATIONS

♦ Erythema
♦ Edema, swelling, or blistering
♦ Nausea and pruritus
♦ Long-term adverse effects:
– Premature aging (xerosis, wrinkles, and mottled skin)
– Lentigines
– Telangiectasia
– Increased skin cancer risk
– Ocular damage if eye protection isn't used

PATIENT TEACHING

♦ Inform the patient that UV light treatments produce a mild sunburn that will help reduce or resolve skin lesions.
♦ Tell the patient to shield exposed areas of skin from sunlight for 8 hours after therapy.
♦ Tell the patient to look for marked erythema, blistering, peeling, or other signs of overexposure 4 to 6 hours after UVB therapy and 24 to 48 hours after UVA therapy; the erythema should disappear within another 24 hours.
♦ Tell the patient that mild dryness and desquamation will occur in 1 or 2 days.
♦ Teach the patient appropriate skin care measures.
♦ Advise the patient to notify the practitioner if overexposure occurs. The practitioner may recommend stopping treatment for a few days, then starting over at a lower exposure level.

DOCUMENTATION

♦ Record the date and time of initial and subsequent treatments, UV wavelength used, and name and dose of oral or topical drugs given.
♦ Record the exact duration of therapy, the distance between the light source and skin, and the patient's tolerance. Note safety measures used such as eye protection.
♦ Describe the skin condition before and after treatment.
♦ Note improvements and adverse reactions, such as increased pruritus, oozing, and scaling.

SELECTED REFERENCES

Park, J.H., et al. "Treatment of Generalized Lichen Nitidus with Narrowband Ultraviolet B," *Journal of the American Academy of Dermatology* 54(3):545-46, March 2006.

Sanders, C.J., et al. "UV Hardening Therapy: A Novel Intervention in Patients with Photosensitive Cutaneous Lupus Erythematosus," *Journal of the American Academy of Dermatology* 54(3):479-86, March 2006.

Thai, T.P., et al. "Effect of Ultraviolet Light C on Bacterial Colonization in Chronic Wounds," *Ostomy/Wound Management* 51(10):32-45, October 2005.

Yelverton, C.B., et al. "Home Ultraviolet B Phototherapy: A Cost-Effective Option for Severe Psoriasis," *Managed Care Interface* 19(1):33-36, 39, January 2006.

Unna's boot

DESCRIPTION

- This commercially prepared, medicated gauze compression dressing wraps around the affected foot and leg.
- It can be used to treat uninfected, nonnecrotic leg and foot ulcers caused by venous insufficiency and stasis dermatitis.
- Alternatively, Unna's paste (gelatin, zinc oxide, calamine lotion, and glycerin) may be applied to the ulcer and covered with lightweight gauze.
- Effectiveness results from compression (bandage) and moisture (paste).

CONTRAINDICATIONS

- Allergy to ingredients used in paste
- Arterial ulcers
- Weeping eczema
- Cellulitis

Scrub sponge with ordered cleaning agent ◆ normal saline solution ◆ commercially prepared gauze bandage saturated with Unna's paste (or Unna's paste and lightweight gauze) ◆ bandage scissors ◆ gloves ◆ elastic bandage to cover Unna's boot ◆ extra gauze for excessive drainage (optional)

- Confirm the patient's identity using two patient identifiers according to facility policy.
- Explain the procedure and provide privacy.
- Wash your hands and put on gloves.
- Assess the ulcer and surrounding skin. Evaluate ulcer size, drainage, and appearance. Perform a neurovascular assessment of the affected foot to ensure adequate circulation.

WARNING *If you don't detect a pulse in the foot, check with the ordering practitioner before applying Unna's boot.*

- Clean the affected area with the sponge and cleaning agent to retard bacterial growth and remove dirt and wound debris, which may create pressure points after you apply the bandage. Rinse with normal saline solution.
- If a commercially prepared gauze bandage isn't ordered (a prepared bandage is impregnated with the paste), spread Unna's paste evenly on the leg and foot; cover with the lightweight gauze.
- Apply three to four layers of paste interspersed with layers of gauze.
- Apply gauze or the prepared bandage in a spiral motion, from just above the toes to the knee. (See *How to wrap Unna's boot.*)
- Cover the heel; the wrap should be snug but not tight. To cover the area completely, make sure each turn overlaps the previous one by one-half the bandage width.
- Continue wrapping the patient's leg up to the knee, using firm, even pressure.
- Stop the dressing 1" (2.5 cm) below the popliteal fossa to prevent irritation when the knee is bent.
- Mold the boot with your free hand as you apply the bandage to make it smooth and even.
- Cover the boot with an elastic bandage to provide compression.

◆ Instruct the patient to remain in bed with his leg outstretched and elevated on a pillow until the paste dries (about 30 minutes).

⚡ **WARNING** *Observe the patient's foot for signs of impairment, such as cyanosis, loss of feeling, and swelling, which indicate the bandage is too tight and must be removed.*

◆ Leave the boot on for 5 to 7 days, or as ordered.

◆ Change the boot weekly or as ordered to assess underlying skin and ulcer healing. Remove the boot by unwrapping the bandage from the knee back to the foot.

SPECIAL CONSIDERATIONS

◆ If the boot is applied over a swollen leg, it must be changed as the edema subsides — if necessary, more frequently than every 5 days.

◆ Don't make reverse turns while wrapping the bandage. This can create excessive pressure areas that may cause discomfort as the bandage hardens.

COMPLICATIONS
◆ Contact dermatitis

PATIENT TEACHING

◆ Explain the procedure to the patient.

◆ Instruct the patient to walk on and handle the wrap carefully to avoid damaging it.

◆ Tell the patient the boot will stiffen but won't be as hard as a cast.

◆ Tell the patient that before bathing, he should cover the boot with a plastic kitchen trash bag sealed at the knee with an elastic bandage to avoid getting the boot wet. A wet boot softens and loses it effectiveness.

◆ Instruct the patient to take a sponge bath if safety is a concern.

DOCUMENTATION

◆ Record the date and time of application and presence of a pulse in the affected foot.

◆ Specify which leg you bandaged; describe skin appearance before and after application.

◆ Name the equipment used (a commercially prepared bandage or Unna's paste and lightweight gauze).

◆ Note an allergic reaction.

SELECTED REFERENCES
Bergan, J.J., and Pascarella, L. "Severe Chronic Venous Insufficiency: Primary Treatment with Sclerofoam," *Seminars in Vascular Surgery* 18(1):49-56, March 2005.

Pascarella, L., et al. "Severe Chronic Venous Insufficiency Treated by Foamed Sclerosant," *Annals of Vascular Surgery* 20(1):83-91, January 2006.

Schaum, K.D. "Unna Boots Versus Multi-layered, Sustained, Graduated High Compression Bandage Systems," *Ostomy/Wound Management* 51(5):28, 30, May 2005.

How to wrap Unna's boot

After cleaning the skin thoroughly, flex the patient's knee. Starting with the foot positioned at a right angle to the leg, wrap the medicated gauze bandage firmly — not tightly — around his foot. Make sure the dressing covers the heel. Continue wrapping upward, overlapping the dressing slightly with each turn. Smooth the boot with your free hand as you go, as shown below.

Stop wrapping about 1" (2.5 cm) below the knee. If necessary, make a 2" (5 cm) slit in the boot just below the knee to relieve constriction that may develop as the dressing hardens.

If drainage is excessive, wrap a roller gauze dressing over the Unna's boot. As the final layer, wrap an elastic bandage in a figure-eight pattern.

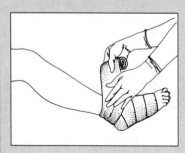

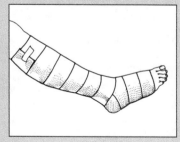

Urinary diversion stoma care

DESCRIPTION

- A urinary diversion stoma provides an alternative route for urine flow when a disorder (such as an invasive bladder tumor) impedes normal drainage.
- It may be indicated for patients with neurogenic bladder, congenital anomaly, traumatic injury to the lower urinary tract, or severe chronic urinary tract infection.
- There are two types of urinary diversion: ileal conduit and continent.
- The devices usually require the patient to wear a urine-collection appliance and to care for the stoma created during surgery. Evaluation by a wound ostomy continence nurse will facilitate site selection and postoperative stoma care.
- Some devices have a semipermeable skin barrier (impermeable to liquid but permeable to vapor and oxygen—essential for maintaining skin integrity).
- Wafer-type barriers may offer more protection against irritation than adhesive appliances.

CONTRAINDICATIONS

- None known

EQUIPMENT

Soap and warm water ◆ waste receptacle (impervious or wax-coated bag) ◆ linen-saver pad ◆ hypoallergenic paper tape ◆ povidone-iodine solution ◆ urine collection container ◆ rubber catheter (usually #14 or #16 French) ◆ ruler ◆ scissors ◆ urine-collection appliance (with or without antireflux valve) ◆ graduated cylinder ◆ cotton-less gauze pads (some rolled, some flat) ◆ washcloth ◆ skin barrier in liquid, paste, wafer, or sheet form ◆ appliance belt ◆ stoma covering (nonadherent gauze pad or panty liner) ◆ two pairs of gloves ◆ adhesive solvent, irrigating syringe, tampon, hair dryer, electric razor, regular gauze pads, vinegar, deodorant tablets (optional)

Commercially packaged stoma care kits are available. In place of soap and water, you can use adhesive remover pads, if available, or cotton gauze saturated with adhesive solvent.

PREPARATION

- Assemble equipment on the patient's overbed table; tape the waste receptacle to the table.
- Confirm the patient's identity using two patient identifiers according to facility policy.
- Provide privacy and wash your hands.
- Measure the diameter of the stoma with a ruler.
- Cut the opening of the appliance with the scissors—it shouldn't be more than ⅛″ to ⅙″ (0.3 to 0.4 cm) larger than the diameter of the stoma.
- Moisten the faceplate of the appliance with a small amount of solvent or water to prepare it for adhesion.
- Performing preliminary steps at the bedside allows you to demonstrate the procedure and show him that it isn't difficult, which will help him relax.

KEY STEPS

- Wash your hands again. Explain the procedure and offer constant reassurance to counteract negative reactions that may be elicited by stoma care.
- Place the bed in low Fowler's position so the patient's abdomen is flat, which eliminates skin folds that could cause the appliance to slip or irritate the skin.
- Put on the gloves and place a linen-saver pad under his side, near the stoma.
- Open the drain valve of the appliance being replaced to empty the urine into the graduated cylinder.
- To remove the appliance, use a washcloth to apply soap and water or adhesive solvent as you push the skin back from the pouch.
- Discard disposable appliances; clean

reuseable ones with soap and luke-warm water and let air-dry.

⚡ **WARNING** *To avoid irritating the stoma, avoid touching it with adhesive solvent. If adhesive remains on the skin, rub it off with a dry gauze pad.*

- To prevent a constant flow of urine onto the skin while changing the appliance, wick the urine with an absorbent, lint-free material.
- If urine has stagnated and has a strong odor, use soap to wash it off. Be sure to rinse to remove an oily residue that could cause the appliance to slip.
- Use water to carefully wash off crystal deposits that may have formed around the stoma.
- Follow your facility's skin care protocol to treat minor skin problems.
- Dry the peristomal area with a gauze pad; moisture will keep the appliance from sticking. Use a hair dryer if you wish.
- Remove hair from the area with scissors or an electric razor to prevent folliculitis, resulting from irritation when the pouch is removed.
- Inspect the stoma to see if it's healing properly and to detect complications. Check the color and appearance of the suture line and examine moisture or drainage. Inspect the peristomal skin for redness, irritation, and intactness.
- Apply the skin barrier. If you apply a wafer or sheet, cut it to fit over the stoma. Remove protective backing and set the barrier aside with the adhesive side up.
- If you apply a liquid barrier (such as Skin-Prep), saturate a gauze pad with it and coat the peristomal skin. Move the gauze in concentric circles outward from the stoma until you've covered an area 2″ (5 cm) larger than the wafer. Let the skin dry for several minutes — it should feel tacky. Gently press the wafer around the stoma, sticky side down, smoothing from the stoma outward.
- If using a barrier paste, open the tube, squeeze out a small amount, then discard it.
- Squeeze a ribbon of paste directly

onto the peristomal skin about ½" (1.5 cm) from the stoma, making a complete circle. Make several more concentric circles outward.

♦ Dip your fingers into lukewarm water and smooth the paste with your fingers until the skin is completely covered from the edge of the stoma to 3" or 4" (7.5 to 10 cm) outward.

♦ The paste should be ¼" to ½" (0.5 to 1.5 cm) thick.

♦ Discard the gloves, wash your hands, and put on new gloves.

♦ Remove and discard the material used for wicking urine.

♦ Place the appliance over the stoma, leaving only a small amount (⅜" to ¾" [1 or 2 cm]) of skin exposed.

♦ Secure the faceplate of the appliance to the skin with paper tape, if recommended. Place a piece of tape lengthwise on each edge of the faceplate so the tape overlaps onto the skin.

♦ Apply the appliance belt. Make sure that it's on a level with the stoma.

⚡ **WARNING** *If applied above or below the stoma, the belt can break the bag's seal or rub or injure the stoma. The belt should be loose enough for you to insert two fingers between the skin and the belt. If it's too tight, it can irritate the skin or cause internal damage.*

♦ Some devices don't require a belt. Instead, the pouch has a ridge that fits over the rim of barrier adhesive and snaps securely into place.

SPECIAL CONSIDERATIONS

♦ When positioned correctly, most appliances remain in place for at least 3 days and for as long as 5 days if no leakage occurs.

♦ After 5 days, the appliance should be changed. With the improved adhesives and pouches available, belts aren't always necessary.

♦ Because urine flows constantly, it accumulates quickly, becoming even heavier than stools.

♦ To prevent the weight of the urine from loosening the seal around the stoma and separating the appliance

from the skin, empty the appliance through the drain valve when it's one-third to one-half full.

♦ Reusable appliances should be washed with soap and lukewarm water, then air-dried to prevent brittleness. Soaking the appliance in vinegar and water or placing deodorant tablets in it can further dissipate stubborn odors.

♦ An acid-ash diet that includes ascorbic acid and cranberry juice may raise urinary acidity, thereby reducing bacterial action and fermentation (the underlying causes of odor). Generous fluid intake also helps reduce odors by diluting urine.

♦ If the patient has a continent urinary diversion, make sure you know how to meet his special needs.

COMPLICATIONS

♦ Bleeding occurring from an ill-fitting appliance, especially with an ileal conduit, because a segment of the intestine forms the conduit

♦ Peristomal skin becoming reddened or excoriated from too-frequent changing or improper placement of the appliance, poor skin care, or allergic reaction to the appliance or adhesive

♦ Constant leakage around the appliance resulting from improper placement of the appliance or from poor skin turgor

PATIENT TEACHING

♦ To encourage a positive attitude, help the patient get used to the idea of caring for the stoma and appliance as though they're natural extensions of himself.

♦ Supply written instructions and provide positive reinforcement after the patient completes each step.

♦ Suggest that the patient perform the procedure in the morning when urine flows most slowly.

♦ Arrange for a visiting nurse or an enterostomal therapist to assist the patient at home.

♦ Help the patient choose between disposable and reusable appliances by explaining the advantages and disadvantages of each.

♦ Emphasize the importance of correct placement and adequate fit, to prevent seepage of urine onto the skin.

♦ Instruct the patient to connect the appliance to a urine-collection container before going to sleep, which prevents the urine from accumulating and stagnating in the appliance.

♦ Teach the patient sanitary and dietary measures that can protect the peristomal skin and control odor that commonly results from alkaline urine, infection, or poor hygiene.

♦ Tell the patient that mucus may be visible in the urine.

♦ Advise the patient about ostomy clubs and the American Cancer Society, who routinely visit hospitals to explain ostomy care and the types of appliances available and to help patients learn to function normally with a stoma.

DOCUMENTATION

♦ Record the appearance and color of the stoma and whether it's inverted, flush with the skin, or protruding.

♦ If it protrudes, note how much. (Normal range is ½" to ¾" [1.5 to 2 cm].)

♦ Record the appearance and condition of the peristomal skin, noting redness or irritation or complaints of itching or burning.

SELECTED REFERENCES
Burch, J. "The Pre- and Postoperative Nursing Care for Patients with a Stoma," *British Journal of Nursing* 14(6):310-18, March-April 2005.
Gray, E.H., et al. "Stoma Care in the School Setting," *Journal of School Nursing* 22(2):74-80, April 2006.
Gray, M., et al. "Counseling Patients Undergoing Urinary Diversion: Does the Type of Diversion Influence Quality of Life?" *Journal of Wound, Ostomy, and Continence Nursing* 32(1):7-15, January-February 2005.

Urine collection

DESCRIPTION

♦ Random urine collection can be done as part of a physical examination, during hospitalization to screen for urinary and systemic disorders, or to screen for drug use.

♦ An indwelling catheter specimen (obtained either by clamping the drainage tube and emptying the accumulated urine into a container or by aspirating a specimen with a syringe) requires sterile collection technique to prevent catheter contamination and urinary tract infection.

♦ The clean-catch midstream specimen method is commonly used in place of random collection because it provides a virtually uncontaminated specimen without the need for catheterization.

♦ Commercial clean-catch kits containing antiseptic towelettes, sterile specimen container with lid and label, and instructions for use in several languages are widely used.

CONTRAINDICATIONS

♦ Genitourinary surgery

EQUIPMENT

RANDOM SPECIMEN

Bedpan or urinal with cover, if necessary ♦ gloves ♦ graduated container ♦ specimen container with lid ♦ label ♦ laboratory request form

CLEAN-CATCH MIDSTREAM SPECIMEN

Soap and water ♦ gloves ♦ graduated container ♦ three sterile 2″ × 2″ gauze pads or sterile cotton balls ♦ povidone-iodine solution ♦ sterile specimen container with lid ♦ label ♦ bedpan or urinal ♦ laboratory request form (if necessary)

INDWELLING CATHETER SPECIMEN

Gloves ♦ alcohol pad ♦ 10-ml syringe ♦ 21G or 22G 1½″ needle ♦ tube clamp ♦ sterile specimen container with lid ♦ label ♦ laboratory request form

KEY STEPS

♦ Confirm the patient's identity using two patient identifiers according to facility policy.

♦ Explain to the patient that you need a urine specimen for laboratory analysis.

♦ Explain the procedure, if necessary, to promote cooperation and prevent accidental disposal of specimens

COLLECTING A RANDOM SPECIMEN

♦ Provide privacy.

♦ Instruct the patient on bed rest to void into a clean bedpan or urinal, or ask the ambulatory patient to void into either one in the bathroom.

♦ Put on gloves.

♦ Pour at least 120 ml of urine into the specimen container, and cap the container securely.

♦ If the patient's urine output must be measured and recorded, pour the remaining urine into the graduated container. Otherwise, discard the urine.

♦ If you spill urine outside the container, clean and dry it to prevent cross-contamination.

♦ After you label the sample container with the patient's name, room number, and date and time of collection, attach the request form and send it to the laboratory immediately.

⚡ **WARNING** *Delayed transport of the specimen may alter test results.*

♦ Clean the graduated container and urinal or bedpan and return them to their proper storage.

♦ Wash your hands to prevent cross-contamination.

♦ Offer the patient a washcloth and soap and water to wash his hands.

COLLECTING A CLEAN-CATCH MIDSTREAM SPECIMEN

♦ Because the goal is a virtually uncontaminated specimen, explain the procedure to the patient.

♦ Provide illustrations to emphasize the correct collection technique.

♦ Tell the patient to remove all clothing from the waist down and to stand in front of the toilet as for urination or, for a female, to sit far back on the toilet seat and spread her legs.

♦ Have the patient clean the periurethral area (tip of the penis or labial folds, vulva, and urethral meatus) with soap and water, then wipe the area three times, each time with a fresh 2″ × 2″ gauze pad soaked in povidone-iodine solution or with the wipes provided in a commercial kit.

♦ Instruct a female patient to separate her labial folds with the thumb and forefinger. Tell her to wipe down one side with the first pad and discard it, wipe the other side with the second pad and discard it, and wipe down the center over the urinary meatus with the third pad and discard it.

♦ Stress the importance of cleaning from front to back to avoid contaminating the genital area with fecal matter.

♦ Tell the female patient to straddle the bedpan or toilet to allow labial spreading. She should continue to keep her labia separated while voiding.

♦ For the uncircumcised male patient, emphasize the need to retract his foreskin to effectively clean the meatus and to keep it retracted during voiding.

♦ Instruct the patient to begin voiding into the bedpan, urinal, or toilet. Without stopping the urine stream, the patient should move the collection container into the stream, collecting about 30 to 50 ml at the midstream portion of voiding, and finish voiding into the bedpan, urinal, or toilet.

♦ Put on gloves before discarding the first and last portions of the voiding; measure the remaining urine in a graduated container for intake and output records, if necessary.

♦ Include the amount in the specimen container when recording the total amount voided.

♦ Take the sterile container from the patient, and cap it securely. Avoid touching the inside of the container or the lid.

- If the outside of the container is soiled, clean it and wipe it dry. Remove gloves and discard them properly. Wash your hands and tell the patient to wash his hands.
- Label the container with the patient's name and room number, name of test, type of specimen, collection time, and suspected diagnosis, if known. Also note whether the patient is menstruating at the time of specimen collection.
- If a urine culture has been ordered, note current antibiotic therapy on the laboratory request form.
- Send the container to the laboratory immediately, or place it on ice to prevent specimen deterioration and altered test results.

COLLECTING AN INDWELLING CATHETER SPECIMEN

- About 30 minutes before collecting the specimen, clamp the drainage tube to allow urine to accumulate.
- Put on gloves.
- If the drainage tube has a built-in sampling port, wipe the port with an alcohol pad.

Aspirating a urine specimen

If the patient has an indwelling urinary catheter in place, clamp the tube distal to the aspiration port for about 30 minutes. Wipe the port with an alcohol pad, and insert a needle and a 20- or 30-ml syringe into the port perpendicular to the tube. Aspirate the required amount of urine, and expel it into the specimen container. Remove the clamp on the drainage tube.

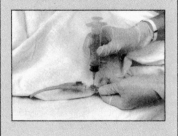

- Uncap the needle on the syringe, and insert the needle into the sampling port at a 90-degree angle to the tubing.
- Aspirate the specimen into the syringe. (See *Aspirating a urine specimen.*)

SPECIAL CONSIDERATIONS

- If the drainage tube doesn't have a sampling port and the catheter is made of rubber, obtain the specimen from the catheter. Other types of catheters will leak after you withdraw the needle.
- Before withdrawing the specimen from a rubber catheter, wipe it with an alcohol pad just above where it connects to the drainage tube.
- Insert the needle into the rubber catheter at a 45-degree angle and withdraw the specimen. Never insert the needle into the shaft of the catheter because you may puncture the lumen leading to the catheter balloon.
- Transfer the specimen to a sterile container, label it, and send it to the laboratory immediately, or place it on ice. If a urine culture is to be performed, be sure to list current antibiotic therapy on the laboratory request form.
- If the catheter isn't made of rubber or has no sampling port, wipe the area where the catheter joins the drainage tube with an alcohol pad; disconnect the catheter, and allow urine to drain into the sterile specimen container.
- Avoid touching the inside of the sterile container with the catheter, and don't touch anything with the catheter drainage tube to avoid contamination.
- When you've collected the specimen, wipe both connection sites with an alcohol pad and join them. Cap the container, label it, and send it to the laboratory immediately, or place it on ice.

⚡ **WARNING** *Make sure you unclamp the drainage tube after collecting the specimen to prevent urine backflow, which can cause bladder distention and infection.*

COMPLICATIONS
- None known

- Use visual aids to describe collection of the specimen, if needed.
- Explain the significance of cleaning the genital area before collecting the specimen.
- Instruct the patient to collect the specimen in a clean container with a tight-fitting lid and to keep it on ice or in the refrigerator (separate from food items) for up to 24 hours.

DOCUMENTATION

- Record the times of specimen collection and transport to the laboratory.
- Specify the test as well as the appearance, odor, color, and unusual characteristics of the specimen.
- If necessary, record the urine volume on the intake and output record.

SELECTED REFERENCES

Alam, M.T., et al. "Comparison of Urine Contamination Rates Using Three Different Methods of Collection: Clean-Catch, Cotton Wool Pad and Urine Bag," *Annals of Tropical Paediatrics* 25(1):29-34, March 2005.

Jenner, R., and Afzalnia, S. "Best Evidence Topic Report. Clean Catch or Bag Specimen in UTI in Non Toilet Trained Children," *Emergency Medicine Journal* 23(3):219-20, March 2006.

Loane, V. "Obtaining Urine for Culture from Non-Potty-Trained Children," *Paediatric Nursing* 17(9):39-42, November 2005.

Shvartzman, P., and Nasri, Y. "Urine Culture Collected from Gel-Based Diapers: Developing a Novel Experimental Laboratory Method," *Journal of the American Board of Family Practice* 17(2):91-95, March-April 2004.

Urine collection, timed

DESCRIPTION

- Hormones, proteins, and electrolytes are excreted in small, variable amounts in urine; specimens for measuring these substances must typically be collected over an extended period to yield quantities of diagnostic value.
- A 24-hour specimen is used most commonly; it provides an average excretion rate for substances eliminated during this period.
- Timed specimens may be collected for shorter periods, such as 2 or 12 hours, depending on specific information needed.
- Check with the laboratory to see what preservatives may be needed in the urine specimen or if a dark collection container is required.

CONTRAINDICATIONS

- None known

Large collection container with a cap or stopper or a commercial plastic container ◆ preservative, if necessary ◆ gloves ◆ bedpan or urinal (if patient doesn't have an indwelling catheter) ◆ graduated container (if patient is on intake and output measurement) ◆ gloves ◆ ice-filled container (if a refrigerator isn't available) ◆ label ◆ laboratory request form ◆ four patient care reminders

- Confirm the patient's identity using two patient identifiers according to facility policy.
- Explain the procedure to the patient and his family, as necessary, to enlist cooperation and prevent accidental disposal of urine during the collection period.
- Emphasize that failure to collect even one specimen during the collection period invalidates the test and requires that it begin again.
- Place patient care reminders over the patient's bed, in his bathroom, on the bedpan hopper in the utility room, and on the urinal or indwelling catheter collection bag. Include his name, room number, date, and collection interval.
- Instruct him to save all urine during the collection period, to notify you after each voiding, and to avoid contaminating the urine with stool or toilet tissue.
- Explain dietary or drug restrictions, and make sure the patient understands and is willing to comply with them.

2-HOUR COLLECTION

- Instruct the patient to drink two to four 8-oz glasses (480 to 960 ml) of water about 30 minutes before collection begins, if possible. After 30 minutes, tell him to void.
- Put on gloves; discard this specimen so the patient starts the collection period with an empty bladder.
- If ordered, give a challenge dose of drug (such as glucose solution or corticotropin), and record the time.
- Offer a glass of water at least every hour during the collection period to stimulate urine production.
- After each voiding, put on gloves and add the specimen to the collection container.
- Instruct the patient to void about 15 minutes before the end of the collection period, if possible, and add this specimen to the collection container.
- At the end of the collection period, remove and discard gloves.

◆ Send the appropriately labeled collection container to the laboratory immediately, along with a properly completed laboratory request form.

12- AND 24-HOUR COLLECTION

◆ Put on gloves and ask the patient to void; discard this urine so he starts the collection period with an empty bladder. Record the time.
◆ After putting on gloves and pouring the first urine specimen into the collection container, add the required preservative.
◆ Refrigerate the bottle or keep it on ice until the next voiding.
◆ Collect all urine voided during the prescribed period. Just before the collection period ends, ask the patient to void again, if possible.
◆ Add this last specimen to the collection container, pack it in ice to inhibit deterioration of the specimen, and remove and discard gloves.
◆ Label the collection container, and send it to the laboratory with a properly completed laboratory request form.

SPECIAL CONSIDERATIONS

◆ Keep the patient well hydrated before and during the test to ensure adequate urine flow.
◆ Before collection of a timed specimen, make sure the laboratory will be open when the collection period ends to help ensure prompt, accurate results.

WARNING *Never store a specimen in a refrigerator containing food or drugs to avoid contamination.*
◆ If the patient has an indwelling catheter in place, put the collection bag in an ice-filled container at his bedside.
◆ If you accidentally discard a specimen during the collection period, you'll need to restart the collection. This may result in an additional day of hospitalization, which may cause the patient personal and financial hardship.
◆ Emphasize the need to save all of the patient's urine during the collection period to everyone involved in his care as well as to family and other visitors.

COMPLICATIONS
◆ None known

PATIENT TEACHING

◆ If the patient must continue collecting urine at home, provide written instructions for the appropriate method.
◆ Explain that the patient can keep the collection container in a brown bag in the refrigerator at home, separate from other refrigerator contents.
◆ Instruct the patient to avoid exercise and ingestion of coffee, tea, or drugs (unless directed otherwise by the practitioner) before the test to avoid altering test results.

DOCUMENTATION

◆ Record the date and intervals of specimen collection and when the container was sent to the laboratory.

SELECTED REFERENCES
Graves, C., et al. "Comparison of Urine Urea Nitrogen Collection Times in Critically Ill Patients," *Nutrition in Clinical Practice* 20(2):271-75, April 2005.
Hellerstein, S., et al. "Timed-Urine Collections for Renal Clearance Studies," *Pediatric Nephrology* 21(1):96-101, January 2006.
Pong, S., et al. "12-Hour versus 24-Hour Creatinine Clearance in Critically Ill Pediatric Patients," *Pediatric Research* 58(1):83-88, July 2005.

Urine glucose and ketone testing

DESCRIPTION

◆ Reagent strip tests are used to monitor urine glucose and ketone levels and to screen for diabetes.

◆ Urine glucose tests are less accurate than blood glucose tests and are used less often because of the increasing convenience of blood self-testing.

◆ Urine ketone tests monitor fat metabolism, help diagnose carbohydrate deprivation and diabetic ketoacidosis, and help distinguish between diabetic and nondiabetic coma.

◆ Glucose oxidase tests (for example, Clinistix, Diastix, and Tes-Tape strips) produce color changes when patches of reagents implanted in handheld plastic strips react with glucose in the patient's urine. Urine ketone strip tests (such as Ketostix and Keto-Diastix) are similar.

◆ Results are read by comparing color changes with a standardized reference chart.

CONTRAINDICATIONS

◆ None known

Specimen container ◆ gloves ◆ glucose or ketone test strips ◆ reference color chart

PREPARATION

◆ When performing all urine tests, wear gloves as barrier protection.

◆ Confirm the patient's identity using two patient identifiers according to facility policy.

◆ Explain the test to the patient; if he's a newly diagnosed diabetic, teach him to perform the test himself.

◆ Check the patient's history for drugs that may interfere with test results.

◆ Before each test, instruct the patient not to contaminate the urine specimen with stool or toilet tissue.

GLUCOSE OXIDASE STRIP TEST

◆ Put on gloves before collecting a specimen for the test, and remove them to record test results.

◆ Instruct the patient to void.

◆ Ask him to drink a glass of water; collect a second-voided specimen after 30 to 45 minutes.

CLINISTIX STRIP TEST

◆ Dip the reagent end of the strip into the urine for 2 seconds.

◆ Tap off excess urine.

◆ Wait exactly 10 seconds, and then compare its color with the color chart on the test strip container.

◆ Ignore color changes that occur after 10 seconds.

◆ Record the result.

DIASTIX STRIP TEST

◆ Dip the reagent end of the strip into the urine for 2 seconds.

◆ Tap off excess urine.

◆ Wait exactly 30 seconds, and then compare the strip's color with the chart on the container.

◆ Ignore color changes that occur after 30 seconds.

◆ Record the result.

TES-TAPE STRIP TEST

◆ Pull about 1½″ (4 cm) of the reagent strip from the dispenser and dip one end about ½″ (0.5 cm) into the specimen for 2 seconds.
◆ Tap off excess urine.
◆ Wait exactly 60 seconds, and then compare the darkest part of the tape with the chart on the dispenser.
◆ If the test result exceeds 0.5%, wait an additional 60 seconds and make a final comparison.
◆ Record the result.

KETONE STRIP TEST

◆ Put on gloves and collect a second-voided midstream specimen.

KETOSTIX STRIP TEST

◆ Dip the reagent end of the strip into the specimen and remove it immediately.
◆ Wait exactly 15 seconds, and then compare the color of the strip with the chart on the container.
◆ Ignore color changes that occur after 15 seconds.
◆ Remove and discard your gloves.
◆ Record the test result.

KETO-DIASTIX STRIP TEST

◆ Dip the reagent end of the strip into the specimen and remove it immediately.
◆ Tap off excess urine.
◆ Hold the strip horizontally to avoid mixing chemicals between the two reagent squares.
◆ Wait exactly 15 seconds, and then compare the color of the ketone part of the strip with the chart on the test strip container.
◆ After 30 seconds, compare the color of the glucose section with the chart.
◆ Record the test results.

SPECIAL CONSIDERATIONS

◆ Keep reagent strips in a closed container in a cool, dry place at a temperature below 86° F (30° C), but don't refrigerate them.
◆ Don't use discolored or outdated strips.

COMPLICATIONS

◆ None known

PATIENT TEACHING

◆ Explain the test to the patient; if newly diagnosed with diabetes, show how to perform the test.
◆ Before each test, instruct the patient not to contaminate the urine specimen with stool or toilet tissue.

DOCUMENTATION

◆ Record test results according to the information on the reagent containers, or use a flowchart designed to record this information.
◆ Indicate whether the practitioner was notified of the test results.
◆ Note the patient's progress in performing the tests.
◆ Record treatments given as a result of the testing.

SELECTED REFERENCES

Emery, S.P., et al. "Twenty-four-hour Urine Insulin as a Measure of Hyperinsulinaemia/Insulin Resistance before Onset of Pre-Eclampsia and Gestational Hypertension," *BJOG: An International Journal of Obstetrics and Gynaecology* 112(11):1479-85, November 2005.

Penders, J., et al. "Quantitative Measurement of Ketone Bodies in Urine Using Reflectometry," *Clinical Chemistry and Laboratory Medicine* 43(7):724-29, 2005.

Wei, O.Y., and Teece, S. "Best Evidence Topic Report. Urine Dipsticks in Screening for Diabetes Mellitus," *Emergency Medicine Journal* 23(2):138, February 2006.

Wilson, L.A. "Urinalysis," *Nursing Standard* 19(35):51-54, May 2005.

Urine specific gravity

DESCRIPTION

- Urine specific gravity measures concentration of urine solutes, which reflects the kidneys' capacity to concentrate urine — among the first functions lost when renal tubular damage occurs.
- It's determined by comparing the weight of a urine specimen with an equivalent volume of distilled water, which is 1.000. Because urine contains dissolved salts and other substances, it's heavier than 1.000.
- Urine specific gravity ranges from 1.003 (very dilute) to 1.035 (highly concentrated); normal values range from 1.010 to 1.025.
- It's measured with a urinometer (a specially calibrated hydrometer designed to float in a cylinder of urine). The more concentrated the urine, the higher the urinometer floats, and the higher the specific gravity.
- Specific gravity may also be measured by a refractometer, which measures the refraction of light as it passes through a urine specimen, or a reagent strip test.
- High specific gravity reflects an increased concentration of urine solutes, which occurs in conditions that cause renal hypoperfusion and may indicate heart failure, dehydration, hepatic disorders, or nephrosis.
- Low specific gravity reflects failure to reabsorb water and concentrate urine, hypercalcemia, hypokalemia, alkalosis, acute renal failure, pyelonephritis, glomerulonephritis, or diabetes insipidus.
- It's commonly measured with a random urine specimen. More accurate measurement is possible with a specimen collected after fluids are withheld for 12 to 24 hours.

CONTRAINDICATIONS

- None known

Calibrated urinometer and cylinder, refractometer, or reagent strips (Multistix) ◆ gloves ◆ specimen container

MEASURING WITH A URINOMETER

- Confirm the patient's identity using two patient identifiers according to facility policy.
- Put on gloves and collect a random urine specimen. Allow the specimen to come to room temperature (71.6° F [22° C]) before testing; this is the temperature at which most urinometers are calibrated.
- Fill the cylinder about three-quarters full of urine; spin the urinometer and drop it into the cylinder.
- When the urinometer stops bobbing, read the specific gravity from the calibrated scale marked directly on the stem of the urinometer.
- Make sure the instrument floats freely and doesn't touch the sides of the cylinder. Read the scale at the lowest point of the meniscus to ensure an accurate reading. (See *Using a urinometer.*)
- Discard the urine; rinse the cylinder and urinometer in cool water.
- Warm water coagulates proteins in urine, making them stick to the instrument.
- Remove gloves and wash your hands to prevent cross-contamination.

MEASURING WITH A REFRACTOMETER

- Put on gloves and collect a random or controlled urine specimen.
- Place a single drop of urine on the refractometer slide.
- Turn on the light and look through the eyepiece to see the specific gravity indicated on a scale. Some instruments use a digital display.
- Discard the urine and clean the equipment.
- Discard your gloves and perform hand hygiene.

MEASURING WITH A REAGENT STRIP

◆ Put on gloves and obtain a random or controlled urine specimen.
◆ Dip the reagent end of the test strip into the specimen for 2 seconds; tap the strip to remove excess urine, and compare the color change with the chart supplied with the kit.
◆ Discard the urine and the specimen container; discard your gloves and wash your hands.

Using a urinometer

With the urinometer floating in a cylinder of urine, position your eye at a level even with the bottom of the meniscus and read the specific gravity from the scale printed on the urinometer:

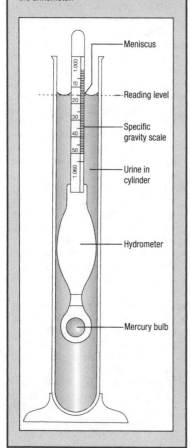

- Meniscus
- Reading level
- Specific gravity scale
- Urine in cylinder
- Hydrometer
- Mercury bulb

SPECIAL CONSIDERATIONS

◆ Test the urinometer in distilled water at room temperature to ensure that its calibration is 1.000.
◆ If necessary, correct the urinometer reading for temperature effects; add 0.001 to your observed reading for every 5.4° F (3° C) above the calibration temperature of 71.6° F (22° C); subtract 0.001 for every 5.4° F below 71.6° F.

COMPLICATIONS

◆ None known

PATIENT TEACHING

◆ Explain the procedure and tell the patient when you'll need the specimen.
◆ Explain why you're withholding fluids and for how long.

DOCUMENTATION

◆ Record the specific gravity, volume, color, odor, and appearance of the collected urine specimen.
◆ Indicate whether the practitioner was made aware of the test results.

SELECTED REFERENCES

Mentes, J.C., et al. "Use of a Urine Color Chart to Monitor Hydration Status in Nursing Home Residents," *Biological Research for Nursing* 7(3):197-203, January 2006.

Oppliger, R.A., et al. "Accuracy of Urine Specific Gravity and Osmolality as Indicators of Hydration Status," *International Journal of Sport Nutrition and Exercise Metabolism* 15(3):236-51, June 2005.

Polat, M., et al. "The Effect of Seasonal Changes on Blood Pressure and Urine Specific Gravity in Children Living in Mediterranean Climate," *Medical Science Monitor* 12(4):CR186-90, April 2006.

Stover, E.A., et al. "Urine Specific Gravity in Exercises Prior to Physical Training," *Applied Physiology, Nutrition, and Metabolism* 31(3):320-27, June 2006.

Vacuum-assisted closure pressure therapy

DESCRIPTION

- Vacuum-assisted closure (VAC) pressure therapy (also known *as negative pressure wound therapy*) is used to enhance delayed or impaired wound healing.
- The device applies localized subatmospheric pressure to draw the edges of the wound toward the center.
- A special dressing is placed in the wound or over a graft or flap, which removes fluids from the wound and stimulates growth of healthy granulation tissue. (See *Understanding VAC pressure therapy*.)
- The procedure is used for acute and traumatic wounds and pressure ulcers or chronic open wounds, such as diabetic ulcers, meshed grafts, and skin flaps.

CONTRAINDICATIONS

- Fistulas that involve organs or body cavities
- Necrotic tissue with eschar
- Untreated osteomyelitis
- Malignant wounds

Waterproof trash bag ◆ goggles ◆ gown, if indicated ◆ emesis basin ◆ normal saline solution ◆ clean gloves ◆ sterile gloves ◆ sterile scissors ◆ linen-saver pad ◆ 35-ml piston syringe with 19G catheter ◆ reticulated foam ◆ fenestrated tubing ◆ evacuation tubing ◆ skin protectant wipe ◆ transparent occlusive air-permeable drape ◆ evacuation canister ◆ vacuum unit

PREPARATION

- Assemble the vacuum-assisted closure device at the bedside.
- Set negative pressure according to the practitioner's order (25 to 200 mm Hg).

- Confirm the patient's identity using two patient identifiers according to facility policy.
- Check the practitioner's order, and assess the patient's condition.
- Explain the procedure, provide privacy, and wash your hands.
- If necessary, put on a gown and goggles to protect yourself from wound drainage and contamination.
- Place a linen-saver pad under the patient to catch spills.
- Position the patient to allow maximum wound exposure, and place the emesis basin under the wound to collect drainage.
- Put on clean gloves; remove the soiled dressing and discard.
- Attach the 19G catheter to the 35-ml piston syringe and irrigate the wound thoroughly using normal saline solution.
- Clean the area around the wound with normal saline solution; wipe intact skin with a skin protectant wipe and allow it to dry.
- Remove and discard your gloves and put on sterile gloves.
- Using sterile scissors, cut the foam to the shape and measurement of the wound. More than one piece may be needed to ensure you get the right size.
- Carefully place the foam in the wound.
- Place the fenestrated tubing into the center of the foam; this delivers negative pressure to the wound.
- Place the transparent occlusive air permeable drape over the foam, enclosing the foam and the tubing together.
- Remove and discard your gloves.
- Connect the free end of the fenestrated tubing to the tubing that's connected to the evacuation canister.
- Turn on the vacuum unit and make sure the patient is comfortable.
- Dispose of drainage, solution, linen-saver pad, and trash bag, and clean or dispose of soiled equipment and supplies according to guidelines.

SPECIAL CONSIDERATIONS

- Change the dressing every 48 hours; try to coordinate dressing changes with the practitioner's visits so he can inspect the wound.
- Measure the amount of drainage every shift.
- Audible and visual alarms alert you if the unit is tipped greater than 45 degrees, the canister is full, the dressing has an air leak, or the canister becomes dislodged.

COMPLICATIONS

- Temporary increase in the patient's pain
- Risk of infection

PATIENT TEACHING

- Explain the procedure to the patient and answer questions, as needed.

DOCUMENTATION

- Document the frequency and duration of therapy.
- Note the amount of negative pressure applied, the size and condition of the wound, and patient's response to treatment.

SELECTED REFERENCES

Clubley, L., and Harper, L. "Using Negative Pressure Therapy for Healing of a Sternal Wound," *Nursing Times* 101(16):44-46, April 2005.

Gibson, K. "Vacuum-Assisted Closure," *AJN* 104(12):16, December 2004.

Malli, S. "Keep a Close Eye on Vacuum-Assisted Wound Closure," *Nursing* 35(7):25, July 2005.

Smith, N. "The Benefits of VAC Therapy in the Management of Pressure Ulcers," *British Journal of Nursing* 13(22):1359-65, December 2004-January 2005.

Understanding VAC pressure therapy

Vacuum-assisted closure (VAC) pressure therapy may be used when a wound fails to heal in a timely manner. It encourages healing by applying localized subatmospheric pressure at the site of the wound. This reduces edema and bacterial colonization and stimulates the formation of granulation tissue

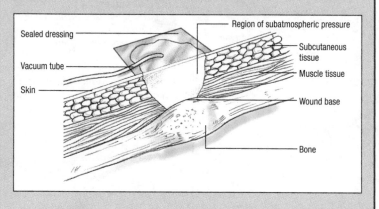

Sealed dressing
Vacuum tube
Skin
Region of subatmospheric pressure
Subcutaneous tissue
Muscle tissue
Wound base
Bone

Vagal maneuvers

DESCRIPTION

- Valsalva's maneuver and carotid sinus massage can slow the heart rate in a patient with sinus, atrial, or junctional tachyarrhythmias.
- The maneuvers are usually performed by a practitioner, but may also be done by a specially prepared nurse under a practitioner's supervision.
- The maneuvers stimulate nerve endings, which respond as they would to an increase in blood pressure, sending a message to the brain stem that stimulates the autonomic nervous system to increase vagal tone and decrease the heart rate.
- For Valsalva's maneuver, the patient holds his breath and bears down, raising his intrathoracic pressure.
- When pressure increase is transmitted to the heart and great vessels, venous return, stroke volume, and systolic blood pressure decrease. Within seconds, the baroreceptors increases heart rate and cause peripheral vasoconstriction.
- When the patient exhales at the end of the maneuver, his blood pressure rises to its previous level. This increase, combined with the peripheral vasoconstriction caused by bearing down, stimulates the vagus nerve, decreasing the heart rate.
- For carotid sinus massage, manual pressure applied to the left or right carotid sinus slows the heart rate.
- Response to carotid sinus massage depends on the particular arrhythmia.
- With sinus tachycardia, the heart rate will slow gradually during the procedure and speed up again after it.
- With atrial tachycardia, the arrhythmia may stop and the heart rate may remain slow because the procedure increases atrioventricular (AV) block.
- With atrial fibrillation or flutter, the ventricular rate may not change; AV block may even worsen.
- With paroxysmal atrial tachycardia, the reversion to sinus rhythm occurs only 20% of the time.
- Nonparoxysmal tachycardia and ventricular tachycardia won't respond.
- Typically vagal maneuvers will either "break" PSVT or have no effect. Conversely, vagal maneuvers will not usually convert atrial flutter to sinus rhythm, but will unmask any hidden flutter waves, thus clarifying the diagnosis.

CONTRAINDICATIONS

- Valsalva's maneuver:
- Severe coronary artery disease
- Acute myocardial infarction
- Hypovolemia
- Carotid sinus massage:
- Cardiac glycoside toxicity
- Cerebrovascular disease
- Carotid surgery

🐾 **WARNING** *Use caution when performing carotid sinus massage on elderly patients, patients receiving cardiac glycosides, and those with heart block, hypertension, coronary artery disease, diabetes mellitus, or hyperkalemia. It may cause arterial pressure to plummet in these patients, although it usually rises quickly afterward.*

Location and technique for carotid sinus massage

Before applying manual pressure to the patient's right carotid sinus, locate the bifurcation of the carotid artery on the right side of the neck. Turn his head slightly to the left and hyperextend the neck, bringing the carotid artery closer to the skin and moving the sternocleidomastoid muscle away from the carotid artery.

Using a circular motion, massage the right carotid sinus between your fingers and the transverse processes of the spine for 3 to 5 seconds. Don't massage for more than 5 seconds to avoid risking life-threatening complications.

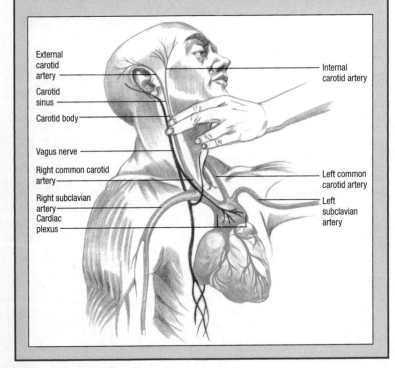

External carotid artery

Carotid sinus

Carotid body

Vagus nerve

Right common carotid artery

Right subclavian artery

Cardiac plexus

Internal carotid artery

Left common carotid artery

Left subclavian artery

EQUIPMENT

Crash cart with emergency drugs and airway equipment ◆ electrocardiogram (ECG) monitor and electrodes ◆ I.V. catheter and tubing ◆ tourniquet ◆ dextrose 5% in water ◆ hair clipping supplies, cardiotonic drugs (optional)

KEY STEPS

◆ Confirm the patient's identity using two patient identifiers according to facility policy.
◆ Explain the procedure to the patient to ease his fears and promote cooperation. Ask him to let you know if he feels light-headed.
◆ Place the patient in a supine position.
◆ Insert an I.V. line, if necessary, to be used if emergency drugs become necessary. Give dextrose 5% in water at a keep-vein-open rate, as ordered.
◆ Prepare the patient's skin, clipping hair if necessary, and attach ECG electrodes.
◆ Adjust the size of the ECG complexes on the monitor so you can see the arrhythmia clearly.
◆ If possible, obtain a rhythm strip before, during, and after the procedure.

VALSALVA'S MANEUVER
◆ Ask the patient to take a deep breath and bear down, as if he were trying to defecate.
◆ If he doesn't feel light-headed or dizzy and, if no new arrhythmias occur, have him hold his breath and bear down for 10 seconds.
◆ If he feels dizzy or light-headed or if you see a new arrhythmia on the monitor—asystole for more than 6 seconds, frequent premature ventricular contractions (PVCs), or ventricular tachycardia or ventricular fibrillation—allow him to exhale and stop bearing down.
◆ After 10 seconds, ask the patient to exhale and breathe quietly.
◆ If the maneuver was successful, the monitor will show his heart rate slowing before he exhales.

CAROTID SINUS MASSAGE
◆ Begin by obtaining a rhythm strip, using the lead that shows the strongest P waves.
◆ Auscultate both carotid sinuses.

⚡ **WARNING** *If you detect bruits, inform the practitioner and don't perform carotid sinus massage.*

◆ If you don't detect bruits, proceed as ordered. (See *Location and technique for carotid sinus massage.*)
◆ Monitor the ECG throughout the procedure.

⚡ **WARNING** *Stop massaging when the ventricular rate slows enough to permit diagnosis of the rhythm. Stop as soon as evidence of a rhythm change appears. Have the crash cart available in case a dangerous arrhythmia occurs.*

◆ If the procedure has no effect within 5 seconds, stop massaging the right carotid sinus and begin to massage the left.
◆ If this also fails, give cardiotonic drugs, as ordered.

SPECIAL CONSIDERATIONS

◆ A brief period of asystole (3 to 6 seconds) and several PVCs may precede conversion to normal sinus rhythm.
◆ If the vagal maneuver succeeded in slowing the patient's heart rate and converting the arrhythmia, continue monitoring him for several hours.
◆ Vagal maneuvers can occasionally cause bradycardia or complete heart block, so monitor the patient's cardiac rhythm closely.

🌸 **AGE FACTOR** *Elderly patients with heart disease are especially susceptible to adverse effects of vagal maneuvers.*

COMPLICATIONS
Valsalva's maneuver
◆ Bradycardia
◆ Decreased cardiac output
◆ Complete heart block
◆ Mobilization of venous thrombi
◆ Asystole
◆ Bleeding

Carotid sinus massage
◆ Ventricular fibrillation
◆ Ventricular tachycardia
◆ Ventricular standstill
◆ Worsening of AV block
◆ Cerebral damage
◆ Stroke

PATIENT TEACHING

◆ Explain the procedure to the patient and answer questions, as needed.

DOCUMENTATION

◆ Record the date and time of the procedure, who performed it, and why it was necessary.
◆ Note the patient's response, complications, and interventions taken.

SELECTED REFERENCES
Barriga, F.J., et al. "Cluster Headache: Orbital Hemodynamic Changes during Valsalva Maneuver," *Headache* 46(2): 298-305, February 2006.

Basaranoglu, G., et al. "The Effects of Valsalva Manoeuvres on Venepuncture Pain," *European Journal of Anaesthesiology* 23(7):591-93, July 2006.

Deepak, S.M., et al. "Ventricular Fibrillation Induced by Carotid Sinus Massage without Preceding Bradycardia," *Europace* 7(6):638-40, November 2005.

Farwell, D.J., and Sulke, A.N. "A Randomised Prospective Comparison of Three Protocols for Head-Up Tilt Testing and Carotid Sinus Massage," *International Journal of Cardiology* 105(3):241-49, December 2005.

Felker, G.M., et al. "The Valsalva Maneuver: A Bedside 'Biomarker' for Heart Failure," *American Journal of Medicine* 119(2):117-22, February 2006.

Vaginal medication insertion

DESCRIPTION
- Vaginal medications include suppositories, creams, gels, and ointments.
- These medications can be inserted as a topical treatment for infection (particularly *Trichomonas vaginalis* and monilial vaginitis) or inflammation, or as a contraceptive.
- Suppositories melt when they contact the vaginal mucosa, and their medication diffuses topically (as effectively as creams, gels, and ointments).
- Vaginal medications usually come with a disposable applicator that enables placement of medication in the anterior and posterior fornices.
- Vaginal administration is most effective when the patient can remain lying down afterward to retain the medication.

CONTRAINDICATIONS
- None known

Patient's medication record and chart ◆ prescribed medication and applicator, if necessary ◆ gloves ◆ water-soluble lubricant ◆ small sanitary pad

PREPARATION
- If possible, plan to insert vaginal medications at bedtime, when the patient is recumbent.
- Verify the order on the patient's medication record by checking it against the practitioner's order.

- Confirm the patient's identity using two patient identifiers according to facility policy.
- Wash your hands, explain the procedure to the patient, and provide privacy.
- Ask the patient to void.
- Ask the patient if she would rather insert the medication herself. If so, provide appropriate instructions. If not, proceed with the following steps.
- Help her into the lithotomy position.
- Expose only the perineum.

INSERTING A SUPPOSITORY
- Remove the suppository from the wrapper, and lubricate it with water-soluble lubricant.
- Put on gloves and expose the vagina.
- With an applicator or the forefinger of your free hand, insert the suppository about 2″ (5 cm) into the vagina. (See *How to insert a vaginal suppository.*)

INSERTING OINTMENTS, CREAMS, OR GELS
- Insert the plunger into the applicator. Then attach the applicator to the tube of medication.
- Gently squeeze the tube to fill the applicator with the prescribed amount of medication.
- Detach the applicator from the tube, and lubricate the applicator.
- Put on gloves and expose the vagina.
- Insert the applicator as you would a small suppository, and administer the medication by depressing the plunger on the applicator.

AFTER VAGINAL INSERTION
◆ Remove and discard your gloves.
◆ Wash the applicator with soap and warm water and store it, unless it's disposable. If the applicator can be used again, label it so that it will be used only for the same patient.
◆ To prevent the medication from soiling the patient's clothing and bedding, provide a sanitary pad.
◆ Help the patient return to a comfortable position, and advise her to remain in bed as much as possible for the next several hours.
◆ Wash your hands thoroughly.

SPECIAL CONSIDERATIONS
◆ Refrigerate vaginal suppositories that melt at room temperature.
◆ Instruct the patient not to wear a tampon after inserting vaginal medication because it would absorb the medication and decrease its effectiveness.
◆ Instruct the patient to avoid sexual intercourse during treatment.

COMPLICATIONS
◆ Local irritation

PATIENT TEACHING
◆ If possible, teach the patient how to insert vaginal medication because she may have to administer it herself after discharge. Give her a patient-teaching sheet if one is available.

DOCUMENTATION
◆ Record the medication administered as well as the time and date.
◆ Note adverse effects and other pertinent information.

SELECTED REFERENCES
Applerloo, M., et al. "Vaginal Application of Testosterone: A Study on Pharmacokinetics and the Sexual Response in Healthy Volunteers," *Journal of Sexual Medicine* 3(3):541-49, May 2006.
das Neves, J., and Bahia, M.F. "Gels as Vaginal Drug Delivery Systems," *International Journal of Pharmaceutics* 318(1-2):1-14, August 2006.
Nyirjesy, P., et al. "The Effects of Intravaginal Clindamycin and Metronidazole Therapy on Vaginal Lactobacilli in Patients with Bacterial Vaginosis," *American Journal of Obstetrics and Gynecology* 194(5):1277-82, May 2006.
Theroux, R. "Factors Influencing Women's Decisions to Self-Treat Vaginal Symptoms," *Journal of the American Academy of Nurse Practitioners* 17(4):156-62, April 2005.

How to insert a vaginal suppository

If the suppository is small, place it in the tip of an applicator. Then lubricate the applicator, hold it by the cylinder, and insert it into the vagina. To ensure the patient's comfort, direct the applicator down initially, toward the spine, and then up and back, toward the cervix (as shown).

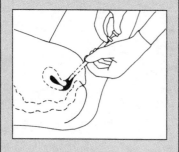

Vascular access device insertion and maintenance

DESCRIPTION

◆ The device consists of a silicone catheter attached to a reservoir, covered with a self-sealing silicone rubber septum that's surgically implanted under local anesthesia; it's used when an external central venous catheter (CVC) isn't desirable for long-term I.V. therapy.

◆ The most common type is a vascular access port (VAP); one- and two-piece units with single or double lumens are available. (See *Understanding VAPs*.)

◆ The two basic types are top entry (most commonly used—Med-i-Port, Port-A-Cath, and Infuse-A-Port), and side entry.

◆ Type and size of lumen depend on the patient's needs.

◆ The device is also used for arterial access or is implanted into the epidural space, peritoneum, or pericardial or pleural cavity.

◆ It delivers intermittent infusions of chemotherapy, fluids, drugs, and blood or it's used to obtain blood.

◆ Implantation and removal of the device require surgery and hospitalization.

◆ Cost makes it worthwhile only for patients who require infusion therapy for at least 6 months.

CONTRAINDICATIONS

◆ Patients who can't tolerate other implanted devices

IMPLANTING A VASCULAR ACCESS PORT

Noncoring needles of appropriate type and gauge with attached extension set tubing (a noncoring needle has a deflected point that slices the port's septum) ◆ VAP ◆ sterile gloves ◆ mask ◆ alcohol pads ◆ povidone-iodine swabs ◆ local anesthetic (lidocaine without epinephrine) ◆ ice pack ◆ 10- and 20-ml syringes ◆ normal saline and heparin flush solutions ◆ I.V. solution ◆ sterile dressings ◆ luer-lock injection cap ◆ adhesive skin closures ◆ suture removal set

GIVING A BOLUS INJECTION

Noncoring needle of appropriate type and gauge with attached extension set ◆ 10-ml syringe filled with normal saline solution ◆ syringe containing the prescribed drug ◆ sterile syringe filled with heparin flush solution (optional)

GIVEING A CONTINUOUS INFUSION

Prescribed I.V. solution or drugs ◆ I.V. administration set ◆ filter, if ordered ◆ noncoring needle of appropriate type and gauge with attached extension set ◆ 10-ml syringe filled with normal saline solution ◆ adhesive tape ◆ sterile 2″×2″ gauze pad ◆ sterile tape ◆ transparent semipermeable dressing ◆ sterile marker ◆ sterile labels

PREPARATION

◆ Confirm the size and type of the device and the insertion site with the practitioner.

◆ Attach the tubing to the solution container, prime the tubing with fluid, fill the syringes with normal saline solution or heparin flush solution, and prime the noncoring needle with extension set.

◆ All priming must be done using strict aseptic technique; all tubing must be free from air.

◆ After you've primed the tubing, recheck all connections for tightness. Make sure that all open ends are covered with sealed caps.

Understanding VAPs

A vascular access port (VAP) is used to deliver intermittent infusions of drugs, chemotherapy, and blood products. Because the device is completely covered by the patient's skin, the risk of extrinsic contamination is reduced. Patients may prefer this type of central line because it doesn't alter body image and requires less routine catheter care.

The VAP consists of a catheter connected to a small reservoir. A septum designed to withstand multiple punctures seals the reservoir.

ACCESSING VAP

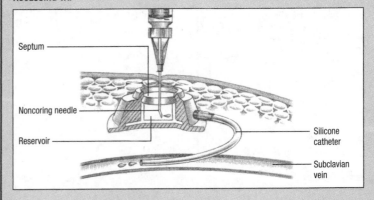

- Label all medication syringes, medication containers, and all solution containers on and off the sterile field.

KEY STEPS

- Wash your hands.

ASSISTING WITH IMPLANTATION

- Reinforce the practitioner's explanation, its benefit, and what's expected during and after implantation.
- The practitioner is responsible for obtaining consent for the procedure, but make sure the written document is signed, witnessed, and on the chart.
- Allay the patient's fears and answer questions about movement restrictions, cosmetic concerns, and management regimens.
- Check the patient's history for hypersensitivity to local anesthetics or iodine.
- The practitioner will surgically implant the VAP, probably using a local anesthetic (similar to insertion of a CVC). He may use a general anesthetic.

PREPARING TO ACCESS THE PORT

- The VAP can be used immediately after placement, although some edema and tenderness may persist for about 72 hours. This makes the device initially difficult to palpate and slightly uncomfortable for the patient.
- Prepare to access the port, following the specific steps for top-entry or side-entry ports.
- Using aseptic technique, inspect the area around the port for signs of infection or skin breakdown.
- Place an ice pack over the area for several minutes to alleviate needle puncture discomfort. Alternatively, give a local anesthetic after cleaning the area.
- Wash your hands. Put on sterile gloves and mask.
- Clean the area with an alcohol pad, starting at the center of the port and working outward with a firm, circular motion over a 4″ or 5″ (10- to 12.5-cm) diameter. Repeat twice.

- Allow the site to dry; then clean the area with povidone-iodine swabs the same way. Repeat twice.
- If facility policy calls for a local anesthetic, check the patient's record for possible allergies. As indicated, anesthetize the insertion site by injecting 0.1 ml of lidocaine (without epinephrine).

ACCESSING A TOP-ENTRY PORT (MOST COMMON APPROACH)

- Palpate the area over the port to find its septum.
- Anchor the port with your nondominant hand. Then, using your dominant hand, aim the needle at the center of the device.
- Insert the needle perpendicular to the port septum.
- Push the needle through the skin and septum until you reach the bottom of the reservoir.
- Check needle placement by aspirating for blood return.
- If you can't obtain blood, remove the needle and repeat the procedure.

⚡ ***WARNING** Inability to obtain blood may indicate sludge build-up (from drugs) in the port reservoir. You may need to use a fibrinolytic agent to free an occlusion. Ask the patient to raise his arms and perform Valsalva's maneuver. If you still don't get a blood return, notify the practitioner. (See* Managing common VAP problems, *page 566. See also* Risks of VAP therapy, *page 567.)*

- Flush the device with normal saline solution.

⚡ ***WARNING** If you detect swelling or the patient reports pain at the site, remove the needle and notify the practitioner.*

ACCESSING A SIDE-ENTRY PORT

- Follow the same procedure as with a top-entry port, except you'll insert the needle parallel to the reservoir instead of perpendicular to it.

GIVING A BOLUS INJECTION

- Attach the 10-ml syringe filled with normal saline solution to the end of the extension set of the noncoring needle and remove all the air.
- Check for blood return; flush the port with normal saline solution, according to facility policy.
- Clamp the extension set and remove the saline syringe.
- Connect the drug syringe to the extension set.
- Open the clamp and inject the drug, as ordered.
- Examine the skin around the needle for signs of infiltration, such as swelling or tenderness. If signs are present, stop the injection and intervene appropriately.
- When the injection is complete, clamp the extension set and remove the drug syringe.
- Open the clamp and flush with 5 ml of normal saline solution after each drug injection to minimize drug incompatibility reactions.
- Flush with heparin solution according to facility policy.

GIVING A CONTINUOUS INFUSION

- Remove all air from the noncoring needle's extension set by priming it with an attached syringe of normal saline solution.
- Flush the port system with normal saline solution; clamp the extension set and remove the syringe.
- Connect the administration set, and secure the connections with sterile tape if necessary.
- Unclamp the extension set and begin the infusion.
- Affix the needle to the skin.
- Examine the site carefully for infiltration. If the patient complains of stinging, burning, or pain at the site, discontinue the infusion and intervene appropriately.
- When the solution container is empty, obtain a new I.V. solution container, as ordered.
- Flush with normal saline solution followed by heparin solution according to facility policy.

(continued)

SPECIAL CONSIDERATIONS

◆ After implantation, monitor the site for signs of hematoma and bleeding.
◆ The incision site requires routine postoperative care for 7 to 10 days.
◆ Assess the implantation site for infection, device rotation, or skin erosion.
◆ No dressing is needed except during infusions or to maintain an intermittent infusion device.
◆ While the patient is hospitalized, a luer-lock injection cap may be attached to the end of the extension set to provide ready access for intermittent infusions.
◆ If the patient is receiving a continuous or prolonged infusion, change the transparent dressing and needle every 7 days.
◆ Gauze dressings should be changed every 48 hours or immediately if compromised.
◆ Change the tubing and solution as you would for a long-term central venous infusion.
◆ If the patient is receiving an intermittent infusion, flush the port periodically with heparin solution. When the VAP isn't being used, flush it every 4 weeks.
◆ If clotting threatens to occlude the VAP, the practitioner may order a fibrinolytic agent to clear the catheter.

⚡ **WARNING** *Because such drugs increase risk of bleeding, fibrinolytic drugs may be contraindicated in patients who have had surgery within the past 10 days, who have active internal bleeding, or who have experienced central nervous system damage, such as infarction, hemorrhage, traumatic injury, surgery, or primary or metastatic disease within the past 2 months.*

COMPLICATIONS
◆ Infection
◆ Thrombus formation
◆ Occlusion

PATIENT TEACHING

◆ Explain the procedures and that the patient will have follow-up visits from a home care nurse to ensure safety and successful treatment.
◆ If the patient will be accessing the port, explain that the most uncomfortable part of the procedure is insertion of the needle into the skin.
◆ Tell the patient that the skin over the port will eventually become desensitized from frequent needle punctures; until then, he may use a topical anesthetic.

◆ Stress the importance of pushing the needle into the port until the patient feels the needle bevel touch the back of the port.
◆ Stress the importance of monthly flushes when no more infusions are scheduled.
◆ Instruct a family member in all aspects of care.

Managing common VAP problems

PROBLEMS AND POSSIBLE CAUSES	NURSING INTERVENTIONS
Inability to flush the device or draw blood	
Kinked tubing or closed clamp	◆ Check tubing or clamp and reposition the patient.
Catheter lodged against vessel wall	◆ Teach the patient to change his position to free the catheter from the vessel wall. ◆ Raise the arm that's on the same side as the catheter. ◆ Roll the patient to his opposite side; have him cough, sit up, or take a deep breath. ◆ Infuse 10 ml of normal saline solution into the catheter. ◆ Regain access to the catheter or vascular access port (VAP) using a new needle.
Incorrect needle placement or needle not advanced through septum	◆ Regain access to the device. ◆ Teach the home care patient to push down firmly on the noncoring needle device in the septum and to verify needle placement by aspirating for blood return.
Clot formation	◆ Assess patency by trying to flush the VAP while the patient changes position. ◆ Notify the practitioner; obtain an order for instillation of a fibrinolytic agent. ◆ Teach the patient to recognize clot formation, to notify the practitioner if it occurs, and to avoid forcibly flushing the VAP.
Kinked catheter, catheter migration, or port rotation	◆ Notify the practitioner immediately. ◆ Tell the patient to notify the practitioner if he has trouble using the VAP.
Inability to palpate the device	
Deeply implanted port	◆ Note portal chamber scar. ◆ Use deep palpation technique. ◆ Ask another nurse to try locating the VAP. ◆ Use a 1½" or 2" (4- or 5-cm) noncoring needle to gain access to the VAP.

DOCUMENTATION

♦ Record your assessment findings and interventions according to facility policy.
♦ Note the type, amount, rate, and duration of the infusion, the appearance of the site, and adverse reactions and nursing interventions.
♦ Record needle and dressing changes for continuous infusions; blood samples obtained, including type and amount; and patient teaching covered.

♦ Document the removal of the infusion needle, the status of the site, the use of the heparin flush, and problems you found and resolved.

SELECTED REFERENCES

Cowley, K. "Make the Right Choice of Vascular Access Device," *Professional Nurse* 19(10):43-46, June 2004.
Gabriel, J., et al. "Vascular Access: Indications and Implications for Patient Care," *Nursing Standard* 19(26):45-52, March 2005.
Mapes, D. "Nurses' Impact in the Choice and Longevity of Vascular Access," *Nephrology Nursing Journal* 32(6):670-74, November-December 2005.
Masoorli, S. "Legal Issues Related to Vascular Access Devices and Infusion Therapy," *Journal of Infusion Nursing* 28(3 Suppl):S18-21, May-June 2005.

Risks of VAP therapy

COMPLICATIONS	SIGNS AND SYMPTOMS	POSSIBLE CAUSES	NURSING INTERVENTIONS
Site infection or skin breakdown	♦ Erythema and warmth at vascular access port (VAP) site ♦ Oozing or purulent drainage at VAP site or pocket ♦ Fever	♦ Infected incision or VAP pocket ♦ Poor postoperative healing	♦ Assess the site daily for redness; note drainage. ♦ Notify the practitioner. ♦ Administer antibiotics, as prescribed. ♦ Apply warm soaks for 20 minutes four times per day. **Prevention** ♦ Teach the patient to inspect for and report redness, swelling, drainage, or skin breakdown at VAP site.
Extravasation	♦ Burning sensation or swelling in subcutaneous tissue	♦ Needle dislodged into subcutaneous tissue ♦ Needle incorrectly placed in VAP ♦ Needle position not confirmed; needle pulled out of septum ♦ Use of vesicant drugs	♦ Stop the infusion. ♦ Notify the practitioner; prepare to administer an antidote, if ordered. ♦ Follow your facility's protocol for removing the needle. **Prevention** ♦ Teach the patient how to gain access to the device, verify its placement, and secure the needle before initiating an infusion.
Thrombosis	♦ Inability to flush VAP or administer infusion	♦ Frequent blood sampling ♦ Infusion of packed red blood cells (RBCs)	♦ Notify the practitioner; obtain an order to administer a fibrinolytic agent as per your facility's policy and procedure. **Prevention** ♦ Flush the VAP thoroughly right after obtaining a blood sample. ♦ Administer packed RBCs as a piggyback with normal saline solution and use an infusion pump; flush with normal saline solution between units.
Fibrin sheath formation	♦ Blocked VAP and catheter lumen ♦ Inability to flush VAP or administer infusion ♦ Inability to withdraw blood despite being able to flush easily ♦ Possibly swelling, tenderness, and erythema in neck, chest, and shoulder	♦ Adherence of platelets to catheter	♦ Notify the practitioner; add heparin (1,000 to 2,000 units) to continuous infusions as ordered. (A fibrinolytic agent may also be ordered.) Follow your facility's policy and procedure. **Prevention** ♦ Use the port only to infuse fluids and drugs; don't use it to obtain blood samples. ♦ Administer only compatible substances through the port.

Venipuncture

OVERVIEW

DESCRIPTION

- Venipuncture involves piercing a vein with a needle and collecting blood in a syringe or evacuated tube to obtain a venous blood sample.
- The procedure is performed using the antecubital fossa, but can be done on a vein in the dorsal forearm, dorsum of the hand or foot, or other accessible location.
- The inner wrist isn't advised because of high risk of damage to underlying structures.
- Laboratory personnel or nurses with proper training perform the procedure.

CONTRAINDICATIONS

- None known

EQUIPMENT

Tourniquet ◆ gloves ◆ syringe or evacuated tubes and needle holder ◆ alcohol or povidone-iodine pads ◆ 20G or 21G needle for the forearm or 25G needle for the wrist, hand, and ankle and for children ◆ color-coded collection tubes containing appropriate additives ◆ labels ◆ laboratory request form ◆ 2″×2″ gauze pads ◆ adhesive bandage

PREPARATION

- If you're using evacuated tubes, open the needle packet, attach the needle to its holder, and select the appropriate tubes.
- If you're using a syringe, attach the appropriate needle to it.
- Choose a syringe large enough to hold all the blood required for the test.
- Label all collection tubes clearly with the patient's name and room number, the practitioner's name, and date and time of collection.

KEY STEPS

- Wash your hands and put on gloves.
- Confirm the patient's identity using two patient identifiers according to facility policy.
- Tell the patient that you're about to take a blood sample; explain the procedure to ease his anxiety and gain cooperation.
- Ask the patient if he's ever felt faint, sweaty, or nauseated when having blood drawn. If he's on bed rest, ask him to lie supine, with his head slightly elevated and his arms at his sides.
- Ask the ambulatory patient to sit in a chair and support his arm securely on an armrest or table.
- Assess his veins to determine the best puncture site. (See *Common venipuncture sites*.)
- Observe the skin for the vein's blue color, or palpate the vein for a firm rebound sensation.
- Tie a tourniquet 2″ (5 cm) proximal to the area chosen.
- By impeding venous return to the heart while still allowing arterial flow, a tourniquet produces venous dilation. If arterial perfusion remains adequate, you'll be able to feel the radial pulse.
- If the tourniquet fails to dilate the vein, have the patient open and close his fist a few times. Then ask him to close his fist as you insert the needle and open it again when the needle is in place.
- Clean the venipuncture site with an alcohol or povidone-iodine pad.
- Don't wipe off the povidone-iodine with alcohol; alcohol cancels the effect of povidone-iodine.
- Wipe in a circular motion, spiraling outward from the site to avoid introducing potentially infectious skin flora into the vessel during the procedure.
- If you use alcohol, apply it with friction for 30 seconds, or until the final pad comes away clean.
- Allow the skin to dry before performing venipuncture.

Common venipuncture sites

These illustrations show the anatomic locations of veins commonly used for venipuncture. The most commonly used sites are on the forearm, followed by those on the hand.

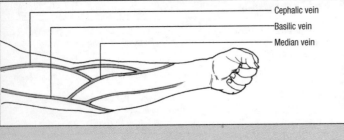

Cephalic vein
Basilic vein
Median vein

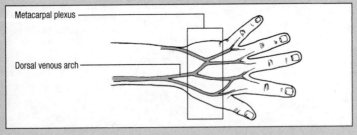

Metacarpal plexus

Dorsal venous arch

- Immobilize the vein by pressing just below the venipuncture site with your thumb and drawing the skin taut.
- Position the needle holder or syringe with the needle bevel up and the shaft parallel to the path of the vein and at a 30-degree angle to the arm.
- Insert the needle into the vein.
- If using a syringe, blood will appear in the hub; withdraw the blood slowly, pulling the plunger of the syringe gently to create steady suction until you obtain the required sample. Pulling the plunger forcibly may collapse the vein.
- If using a needle holder and an evacuated tube, grasp the holder securely to stabilize it in the vein; push down on the collection tube until the needle punctures the rubber stopper. Blood will flow into the tube automatically.
- Remove the tourniquet as soon as blood flows adequately to prevent stasis and hemoconcentration, which can impair test results.

  ⬥ **WARNING** *If flow is sluggish, leave the tourniquet in place longer, but always remove it before withdrawing the needle. Don't leave the tourniquet on longer than 3 minutes.*
- Continue to fill the required tubes, removing one and inserting another.
- Rotate each tube as you remove it to help mix the additive with the sample.
- After you've drawn the sample, place a gauze pad over the puncture site, and slowly remove the needle from the vein.
- When using an evacuated tube, remove it from the needle holder to release the vacuum before withdrawing the needle from the vein.
- Apply gentle pressure to the puncture site for 2 or 3 minutes or until bleeding stops to prevent extravasation into the surrounding tissue, which can cause a hematoma.
- After bleeding stops, apply an adhesive bandage.
- If you've used a syringe, transfer the sample to a collection tube.
- Detach the needle from the syringe, open the collection tube, and empty the sample into the tube, being careful to avoid foaming, which can cause hemolysis.
- Check the venipuncture site to see if a hematoma has developed; if it has, apply pressure until you are sure the bleeding has stopped.
- Discard syringes, needles, and used gloves in appropriate containers.

SPECIAL CONSIDERATIONS

- Safety-engineered blood collection sets are recommended to prevent needle sticks.
- Never draw a venous sample from an arm or leg that's already being used for I.V. therapy or blood administration; this may affect test results.

  ⬥ **WARNING** *Don't collect a venous sample from an infected site; this may introduce pathogens into the vascular system. Avoid drawing blood from edematous areas, arteriovenous shunts, or sites of previous hematoma or vascular injury.*
- If the patient has large, distended, highly visible veins, perform venipuncture without a tourniquet to minimize risk of hematoma formation.
- If he has a clotting disorder or is receiving anticoagulant therapy, maintain firm pressure on the venipuncture site for at least 5 minutes after withdrawing the needle to prevent hematoma formation.
- Avoid using veins in the patient's legs for venipuncture, if possible, because this increases the risk of thrombophlebitis. Some facilities require a practitioner's order to collect blood from a leg or foot vein. Check the policy at your facility.

  ⬥ **AGE FACTOR** *Use pediatric tubes for collecting specimens on infants and children; the volumes are less than volumes collected on adults. Pediatric tubes may also be used in elderly patients or others with low blood volumes as indicated. Check facility policy.*

COMPLICATIONS
- Hematoma at needle insertion site
- Infection from poor technique

PATIENT TEACHING

- Explain the procedure to ease the patient's anxiety and gain cooperation.

DOCUMENTATION

- Record the date, time, and site of venipuncture.
- Note the name of the test and the time the sample was sent to the laboratory.
- Record the amount of blood collected and the patient's temperature.
- Document adverse reactions to the procedure.

SELECTED REFERENCES

Higgins, D. "Venipuncture," *Nursing Times* 100(39):30-31, September-October 2004.

Melhuish, S., and Payne, H. "Nurses' Attitudes to Pain Management during Routine Venepuncture in Young Children," *Paediatric Nursing* 18(2):20-23, March 2006.

Rosenthal, K. "Tips for Venipuncture in Children," *Nursing* 35(12):31, December 2005.

Thurgate, C., and Heppell, S. "Needle Phobia—Changing Venepuncture Practice in Ambulatory Care," *Paediatric Nursing* 17(9):15-8, November 2005.

Ventricular assist device

OVERVIEW

DESCRIPTION
◆ A ventricular assist device (VAD) is used for temporary life-sustaining treatment of a failing heart; it diverts systemic blood flow from a diseased ventricle into a centrifugal pump.
◆ The VAD temporarily reduces ventricular work, allowing the myocardium to rest, and contractility to improve.
◆ The VAD is used to assist the left or right ventricle, or both. (See *VAD: Help for the failing heart.*)
◆ Candidates for VAD include those with massive myocardial infarction, irreversible cardiomyopathy, acute myocarditis, inability to be weaned from cardiopulmonary bypass, valvular disease, bacterial endocarditis, and heart transplant rejection.
◆ The device may also be used in those awaiting a heart transplant.

CONTRAINDICATIONS
◆ None known

EQUIPMENT

The VAD is inserted in the operating room.

KEY STEPS

◆ Before surgery, food and fluid intake must be restricted and cardiac function must be continuously monitored (using an electrocardiogram, a pulmonary artery catheter, and an arterial line).
◆ Before sending the patient to the operating room, make sure that he has signed a consent form.
◆ If time permits, clip hair on the patient's chest and scrub it with an antiseptic solution.
◆ When he returns from surgery, give analgesics, as ordered.
◆ Frequently monitor vital signs, intake, and output.
◆ Keep the patient immobile to prevent accidental extubation, contamination, or disconnection of the VAD.
◆ Monitor pulmonary artery pressures.
◆ If you've been prepared to adjust the pump, maintain cardiac output at about 5 to 8 L/minute, central venous pressure at about 8 to 16 mm Hg, pulmonary capillary wedge pressure at about 10 to 20 mm Hg, mean arterial pressure at greater than 60 mm Hg, and left atrial pressure between 4 and 12 mm Hg.
◆ Monitor the patient for signs and symptoms of poor perfusion and ineffective pumping, including arrhythmias, hypotension, slow capillary refill, cool skin, oliguria or anuria, confusion, anxiety, and restlessness.
◆ Give heparin, as ordered, to prevent clotting in the pump head and thrombus formation.
◆ Check for bleeding, especially at the operative sites.
◆ Monitor laboratory studies, as ordered, especially complete blood count and coagulation studies.
◆ Assess the incisions and the cannula insertion sites for signs of infection. Monitor the patient's white blood cell count and differential daily, and take rectal or core temperatures every 4 hours.
◆ Change the dressing over the cannula sites daily or according to facility policy.
◆ Provide supportive care, including range-of-motion exercises and mouth and skin care.

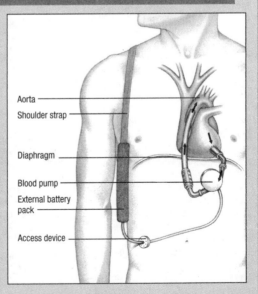

VAD: Help for the failing heart

A ventricular assist device (VAD) functions like an artificial heart. The major difference is that the VAD assists the heart instead of replacing it. The VAD can aid one or both ventricles. The pumping chambers themselves aren't usually implanted in the patient.

A permanent VAD is implanted in the patient's chest cavity, although it still provides only temporary support. The device receives power through the skin by a belt of electrical transformer coils (worn externally as a portable battery pack). It can also operate off an implanted, rechargeable battery for up to 1 hour at a time.

- Aorta
- Shoulder strap
- Diaphragm
- Blood pump
- External battery pack
- Access device

SPECIAL CONSIDERATIONS

◆ If ventricular function fails to improve within 4 days, the patient may need a transplant. If so, provide psychological support for the patient and family as they endure referral.
◆ You may also initiate the transplant process by contacting the appropriate agency.
◆ The psychological effects of the VAD can produce stress in the patient, his family, and his close friends. If appropriate, refer them to other support personnel.

COMPLICATIONS

◆ Damaged blood cells
◆ Thrombus formation
◆ Pulmonary embolism
◆ Stroke

PATIENT TEACHING

◆ Explain to the patient before surgery that food and fluid intake must be restricted and that you'll continuously monitor cardiac function.

DOCUMENTATION

◆ Note the patient's condition following insertion of the VAD.
◆ Document pump adjustments as well as complications and interventions.

SELECTED REFERENCES

Helton, T.J., et al. "Haemodynamic Monitoring with a Left Ventricular Assist Device," *Heart* 91(10):1261, October 2005.

Hipkins, M., et al. "Care of Patients with Heart Failure and the Use of Ventricular Assist Devices," *Professional Nurse* 19(12):34-36, August 2004.

Lietz, K., and Miller, L.W. "Will Left-Ventricular Assist Device Therapy Replace Heart Transplantation in the Foreseeable Future?" *Current Opinion in Internal Medicine* 4(3):291-96, June 2005.

Sample, S. "Technology Today: Left Ventricular Assist Devices," *RN* 68(11): 46-51, November 2005.

Stahovich, M., et al. "Management of Adult Patients with a Left Ventricular Assist Device," *Rehabilitation Nursing* 29(3):100-03, May-June 2004.

Volume-control set

DESCRIPTION

◆ A volume-control set utilizes an I.V. line with a graduated chamber that delivers precise amounts of fluid and shuts off when the fluid is exhausted, preventing air from entering the I.V. line.

◆ The set may be used as a secondary line in adults for intermittent infusion of drugs.

⚙ *AGE FACTOR A volume-control set is used as a primary line in children for continuous infusion of fluids or drug.*

CONTRAINDICATIONS

◆ None known

EQUIPMENT

Volume-control set ◆ I.V. pole (for setting up a primary I.V. line) ◆ I.V. solution ◆ 20G to 22G 1″ needle or needle-free adapter ◆ alcohol pads ◆ drug in labeled syringe ◆ tape ◆ label

KEY STEPS

PREPARATION

◆ Various models of volume-control sets are available; each consists of a graduated fluid chamber (120 to 250 ml) with a spike and a filtered air line on top and administration tubing underneath.

◆ Floating-valve sets have a valve at the bottom that closes when the chamber empties; membrane-filter sets have a rigid filter at the bottom that, when wet, prevents the passage of air.

◆ Ensure the sterility of all equipment and inspect it carefully to ensure the absence of flaws.

◆ Take the equipment to the patient's bedside.

◆ Wash your hands.

◆ Confirm the patient's identity using two patient identifiers according to facility policy.

◆ Explain the procedure to the patient.

◆ If an I.V. line is already in place, check its insertion site for signs of infiltration and infection.

◆ Remove the volume-control set from its box and close all clamps.

◆ Remove the protective cap from the volume-control set spike, insert the spike into the I.V. solution container, and hang the container on the I.V. pole.

◆ Open the air vent clamp and close the upper slide clamp.

◆ Open the lower clamp on the I.V. tubing, slide it upward until it's slightly below the drip chamber, and close the clamp.

◆ If using a valve set, open the upper clamp until the fluid chamber fills with about 30 ml of solution; close the clamp and carefully squeeze the drip chamber until it's one-half full.

◆ If using a volume-control set with a membrane filter, open the upper clamp until the fluid chamber fills with about 30 ml of solution, then close the clamp.

◆ Open the lower clamp and squeeze the drip chamber flat with two fingers of your opposite hand.

WARNING *If you squeeze the drip chamber with the lower clamp closed, you'll damage the membrane filter.*

◆ Keeping the drip chamber flat, close the lower clamp. Release the drip chamber so it fills halfway.
◆ Open the lower clamp, prime the tubing, and close the clamp.
◆ To use the set as a primary line, insert the distal end of the tubing into the catheter or needle hub. To use as a secondary line, attach a needle to the adapter on the volume-control set.
◆ Wipe the Y-port of the primary tubing with an alcohol pad, and insert the needle and tape the connection.
◆ If you're using a needle-free system, attach the distal end of the tubing to the Y-port of the primary tubing, following the manufacturer's instructions.
◆ To add the drug, wipe the injection port on the volume-control set with an alcohol pad, and inject the drug.
◆ Label the chamber with the drug, dose, and date.

WARNING *Don't write directly on the chamber because the plastic absorbs ink.*

◆ Open the upper clamp, fill the fluid chamber with the prescribed amount of solution, and close the clamp. Rotate the chamber to mix the drug.
◆ Turn off the primary solution (if present) or lower the drip rate to maintain an open line.
◆ Open the lower clamp on the volume-control set, and adjust the drip rate as ordered.
◆ After completion of the infusion, open the upper clamp and let 10 ml of I.V. solution flow into the chamber and through the tubing to flush them.
◆ If using the volume-control set as a secondary I.V. line, close the lower clamp and reset the flow rate of the primary line.
◆ If using the set as a primary I.V. line, close the lower clamp, refill the chamber to the prescribed amount, and begin the infusion again.

SPECIAL CONSIDERATIONS

◆ Always check compatibility of the drug and the I.V. solution.
◆ If using a membrane-filter set, avoid giving any suspensions, lipid emulsions, blood, or blood components through it.
◆ If using a floating-valve set, the diaphragm may stick after repeated use. If it does, close the air vent and upper clamp, invert the drip chamber, and squeeze it. If the diaphragm opens, reopen the clamp and continue to use the set.
◆ If the drip chamber of a floating-valve diaphragm set overfills, immediately close the upper clamp and air vent, invert the chamber, and squeeze excess fluid from the drip chamber back into the graduated fluid chamber.

COMPLICATIONS
◆ None known

PATIENT TEACHING

◆ Explain the procedure to the patient and answer questions, as needed.

DOCUMENTATION

◆ Record the amount and type of drug you added to the volume-control set.
◆ Note the amount of fluid used to dilute it.
◆ Document the date and time of infusion.

SELECTED REFERENCES

Husch, M., et al. "Insights from the Sharp End of Intravenous Medication Errors: Implications for Infusion Pump Technology," *Quality & Safety in Health Care* 14(2):80-86, April 2005.
Jacobs, B. "Pump Away High-Risk Infusion Errors," *Nursing Management* 36(12):40-44, December 2005.
Rohman, C. "Smart Pump Implementation: One Hospital's Story," *Nursing Management* 36(6):49-51, June 2005

Walkers

DESCRIPTION

- Walkers provide greater stability and security than other ambulatory aids; they're recommended for the patient with insufficient strength and balance to use crutches or a cane or with weakness requiring frequent rest periods.
- Attachments for standard walkers and modified walkers, such as platforms for injured or arthritic arms, help meet special needs.
- A standard walker is used by a patient with unilateral or bilateral weakness or an inability to bear weight on one leg; it requires arm strength and balance. With practitioner's approval, wheels may be placed on the front legs of the standard walker to allow the extremely weak or poorly coordinated patient to roll the device forward, instead of lifting it. Wheels may be a safety hazard, however.
- A stair walker is for the patient who must negotiate stairs without bilateral handrails. It requires good arm strength and balance. Its extra set of handles extends toward the patient on the open side.
- A rolling walker is for the patient with very weak legs. It has four wheels and may have a seat.
- A reciprocal walker is for the patient with very weak arms. It allows one side to be advanced ahead of the other.

CONTRAINDICATIONS

- None known

Walker ♦ platform or wheel attachments, as necessary

PREPARATION

- Obtain the appropriate walker with the advice of a physical therapist, and adjust it to the patient's height. His elbows should be flexed at a 15-degree angle when standing comfortably within the walker with his hands on the grips.
- To adjust the walker, turn it upside down, and change the leg length by pushing in the button on each shaft and releasing when the leg is in the correct position.
- Make sure the walker is level before the patient attempts to use it.

- Help the patient stand within the walker, and instruct him to hold the handgrips firmly and equally.
- Stand behind him, closer to the involved leg.
- If he has one-sided leg weakness, tell him to advance the walker 6″ to 8″ (15 to 20 cm) and to step forward with the involved leg and follow with the uninvolved leg, supporting himself on his arms.
- Encourage him to take equal strides.
- If he has equal strength in both legs, instruct him to advance the walker 6″ to 8″ and to step forward with either leg.
- If he can't use one leg, tell him to advance the walker 6″ to 8″ and to swing onto it, supporting his weight on his arms.
- If the patient is using a wheeled or stair walker, reinforce the physical therapist's instructions. Stress the need for caution when using a stair walker.

SPECIAL CONSIDERATIONS

◆ If the patient starts to fall, support his hips and shoulders to help maintain an upright position if possible. If unsuccessful, ease him slowly to the closest surface — bed, floor, or chair.

COMPLICATIONS
◆ None known

PATIENT TEACHING

◆ Teach the patient how to use a chair safely. (See *Teaching safe use of a walker*.)
◆ Teach the patient the two-point gait: Instruct him to stand with his weight evenly distributed between his legs and the walker. Tell him to simultaneously advance the walker's right side and his left foot, and then advance the walker's left side and his right foot.
◆ Teach the patient the four-point gait: Instruct him to evenly distribute his weight between his legs and the walker. Tell him to move the right side of the walker forward, and then move his left foot forward. Instruct him to move the left side of the walker forward, and then his right foot forward.

DOCUMENTATION

◆ Record the type of walker and attachments used.
◆ Document the distance walked and the patient's tolerance of ambulation.

SELECTED REFERENCES
Bateni, H., et al. "Can Use of Walkers or Canes Impede Lateral Compensatory Stepping Movements?" *Gait & Posture* 20(1):74-83, August 2004.
Bateni, H., and Maki, B.E. "Assistive Devices for Balance and Mobility: Benefits, Demands, and Adverse Consequences," *Archives of Physical Medicine and Rehabilitation* 86(1):134-45, January 2005.
"Stepping Out: How to Select a Walking Device," *Johns Hopkins Medical Letter Health After 50* 17(9):6-7, November 2005.
Youdas, J.W., et al. "Partial Weight-Bearing Gait Using Conventional Assistive Devices," *Archives of Physical Medicine and Rehabilitation* 86(3):394-98, March 2005.

Teaching safe use of a walker

SITTING DOWN
◆ Tell the patient to stand with the back of his stronger leg against the front of the chair, his weaker leg slightly off the floor, and the walker directly in front.
◆ Tell him to grasp the armrests on the chair one arm at a time while supporting most of his weight on the stronger leg. (In these illustrations, the patient has left leg weakness.)
◆ Tell the patient to lower himself into the chair and slide backward. After he's seated, he should place the walker beside the chair.

GETTING UP
◆ After the patient brings the walker to the front of his chair, tell him to slide forward in the chair. Placing the back of his stronger leg against the seat, he should advance the weaker leg.
◆ With both hands on the armrests, the patient can push himself to a standing position. Supporting himself with the stronger leg and the opposite hand, he should grasp the walker's handgrip with his free hand.
◆ Then have the patient grasp the free handgrip with his other hand.

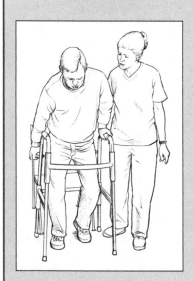

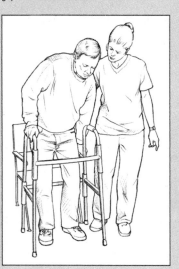

Wound dehiscence and evisceration

OVERVIEW

DESCRIPTION
- Surgical wounds usually heal well; however, edges of a wound may fail to join or may separate even after they seem to be healing normally.
- This may lead to more serious complications of evisceration, in which a portion of the viscera (usually a bowel loop) protrudes through the incision.
- Evisceration can lead to peritonitis and septic shock.
- Dehiscence and evisceration are most likely to occur 6 or 7 days after surgery, when sutures may have been removed and the patient can cough easily and breathe deeply — which strain the incision. (See *Recognizing dehiscence and evisceration*.)
- Conditions are caused by:
- poor nutrition (from inadequate intake or condition such as diabetes mellitus)
- chronic pulmonary or cardiac disease and metastatic cancer, because the injured tissue doesn't get needed nutrients and oxygen
- localized wound infection may limit closure, delay healing, and weaken the incision
- stress on the incision from coughing or vomiting may cause abdominal distention or severe stretching. (A midline abdominal incision, for instance, poses a high risk of wound dehiscence.)

CONTRAINDICATIONS
- None known

EQUIPMENT

Two sterile towels ◆ 1 L of sterile normal saline solution ◆ sterile irrigation set, including a basin, a solution container, and a 50-ml catheter-tip syringe ◆ several large abdominal dressings ◆ sterile, waterproof drape ◆ linen-saver pads ◆ sterile gloves

RETURN TO THE OPERATING ROOM
All previous equipment ◆ I.V. administration set and I.V. fluids ◆ equipment for nasogastric (NG) intubation ◆ sedative, as ordered ◆ suction apparatus

KEY STEPS

- Provide reassurance and support to ease the patient's anxiety.
- Tell the patient to stay in bed. If possible, stay with him while someone else notifies the practitioner and collects the necessary equipment.
- Place a linen-saver pad under the patient to keep sheets dry when you moisten the exposed viscera.
- Using sterile technique, unfold a sterile towel to create a sterile field.
- Open the package containing the irrigation set, and place the basin, solution container, and 50-ml syringe on the sterile field.
- Open the bottle of normal saline solution and pour about 400 ml into the solution container. Also pour about 200 ml into the sterile basin.
- Open several large abdominal dressings and place them on the sterile field.
- Put on the sterile gloves and place one or two of the large abdominal dressings into the basin to saturate them with normal saline solution.
- Place the moistened dressings over the exposed viscera; place a sterile, waterproof drape over the dressings to prevent the sheets from getting wet.
- Moisten the dressings every hour by drawing normal saline solution into a syringe and squirting solution on the dressings.
- When you moisten the dressings, inspect the color of the viscera.

⚡ **WARNING** *If the viscera appears dusky or black, notify the practitioner immediately. With its blood supply interrupted, a protruding organ may become ischemic and necrotic.*

- Keep the patient on absolute bed rest in low-Fowler's position (no more than 20 degrees' elevation) with his knees flexed to prevent injury and reduce stress on an abdominal incision.

⚡ **WARNING** *Don't allow the patient to have anything by mouth, to decrease risk of aspiration during surgery.*

- Monitor the patient's pulse, respirations, blood pressure, and temperature every 15 minutes to detect shock.
- If necessary, prepare him to return to the operating room. After gathering the appropriate equipment, start an I.V. infusion, as ordered.
- Insert an NG tube and connect it to continuous or intermittent low suction, as ordered.
- Give preoperative drugs to the patient as ordered.
- Depending on circumstances, some of these procedures may not be done at the bedside.
- NG intubation may make the patient gag or vomit, causing further evisceration; the practitioner may choose to have the NG tube inserted in the operating room with the patient under anesthesia.
- Continue to reassure the patient while you prepare him for surgery.
- Make sure the patient signed a consent form and the operating room staff has been informed about the procedure.

- If you're caring for a postoperative patient who's at risk for poor healing, make sure he gets an adequate supply of protein, vitamins, and calories. Monitor his dietary deficiencies; discuss problems with the practitioner and dietitian.
- When changing wound dressings, always use sterile technique.
- Inspect the incision with each dressing change; if you recognize early signs of infection, start treatment before dehiscence or evisceration can occur.
- If local infection develops, clean the wound as necessary to eliminate a buildup of purulent drainage.
- Make sure bandages aren't so tight that they limit blood supply to the wound.

COMPLICATIONS
- Infection
- Peritonitis
- Septic shock
- Necrosis

- Explain the procedures and reassure the patient before surgery.

- Note when the problem occurred.
- Record the patient's activity preceding the problem.
- Document the patient's condition and the time the practitioner was notified.
- Describe the appearance of the wound or eviscerated organ; the amount, color, consistency, and odor of drainage; and nursing actions taken.
- Record vital signs, the patient's response to the incident, and the practitioner's actions.
- Change the care plan to reflect nursing actions needed to promote proper healing.

SELECTED REFERENCES
Banwell, P.E., et al. "Treatment of Dehisced and Infected Wounds," *Journal of Wound Care* 14(3):110, March 2005.
Moz, T. "Wound Dehiscence and Evisceration," *Nursing* 34(5):88, May 2004.
Penn, E., and Rayment, S. "Management of a Dehisced Abdominal Wound with VAC Therapy," *British Journal of Nursing* 13(4):194-201, February-March 2004.

Recognizing dehiscence and evisceration

In wound dehiscence, the layers of the surgical wound separate. With evisceration, the viscera (in this case, a bowel loop) protrude through the surgical incision.

WOUND DEHISCENCE

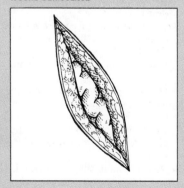

EVISCERATION OF BOWEL LOOP

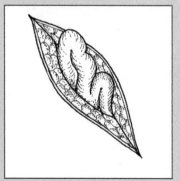

Wound irrigation

DESCRIPTION

◆ Wound irrigation cleans tissues and flushes cell debris and drainage from an open wound.

◆ A commercial wound cleanser helps the wound heal properly from the inside tissue layers outward to the skin surface and prevents premature surface healing over an abscess pocket or infected tract.

◆ Strict sterile technique is required.

◆ After irrigation, open wounds are usually packed to absorb additional drainage.

CONTRAINDICATIONS

◆ None known

Waterproof trash bag ◆ linen-saver pad ◆ emesis basin ◆ clean gloves ◆ sterile gloves ◆ goggles ◆ gown, if indicated ◆ prescribed irrigant such as sterile normal saline solution ◆ sterile water ◆ soft rubber or plastic catheter ◆ sterile container ◆ materials as needed for wound care ◆ sterile irrigation and dressing set ◆ commercial wound cleanser ◆ 35-ml piston syringe with 19G needle or catheter ◆ skin protectant wipe

PREPARATION

◆ Assemble the equipment in the patient's room.

◆ Check the expiration date on each sterile package and inspect for tears.

◆ Check the sterilization date and the date that each bottle of irrigating solution was opened; don't use a solution that's been open longer than 24 hours.

◆ Using aseptic technique, dilute the prescribed irrigant to the correct proportions with sterile water or normal saline solution, if necessary.

◆ Let the solution stand until it reaches room temperature, or warm it to 90° to 95° F (32.2° to 35° C).

◆ Position the waterproof trash bag to avoid reaching across the sterile field or the wound when disposing of soiled items. Turn down the top of the trash bag to provide a wide opening, preventing contamination by touching the bag's edge.

◆ Check the practitioner's order, and assess the patient's condition.

◆ Confirm the patient's identity using two patient identifiers according to facility policy.

◆ Identify allergies, especially to povidone-iodine or other topical solutions or drugs.

◆ Explain the procedure to the patient, provide privacy, and position him for the procedure.

◆ Place the linen-saver pad under him to catch spills.

◆ Place the emesis basin below the wound so irrigating solution flows from the wound into the basin.

◆ Wash your hands and put on gloves.

◆ Put on a gown to protect yourself from wound drainage and contamination.

◆ Remove the soiled dressing; discard the dressing and gloves in the trash bag.

◆ Establish a sterile field with the equipment and supplies you'll need for irrigation and wound care.

◆ Pour the prescribed amount of irrigating solution into a sterile container so you won't contaminate your sterile gloves later by picking up unsterile containers.

◆ Put on sterile gloves, gown, and goggles, if indicated.

◆ Fill the syringe with irrigating solution; connect the catheter to the syringe.

◆ Instill a slow, steady stream of irrigating solution into the wound until the syringe empties. (See *Irrigating a deep wound.*)

◆ Make sure solution reaches all areas of the wound and flows from the clean to the dirty area of the wound to prevent contamination of clean tissue.

◆ Refill the syringe, reconnect it to the catheter, and repeat irrigation.

◆ Continue to irrigate the wound until you've given the prescribed amount of solution or until the solution returns clear.

◆ Note the amount of solution used.

- Remove and discard the catheter and syringe.
- Keep the patient positioned to allow further wound drainage into the basin.
- Clean the area around the wound with normal saline solution; wipe intact skin with a skin protectant wipe and allow it to dry to help prevent skin breakdown and infection.
- Pack the wound, if ordered, and apply a sterile dressing.
- Remove and discard your gloves and gown.
- Properly dispose of drainage, solutions, and trash bag, and clean or dispose of soiled equipment and supplies.

⚠ **WARNING** *To prevent contamination of other equipment, don't return unopened sterile supplies to the sterile supply cabinet.*

SPECIAL CONSIDERATIONS

- Try to coordinate wound irrigation with the practitioner's visit so he can inspect the wound.
- Use only the irrigant specified by the practitioner; others may be erosive or otherwise harmful.
- Follow your facility's policy and Centers for Disease Control and Prevention guidelines concerning wound and skin precautions.
- Irrigate with a bulb syringe only if a piston syringe is unavailable. Use a bulb syringe cautiously because it doesn't deliver enough pressure to adequately clean the wound. If the wound is small or not particularly deep, you may use just the syringe for irrigation.

COMPLICATIONS
- Infection
- Excoriation
- Increased pain
- Wound trauma

PATIENT TEACHING

- If the wound must be irrigated at home, teach the patient or a family member how to do it using strict aseptic technique. Provide written instructions.
- Ask for a return demonstration of the proper technique.
- Arrange for home health supplies and nursing visits, as appropriate.
- Urge the patient to call the practitioner if signs of infection occur.

DOCUMENTATION

- Record the date and time of irrigation and the amount and type of irrigant.
- Note appearance of the wound and sloughing tissue or exudate.
- Document the amount of solution returned.
- Record skin care performed around the wound and dressings applied.
- Note the patient's tolerance of the treatment.

SELECTED REFERENCES
Al-Ramahi, M., et al. "Saline Irrigation and Wound Infection in Abdominal Gynecologic Surgery," *International Journal of Gynaecology and Obstetrics* 94(1):33-36, July 2006.

Draeger, R.W., and Dahners, L.E. "Traumatic Wound Debridement: A Comparison of Irrigation Methods," *Journal of Orthopaedic Trauma* 20(2):83-88, February 2006.

Todkar, M. "Comparison of Soap and Antibiotic Solutions for Irrigation of Lower-Limb Open Fracture Wounds," *Journal of Bone and Joint Surgery* 88(2):452, February 2006.

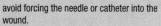

Irrigating a deep wound

When preparing to irrigate a wound, attach a 19G needle or catheter to a 35-ml piston syringe. This setup delivers an irrigation pressure of 8 psi, which is effective in cleaning the wound and reducing risk of trauma and wound infection. To prevent tissue damage or, in an abdominal wound — intestinal perforation — avoid forcing the needle or catheter into the wound.

Irrigate the wound with gentle pressure until the solution returns clean. Position the emesis basin under the wound to collect remaining drainage.

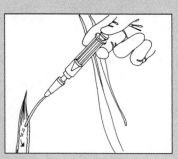
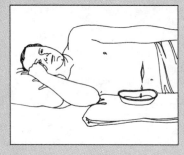

Wound management, surgical

DESCRIPTION

- Wound management procedures help to prevent infection by stopping pathogens from entering the wound.
- These procedures promote patient comfort and protect the skin surface from maceration and excoriation caused by contact with irritating drainage.
- They also allow you to measure wound drainage to monitor healing and fluid and electrolyte balance.
- There are two primary methods of wound management: dressing and pouching.
- Dressing is preferred unless caustic or excessive drainage is compromising skin integrity.
- Lightly seeping wounds with drains and wounds with minimal purulent drainage can be managed with packing and gauze dressings.
- Some wounds, such as those that become chronic, may require an occlusive dressing.
- A wound with copious, excoriating drainage calls for pouching to protect the surrounding skin.
- If your patient has a surgical wound, monitor him and choose the appropriate dressing.
- Use the color of the wound to help determine which type of dressing to apply. (See *Tailoring wound care to wound color*.)
- These procedures require sterile technique and sterile supplies to prevent contamination. Be sure to change the dressing often enough to keep the skin dry.

CONTRAINDICATIONS

- None known

EQUIPMENT

Waterproof trash bag ◆ clean gloves ◆ sterile gloves ◆ gown and face shield or goggles, if indicated ◆ sterile 4″ × 4″ gauze pads ◆ large absorbent dressings, if indicated ◆ sterile cotton-tipped applicators ◆ sterile dressing set ◆ povidone-iodine swabs ◆ topical drug, if ordered ◆ adhesive or other tape ◆ soap and water ◆ skin protectant; nonadherent pads; collodion spray or acetone-free adhesive remover; sterile normal saline solution; graduated container; Montgomery straps, a fishnet tube elasticized dressing support, or a T-binder (optional)

WOUND WITH A DRAIN

Sterile scissors ◆ sterile 4″ × 4″ gauze pads without cotton lining ◆ sump drain ◆ ostomy pouch or another collection bag ◆ sterile precut tracheostomy pads or drain dressings ◆ adhesive tape (paper or silk tape if patient is hypersensitive) ◆ surgical mask

POUCHING A WOUND

Collection pouch with drainage port ◆ sterile gloves ◆ skin protectant ◆ sterile gauze pads

PREPARATION

- Assess the patient's condition and identify his allergies, especially to adhesive tape, povidone-iodine or other topical solutions, or drugs.
- Assemble the equipment in his room.
- Check the expiration date on each sterile package, and inspect for tears.
- Put the waterproof trash bag near the patient, to avoid reaching across the sterile field or the wound when disposing of soiled items.
- Turn down the top of the trash bag to provide a wide opening and prevent contamination of instruments or gloves by touching the bag's edge.

Tailoring wound care to wound color

If your patient has an open wound, you can assess how well it's healing by inspecting its color, which you can then use to guide management of the wound.

RED WOUNDS

Red indicates normal healing. When a wound begins to heal, a layer of pale pink granulation tissue covers the wound bed. As it thickens, it becomes beefy red.

Cover a red wound, keep it moist and clean, and protect it from trauma. Use a transparent dressing (such as Tegaderm or Op-site), a hydrocolloidal dressing (such as DuoDerm), or a gauze dressing moistened with sterile normal saline solution or impregnated with petroleum jelly or an antibiotic.

YELLOW WOUNDS

Yellow is the color of exudate produced by microorganisms in an open wound. Exudate usually appears whitish yellow, creamy yellow, yellowish green, or beige. Water content influences shade: Dry exudate appears darker.

If the wound is yellow, clean it and remove exudate, using high-pressure irrigation; then cover it with a moist dressing. Use absorptive products (for example, Debrisan beads and paste) or a moist gauze dressing with or without an antibiotic. You may also use hydrotherapy with whirlpool or high-pressure irrigation.

BLACK WOUNDS

Black, the least healthy color, signals necrosis. Dead, avascular tissue slows healing and provides a site for microorganisms to proliferate.

You should debride a black wound. After removing dead tissue, apply a dressing to keep the wound moist and guard against external contamination. As ordered, use enzyme products, surgical debridement, hydrotherapy with whirlpool or high-pressure irrigation, or a moist gauze dressing.

MULTICOLORED WOUNDS

You may note two or even all three colors in a wound. In this case, classify the wound according to the least healthy color present. For example, if his wound is red and yellow, classify it as a yellow wound.

- Check the practitioner's order for specific wound care and drug instructions. Note the location of surgical drains to avoid dislodging them during the procedure.
- Confirm the patient's identity using two patient identifiers according to facility policy.
- Explain the procedure to the patient to lessen his fear and gain his cooperation.
- Provide the patient with privacy, position him as necessary, and expose the wound site.
- Wash your hands and put on a gown, clean gloves, and a face shield, if necessary.
- Loosen the soiled dressing by holding the patient's skin and pulling the tape or dressing toward the wound. This protects the newly formed tissue and prevents stress on the incision.
- Moisten the tape with acetone-free adhesive remover, if necessary, to make tape removal less painful (particularly if the skin is hairy).

WARNING *Don't apply solvents to the incision; they can contaminate the wound.*

- Slowly remove the soiled dressing.
- If the gauze adheres to the wound, loosen the gauze by moistening it with sterile normal saline solution.
- Observe the dressing for amount, type, color, and odor of drainage.
- Discard the dressing and gloves in the waterproof trash bag.

CARING FOR THE WOUND

- Wash your hands.
- Establish a sterile field with the equipment and supplies you'll need for suture-line care and dressing change, including a sterile dressing set and povidone-iodine swabs.
- If the practitioner has ordered ointment, squeeze the needed amount onto the sterile field.
- If using an antiseptic from an unsterile bottle, pour the antiseptic cleaning agent into a sterile container so you won't contaminate your gloves.

- Put on sterile gloves.
- Saturate the sterile gauze pads with the prescribed cleaning agent.

WARNING *Avoid using cotton balls. They may shed fibers in the wound, causing irritation, infection, or adhesion.*

- If ordered, obtain a wound culture; then proceed to clean the wound.
- Pick up the moistened gauze pad or swab and squeeze out excess solution.
- Working from the top of the incision, wipe once to the bottom, and then discard.
- Wipe a second moistened pad from top to bottom in a vertical path next to the incision.
- Continue to work outward from the incision in lines running parallel to it.
- Always wipe from the clean area toward the less clean area (usually from top to bottom).
- Use each gauze pad or swab for only one stroke.
- The suture line is cleaner than adjacent skin and the top of the suture line is usually cleaner than the bottom where drainage collects.
- Use sterile cotton-tipped applicators for efficient cleaning of tight-fitting wire sutures, deep and narrow wounds, or wounds with pockets.
- Wipe only once with each applicator.
- If the patient has a surgical drain, clean the drain's surface last.
- Moist drainage promotes bacterial growth; the drain is considered the most contaminated area. Clean skin around the drain by wiping in half or full circles from the drain site outward.
- Clean all areas of the wound to wash away debris, pus, blood, and necrotic material. Try not to disturb sutures or irritate the incision.
- Clean to at least 1″ (2.5 cm) beyond the end of the new dressing. If you aren't applying a new dressing, clean to at least 2″ (5 cm) beyond the incision.
- Check to make sure the edges of the incision are lined up properly, and check for signs of infection (heat, redness, swelling, induration, and odor), dehiscence, or evisceration.

WARNING *If you see infection or the patient reports pain at the wound, notify the practitioner.*

- Irrigate the wound, as ordered.
- Wash skin surrounding the wound with soap and water, and pat dry using a sterile 4″ × 4″ gauze pad.

WARNING *Avoid oil-based soap; it may interfere with pouch adherence. Apply prescribed topical drug.*

- Apply a skin protectant, if needed.
- If ordered, pack the wound with gauze pads or strips folded to fit, using a sterile forceps.

WARNING *Avoid using cotton-lined gauze pads. Cotton fibers can adhere to the wound surface and cause complications.*

- Pack the wound using the wet-to-damp method. Soaking the packing material in solution and wringing it out so it's slightly moist provides a moist wound environment that absorbs debris and drainage. Removing the packing won't disrupt new tissue.

WARNING *Don't pack the wound tightly. You may damage the wound.*

APPLYING A FRESH GAUZE DRESSING

- Place sterile 4″ × 4″ gauze pads at the center of the wound, and move progressively outward to the edges of the wound site.
- Extend the gauze at least 1″ (2.5 cm) beyond the incision in each direction, and cover the wound evenly with enough sterile dressings (usually two or three layers) to absorb drainage until the next dressing change.
- Use large absorbent dressings to form outer layers, if needed, to provide greater absorbency.
- Secure the dressing's edges to the patient's skin with strips of tape to maintain sterility of the wound site, or secure the dressing with a T-binder or Montgomery straps to prevent skin excoriation, which may occur with repeated tape removal necessitated by frequent dressing changes.

(continued)

- If the wound is on a limb, secure the dressing with a fishnet tube elasticized dressing support.
- Make sure the patient is comfortable.
- Properly dispose of the solutions and trash bag. Clean or discard soiled equipment and supplies according to facility policy.

⚡ **WARNING** *If the patient's wound has purulent drainage, don't return unopened sterile supplies to the sterile supply cabinet; this could cross-contaminate other equipment.*

DRESSING A WOUND WITH A DRAIN

- Prepare a drain dressing by using sterile scissors to cut a slit in a sterile 4″×4″ gauze pad.
- Fold the pad in half; then cut inward from the center of the folded edge.
- Don't use a cotton-lined gauze pad. Cutting the gauze opens the lining and releases cotton fibers into the wound.
- Prepare a second pad the same way, or use commercially precut gauze.
- Press one folded pad close to the skin around the drain so that the tubing fits into the slit. Press the second folded pad around the drain from the opposite direction so that the two pads encircle the tubing.
- Layer as many uncut sterile 4″×4″ gauze pads or large absorbent dressings around the tubing as needed to absorb expected drainage. Tape the dressing in place, or use a T-binder or Montgomery straps.

POUCHING A WOUND

- If the patient's wound is draining heavily, or if drainage may damage surrounding skin, apply a pouch.
- Measure the wound. Cut an opening 3/8″ (0.3 cm) larger than the wound in the facing of the collection pouch.
- Apply a skin protectant as needed.
- Plan to position the pouch's drainage port so that gravity facilitates drainage.
- Make sure the drainage port at the bottom of the pouch is closed firmly to prevent leaks.
- Gently press the contoured pouch opening around the wound, starting at its lower edge, to catch drainage.
- To empty the pouch, put on gloves and a face shield or mask and goggles to avoid splashing.
- Insert the pouch's bottom one-half into a graduated biohazard container, and open the drainage port. Note the color, consistency, odor, and amount of fluid.
- If ordered, obtain a culture specimen and send it to the laboratory immediately.
- Remember to follow Centers for Disease Control and Prevention standard precautions when handling infectious drainage.
- Wipe the bottom of the pouch and drainage port with a gauze pad and reseal the port.
- Change the pouch only if it leaks or fails to adhere.

- If the patient has two wounds in the same area, cover each wound separately with layers of sterile 4″×4″ gauze pads. Cover each site with a large absorbent dressing secured to the patient's skin with tape.
- Don't use a single large absorbent dressing to cover both sites because drainage quickly saturates a pad, promoting cross-contamination.
- Don't pack the wound too tightly.
- Avoid overlapping damp packing onto surrounding skin because it macerates the intact tissue.
- To save time when dressing a wound with a drain, use precut tracheostomy pads or drain dressings to fit around the drain.
- If the patient is sensitive to adhesive tape, use paper or silk tape.
- Use a surgical mask to cradle a chin or jawline dressing.
- If ordered, use a collodion spray or similar topical protectant instead of a gauze dressing.
- If a sump drain isn't adequately collecting wound secretions, reinforce it with an ostomy pouch or another collection bag.
- Use waterproof tape to strengthen a spot on the front of the pouch near the adhesive opening; then cut a small "X" in the tape. Feed the drain catheter into the pouch through the "X" cut.
- Seal the cut around the tubing with more waterproof tape; then connect the tubing to the suction pump.
- If you use more than one collection pouch for a wound or wounds, record drainage volume separately for each pouch.
- Avoid using waterproof material over the dressing.
- Many practitioners prefer to change the first postoperative dressing themselves to check the incision; don't change the first dressing unless you have specific instructions.

- If you have no such order and drainage comes through the dressings, reinforce the dressing with fresh sterile gauze. Request an order to change the dressing, or ask the practitioner to change it as soon as possible.
- A reinforced dressing shouldn't remain in place longer than 24 hours because it's a medium for bacterial growth.
- For the recent postoperative patient or a patient with complications, check the dressing every 15 to 30 minutes or as ordered. For the patient with a properly healing wound, check the dressing at least once every 8 hours.
- If the dressing becomes wet from the outside, replace it as soon as possible to prevent wound contamination.

COMPLICATIONS
- Allergic reaction
- Skin redness, rash, or excoriation
- Infection
- Skin tears

PATIENT TEACHING
- Teach the patient wound care methods for use after discharge.
- Stress the importance of using aseptic technique.
- Teach the patient how to check the wound for infection and other complications.
- Show the patient how to change dressings.
- Give the patient written instructions for procedures to be performed at home.

DOCUMENTATION
- Note special or detailed wound care instructions and pain management steps on the care plan.
- Note the date, time, and type of wound management procedure.
- Record the amount of soiled dressing and packing removed.
- Document wound appearance (including size, condition of margins, and presence of necrotic tissue) and odor (if present).
- Note the type, color, consistency, and amount of drainage (for each wound); the presence and location of drains.
- Note additional procedures, such as irrigation, packing, or application of a topical drug.
- Document the type and amount of new dressing or pouch applied.
- Record the patient's tolerance of the procedure.

SELECTED REFERENCES
Harvey, C. "Wound Healing," *Orthopaedic Nursing* 24(2):143-57, March-April 2005.
Hoban, V. "Wound Care: What Every Nurse Should Know," *Nursing Times* 101(12):20-22, March 2005.
Worley, C.A. "Assessment and Terminology: Critical Issues in Wound Care," *Dermatology Nursing* 16(5):451-52, 457, October 2004.

Wound management, traumatic

OVERVIEW

DESCRIPTION
- Wounds include abrasions, lacerations, puncture wounds, and amputations:
- abrasion: the skin is scraped, with partial loss of skin surface
- laceration: the skin is torn and has jagged, irregular edges; the severity of a laceration depends on its size, depth, and location
- puncture wound: occurs when a pointed object penetrates the skin
- traumatic amputation: involves removal of part of the body, a limb, or part of a limb.
- Assess the patient's ABCs: airway, breathing, and circulation; a patent airway and pumping heart take first priority.
- When ABCs are stabilized, control bleeding by applying firm, direct pressure and elevating the extremity.
- If bleeding continues, you may need to compress a pressure point.
- Assess the condition of the wound. Management and cleaning technique usually depend on specific type of wound and degree of contamination.

CONTRAINDICATIONS
- None known

EQUIPMENT

Sterile basin ◆ normal saline solution ◆ sterile 4″ × 4″ gauze pads ◆ sterile gloves ◆ clean gloves ◆ dry sterile dressing, nonadherent pad, or petroleum gauze ◆ linen-saver pad ◆ scissors ◆ towel ◆ goggles ◆ mask ◆ gown ◆ 50-ml catheter-tip syringe ◆ surgical scrub brush ◆ antibacterial ointment ◆ porous tape ◆ sterile forceps ◆ sutures and suture set ◆ hydrogen peroxide (optional)

PREPARATION
- Place a linen-saver pad under the area to be cleaned and remove clothing covering the wound.
- If necessary, clip hair around the wound with scissors.
- Assemble needed equipment at the patient's bedside.
- Fill a sterile basin with normal saline solution.
- Make sure the treatment area has enough light to allow close observation of the wound.
- Depending on the nature and location of the wound, wear sterile or clean gloves to avoid spreading infection.

KEY STEPS

- Check the patient's medical history for previous tetanus immunization and, if needed and ordered, arrange for immunization.
- Administer medication for pain, if ordered.
- Wash your hands.
- Use appropriate protective equipment, such as a gown, gloves, mask, and goggles, if spraying or splashing of body fluids is possible.

ABRASION
- Flush the scraped skin with normal saline solution.
- Remove dirt or gravel with a sterile 4″ × 4″ gauze pad moistened with normal saline solution. Rub in the opposite direction from which the dirt or gravel became embedded.
- If the wound is extremely dirty, use a surgical brush to scrub it.
- Allow a small wound to dry and form a scab. A larger wound may need to be covered with a nonadherent pad or petroleum gauze and a light dressing.
- Apply antibacterial ointment if ordered.

LACERATION
- Moisten a sterile 4″ × 4″ gauze pad with normal saline solution and clean the wound, working outward from its center to about 2″ (5 cm) beyond its edges.
- Discard the soiled gauze pad and use a fresh one as necessary until the wound is clean.
- If the wound is dirty, irrigate with a 50-ml catheter-tip syringe and normal saline solution.
- Help the practitioner suture the wound edges using the suture kit, or apply sterile strips of porous tape.
- Apply prescribed antibacterial ointment to help prevent infection.
- Apply a dry sterile dressing over the wound to absorb drainage and help prevent bacterial contamination.

PUNCTURE WOUND

◆ If the wound is minor, allow it to bleed for a few minutes before cleaning it.
◆ For a larger puncture wound, irrigate it before applying a dry dressing.
◆ Stabilize an embedded foreign object until the practitioner can remove it.
◆ Clean the wound as you would clean a laceration.

AMPUTATION

◆ Apply a gauze pad moistened with normal saline solution to the amputation site. Elevate the affected part, and immobilize it for surgery.
◆ Recover the amputated part, and prepare it for transport to a facility where microvascular surgery is performed.

SPECIAL CONSIDERATIONS

◆ When irrigating a traumatic wound, avoid using more than 8 psi of pressure. High-pressure irrigation can seriously interfere with healing, kill cells, and allow bacteria to infiltrate the tissue.
◆ Use normal saline solution or hydrogen peroxide; its foaming action facilitates debris removal. Peroxide should never be instilled into a deep wound because of risk of embolism from evolving gases.
◆ Solutions such as hydrogen peroxide or sodium hypochlorite may damage tissue and delay healing.
◆ Rinse your hands well after using hydrogen peroxide.

WARNING *Avoid cleaning a traumatic wound with alcohol; it causes pain and tissue dehydration. Avoid using antiseptics for wound cleaning; they can impede healing. Never use a cotton ball or cotton-filled gauze pad to clean a wound; cotton fibers left in the wound can cause contamination.*

◆ After a wound has been cleaned, the practitioner may want to debride it to remove dead tissue and reduce risks of infection and scarring. If this is to be done, pack the wound with gauze pads soaked in normal saline solution until debridement.
◆ Observe for signs and symptoms of infection, such as warm red skin at the site or purulent discharge. Infection of a traumatic wound can delay healing, increase scar formation, and trigger systemic infection such as septicemia.
◆ Observe dressings. If edema is present, adjust the dressing to avoid impairing circulation to the area.

COMPLICATIONS

◆ Temporary increase in the patient's pain during cleaning and care of traumatic wounds
◆ Further disruption of tissue integrity during excessive, vigorous cleaning

PATIENT TEACHING

◆ Explain the procedures to the patient and answer questions, as needed.

DOCUMENTATION

◆ Document the date and time of the procedure.
◆ Record wound size and condition, drug administration, and specific wound care measures.
◆ Document patient teaching.

SELECTED REFERENCES

Chavez, B. "Making the Case for Using a Silicone Dressing in Burn Wound Management," *Ostomy/Wound Management* 51(11A Suppl):17-18, November 2005.

Clontz, A.S., et al. "Trauma Nursing: Amputation," *RN* 67(7):38-43, July 2004.

Eckert, K.L. "Penetrating and Blunt Abdominal Trauma," *Critical Care Nursing Quarterly* 28(1):41-59, January-March 2005.

Hoban, V. "Wound Care: What Every Nurse Should Know," *Nursing Times* 101(12):20-22, March 2005.

Worley, C.A. "Assessment and Terminology: Critical Issues in Wound Care," *Dermatology Nursing* 16(5):451-52, 457, October 2004.

Z-track injection

DESCRIPTION

- The Z-track method of I.M. injection prevents leakage, or tracking, into the subcutaneous tissue.
- It's typically used to administer drugs that irritate and discolor subcutaneous tissue, primarily iron preparations, such as iron dextran.
- It may also be used in elderly patients who have decreased muscle mass.
- Lateral displacement of the skin during injection helps seal the drug in the muscle.
- The procedure requires careful attention to technique because leakage into subcutaneous tissue can cause patient discomfort and may permanently stain some tissues.

CONTRAINDICATIONS

- None known

Patient's medication record and chart ◆ two 20G 1¼" to 2" needles ◆ prescribed medication ◆ gloves ◆ 3- to 5-ml syringe ◆ two alcohol pads

PREPARATION

- Verify the order on the patient's medication record by checking it against the practitioner's order.
- Wash your hands.
- Make sure the needle you're using is long enough to reach the muscle. Generally, a 200-lb (90.7-kg) patient requires a 2" needle; a 100-lb (45.4-kg) patient requires a 1¼" to 1½" needle.
- Attach one needle to the syringe and draw up the prescribed medication.

- Then draw 0.2 to 0.5 cc of air (depending on facility policy) into the syringe.
- Remove the first needle and attach the second to prevent tracking the medication through the subcutaneous tissue as the needle is inserted

Displacing the skin for Z-track injection

By blocking the needle pathway after injection, the Z-track technique allows you to give an I.M. injection while minimizing risk of subcutaneous irritation and staining.

Before the procedure, the skin, subcutaneous fat, and muscle lie in their normal positions.

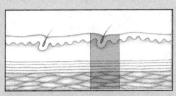

To begin, put your finger on the skin surface and pull the skin and subcutaneous layers out of alignment with underlying muscle. You should move the skin about ½" (1 cm).

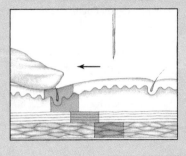

Insert the needle at a 90-degree angle at the site where you initially placed your finger. Inject the drug and withdraw the needle.

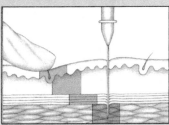

Remove your finger from the skin surface, allowing the layers to return to their normal positions. The needle track (shown by the dotted line) is now broken at the junction of each tissue layer, trapping the drug in the muscle.

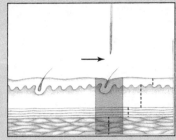

KEY STEPS

- Confirm the patient's identity using two patient identifiers according to facility policy.
- Explain the procedure and provide privacy.
- Place the patient in the lateral position, exposing the gluteal muscle to be used as the injection site. The patient may also be placed in the prone position.
- Clean an area on the upper outer quadrant of the patient's buttock with an alcohol pad.
- Put on gloves.
- Displace the skin laterally by pulling it away from the injection site. (See *Displacing the skin for Z-track injection.*)
- Insert the needle into the muscle at a 90-degree angle.
- Aspirate for blood return; if none appears, inject the drug slowly, followed by the air.
- Injecting air after the drug helps clear the needle and prevents tracking the medication through subcutaneous tissues as the needle is withdrawn.
- Wait 10 seconds before withdrawing the needle to ensure dispersion of the medication.
- Withdraw the needle slowly.
- Release the displaced skin and subcutaneous tissue to seal the needle track.
- **WARNING** *Don't massage the injection site or allow the patient to wear a tight-fitting garment over the site; it could force the medication into subcutaneous tissue.*
- Encourage the patient to walk or to move about in bed to facilitate absorption of the drug from the injection site.
- Discard the needles and syringe in an appropriate sharps container. To avoid needle-stick injuries, don't recap needles.
- Remove and discard your gloves.

SPECIAL CONSIDERATIONS

- Don't inject more than 5 ml of solution into a single site using the Z-track method.
- Alternate gluteal sites for repeat injections.
- Encourage the patient to relax the muscles you'll be injecting because injections into tense muscle are more painful than usual and may bleed more.
- If the patient is on bed rest, encourage active range-of-motion (ROM) exercises or perform passive ROM exercises to facilitate absorption from the injection site.
- I.M. injections can damage local muscle cells, causing elevated serum enzyme levels (for example, of creatine kinase) that can be confused with the elevated enzyme levels resulting from damage to cardiac muscle, as in myocardial infarction. If measuring enzyme levels is important, suggest that the practitioner switch to I.V. administration and adjust dosages accordingly.

COMPLICATIONS

- Discomfort and tissue irritation from drug leakage into subcutaneous tissue
- Medication absorption interference due to failure to rotate sites in patients who require repeated injections
- Unabsorbed medication build up in deposits (can reduce desired pharmacologic effect and lead to abscess formation or tissue fibrosis)

PATIENT TEACHING

- Explain the procedure to the patient and answer questions, as needed.

DOCUMENTATION

- Record the medication, dosage, date, time, and site of injections on the patient's medication record.
- Note the patient's response to the injected drug.

SELECTED REFERENCES

Donaldson, C., and Green, J. "Using the Ventrogluteal Site for Intramuscular Injections," *Nursing Times* 101(16):36-38, April 2005.

Higgins, D. "Practical Procedures. IM Injection," *Nursing Times* 100(45):36-37, November 2004.

Pullen, R.L., Jr. "Administering Medication by the Z-track Method," *Nursing* 35(7):24, July 2005.

Wynaden, D., et al. "Establishing Best Practice Guidelines for Administration of Intra Muscular Injections in the Adult: A Systematic Review of the Literature," *Contemporary Nurse* 20(2): 267-77, December 2005

Index

i refers to an illustration; t refers to a table.

---

i refers to an illustration; t refers to a table.

i refers to an illustration; t refers to a table.

i refers to an illustration; t refers to a table.

Humidifiers, 244-245
  types of, 244-245
  uses for, 244
Hydraulic lift transfer, 528-529, 528i
Hydrocolloid dressing, applying, to
    pressure ulcer, 404
Hydrogel dressing, applying, to pres-
    sure ulcer, 405
Hydrotherapy, 246-247
  mechanical debridement and,
    310, 311
  positioning patient for, 247i
  uses for, 246
Hyperthermia-hypothermia blanket,
    248-249
  uses for, 248
Hypocalcemia as transfusion reaction
    cause, 534t
Hypothermia as transfusion reaction
    cause, 534t

I

Ice bag or collar, applying, 128, 129
Ice massage, reducing pain with, 128
Ileal pouch. See Continent ileostomy
    care.
Ileostomy care, 130-131. See also Conti-
    nent ileostomy care.
  applying or changing pouch in,
    130-131
  emptying pouch in, 131
  fitting pouch and skin barrier in, 130
Ilizarov fixator, 202
  patient teaching for, 203
  special considerations for, 203
Immunosuppressive therapy, neutro-
    penic precautions for, 348-349
Impaired swallowing and aspiration
  blue dye test for, 251
  endotracheal tubes and, 251
  esophageal dysphagia and, 250-251
  oropharyngeal dysphagia and, 250
  in patient with feeding tube, 251
  precautions for, 250-251
  strategies for, 250
  supervision and, 250
  tracheostomies and, 251
Impetigo, contact precautions for,
    136-137, 137t
Incentive spirometry, 252-253
  candidates for, 252
  purpose of, 252

Incontinence management, 254-255
  fecal, 254-255
  pelvic floor muscle exercises for, 255
  urinary, 254
Induction chemotherapy, 112
Infant, cardiopulmonary resuscitation
    in, 82-83
Influenza, droplet precautions for,
    152-153, 153t
Informed consent, obtaining, 403
Injection
  heparin, 475
  insulin, 475
  intradermal, 270-271
  intramuscular, 272-273
  intrathecal, 192
  I.V. bolus, 282-283
  subcutaneous, 474-475
  Z-track, 586-587, 586i
Insulin drugs, mixing, in syringe, 3
Insulin injection, 475
Intermittent infusion device
  advantages of, 256, 258
  converting I.V. line to, 258i
  drug administration and, 256-257
  inserting, 258-259
Intermittent positive-pressure breath-
    ing, 260-261
  uses for, 260
Internal fixation, 262-263
  advantages of, 262
  devices for, 262i
  uses for, 262
Intra-aortic balloon counterpulsation,
    264-267
  discontinuing, 267
  indications for, 264
  interpreting waveforms in, 265i
  monitoring patient after insertion
    of, 266
  percutaneous insertion of, 265-266
  preparing for insertion of, 264-265
  purpose of, 264
  surgical insertion of, 266
  weaning patient from, 266-267
Intra-arterial pressure monitoring.
    See Arterial pressure monitoring,
    invasive.
Intracranial pressure monitoring,
    268-269
  basic systems for, 268
  indications for, 268
  purpose of, 268

Intradermal injection, 270-271
  sites for, 270, 270i
  technique for administering, 271i
    to pediatric patient, 155
  uses for, 270
Intramuscular injection, 272-273
  administering, to pediatric patient,
    155
  choosing site for, 157i, 272
  modifying, for geriatric patient, 162
  uses for, 272
Intraosseous infusion, 274-275
  indications for, 274
  mechanics of, 274i
  purpose of, 274
  sites for, 274
Intrapleural administration, 276-277
  drugs commonly given by, 276
  inserting catheter for, 276
  inserting chest tube for, 276-277
  uses for, 276
Intrathecal injections, 192
Iontophoresis, 278-279
  benefits of, 278
  delivery device for, 279i
Irrigating enema. See Enema adminis-
    tration.
Isolation equipment
  putting on, 280, 280i
  removing, 280, 281i
Isolator blood-culturing system, 47
I.V. bolus injection, 282-283
  administering, with intermittent
    infusion device, 256-257
  ready injectable medication for, 282
  through existing I.V. line, 283
  through venous access port, 283
  uses for, 282
I.V. flow rate
  calculating and setting drip rate
    for, 284
  expression of, 284
  managing deviations in, 285t
  manual control of, 284-285
  regulators for, 284
  time tape for, 284
I.V. glucose tolerance test, 48
I.V. line
  converting, to intermittent infusion
    device, 258i
  existing, giving bolus injection
    through, 283

i refers to an illustration; t refers to a table.

Mumps, droplet precautions for, 152-153, 153t
Muslim, beliefs and practices of, 456t
Mycoplasma pneumoniae infection, droplet precautions for, 152-153, 153t

N

Narrowed pulse pressure, 50
Nasal aerosol, using, 324, 325
Nasal care in burn injury, 63. *See also* Burns.
Nasal drug instillation, 324-325
  drugs used for, 324
  positioning patient for, 324i
Nasal irrigation, 326-327
  with bulb syringe, 326
  concluding, 327
  indications for, 327
  with oral irrigating device, 326
  positioning patient for, 327
  purpose of, 327
Nasal packing, 328-329
  for anterior bleeding, 328-329
  for posterior bleeding, 329
  purpose of, 328
Nasal spray, using, 324-325
Nasoenteric-decompression tube
  assisting with insertion of, 332-333
  clearing obstruction in, 331
  performing care for, 330-331
  removing, 333
  types of, 332i
  uses for, 332
Nasogastric tube
  common types of, 338
  ensuring proper placement of, 338-339
  inserting, 338
  instilling drugs through, 336-337, 337i
  instilling solution through, 335
  irrigating, 334-335
  monitoring comfort and condition of patient with, 335
  removing, 339
  suction devices for, 334i
  uses for, 338
Nasopharyngeal airway
  caring for, 340-341
  inserting, 340, 340i, 341
  purpose of, 340
  uses of, 340

Nasopharyngeal specimen collection, 481, 481i
Nebulizer therapy, 342-343
  with in-line nebulizer, 242, 243
  with large-volume nebulizer, 342
  with small-volume nebulizer, 342
  with ultrasonic nebulizer, 342, 343
  uses for, 342
Negative-pressure ventilator, 314
Negative pressure wound therapy. *See* Vacuum-assisted closure pressure therapy.
Neisseria meningitidis disease, invasive, droplet precautions for, 152-153, 153t
Neoadjuvant chemotherapy, 112
Nephrostomy, urinary diversion and, 344i
Nephrostomy tube
  changing dressing for, 344-345
  irrigating, 345
  purpose of, 344
Neurologic vital sign assessment, 346-347
  assessing level of consciousness and orientation in, 346
  checking accommodation in, 347
  evaluating motor function in, 347
  examining pupils and eye movement in, 346
  Glasgow Coma Scale and, 346t
  purpose of, 346
  testing consensual light response in, 346-347
  testing direct light response in, 346
  warning postures and, 347i
Neutropenic precautions, 348-349
  conditions and treatments that require, 348t
  types of, 348
Nitroglycerin ointment, applying, 518i
Nose drops, instilling, 324, 324i, 325

O

OASIS-B1, 222
Obstructed airway. *See* Airway obstruction with foreign body.
Ocular medication disk, 206, 207
Oil bath, 486
Ommaya reservoir
  benefits of, 352
  drug infusion through, 352-353
  implantation of, 352

Ommaya reservoir *(continued)*
  mechanics of, 353i
  purpose of, 352
  uses for, 352
Open reduction-internal fixation. *See* Internal fixation.
Oral drug administration, 354-355
  drug forms used in, 354
  measuring liquid drugs for, 354i
Oral glucose tolerance test, 48
Oral irrigating device, mouth care and, 320
Oral medication, administering
  to infant, 154-155
  to older child, 155
  to toddler, 155
Oral temperature assessment, 484, 485
Organ donation, 165
Oronasopharyngeal suction, 356-357
  inserting catheter for
    through mouth, 356
    through nose, 356
  removing secretions with, 356-357
  uses for, 356
Oropharyngeal airway
  caring for, 358-359
  inserting, 358, 359i
  purpose of, 358
  removing, 358
Oropharyngeal handheld inhalers, 360-361
  metered-dose, 360
  nasal, 360-361
  purpose of, 360
  turbo-inhaler, 360, 361
Orthodox Presbyterian, beliefs and practices of, 456t
Orthostatic hypotension as adverse drug reaction, 163
Outcome and Assessment Information Set, 222
Overbed cradle, 34, 35
Oxygen administration, 362-363
  candidates for, 362
  determining effectiveness of, 362
  in home setting, 363
  uses for, 362
Oxygen affinity for hemoglobin, increased, as transfusion reaction cause, 534t
Oxygen concentrator in home setting, 363
Oxygen tank in home setting, 363

---

i refers to an illustration; t refers to a table.

i refers to an illustration; t refers to a table.

---

i refers to an illustration; t refers to a table.

i refers to an illustration; t refers to a table.

---

i refers to an illustration; t refers to a table.

i refers to an illustration; t refers to a table.

Widened pulse pressure, 50
Wound color, wound care and, 580
Wound dehiscence and evisceration,
        576-577, 577i
    causes of, 576
Wound irrigation, 578-579, 579i
    purpose of, 578
Wound management
    surgical, 580-583
    traumatic, 584-585
Wound specimen collection, 481, 483i
Wrong site surgery, risk factors for, 476

X
Xenograft burn dressing, 64t

Y
Yellow wounds, caring for, 580

Z
Zoster, contact precautions for,
        136-137, 137t
Z-track injection, 586-587
    advantages of, 586
    displacing skin for, 586i
    uses for, 586

i refers to an illustration; t refers to a table.